Prevention and Management of Complications in Minimally Invasive Surgery

Prevention and Management of Complications in Minimally Invasive Surgery

Raymond J. Lanzafame, M.D., F.A.C.S.
Associate Professor of Surgery
University of Rochester School of Medicine
Director, Laser Center
Rochester General Hospital
Rochester, New York

IGAKU-SHOIN New York • Tokyo

Published and distributed by

IGAKU-SHOIN Medical Publishers, Inc.
One Madison Avenue, New York, New York 10010

IGAKU-SHOIN Ltd.,
5-24-3 Hongo, Bunkyo-ku, Toyko 113-91

Library of Congress Cataloging-in-Publication Data

Prevention and management of complications in minimally invasive surgery / [edited by] Raymond J. Lanzafame.
p. cm.
Includes bibliographical references and index.
1. Endoscopic surgery—Complications. I. Lanzafame, Raymond J.
[DNLM: 1. Surgery, Laparoscopic—methods. 2. Surgery, Minimally Invasive—methods. 3. Surgery, Minimally Invasive—instrumentation.
WO 500 P944 1996]
RD33.53.P736 1996
617—dc20
DNLM/DLC
for Library of Congress 96-1928
CIP

ISBN: 0-89640-296-7 (New York)
ISNB: 4-260-14296-8 (Tokyo)

Printed and bound in Hong Kong
10 9 8 7 6 5 4 3 2 1

Dedication

This book is dedicated to my children, Karen and Mark, and my wife, Pat, for their love, support, and understanding as the many hours needed to assemble this text passed; to my staff, who gathered, forwarded, and sought materials long since promised; and to students of surgery of all ages that their continuous quest for knowledge continues to heal.

Raymond J. Lanzafame

Preface

The meteoric rise of laparoscopic cholecystectomy from its humble beginnings in 1987 in France to its acceptance as the standard of care for symptomatic cholelithiasis in 1992 has spawned a revolution in surgery. This has encouraged surgeons to pursue the application of minimally invasive surgical techniques to a variety of other disease processes and to think of closed rather than open surgery. The magnitude of this revolution is arguably unparalleled since the introduction of general anesthesia in the nineteenth century. Laparoscopic surgical techniques continue to evolve, and their merit continues to be assessed. The rapid ongoing development of an everchanging arsenal of instruments and accessories enhances our ability to accomplish a variety of complex maneuvers with these newfound surgical skills.

While laparoscopic cholecystectomy is performed by the vast majority of surgeons, considerable controversy surrounds the advisability of using minimally invasive techniques for routine use in appendectomy, colectomy, herniorrhaphy, and various oncologic procedures. The superiority of procedures such as laparoscopic fundoplication and vagotomy to their open counterparts has been demonstrated in the management of gastroesophageal reflux, particularly in the hands of the experienced surgeon. Laparoscopy and thoracoscopy may eventually replace laparotomy and thoracotomy for exploration or diagnosis.

Although many of the so-called advanced procedures have not been embraced and accepted as rapidly as laparoscopic cholecystectomy within the surgical community, there is little question that minimally invasive surgical techniques will represent an increasingly important component of the surgeons' repertoire as we move into the twenty-first century. The lesson of laparoscopic cholecystectomy has been that new techniques require diligence, patience, and continued acquisition of skills. Sound judgment and experience must prevail over bravado. Meticulous attention to detail is necessary in order to prevent complications or avert disaster. Enthusiasm for minimally invasive procedures must be tempered with the realization that no procedure is immune from complications and that minimally invasive surgical procedures may be associated with significant complications.

The purpose of *The Prevention and Management of Complications in Minimally Invasive Surgery* is to provide the reader with a clear understanding of the factors involved in the development of complications during laparoscopic surgery, as well as the pitfalls which can be avoided. An expert panel of contributors has been assembled to provide a cogent overview of minimally invasive surgical techniques for the thorax, abdomen, and pelvis. In addition, we have included chapters on the application of these techniques in other areas, such as plastic and reconstructive surgery and the direction that minimally invasive surgical techniques may take in the future. We have attempted to identify real and/or potential complications, as well as their current management. These details should be regarded as guidelines and suggestions rather than absolute surgical dogma. The reader should also recognize that the minimally invasive surgical revolution has brought lasting change to patient care, and that it is likely that traditional specialty boundaries will continue to blur as these techniques evolve and are refined in the future. The general surgeon should understand the basic principles and management of abdominal and pelvic diseases and their complications, and should feel comfortable in the management of diseases of the uterus, ovary, or bladder. The gynecologist should similarly be conversant with the management of iatrogenic injury to the bowel or have the ability to treat disease which may involve contiguous structures. This is not to imply that sound judgment and intraoperative consultation are no longer necessary. Rather, it suggests that we must consider surgery and the management of surgical problems or complications more holistically.

The current surgeon in training is in many ways more fortunate than the surgeon already in practice, as many of the skills and experience needed to perform these minimally invasive procedures are accrued more rapidly by the house officer than by the attending mentor. We must all recognize that learning does not cease with the completion of residency but is an ongoing process. Our ultimate goal is to improve the care of our patients and to have the information which, when coupled with skill and experience, will allow us to avoid complications in the future.

Raymond J. Lanzafame, M.D., F.A.C.S.

Contributors

Riccardo Annibali, M.D.
Ospedale Valduce
Como, Italy

Edward J. Brennan, Jr., M.D.
Department of Surgery
Minimally Invasive Surgical Training Institute (MISTI)
Baltimore, Maryland

Jeffrey B. Comitalo, M.D.
Associate in General Surgery
Guthrie Clinic, Ltd.
St. Joe's Hospitals
Arnot-Ogden Hospital
Elmira, New York

John D. Corbitt, Jr., M.D., F.A.C.S.
Attending Surgeon
John F. Kennedy Medical Center
Atlantis, Florida

Leon Daykhovsky, M.D.
Assistant Director, Laser Research Center
Cedars-Sinai Medical Center
Clinical Instructor in Surgery
University of California
Los Angeles, California
Clinical Instructor in Surgery
Wadsworth Veterans Administration Hospital
Los Angeles, California

Utpal S. Desai, M.D.
Resident in Surgery
University of Miami
Jackson Memorial Hospital
Miami, Florida

George S. Ferzli, M.D., F.A.C.S.
Director, Laparoendoscopic Surgery
Department of Laparoendoscopic Surgery
Staten Island University Hospital
Staten Island, New York

Robert J. Fitzgibbons, Jr., M.D., F.A.C.S.
Professor of Surgery
Department of Surgery
Creighton University School of Medicine
Omaha, Nebraska

Kenneth L. Franco, M.D.
Associate Professor
Department of Surgery
Division of Cardiothoracic Surgery
Yale University School of Medicine
New Haven, Connecticut

W. Peter Geis, M.D., F.A.C.S.
Chief, Division of Minimally Invasive Surgery
Director, Minimally Invasive Surgical Training Institute
St. Joseph Hospital
Towson, Maryland

Leo A. Gordon, M.D., F.A.C.S.
Attending Surgeon
Cedars-Sinai Medical Center
Los Angeles, California

Frederick L. Greene, M.D., F.A.C.S.
Professor of Surgery
Division of General Surgery
University of South Carolina
Columbus, South Carolina

Fred Marion Howard, M.D., F.A.C.O.G.
Assistant Professor of Obstetrics and Gynecology
University of Rochester School of Medicine and Dentistry
Associate Chief of Obstetrics and Gynecology
Rochester General Hospital
Rochester, New York

Rao R. Ivatury, M.D., F.R.C.S.
Professor of Surgery
New York Medical College
Director of Trauma, Co-Director Surgical Intensive Care Unit (*SICU*)
Department of Surgery
Lincoln Medical and Mental Health Center
Bronx, New York

Namir Katkhouda, M.D.
Associate Professor of Surgery
Chief Division of Outpatient and Minimally Invasive Surgery
Director Minimally Invasive Surgery Program and Center
USC Healthcare Consulting Center
Los Angeles, California

Michael S. Kavic, M.D.
Ohio Valley General Hospital
St. Francis General Hospital Medical Center
Sewickley Valley Hospital
Visiting Assistant Professor of Surgery
Northeastern Ohio Universities College of Medicine
St. Elizabeth Hospital Medical Center
McKees Rock, Pennsylvania

Louis R. Kavoussi, M.D.
Associate Professor of Urology
Director, Division of Endourology
The James Buchanan Brady Urological Institute
The Johns Hopkins University School of Medicine
Chief, Department of Urology
Johns Hopkins Bayview Medical Center
Baltimore, Maryland

Raymond J. Lanzafame, M.D., F.A.C.S.
Associate Professor of Surgery
University of Rochester School of Medicine
Director, Laser Center
Rochester General Hospital
Rochester, New York

C.Y. Liu, M.D.
Director, Chattanooga Women's Laser Center
Chattanooga, Tennessee

Jeffrey M. Marks, M.D.
The Mount Sinai Medical Center
Assistant Professor
Department of Surgery
Case Western Reserve University School of Medicine
Cleveland, Ohio

Stacey L. Mazzacco, M.D.
Surgical Research Fellow
Department of Surgery
Division of Vascular Surgery
Temple University
Philadelphia, Pennsylvania

Robert McManus, M.D., F.A.C.S., F.A.C.C., F.A.C.C.P.
Associate Clinical Professor of Surgery
Medical College of Wisconsin
Columbia Hospital
Medical Associates Health Center
Milwaukee Medical Clinic
Milwaukee, Wisconsin

Jean Mouiel, M.D.
Department of Surgery
University of Nice School of Medicine
Nice, France

Camran Nezhat, M.D.
Co-Director, Stanford Endoscopy Center for Training and Technology
Clinical Professor
Department of Surgery
Department of Gynecology and Obstetrics
Stanford University School of Medicine
Palo Alto, California
Center for Special Pelvic Surgery
Atlanta, Georgia

Ceana H. Nezhat, M.D.
Clinical Professor of Gynecology and Obstetrics
Stanford University School of Medicine
Palo Alto, California
Center for Special Pelvic Surgery
Atlanta, Georgia, and
Palo Alto, California

Farr Nezhat, M.D.
Clinical Professor of Gynecology and Obstetrics
Stanford University School of Medicine
Palo Alto, California
Center for Special Pelvic Surgery
Atlanta, Georgia, and Palo Alto, California

Douglas O. Olsen, M.D., F.A.C.S.
Assistant Clinical Professor of Surgery
Vanderbilt University Medical Center
Nashville, Tennessee

Michael O'Reilly, M.D., F.A.C.S.
General Surgeon
Advanced Laparoscopic Training Center
Promina Kennestone Hospital
Marietta, Georgia

Adrian Ortega, M.D.
Department of Surgery
University of Southern California
School of Medicine
Los Angeles, California

Ralph P. Pennino, M.D.
Clinical Assistant Professor of Surgery
Department of Surgery
Division of Plastic Surgery
University of Rochester School of Medicine and Dentistry
Rochester General Hospital
Rochester, New York

Joseph B. Petelin, M.D., F.A.C.S.
Clinical Assistant Professor of Surgery
Department of Surgery
University of Kansas School of Medicine
Shawnee Mission, Kansas

Joseph J. Pietrafitta, M.D., F.A.C.S.
Department of Surgery
Abbott Northwestern Hospital
Minneapolis, Minnesota

Jeffrey Ponsky, M.D., F.A.C.S.
Director, Department of Surgery
The Mount Sinai Medical Center
Professor and Vice Chairman
Department of Surgery
Case Western Reserve University School of Medicine
Cleveland, Ohio

Thomas H. Quinn, M.D, Ph.D.
Associate Professor of Anatomy
Department of Biomedical Sciences
Creighton University School of Medicine
Omaha, Nebraska

Eddie Joe Reddick, M.D.
Tennessee Tunesmith International
Brentwood, Tennessee

Ardith Ryberg, M.D., Ph.D.
Laparoscopic Surgical Research Fellow
Department of Surgery
Creighton University School of Medicine
Omaha, Nebraska

Barry A. Salky, M.D., F.A.C.S.
Dr. Robert and Evelyn Turell Professor of Endoscopic Surgery
Professor of Surgery
Chief, Division of Laparoscopic Surgery
The Mount Sinai Medical Center
The Mount Sinai Hospital
Mount Sinai School of Medicine
New York, New York

Juan A. Sanchez, M.D.
Assistant Professor of Surgery
Division of Cardiothoracic Surgery
University of Kentucky
Lexington, Kentucky

William B. Saye, M.D., F.A.C.O.G., F.A.C.S.
President, Advanced Laparoscopy Training Center
Marietta, Georgia

Peter G. Schulam, M.D., Ph.D.
Research Associate
The James Buchanan Brady Urological Institute
The Johns Hospkins University School of Medicine
Baltimore, Maryland

Leonard S. Schultz, M.D., F.A.C.S.
Clinical Assistant Professor of Surgery
University of Minnesota
Abbott Northwestern Hospital
Minneapolis, Minnesota

Daniel S. Seidman, M.D.
Clinical Fellow
Department of Gynecology and Obstetrics
Stanford University School of Medicine
Stanford, California

Stephen J. Shapiro, M.D., F.A.C.S.
Assistant Clinical Professor of Surgery
UCLA School of Medicine
Los Angeles, California
Attending Surgeon
Cedars-Sinai Medical Center
Los Angeles, California

Ronald J. Simon, M.D., F.A.C.S.
Assistant Professor of Surgery
Albert Einstein College of Medicine
Director of Trauma, SICU
Bronx Municipal Hospital Center
Bronx, New York

Robert D. Tucker, M.D., Ph.D.
Associate Professor
Department of Pathology
University of Iowa
Iowa City, Iowa

C. Randle Voyles, M.D.
Clinical Associate Professor
Department of Surgery
University of Mississippi
Jackson, Mississippi

Donald Waldrep, M.D.
Department of Surgery
University of Southern California
School of Medicine
Los Angeles, California

John V. White, M.D., F.A.C.S.
Professor of Surgery
Director of Surgical Research
Temple University Hospital
Department of Surgery
Philadelphia, Pennsylvania

Contents

Prevention and Management of Complications in Minimally Invasive Surgery

section one

Basic Techniques and Technologies

chapter one

Basic Techniques and Equipment for Laparoscopy

Barry A. Salky

Therapeutic laparoscopy has made many strides since Mouret performed the first laparoscopic cholecystectomy in March 1987. If anything, it has made all general surgeons more aware of basic techniques which are needed for safe entrance into the abdominal cavity. The early laparoscopic (therapeutic) literature is replete with articles describing the devastating effects of poor technique when utilizing this technology. Therefore, it is appropriate that this first chapter deal with basic techniques and equipment.

While there are as many techniques as there are surgeons, this author will describe his own, which has evolved from the performance of more than 2500 procedures.

LOCAL ANESTHESIA

We have performed 850 diagnostic laparoscopies, of which 81% were under local anesthesia. The completion of laparoscopy under local anesthesia requires different techniques than most surgeons employ.

Initial Port Placement Site

The author prefers to use a Veress needle approach in the unoperated abdomen. The usual sites for initial puncture are depicted in Figure 1.1. Because many diagnostic procedures involve the liver, the immediate periumbilical area is avoided because of the potential for injuring collateral vessels in portal hypertension. The right upper quadrant is also avoided, as it is the thickest part of the abdominal wall. Unless there has been previous surgery in the area, the ideal incision is 2.5 cm above and 2.5 cm to the left of the umbilicus. The epigastric vessels run vertically about 3 cm off the midline and therefore are avoided. Using a 25-gauge needle, a generous wheal of skin is anesthetized with 0.5% Marcaine (Fig. 1.2), as most of the somatic afferent sensory pain fibers are in the dermis. The area under the wheal is injected in a cone-shaped fashion with the apex of the cone, the skin, and the base the parietal peritoneum (Fig. 1.3). The base should measure approximately 2 to 2.5 cm in diameter. With practice, each layer of the abdominal wall can be felt by the needle during injection. The total amount of local anesthesia placed at the initial puncture site is no more than 15 cc. If the Hasson technique is preferred, the same principles apply, except that infiltration is performed layer by layer under direct vision. The same precautions should be taken as under general anesthesia, that is, previous scars should be avoided.

Veress Needle Insertion

The most important aspect of safe insertion under local anesthesia is patient education in advance of the procedure. Each patient is told about the operating room environment, the needle sticks, and the small incisions. The more tense and stretched the abdominal wall, the easier the entry into the abdominal cavity. Therefore, the patient is instructed the keep the back flat and to push out with the abdominal wall at the same time (Fig. 1.4). The author prefers that no sedation be given beforehand, especially in elderly patients. Small amounts of intravenous sedation can make the patient unable to push out the abdominal wall. A sharp Veress

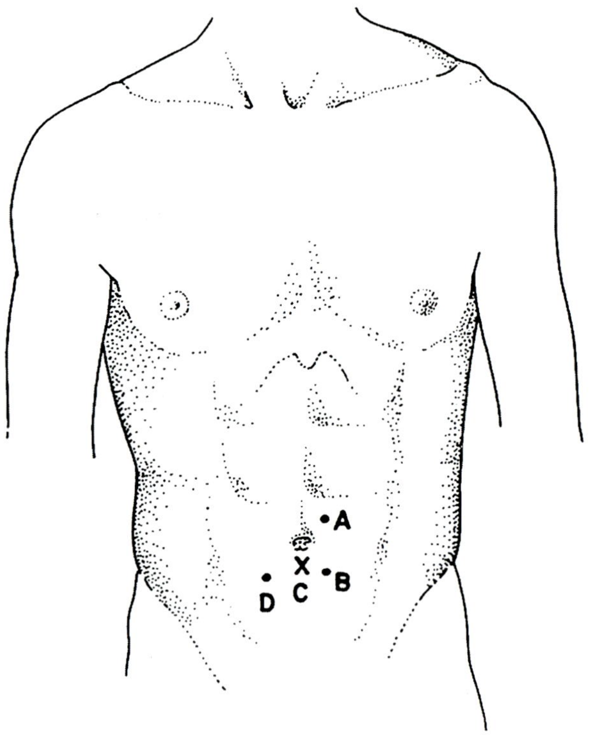

Figure 1.1. The author's preference is site A, however, sites A, B, C and D are safe for puncture.

needle is mandatory. After the skin incision is made and the subcutaneous fat is separated down to the fascia, the Veress needle is placed perpendicular to the fascia. The patient is then asked to push out and tense the abdominal muscles. Two distinct "pops" are felt as the Veress needle traverses the anterior and posterior fascia-peritoneum layers. The needle is never advanced farther than the layer where the second pop occurs. If the local anesthesia has been appropriately placed, this maneuver will not be felt by the patient. The needle is filled with saline. The meniscus of fluid will disappear into the needle when the patient takes a deep breath, confirming the proper intra-abdominal location of the Veress needle.

Insufflation

This author recommends the use of nitrous oxide (N_2O), under local anesthesia, not carbon dioxide (CO_2). CO_2 will combine with the peritoneal fluid to form carbonic acid. This is irritating to the parietal peritoneum and will cause abdominal and shoulder pain (referred from the phrenic nerve). N_2O is inert and better tolerated than CO_2. Absorption from the peritoneum is minimal, and it does not contribute to anesthesia. N_2O is not combustible, but it will support combustion. Therefore, as long as there has been no bowel injury, electrocautery is safe to use in the presence of N_2O.

Figure 1.2. I prefer a vertical incision to avoid the epigastric vessels. The umbilicus is to the left, and the head of the patient is to the right.

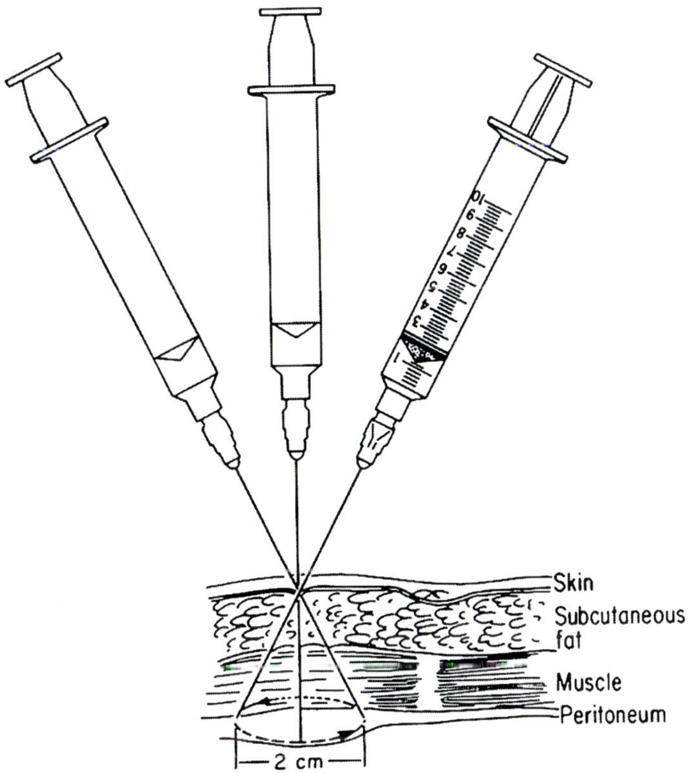

Figure 1.3. Local anesthesia is placed in a cone-shaped fashion with the base at the peritoneum.

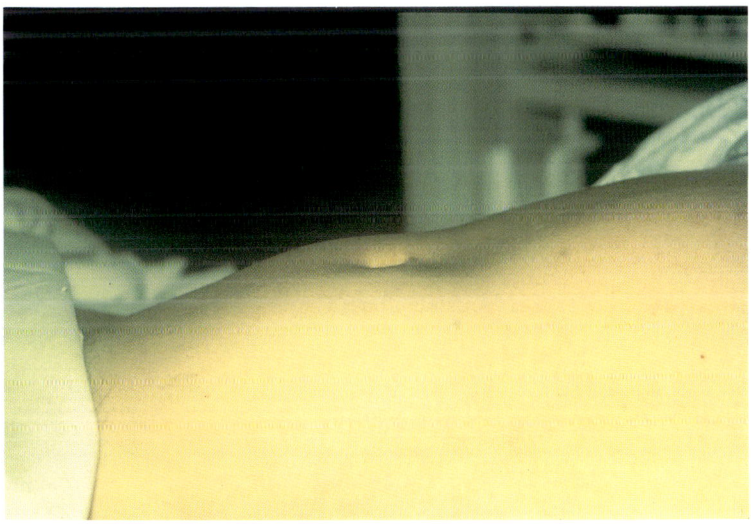

Figure 1.4. This side view demonstrates the patient pushing out the abdomen, while keeping the back flat. Some patients find this difficult to accomplish. Therefore, all patients practice this maneuver before coming to the operating room.

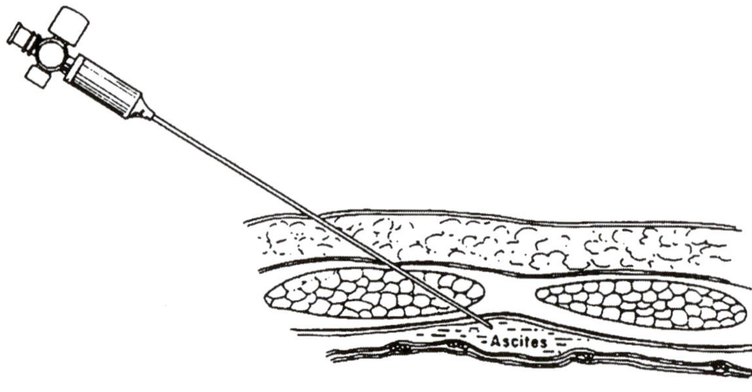

Figure 1.5. The relatively parallel position of the Veress needle to the abdominal wall is shown.

Reflex bradycardia will occur if the patient is insufflated too quickly or excessively. Therefore, the author recommends insufflation at a rate of 1 L/min (low flow rate) and a low volume of gas. Muscular abdominal walls require less gas (young patients) and flaccid muscular walls more gas (elderly patients). In general, it is unusual to need more than 2 L of gas to perform a proper diagnostic laparoscopy under local anesthesia. In the presence of ascites, a slightly different technique should be utilized. After the Veress needle is inserted into the abdomen, it should be placed parallel to the abdominal wall (Fig. 1.5). A small cupola of gas is formed before the needle is placed in a more perpendicular position. Do not insufflate the gas directly into the ascitic fluid, as large, "soapy" bubbles will form, making laparoscopic examination of the abdomen difficult or impossible.

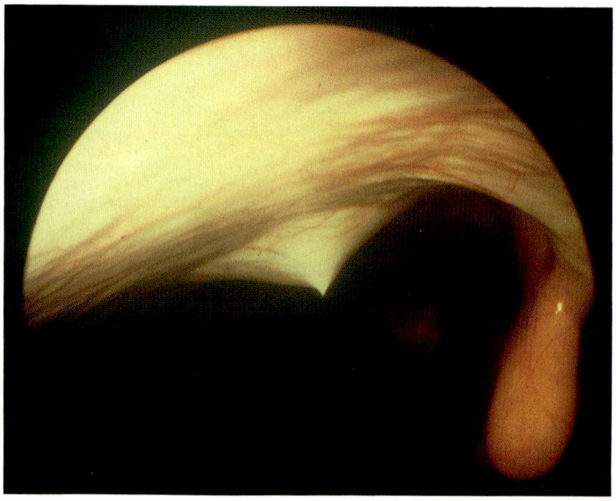

Figure 1.6. This laparoscopic view of the upper right quadrant shows the wheal produced by the injection of local with a 25 gauge needle. The round ligament is to the right.

Ancillary Trocar Sites

If multiple accessory trocars are needed, they are placed under direct vision. The injection of local anesthesia is straightforward once the telescope is in place. Figure 1.6 demonstrates the appropriately sized peritoneal wheal of local anesthesia. All injections are performed with a 25-gauge needle. Discomfort will be minimized if the infiltration is performed slowly. Once the local anesthesia is placed, the patient is again asked to push out and tense the abdominal muscles. If the trocars are sharp, penetration of the abdominal wall is easy to accomplish. If the surgeon is gentle with the laparoscopic manipulations, he or she will be amazed at what can be performed under local anesthesia.

GENERAL ANESTHESIA

The techniques of entry into the abdominal cavity are multiple, but safety is the major concern of all general surgeons performing laparoscopic surgery. There are three ways of entering the abdomen: blind puncture (Veress needle), Hasson trocar, and direct entry with a shielded trocar.

Blind Puncture

Multiple entry sites are available, depending on previous surgery and body habitus. The most common location is periumbilical. In the unoperated abdomen, the author prefers to use the infraumbilical fold. It is the thinnest portion of the abdominal wall, and separation of the peritoneum from the posterior fascia is uncommon at this location. The incision is either transverse or vertical, depending on the shape of the umbilicus. It is important to separate the subcutaneous fat down to the midline fascia to allow unrestricted placement of the Veress needle. Unless the surgical procedure is in the pelvis, a Foley catheter is not inserted routinely. The patient is instructed to void immediately before coming to the holding area, and the urinary bladder is palpated before Veress needle insertion. The author has had no bladder perforations. If the surgery is in the lower abdomen, a Foley catheter is placed. An oral-gastric tube is placed in the stomach to provide decompression. The needle is held in the dominant hand, and the abdominal wall is elevated with the other. If an assistant is present, he or she elevates the other side of the abdominal wall. If there is no assistant, the operator grasps the lower midline of the abdominal wall and elevates it. The Veress needle is placed perpendicular to the fascia and inserted until a pop is heard. The needle is not advanced farther. The needle is checked for proper placement with saline, as described earlier. In the thin patient, extreme care must be taken regarding depth of penetration of the needle. The bifurcation of the aorta and the iliac vessels are at risk in this patient. Elevation of the abdominal wall with towel clips on the skin is not employed, as it increases the separation of subcutaneous fat and the underlying abdominal wall musculature. In laparoscopic cholecystectomy, the author commonly uses the right upper fold of the umbilicus. This area is used if the patient is extremely obese or if there is a long distance between the right costal margin and the umbilicus.

In many European centers, the initial puncture is made in the left upper quadrant just below the costal margin. This is a relatively thin portion of the abdominal wall, and there is little separation of the peritoneum from the posterior fascia. The surgeon must be sure that the stomach is adequately decompressed and that there is no hepatosplenomegaly.

Hasson Technique

The Hasson method of entry into the abdominal cavity was developed to decrease the incidence of intestinal and vascular injury during laparoscopic procedures. It was originally developed for gynecological use. It must be said that the incidence of intestinal injury is the same with Hasson and blind puncture. However, the incidence of major vascular injury is less with the Hasson technique. This author has had no major vascular injuries using the blind puncture method. The most common location of entry with this technique is the infraumbilical area, but it may be anywhere on the abdominal wall. Hasson technique should not be used directly over a previous incision, including the infraumbilical area.

Under direct vision, the midline fascia and umbilical interface are identified. The fascia is opened either transversely or vertically. Staying in the midline, the preperitoneal fat is separated and the peritoneum is opened. A finger is inserted and rotated around the undersurface of the peritoneum to confirm the proper position. Sutures are placed through the fascia and peritoneum. The Hasson trocar is inserted, with the olive placed in the peritoneal cavity. The wings of the trocar are fixed in place with the previously placed sutures. High-flow insufflation may commence immediately.

Direct Puncture

Some surgeons employ direct access into the peritoneal cavity with a shielded trocar. They report this to be a safe and rapid technique with the same incidence of injury as the blind puncture. The problem is that when an injury occurs, it will be secondary to the use of a 10/11-mm trocar, not a 14-gauge needle. For this reason, this author does not recommend its use.

INSUFFLATION

Intra-abdominal pressure does not exceed 14 mmHg in any laparoscopic procedure. In fact, most procedures can be performed under appropriate vision with pressures in the 10 to 12 mmHg range. We have had no instance of spontaneous pneumoperitoneum. Insufflation is begun at a rate of 1 L/min unless entry was performed with Hasson technique. Two or three cycles of the insufflator on low flow with appropriate low pressures (3–6 mmHg) are adequate before changing to high flow (6 L/min or more). During this part of the procedure, the surgeon must observe even distribution of gas in the peritoneal cavity and maintenance of low pressure. Any adverse reactions by the patient require prompt removal of the pneumoperitoneum and evaluation of the cause. Do not maintain pneumoperitoneum while the anesthesiologist is trying to figure out the problem. This author has had no experience with abdominal suspension devices.

EQUIPMENT FOR LAPAROSCOPY

In the early days of therapeutic laparoscopy, availability of appropriate instrumentation was limited. That is not the situation today. A multitude of companies offer an enormous variety of equipment. The selection of equipment and instrumentation should be based on the types of procedures being performed, the familiarity of the surgeon with the instruments, and the budget. The following discussion is related to the author's personal preferences.

Video and Monitor

One-chip and three-chip cameras provide superb image resolution, which is required for laparoscopic surgery. The surgeon must be thoroughly familiar with the mechanics of operation with whatever camera is used. There is nothing more frustrating than to have technical problems in producing the image, making it impossible to perform surgery. The surgeon must be able to troubleshoot. Repeated sterilization of the camera will decrease longevity. Therefore, I cover the camera with a plastic sheath. We have been very satisfied with the Olympus OTV-S4 (single-chip) camera. However, there are other brands which are equally good.

The high-resolution television monitor should have 700 lines per square inch. The size of the screen (13 or 20 in.) depends on the surgeon's preference. I prefer a 13-in. monitor and have been very satisfied with the Sony product.

Videocassette Recorder

A major advantage of laparoscopic surgery is the ability to videotape the procedure. This teaching tool has been instrumental in the advancement of laparoscopic surgery. We require videotaping of all laparoscopic procedures, and we use the tapes for teaching purposes to improve skills. Videotaping is especially valuable when complications arise. Many formats and sizes of VCRs are available. To produce high-quality teaching tapes from the videos, I recommend the use of either 3/4-in. (U-matic) or Hi-8. These two formats allow professional-quality reproduction. If the tapes will be used purely for review of the procedure, then any 1/2-in. VHS system is adequate.

LAPAROSCOPE

Every laparoscopic surgeon should be familiar with 0, 30, and 45 degree telescopes. Many of the more advanced procedures are facilitated with angled telescopes. The more common procedures allow the surgeon to become familiar with angled telescopes. It can be frustrating to use an angled laparoscope for the first time when performing a new procedure. As laparoscopic cholecystectomy is the most common procedure performed, it makes sense to use an angled scope occasionally for this surgery. No specific tricks are involved. It is just a matter of getting used to using them.

Light Source

The light source should be compatible with the video camera and laparoscope. The minimal amount of wattage produced should be 300 watts. An iris cable adapter from the light source to the video camera allows the proper amount of light for imaging. Without its connection, there will be too much glare from the image to be visualized properly. The adapter should be checked before beginning each surgery. I recommend a light source with a lamp life indicator as well. Correcting poor-quality image on the monitor may be as simple as replacing a bulb.

Insufflator

A high-flow insufflator is mandatory for therapeutic laparoscopy. Six- 9-, and 15-L/min machines are available. I have found that a properly functioning 6 L/min insufflator is adequate for both basic and advanced procedures. Minor leaks are easily compensated for by this machine. Maximum pressure is never set above 14 mmHg. A function noise alarm should be present on the insufflator to warn of high pressure. There have been reports of reversed flow of bodily fluids into the insufflation tubing. This occurs when intra-abdominal pressure exceeds insufflator pressure. It is more common when the reserve gas tank is low or empty. Therefore, a trap valve should be used on the tubing to prevent contamination of the insufflator. The pressure in the reserve gas tank should be checked before each surgery, and the tank should be replaced as necessary.

Instrumentation

A variety of instruments are available for therapeutic laparoscopy. In general, the surgeon's preference is key here. Each instrument should be checked for function, insulation, and cleanliness before use. Because of cost limits, most surgeons utilize a combination of reusable and disposable equipment. It is a good idea to have a regularly scheduled maintenance check on all reusable equipment. This will increase the longevity of the instruments and is cost effective. This check includes the periodic sharpening of reusable scissors.

The use of 5- or 10-mm instruments will be dictated by the procedure and the surgeon's preference. However, for basic instrumentation there are both ratcheted and nonratcheted graspers, straight and angled dissectors (Maryland type), and curved and straight scissors.

A high pressure irrigation system is helpful in many of the difficult laparoscopic procedures, along with a functioning aspiration system. There are many on the market; I have found the Cabot system to be exceptional. There are 10-mm suction ports available for clot extraction as well.

There are many tip designs for the electrocautery hook instruments. The choice depends on the surgeon's preference. A variation is the spatula (knife) electrode, which this author finds useful for dissection of the gallbladder from the liver bed.

SUMMARY

Inherent in the ability to perform laparoscopic procedures well is the use of two-handed technique. The more advanced the procedure, the more necessary is the use of two hands. It is critical for the surgeon to develop these skills in the more common procedures performed. There is no substitute for practice in an inanimate trainer before taking these techniques to the operating room. Included in these skills are suturing and knot tying techniques, both intra- and extracorporeally. Mastering these tasks will increase the safety of laparoscopic surgery and decrease the necessity of conversion in most situations.

chapter two

Basic Techniques in Thoracoscopy

Kenneth L. Franco

Thoracoscopy was first described by Jacobaeus, a Swedish physician, in 1910.[1] The technique was limited mainly to pleural disease and collapse therapy for tuberculosis. Enthusiasm for the technique awaited improvements in video endoscopic surgical equipment and a growing interest in minimally invasive surgical approaches. In the 1980s, the development of laparoscopic cholecystectomy caused a resurgence of interest in video-assisted procedures involving the thoracic cavity. Further advances awaited the development of the endoscopic stapler, and newer instruments are being designed specifically for video thoracoscopy.

INSTRUMENTATION

A vast array of disposable and reusable endoscopic surgical instruments are available from a large number of manufacturers; representative samples will be discussed here (Table 2.1). The field is evolving so rapidly that new instruments are being developed every month. The major components of instrumentation include video equipment, staplers, and thoracic instruments such as lung clamps, retractors, scissors, and lasers. A typical setup of video equipment for thoracoscopy includes a large-screen video monitor, a light source, a video recorder, and a printer for still photography. A second video monitor facilitates the operation by allowing both the surgeon and the first assistant to look directly at a monitor without having to turn away from the surgical field (Fig. 2.1).

Most thoracic surgeons use a 0^0 10-mm rigid operating thoracoscope with a 5-mm biopsy channel (Fig. 2.2), but 30^0 scopes are available which permit a more complete view of the thoracic cavity. Initially, trocar cannulas designed for laparoscopy were used to access the pleural space, but they have sharp ends that could injure the lung. Modified trocar cannulas or ports have been developed which consist simply of a bullet-tipped plastic obturator that facilitates passage of the cannula through the chest wall. The outer end of the cannula is covered by a thin plastic diaphragm that stabilizes the position of the thoracoscope but can be easily removed if desired. Trocar cannulas are available in several sizes to accommodate different instruments.

Endoscopic GIA staplers that cut between two rows of staples have been developed and are available in 30- and 60-mm lengths (Fig. 2.3). They are disposable, multi-fire instruments similar to those designed for open procedures and provide excellent hemostasis and closure of air leaks. A number of lung clamps have been developed which facilitate peripheral wedge resections, which is one of the more common indications for thoracoscopic surgery (Fig. 2.4). In addition, scissors are available which incorporate an attachment for electrocautery so that it is possible to cut and cauterize simultaneously (Fig. 2.5). The availability of a Nd:YAG laser can be helpful in the resection of a peripheral lung nodule.[2] All of these instruments give the thoracic surgeon the necessary tools to perform safe video thoracoscopic procedures, as is done through an open thoracotomy.

OPERATIVE SETUP AND SURGICAL TECHNIQUE

All thoracoscopic procedures are performed in the operating room, which allows the thoracic surgeon to convert immediately to an open thoracotomy if necessary. All procedures are performed under general anes-

Table 2.1. Recommended Equipment for Thoracoscopy

General anesthesia
Double-lumen endotracheal tube or bronchial blocker
Thoracotomy instrument tray
Light source and cable
Video monitor ×2
Videocassette recorder
Trocar/cannulas
Telescopes (10 mm, 0^{0})
Babcock clamp
Duval clamp
Scissors
Endo-GIA stapler
Endoclip applicator
Electrocautery unit
Nd:YAG laser
Antifog solution
Adequate suction

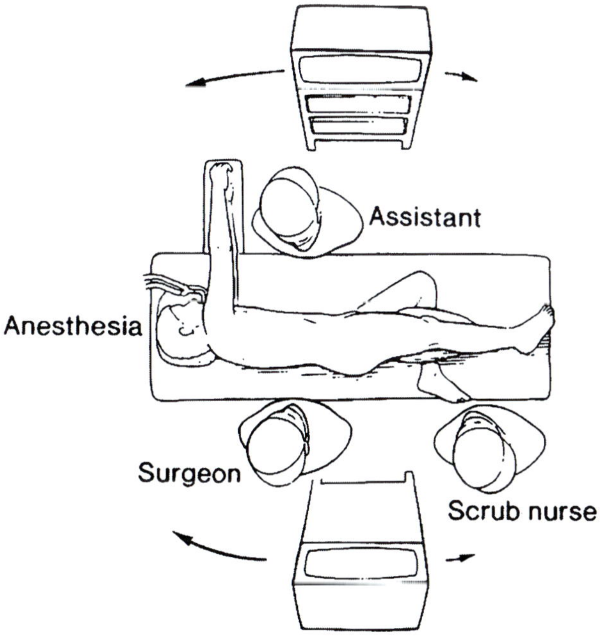

Figure 2.1. Standard operating room setup for thoracoscopic procedures. (From Miller DL, Allen MS: Set-up and present indications for video assisted thoracic surgery. *Semin Thorac Cardiovasc Surg* 5:280–283, 1993. Reprinted with permission from W.B. Saunders Co.)

thesia using a double-lumen endotracheal tube or bronchial blocker. After the induction of general anesthesia, the patient is placed in a full lateral decubitus position and the thorax is surgically prepared in case conversion to an open thoracotomy is necessary.

Placement of incisions depends on the location of the pathology and the procedure planned. The initial trocar placement is usually in the fifth or sixth intercostal space in the midaxillary line, which provides an unobstructed view of the entire hemithorax[3] (Fig. 2.6).

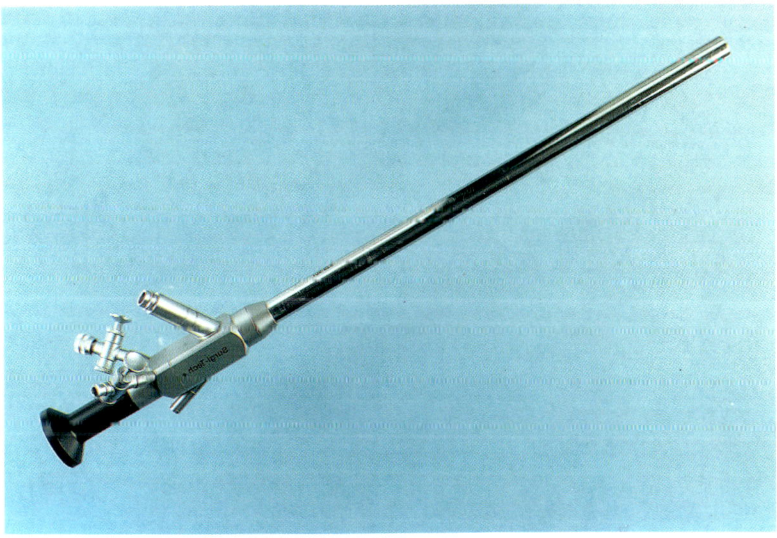

Figure 2.2. Rigid operating thoracoscope (0^{0}, 10-mm) with a 5-mm biopsy channel. (Courtesy of Surgimedics.)

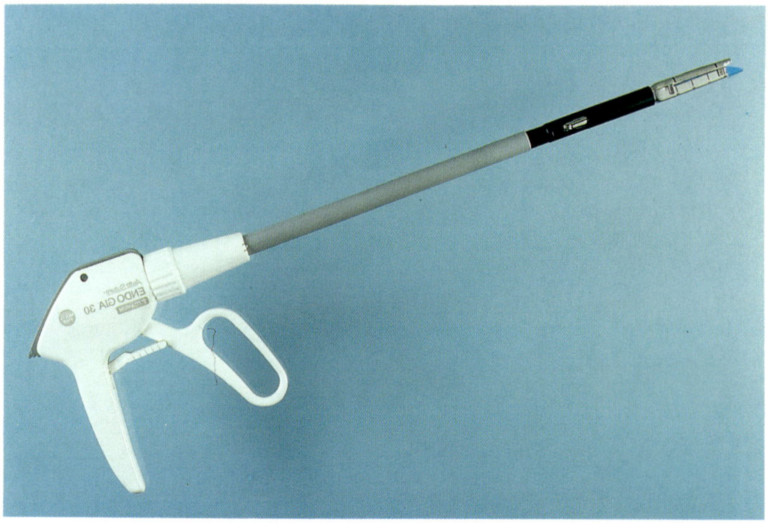

Figure 2.3. Endoscopic GIA stapler. (Courtesy of United States Surgical Corporation.)

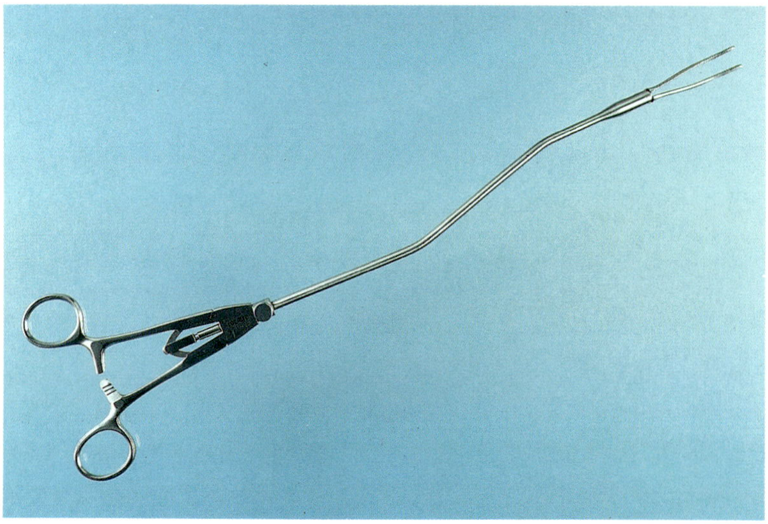

Figure 2.4. Thoracoscopic Duval clamp. (Courtesy of Surgimedics.)

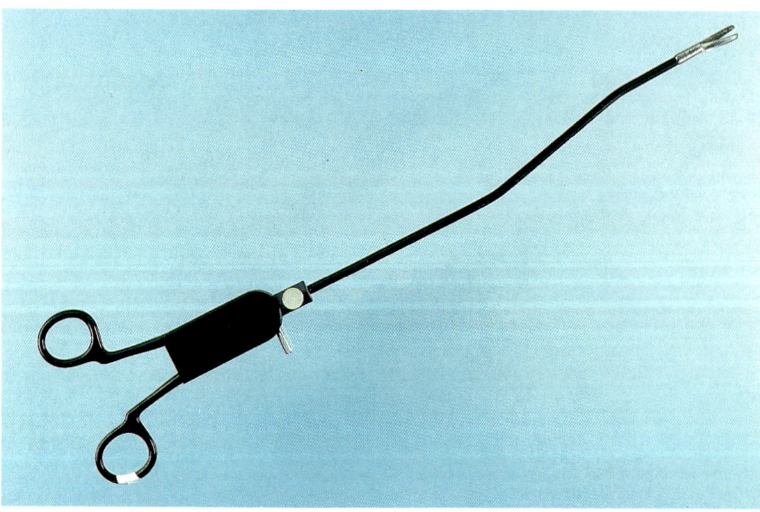

Figure 2.5. Straight thoracoscopic dissecting scissor with cautery. (Courtesy of Surgimedics.)

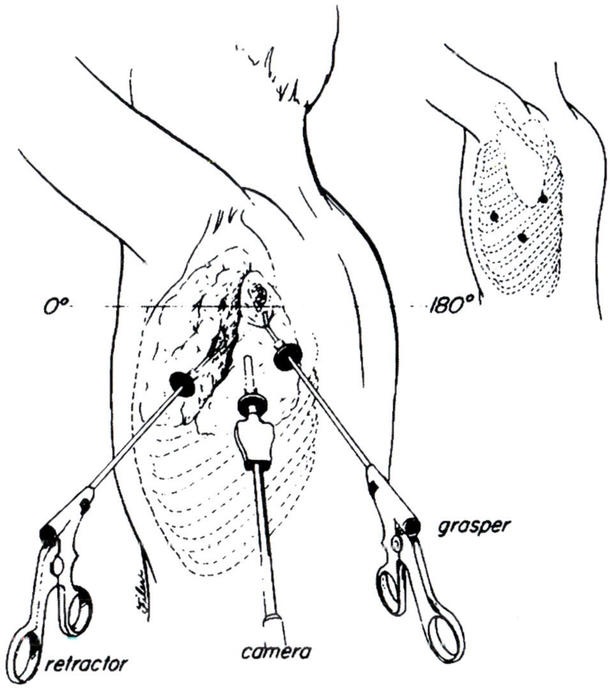

Figure 2.6. Typical positioning of thoracoscopic instruments and camera for resection of pulmonary nodule. (From Ref. 3. Reprinted with permission from W.B. Saunders Co.)

A 10-mm incision is made and dissection performed through the subcutaneous tissue and intercostal muscle with a hemostat until the pleural cavity is entered. The pleura is entered bluntly and probed with a finger to make sure that the pleural surfaces are not fused and the lungs are dropped away to allow free access for trocar insertion. A cylindrical trocar used as a camera port is placed in the chest wall. After the thoracoscopic lens is warmed and covered with defogging solution, the thoracoscope is introduced through the sleeve and the pleural space is explored (Fig. 2.7).

Subsequent incisions are made and additional trocars are placed under direct visualization to ensure that no injury occurs to intrathoracic organs. The number of additional trocars depends on the procedure, ranging from one to four. Optimal positioning of subsequent trocars includes placement at the widest angle possible so that the largest angle for retraction is obtained, instruments do not interfere with one another, and the field of vision is not obscured by instruments.[4] An attempt should be made to keep trocar incisions in line with the standard thoracotomy incision so that if opening is required, the incisions can be incorporated into one. The surgeon should attempt to keep the pathology and instruments between the camera and monitor so that, when the operation is watched on the monitor, the instruments move as expected and not in a mirror image or reverse fashion.

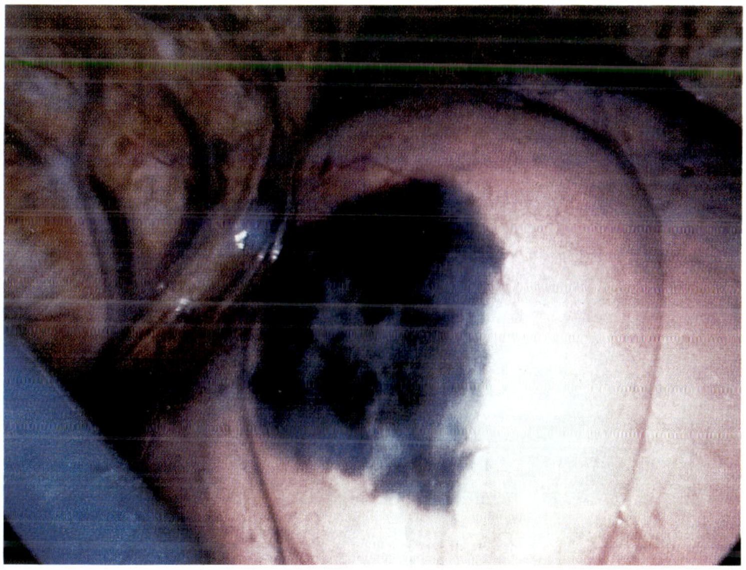

Figure 2.7. Thoracoscopic appearance of melanoma in the lung. (From Mack MJ, Acuff TE, Hazelrigg SR, et al: Video thoracoscopy in thoracic surgery. *Surg Rounds* 10:831–838, 1993. Reprinted with permission from Romaine Pierson Publishers.)

When the procedure is completed, a chest tube is inserted through one of the trocar sites and all sites are closed with absorbable suture.

INDICATIONS

Many surgical procedures performed via an open thoracotomy can now be done thorascoscopically, but current indications are limited because no long-term results of thoracoscopic surgery have been reported.[5] Any operation done through a thoracoscope must be performed as safely as it can via a thoracotomy because the goals of the two procedures should be the same. Short-term benefits should not be exchanged for a poor long-term outcome. The advantages of minimally invasive surgery of the chest include decreased pain, shortened hospital stay, faster return to work, and smaller incisions for the patient. These advantages must be weighed against the present limitations of thoracoscopy, which include the need for a learning curve, increased costs and operating time, evolution of instrumentation, inability to palpate lung tissue, the potential for hemorrhage and lack of vascular control, and the potential for tumor seeding.[6]

The present indications for thoracoscopy are shown in Table 2.2. The most common indications include wedge resection of an indeterminate pulmonary nodule or for diffuse interstitial lung disease, pleural effusions, and recurrent pneumothorax. The thoracic surgeon is frequently asked to participate in the diagnostic evaluation of an indeterminate pulmonary nodule when less invasive means are unsuccessful. This approach is justified because 40–50% of all peripheral nodules are malignant, with the majority of these being primary bronchogenic carcinoma.[7] The nodule should have a smooth border, be less than 3 cm in diameter, be located in the outer third of the lung, and have no endobronchial extension.[8] Preoperative localization procedures can be used if difficulty is expected in localizing the lesion at the time of thoracoscopy (Fig. 2.8). Thoracoscopy is ideal for patients with diffuse interstitial lung disease who need a lung biopsy.[9] It provides improved visualization of the entire thoracic cavity and permits biopsy of any segment of the lung. Patients with progressive respiratory insufficiency are not ideal candidates for thoracoscopy and are best served by a limited thoracotomy.

Thoracoscopy can be very helpful in the treatment of pleural effusions and appears to be well tolerated by these patients. The ability to drain the pleural space completely, achieve pleural symphysis, and distribute a sclerosing agent such as talc evenly on all pleural surfaces enables one to manage this difficult problem and prevent recurrences.

Table 2.2. Indications for Thoracoscopy

Pleura
- Effusion
- Empyema
- Hemothorax
- Chylothorax
- Tumor biopsy—mesothelioma
- Pleurodesis

Lung
- Blebs or bullae
- Lung biopsy
- Indeterminate nodule

Mediastinum
- Mass
- Thymectomy for myasthenia gravis
- Pericardial effusion
- Stage lung cancer
- ligate PDA
- AICD
- Sympathectomy

Esophagus
- Myotomy
- Fundoplication
- Vagotomy
- Esophageal cancer staging
- Esophagectomy

Thoracoscopy has become the procedure of choice for managing recurrent spontaneous pneumothorax.[10] It is easy to excise or obliterate an apical bleb with an endoscopic stapler. In addition, the entire lung can be examined easily for other sites of possible air leak. However, although this procedure causes less postoperative pain, it is still recommended only for recurrent pneumothoraces or first-time, spontaneous pneumothoraces that have a continued air leak beyond 7 days.

Many centers with experience in thoracoscopic procedures have extended the indications to those involving the mediastinum, pericardium, autonomic ganglia, and esophagus. It is important that those performing thoracoscopy be trained to use open techniques. In the future, as experience is gained and as instruments are improved, further advances will occur.

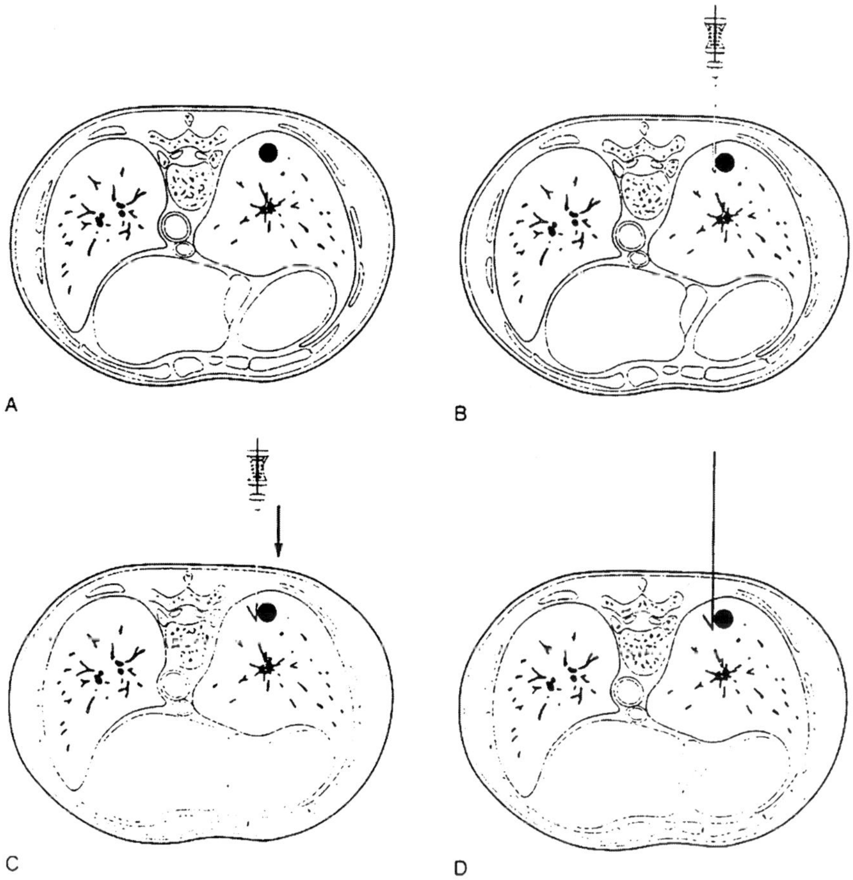

Figure 2.8. Placement of the localization wire to aid in the thoracoscopic resection of lung nodule. (A) Location of nodule (B) insertion of cannula (C) insertion of hookwire through cannula (D) cannula has been withdrawn and the hook wire remains. (From Nosher JL, Gribbin CE, Caccavale RJ: Radiologic localization of lung parenchymal nodules. *Chest Clin North Am* 3:337–344, 1993. Reprinted with permission from W.B. Saunders Co.)

REFERENCES

1. Jacobaeus HC: Possibility of the use of the cystoscope for investigation of serous cavities. *Munch Med Wocheuschr* 59:2090–2092, 1910.
2. Landreneau RJ, Hazelrigg SR, Johnson JA, et al: Neodymium. Yttrium-aluminum garnet laser as-sisted pulmonary resections. *Ann Thorac Surg* 51:973–978, 1991.
3. Landreneau RJ, Mack MJ, Hazelrigg SR, et al: Thoracoscopic management of benign pulmonary lesions. *Chest Clin North Am* 3:249–262, 1993.
4. Landreneau RJ, Mack MJ, Hazelrigg SR, et al: Video-assisted thoracic surgery: Basic technical concepts and intercostal approach strategies. *Ann Thorac Surg* 54:800–807, 1992.
5. Miller JL: Therapeutic thoracoscopy. New horizons for an established procedure. *Ann Thorac Surg* 52:1036–1037, 1991.
6. Page RD, Jeffrey RR, Donnelly RJ: Thoracoscopy—A review of 121 consecutive surgical procedures. *Ann Thorac Surg* 48:66–70, 1989.
7. Lillington GA: Pulmonary nodules. Solitary and multiple. *Clin Chest Med* 3:369–367, 1982.
8. Miller DL, Allen MS, Trastek VF, et al: Videothoracoscopic wedge excision of the lung. *Ann Thorac Surg* 54:410–414, 1992.
9. Miller DL, Allen MS, Trastek VF, et al: Thoracoscopic wedge excision for diffuse interstitial lung disease. *Chest* 102:169–174, 1992.
10. Hazelrigg SR, Landreneau RJ, Mack MJ, et al: Thoracoscopic stapled resection for spontaneous pneumothorax. *J Thorac Cardiovasc Surg* 105:389–393, 1993.

chapter three
Trocars and Insertion Techniques to Avoid Injury

Leon Daykhovsky
Stephen J. Shapiro
Leo A. Gordon

The goal of this chapter is to discuss the step-by-step techniques necessary for the safe and reliable transabdominal placement of the pneumo-needle and trocars for laparoscopic surgery.

The first step in laparoscopic surgery is the creation of the pneumoperitoneum. To achieve this, every surgeon who engages in laparoscopic surgery should carefully and meticulously learn these steps for the insertion of the pneumo-needle and trocars. The time spent learning to create a safe pneumo-peritoneum will help the surgeon avoid unnecessary injury during the initial steps of laparoscopic surgery.

During the last 5 years, our group has performed thousands of laparoscopic procedures. We are interested in sharing our experiences with our colleagues in the hope of helping to make this technique safe and reliable for all patients. In recent years, reusable, semi-reusable, and disposable instruments have been utilized to perform the initial step of laparoscopy.

PNEUMO-NEEDLES

The reusable pneumo-needle consists of a sharp, 12-cm-long, hollow, spring-loaded needle, a blunt stylette, and a stopcock.

During the introduction of the needle, the underlying soft tissue pushes the shaft of the needle. At the time of perforation of the fascia, the stylette pushes forward with a characteristic metal click. The blunt stylette protects the underlying viscera from perforation. Two metal clicks can usually be heard. The first one occurs during penetration of the fascia. The second one occurs during penetration of the peritoneum.

Prior to insertion of the needle, the surgeon should inspect this instrument. Special attention should be paid to the following:

1. Sharpness of the needle.
2. Action of the blunt obturator.
3. Patency of the inner channel.

The usual length of the pneumo-needle is 12 cm. However, for morbidly obese patients, longer pneumo-needles (14 and 16 cm) are available.

One drawback of the reusable pneumo-needle is the multiple parts, which the nurse must disassemble after every surgery for washing, cleaning, and lubrication. After multiple uses, the sharp distal end of the needle can become dull. This may cause trauma during insertion. Many types of disposable pneumo-needles are also available. Their main advantage is that they are always sharp, do not require handling, and are relatively inexpensive.

Semidisposable pneumo-needles have been specifically designed to offset the above disadvantage. These combine an extremely sharp, disposable needle with a reusable spring-loaded, blunt stylette.

TROCARS

For many years, the trocars used during laparoscopic surgery were reusable instruments. These trocars had multiple parts which required assembly and disassembly before and after each surgery. Disposable and semi-disposable trocars have been introduced in recent years. The main advantage of these instruments is the stylette, which is designed with special features. As a safety feature, the sharp distal end is retracted or protected by a specially designed sleeve or shield.

The trocar is composed of three main parts: the stylette, canula, and valve. There are three main valve designs: trumpet, trap door, and ball valve. The distal end of the stylette of the reusable trocar is extremely sharp, with a conical or pyramidal shape. In a disposable trocar, the stylette is protected by the specially designed shields, which are retracted backward during the introduction of the trocar.

Advantages and Disadvantages

The advantage of the reusable trocar is its relatively low cost. The disadvantages are no safety shield, multiple parts, and the considerable labor required for cleaning, assembly, disassembly, and maintenance.

Disposable trocars are relatively affordable. Their stylettes are always sharp, and they are protected by a specially designed shield. They require no maintenance. The main disadvantages of disposable trocars are their expense and concerns about their environmental impact.

CREATION OF THE PNEUMOPERITONEUM

Careful physical examination of the patient is required prior to laparoscopic surgery in order to identify any abnormalities. Variable position of the spine and rib cage, as well as scars on the surface of the abdominal cavity, must be considered. Special attention should be paid to patients with scoliosis and kyphosis, as well as to malnourished patients. In these groups of patients, the aorta and the inferior vena cava are positioned very close to the abdominal wall. The introduction of the pneumo-needle or trocars should take into consideration these anatomic points. When operating on morbidly obese patients, long or extra-long trocars should be used.

The patient is positioned on the operating table in the supine position. Insertion of a nasogastric tube and a urinary catheter decompresses the stomach and bladder. An 11-blade scalpel is used to perform a supra- or infraumbilical incision. The underlying subcutaneous tissue is dissected with a mosquito-type dissector. If bleeding occurs from a subcutaneous vessel, it should be coagulated. Prior to insertion of the pneumo-needle, the operator and assistant must lift the abdominal wall near the incision site. The operator can then drive the needle through the fascia, with the needle firmly positioned between the thumb and index finger. The assistant should perform a two-step test to verify the proper position of the pneumo-needle.

Test 1

A 10-cc syringe with saline solution is attached to the lock of the pneumo-needle. The plunger is withdrawn. Usually one or two bubbles of air will appear in the chamber or the syringe. If there is blood, bile, intestinal contents, or urine in the chamber, the needle should be repositioned. These findings indicate an injury to an adjacent organ. It is mandatory that suspected areas of injury be inspected at the beginning of laparoscopy.

Test 2

In the "hanging drop" test, a 10-cc syringe is attached and a drop of saline solution is positioned in the proximal end of the pneumo-needle. The negative pressure created by the movement of the diaphragm will suck the solution into the channel of the needle shaft. In cases where the surgeon is not satisfied with the performance of the test, the pneumo-needle should be withdrawn and repositioned, repeating all steps.

After properly positioning the pneumo-needle, a CO_2 line should be attached to the needle and the flow of CO_2 gas begun. The insufflator is supposed to deliver 1 L of CO_2 gas per minute. At this rate of flow, the abdominal pressure should be less than 6 mmHg. If the pressure is higher, insufflation should be stopped at once and the needle repositioned. During all of these manipulations, the surgeon must be careful not to misplace the pneumo-needle by accidental movement. After the insufflation of 1 L of CO_2, dullness over the upper right quadrant will disappear. This can be easily checked by percussion. When the pressure in the peritoneal cavity reaches the maximal preset pressure of 15 mmHg, most insufflators will automatically stop. It is usually necessary to have 5 to 7 L of CO_2 to reach 15 mmHg pressure. The insufflator should be checked prior to laparoscopic surgery. The CO_2 tanks attached to the insufflator should be filled with CO_2 gas and the alarm device checked prior to surgery.

There are several possible reasons for high-pressure readings on the CO_2 insufflator:

1. The inner channel of the pneumo-needle is obstructed.
2. The needle is jammed into tissue or against the tissue.
3. The CO_2 line is obstructed.

If high-pressure readings occur, the surgeon should do the following: Check the tubing of the CO_2 line. Rotate and slightly withdraw the needle. Lightly elevate the abdominal wall. Attach a 10-cc solution-filled syringe and irrigate through the needle. The surgeon should be thoroughly convinced that he or she has established an adequate pneumoperitoneum prior to the insertion of the trocar. The time spent on careful creation of a pneumoperitoneum ensures safe insertion of the first trocar.

OPEN HASSON TECHNIQUE FOR DEVELOPING A PNEUMOPERITONEUM

The open technique requires a minilaparotomy with the direct insertion of a specially designed trocar. A 2-cm incision is made in the fascia. A suture is placed on either side of the fascial incision. As soon as the trocar is inserted into the peritoneal cavity, the trocar can be tightened against the fascia and the preplaced sutures. The CO_2 line should then be attached to the trocar and the insufflation begun. This technique has been adopted by many medical centers throughout the country. It is especially recommended when insertion of the Veress needle is difficult or cannot be achieved. Prior abdominal surgery is the most frequent indication for using the Hasson method.

Insertion of the Trocar

As soon as the pneumoperitoneum has been safely established, the surgeon should inspect the trocar prior to its insertion. The pneumo-needle should be withdrawn and the flow of CO_2 gas turned off.

The safety shield of the trocar, if present, should be checked. The trocar should be positioned in the dominant hand in such a way that its proximal part lies in the palm. The index finger should be extended over the shaft of the trocar. The surgeon should then move the trocar perpendicular to the fascia, using a twisting motion. An alternative to this technique is to use two hands. The dominant hand should hold the housing of the trocar, and the nondominant hand should grasp the shaft of the trocar. The nondominant hand acts as a brake, adding control to the trocar insertion. Attention should be paid to the size of the incision. If the incision is too tight, extra force will be required to insert the trocar. This can lead to a loss of control as the trocar penetrates the fascia.

Too large an incision can cause continuous leakage of the CO_2, and a drop in the pneumoperitoneum and eventual dislodgement of the trocar during the procedure may occur. To avoid complications arising from dislodgement, some manufacturers have designed trocar stabilizers. These stabilizers preload on the barrel of the trocar. We have found that specially designed adhesive discs, preloaded prior to insertion of the trocar are extremely useful.

The effectiveness of disposable trocars has been proven in thousands of laparoscopic cases. Newly designed safety shields may minimize trauma to the underlying visceral structures. During insertion of the first trocar, the following events should occur:

1. The underlying subcutaneous tissue, fascia, and peritoneum create a pressure on the safety shield, which will be automatically withdrawn. The naked blade of the trocar will face the fascia and peritoneum.
2. When perforation of the peritoneum has occurred, the pressure of adjacent structures will decrease and the safety shield will slide over the distal end of the trocar, protecting the visceral organs from injury.
3. The stylette will be removed. At this time, the CO_2 line tubing can be reattached to the stopcock of the trocar. The average drop in pressure during this procedure should be around 5–6 mmHg, which will be easily reestablished within a few seconds.

Insertion of Additional Trocars

Once the first trocar has been inserted, additional trocars are placed under direct visual control. This provides safety and accuracy. The following should be observed:

1. Additional trocars should be placed under direct visual control. To achieve sufficient visual control, the laparoscope should be positioned to allow a wide-angle view of the selected penetration site.

2. In nonobese patients, translumination can be very helpful in detecting blood vessels near sites of trocar insertion.
3. Avoid scar tissue during the insertion of trocars.
4. Consider the course of the inferior epigastric artery and vein. They run parallel to the rectus abdominus sheath.
5. Using the index finger, apply pressure on the anterior wall of the abdominal cavity at the site of future trocar placement. Identify the site of trocar placement using the laparoscopic view. Make sure that there is no attachment of visceral organs (i.e., adhesions) to the site of insertion of the remaining trocars.

General rules for trocar placement include the following:

1. Place trocars as far as possible from one another to avoid "sword fighting" with the instruments inserted through the trocars.
2. Use large-bore trocars, (10–12 mm in diameter). These trocars free the surgeon from limitations and enable the utilization of large instruments necessary during the surgery.

Assuming that sites have been selected for trocar placement, the following steps are recommended:

1. Perform a skin incision of 11–12 mm (for large trocars).
2. Spread the subcutaneous tissue with a mosquito-type dissector.
3. Press the fascia with the dissector to verify a safe site for trocar placement under laparoscopic guidance.
4. Inspect the trocar as described.
5. Aim the sharp tip of the trocar toward a space unoccupied by viscera.
6. Withdraw the stylette of the trocar. Adjust the trocar-retaining device or adhesive trocar seal.

Problems during Trocar Insertion

Leakage of CO_2 gas around the trocar site

This problem can occur as a result of a large incision, excessive dissection of subcutaneous tissue, or a discrepancy between the outer diameter of the trocar and the incision. Leakage can be detected by injecting saline solution into the incision around the trocar. Bubbling of the solution will indicate leakage. With CO_2 insufflator pressure of 15 mmHg, minor leakage can be ignored. More significant leaks should be corrected.

This can be done in several ways. The trocar can be replaced with one having a larger diameter. One can also utilize a retaining device which can be preloaded prior to insertion. This device has an adhesive cup which can seal trocar sites and protect them from leakage. If these solutions are ineffective, trocar site cutaneous incisions can be enlarged, subcutaneous tissue dissected, the fascia exposed, and a peritoneal suture placed on the fascia. Tying a suture around the trocar shaft can also eliminate leakage of CO_2. If the leakage is not from the origin of the trocar site, careful inspection of trocar valves, stopcocks, and CO_2 line tubing should be performed. A malfunctioning trocar or damaged CO_2 line tubing should be replaced immediately.

Bleeding from the trocar site

External bleeding from the trocar site can occur during the skin incision and dissection of the subcutaneous tissue. In this case, vessels should be isolated and coagulated with the electrocautery prior to insertion of the trocar.

Internal bleeding

Internal bleeding can be detected as blood dripping from the shaft of the trocar or as a growing hematoma around the trocar insertion site. If the bleeding continues, a puncture closure device can be used to place a suture around the trocar site (Fig. 3.1). The trocar can then be withdrawn and placed at a new site.

Alternatively, a large Foley catheter can be inserted through the trocar into the abdominal cavity, and the balloon at its distal end can be inflated. Pulling on the Foley catheter will approximate the balloon with the inner site of the trocar puncture wound. It will serve as a compressive device and will stop the bleeding. The trocar can be moved over the shaft of the Foley catheter, and a heavy clamp can then be placed over the end of the catheter. This enables the proximal end of the catheter to be cut off, releasing the trocar. To continue laparoscopic surgery, the inflated Foley catheter should be left at the site of the trocar puncture wound. At the end of the procedure, the clamp can be removed, the Foley catheter withdrawn, and the trocar wound carefully inspected. If the bleeding continues, the surgical wound should be increased, and careful inspection and dissection of the damaged blood vessels should be performed. The vessel should be ligated and the wound closed.

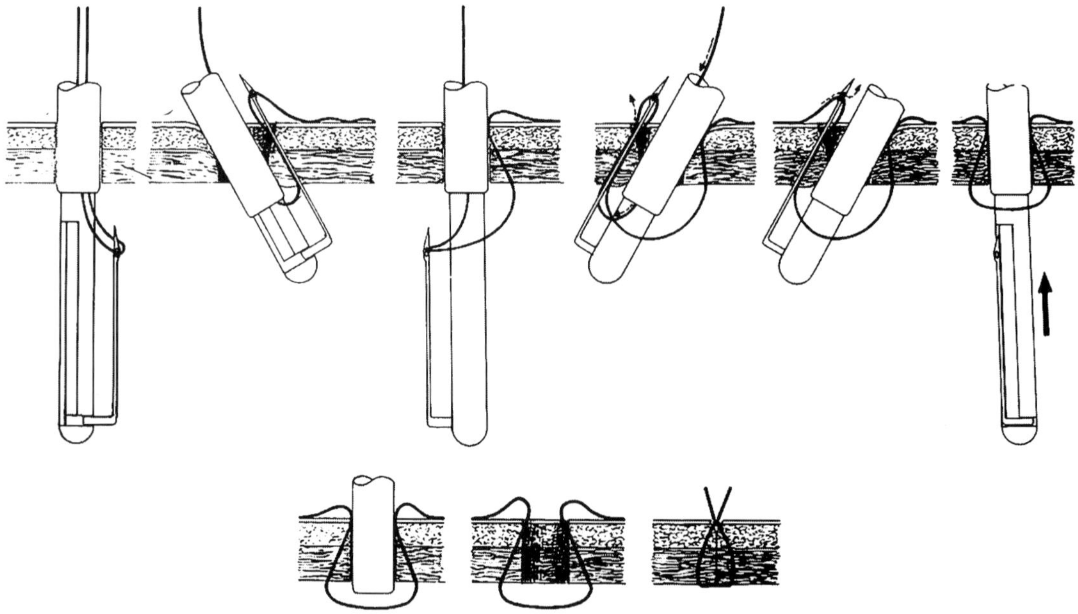

Figure 3.1. This figure depicts a step by step process for trocar wound closure, utilizing an "exit" puncture closure device. (Advanced Surgical, Inc., Princeton, N.J.)

If substantial bleeding occurs from a trocar site, a straight needle with a heavy suture can be guided through the abdominal wall into the peritoneal cavity. Using a laparoscopic needle holder, through-and-through sutures can be placed through the abdominal wall at the trocar site. Applying pressure on the suture can help stop or control the bleeding.

Laparoscopic assessment of all trocar sites is essential, no matter what control technique is used.

Perforation of visceral organs

Perforation of visceral organs most often occurs during the initial steps of blind insertion of the pneumo-needle and first trocar. Meticulous inspection of the areas of trocar insertion should be performed. Signs of visceral perforation include the following:

1. Fecal or bile contamination of the distal end of the stylette.
2. Fecal or bile staining in an area along the path of trocar insertion.
3. The smell of intestinal contents coming from the trocar.
4. Enlargement of the intestinal lumen due to the flow of CO_2 into the intestines.

Major vascular injury can result from insertion of the first blind trocar or of the pneumo-needle. If an injury does occur, these instruments should be left in place and rapid laparotomy performed. Hemostasis should be obtained by occlusion of the injured vessel with soft, atraumatic clamps. At the time of laparotomy, careful inspection of the gastrointestinal tract should be performed, paying special attention to the potential for through-and-through visceral or vascular injuries. Often the only indication of a major vascular injury is a subtle mesenteric hematoma or transient hypotension. Both should be investigated.

Gas embolism

Gas embolism is rare in laparoscopic surgery. When it occurs, it is most commonly due to direct insufflation of CO_2 gas into a vessel or organ during placement of the pneumo-needle or trocar. A low flow of CO_2 gas insufflation through the pneumo-needle is recommended at the beginning of a procedure. This can help minimize the risk of gas embolism and aid early detection of such complications.

Gas embolism is indicated by arrhythmia with a characteristic Mill-Wheel murmur. This typical murmur can be heard at the left parasternal border. If this condition is present, insufflation of CO_2 gas should be stopped. The patient should be placed in the left lateral decubitus position, with the operating table placed in the steep Trendelenburg position. This will allow a bolus of CO_2 gas to pass from the right atrium into the right ventricle. The sudden onset of a new murmur during laparoscopic surgery represents an anesthetic emergency. All anesthesiologists should be familiar with the treatment of this condition.

Trocar Removal

At the end of a laparoscopic procedure, trocars are removed under visual control. Prior to removal, a puncture wound closure device may be inserted through the shaft of the trocar. Its needle is activated and guided through the layers of the abdominal wall. Large suture material is used for this procedure. Closure of the fascia after removal of trocars is extremely important to avoid trocar site hernias.

CONCLUSION

Placement of the pneumo-needle and initial trocar is the first step in most laparoscopic procedures. The concerns and techniques outlined above will help ensure the safe placement of these basic laparoscopic devices.

BIBLIOGRAPHY

Berci G: Instrumentation, rigid endoscopes. In Berci G, (ed.): *Endoscopy*. New York, Appleton-Century-Crofts, 1976, pp 5–74.

Phillips E, Daykhovsky L, Carroll B: Laparoscopic cholecystectomy: Instrumentation and technique. *J Laparoendosc Surg* 1:1–15, 1990.

Gaskin TA, Isobe JH, Mathews JL, et al: Laparoscopy and the general surgeon. *Surg Clin North Am* 71(5):1085–1097, 1991.

Hasson HM. Modified instrument and method for laparoscopy. *Am J Obstet Gynecol* 110:886–887, 1971.

Hulka JF: *Textbook of Laparoscopy*. Orlando, FL, Grune and Stratton, 1985, pp 1–88.

Semm K: *Operative Manual for Endoscopic Abdominal Surgery*. Chicago, Year Book Medical, 1987, pp 1–254.

Veress J: Neues Instrument zur Ausfuhrung von Brust oder Bauchpunktionen. *Dtsch Med Wochschr* 41: 1480, 1938.

chapter four

Safe Use of Electrosurgical Devices During Minimally Invasive Surgery

C. Randle Voyles
Robert D. Tucker

Though a wide variety of energy sources have been used in laparoscopy, monopolar electrosurgery remains the gold standard. Monopolar electrosurgery had been used in open procedures for several decades before it was used in laparoscopic tubal fulguration in the early 1970s. Unfortunately, the early complications with the laparoscopic use of monopolar electrosurgery were not adequately explained. Gynecologic surgeons switched to bipolar electrosurgery rather than resolve the potential problems with monopolar devices.[1] As laparoscopic techniques became more advanced, a more effective energy source was required and gynecologists adopted laser technology. Largely as a result, general surgeons initiated laparoscopic cholecystectomy with laser devices in the United States but switched back to monopolar electrosurgery because of documented benefits in efficacy and costs. Fortunately, the potential complications of monopolar electrosurgery recognized in the early 1970s can be eliminated by education and relatively inexpensive engineering solutions.

When electrosurgery is used during open operations, surgeons do not necessarily require an in-depth knowledge of electrosurgery to use the energy source effectively. Few complications are directly attributable to limitations of the energy source during open procedures. If electrical energy is inadequate for hemostasis, the surgeon can simply place a finger on a bleeder until a suture or clip is placed. The entire surgical electrode is within the view of the surgeon and staff during laparotomy, and the previous problems with pad site and alternate site burns have been eliminated with isolated generators and electronic monitoring of the return pad. One misunderstood injury is the burn that the surgeon may occasionally receive while "buzzing" a hemostat; most surgeons relate the burn to a hole in the glove rather than an avoidable high-voltage, capacitively coupled current.[2]

Several problems are inherent in the use of any energy source during laparoscopy. First, as a result of minimal invasion, the surgeon must rely more heavily on the energy source for hemostasis and cutting than in open operations. No longer can the surgeon place a finger on a bleeder or rapidly place a suture for better hemostasis. In addition, relatively minor bleeding—which is a minor nuisance with open operations—may completely obscure the laparoscopic view and prevent safe dissection. As a result of the conductive properties of blood or saline, laparoscopic control of the energy may be less precise than during a comparable open procedure where a dry operative field is more readily maintained. Overzealous application of energy in a wet field will distort the anatomic planes. In spite of the tremendous advances in videoscopic surgery, the surgeon still has less tactile feedback and less depth and color perception on the two-dimensional screen than in most open procedures. Thus, it is important that the laparoscopic surgeon learn to use the energy source optimally to improve precision of application as well as to avoid unnecessary tissue injury. A better understanding of the science should improve the art of delivery.

Another problem inherent in the laparoscopic use of monopolar electrosurgery is that the surgical electrode is not completely within the surgeon's view during use. The active tip can be viewed, but the shaft of the electrode may be lying on the colon outside the view of the scope. In the absence of surveillance, it is possible to have a tiny defect in the insulation that could deliver 100% of the current to nontarget tissue. In addition, most instruments (especially the articulating scissors and grasper-dissectors) have been designed with a great deal of exposed metal in the distal tip; at best, the instrument will "ground out" on nontarget tissue, but it is also possible for the bowel or bile duct to be burned outside the immediate view of the scope. It is also possible for the exposed metal to be in contact with other conductive instruments (the laparoscope), which could then transfer 100% of the current to tissue outside the visualized field.

Finally, the electrodes that deliver energy to the target tissue are inserted through other conductive tubes, such as cannulas, suction irrigation devices, or operating laparoscopes. In certain situations, up to 70% of the current can be transferred through completely intact insulation to the outer conductor through a process called *capacitive coupling*.

In this chapter, we present the basic concepts of radiofrequency electrical energy that are essential for a better understanding of the art of application, as well as the avoidance of complications. Unfortunately, these topics were not given appropriate consideration in early laparoscopic training courses and have often been poorly understood by instrument manufacturers. While the topics are occasionally complex and have been debated in multiple formats, the common "take-home message" is that the complications associated with monopolar electrosurgery can be essentially eliminated or avoided by surgical education, conductive cannulas, and active electrode monitoring.[3–6]

INCIDENCE OF COMPLICATIONS WITH MONOPOLAR ELECTROSURGERY

The incidence of complications related to the use of electrosurgery is unknown. However, the potential mechanisms of electrosurgical injury can be readily demonstrated in a laboratory model. When complications occur, it is generally impossible to reconstruct the precise mechanism of injury.[7,8] For example, a bowel injury and peritonitis may be related to thermal injury from either direct or stray currents, but how can we exclude a mechanical injury such as a trocar puncture? Specific histologic changes within injured intestine may offer a clue if the specimen is removed early in the postoperative course.[9] However, the intestine is often not excised or the histologic changes may be altered by local infection. Further confusion exists because injuries and complications are often underreported; triumphs are presented more readily than failures, particularly if the underlying mechanism is poorly understood. Finally, unexpected and unexplained complications often lead to litigation, which may delay discussion in formal surgical meetings.

A recent analysis completed by 31 insurance companies associated through the Physician Insurers Association of America (PIAA) may offer some insight into the nature of the problem.[10] The PIAA study included data from 615 claims associated with laparoscopy. Significantly, *the vast majority of injuries were not recognized during the laparoscopic procedure*. For this reason, it is virtually impossible to determine the precise cause of injury. Thus, it is extremely important that *potential* mechanisms of injury be outlined so that preventive measures be taken.

Another observation of the PIAA study was that *the percentage of claims closed with an indemnity payment was higher with laparoscopy* than with formerly used open procedures. By conjecture, delayed treatment of potentially preventable injuries is likely the leading explanation for this situation. As a result of the increased claims, malpractice insurance premiums have increased for laparoscopic surgeons in some states. In addition, the American Trial Lawyers Association has formed a Laparoscopic Litigation Group for aggressive action in this area. Certain complications may occur with any operation, but the delays in recognition, diagnosis, and treatment increase not only the morbidity but also the exposure to litigation. Any patient who is not making daily progress early after laparoscopic surgery should be carefully evaluated for a possible missed laparoscopic injury. Since missed injuries are a common denominator of laparoscopic litigation, it is in the best interest of the patient, surgeon, hospital, insurer, product manufacturer, and our health care system to define and eliminate any potential mechanism of injury—electrosurgical or otherwise.

THE ART AND SCIENCE OF MONOPOLAR ELECTROSURGERY

The goal of electrosurgery is to develop a specific tissue effect (desiccation, cutting, etc.) by directing a variety of electrical currents through the target tissue without causing damage to nontarget tissues. The tissue effects of monopolar electrosurgery are provided by an alternating current with a frequency of around 500,000 cycles per second (CPS) (compared to 60 cps in the electrical current of your home); the high frequency (radio frequency) will minimize neuromuscular stimulation, as discovered by the French almost 100 years ago. Lower-frequency currents may develop with intermittent arcing to metal devices such as clips, instruments, cannulas, or the laparoscope (see below).

Most simply, the art and science of electrosurgery are based on controlling tissue temperatures associated with the high-frequency current. Tissue temperatures vary with the current density in the path between the active surgical electrode and the return pad. The scientific basis of local tissue heating at the electrode–tissue interface (or any other point in the circuit) is outlined in the following formula:

$$\text{temp change} = (I^2/r^4)Rt$$

where I = current, r = radius of tissue electrode contact, R = tissue resistance, and t = time. As outlined, the most important determinant of local tissue heating is the radius of electrode contact. The good technical surgeon is proficient at maintaining a high current density by controlling the radius of electrode contact. Points in the circuit with a very low power density (i.e., the dispersive return pad or perhaps the all-metal trocar-cannula with inadvertent electrode contact) have a minimal temperature change in tissue during electrode activation. Appropriate tension and countertension alter tissue resistance, in addition to increasing current density at the electrode–tissue interface.

The surgeon may select varying waveforms from the generator. The "coag" waveform provides interrupted bursts of high-voltage current, whereas the "cut" waveform has a continuous, uninterrupted waveform at a low voltage (Fig. 4.1). The higher voltage of the coag waveform will "drive" an electrical charge deeper into the tissue or arc for a longer distance to target tissue. For the same power settings, the coag mode provides a high-voltage, low-amperage current, as opposed to the cut mode, which provides a high-amperage, low-voltage current. With most modern generators, the surgeon selects the wattage, but the voltage and amperage vary during application of energy; the voltage increases automatically as tissue is desiccated (and current decreases) or if the generator is activated thereby creating an open circuit (electrode not touching tissue: a high-voltage condition).

$$\text{wattage} = \text{voltage} \times \text{current}$$

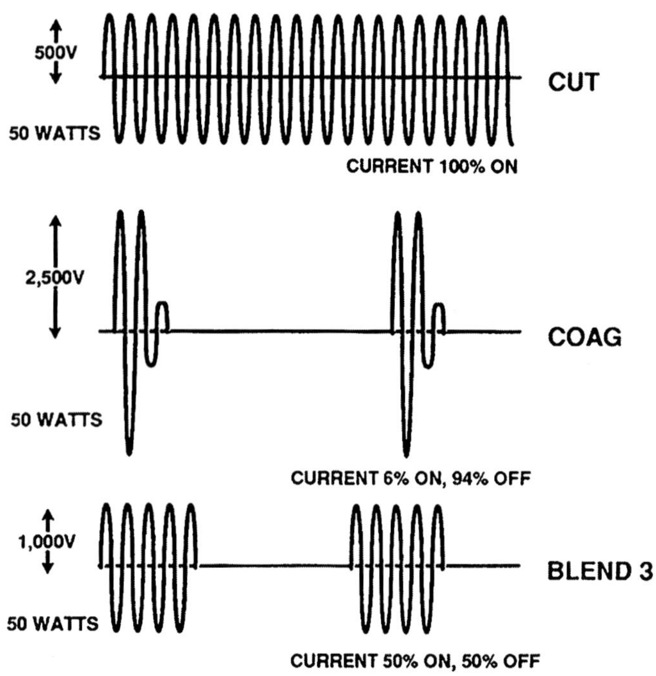

Figure 4.1. Diagram of cut, coag, and blend currents at 50 watts.

Higher voltage conditions are desirable in certain situations, as high voltage leads to longer arcs when noncontact techniques are used and deeper penetration of the electrical charge when contact techniques are used. Though hemostasis may be improved with higher voltage, the higher voltage also increases the surrounding electromagnetic field and the risk of injury with insulation breakdown or induced currents around the electrodes.

The specific tissue effects with monopolar electrosurgery vary according to the generator, generator settings, electrode design, and surgical techniques.

Fulguration is a technique that provides superficial desiccation of tissue by arcing current from the electrode to the nearby tissue. The most effective fulguration occurs with a high-voltage generator operated in the coag mode, since higher voltages generate longer arcing to tissue. Note that the maximum voltage of the coag mode varies by manufacturer as well as by generator. The superficial tissue effect occurs because tissue contact is not made and some of the energy is dissipated in the "lightning." After the first "bolt" strikes a specific tissue point, that tissue is desiccated and loses its conductivity. Thus, the next bolt strikes the next most conductive area. Fulguration is quite useful but also increases the risk of insulation failure and capacitive coupling as high-voltage waveforms are used. While spray fulguration may be enhanced with the use of argon gas, caution is advised because acutely elevated intra-abdominal pressures and hypotension have been reported as a result of the instilled gas.

Contact desiccation occurs when the electrode is activated in contact with tissue, providing excellent hemostasis as successive layers of tissue are desiccated. As the superficial tissue is desiccated, the voltage of the generator increases to facilitate deeper tissue effects. Contact desiccation leads to the development of an eschar, which may be desirable in some settings but may distort anatomic planes. With *broad* contact between the electrode and tissue, desiccation without cutting will occur with either the cut or coag mode. Desiccation in the cut mode takes a bit longer than in the coag mode but is associated with lower voltage (leading to a smaller electromagnetic field and less potential for insulation breakdown or induced currents) and perhaps a more superficial tissue effect. If the power density is high enough, a tissue-cutting effect may be achieved with either the cut or coag mode.

The optimal cutting tissue effect (vaporization) is provided by the cut mode with a fine electrode edge or needle near but not touching tissue. Given ample power density, there will be immediate heating and boiling of intracellular contents by the uninterrupted waveform. The "exploding" cells will produce a cutting effect or vaporization. When the electrode is held near the tissue but not in contact, hemostais is poor, as superficial cells are vaporized without significant desiccation of deeper tissue.

Coaptive coagulation occurs when tissue is compressed within a grasper and current is applied; excellent desiccation occurs with the development of a "collagen weld" of the compressed tissue. This tissue effect can be obtained with either the cut or coag mode. The advantage of the cut mode is that there is less voltage.

With any of the above electrosurgical techniques, good tension and countertension are essential. Appropriate tension reduces the radius of tissue–electrode contact and separates the treated tissue to reveal the next tissue plane.

POTENTIAL PROBLEMS WITH MONOPOLAR ELECTROSURGERY

As stated earlier in this chapter, the true incidence of electrosurgical injuries is unknown. Significant injuries related to monopolar electrosurgery are likely to increase as surgeons pursue more aggressive laparoscopic procedures. Because of the difficulties of retrospectively studying the characteristics and mechanisms of bowel injury during laparoscopy, it is important to categorize potential mechanisms of energy transfer in order to prevent injuries. As will be shown, most bowel injuries can be avoided with education and relatively simple engineering advances.

Electrosurgical injuries within the view of the laparoscope are related to surgical technique and, accordingly, could be reduced with education. The ability to apply science to achieve a specific tissue effect is an art. Poor technique may be manifested by a higher incidence of subhepatic bile leaks or abscess, uncontrolled bleeding or transfusions, and ductal injury. Lesser manifestations may be related to prolonged operating time, more patient discomfort, and increased costs of the procedure. The dissection of tissue planes and adhesions around the bowel creates a much less forgiving scenario than freeing the gallbladder from its bed in the liver or bipolar fulguration of the fallopian tubes.

Electrosurgical injuries outside the view of the scope may occur because of three different types of "stray

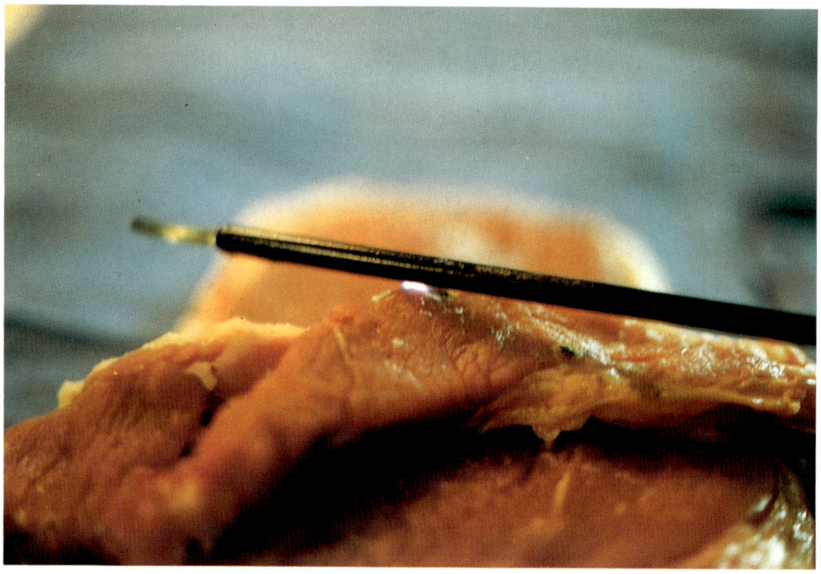

Figure 4.2. Defective insulation with burn outside the view of the laparoscope.

energy": insulation failure, capacitive coupling, and direct coupling. Burns at the return pad site (the most common electrosurgical injury 15 years ago) have been virtually eliminated by dynamic electronic monitoring of adequacy of skin-to-return pad interface.

Insulation Failure

Insulation defects in the shaft of electrodes can be due to mechanical trauma, repeated heating through the use or sterilization, manufacturing flaws, and capacitively coupled meltdown (Fig. 4.2). Insulation failure is frequent and represents one of the most common reasons that instruments are returned to the manufacturer.

The hazard of insulation failure depends on the location of the point of failure (Fig. 4.3). Exposed metal in the handle of the instrument (zone 4) may burn the surgeon. The tips of most articulating electrodes (scissors and atraumatic grasper-dissectors) are incompletely insulated and have several centimeters of exposed metal that may cause injury to nontarget tissue (on the liver during laparoscopic cholecystectomy), with a loss of efficacy at the target tissue. A defect in the shaft of the electrode (zone 2) may cause a nondetectable injury to bowel outside the view of the surgeon.

The signs of insulation failure within zone 3 (within the cannula) depend on whether a metal or plastic cannula is used. If a metal cannula is used, there is often current flow from the metal of the electrode to the metal of the cannula; the resulting arcing of the current creates a lower-frequency current (referred to as a *demodulated frequency*) which can be as low as a few cycles per second. With this lower frequency, there may be neuromuscular stimulation[11] with jerking of the abdominal wall or diaphragm, but a distinct pattern of video interference (*lightning artifact*) is common when current arcs from metal. These indirect signs of

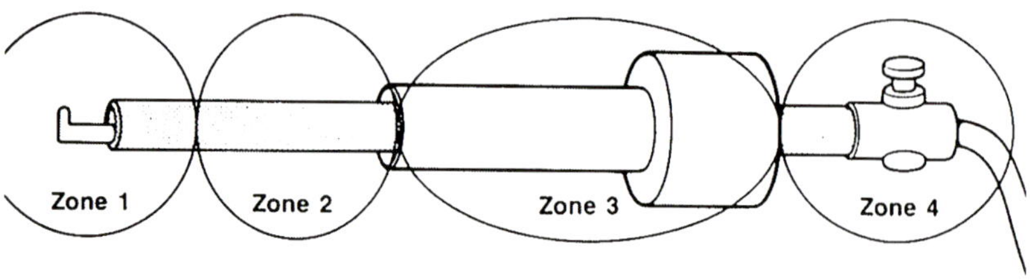

Figure 4.3. Zones of insulation failure.

insulation failure may suggest to the informed surgeon that insulation failure exists. Unfortunately, most surgeons are not knowledgeable about the indirect signs of insulation failure. Since there are no clues to insulation failure if the electrode is within a plastic cannula, the utility of metal cannulas is apparent. Plastic anchoring devices over a metal cannula must be avoided; they will insulate the abdominal wall at the expense of the viscera.

All forms of conventional insulation are based on a passive system with layers of nonconductors around the electrode. Defects in insulation may deliver 100% of the current to tissue outside the field of view of the surgeon and yet remain imperceptible to visual inspection. A new concept of insulation is based on dynamic electronic monitoring of insulation integrity (Electroscope, Boulder, CO). Continuous monitoring (of existing electrodes by an overlying Electroshield or by new instruments with a fully integrated monitoring system) guarantees that energy is being delivered only in zone 1.

Capacitive Coupling

Capacitive coupling is a mechanism whereby electrical current in the electrode induces a current in nearby conductors (unintended) despite other intact insulation. Some degree of capacitive coupling occurs with all standard monopolar electrosurgical instruments. Whether or not the stray energy of capacitive coupling causes any clinical injury depends on (1) the total amount of current transferred and (2) the concentration of the current (i.e., the power density) as it makes its way back to the patient return electrode (inappropriately referred to as the *ground pad*).

Capacitive coupling is increased by higher voltages. The low-voltage cut mode exhibits less capacitive coupling than the coag mode. Low-voltage generators (such as the Valleylab SSE2L) exhibit very little coupling compared to high voltage generators (Valleylab Force 2, 4B, or 40). However, higher-voltage generators are useful because they offer more effective cutting and desiccation. Surgeons must recognize that open-circuit activation (electrode not touching tissue) increases voltage and capacitive coupling dramatically. On the one hand, one should try to limit noncontact activation of the generator and use as low wattage as possible. On the other hand, the use of high-voltage generators in the open-circuit coag mode provides a useful tissue effect if the potential hazards are recognized and controlled.

Four conditions exist in which capacitive coupling can cause enough current to cause an injury:

1. A hybrid cannula (a metal cannula sheath within a plastic tissue anchor) creates a condition whereby current is induced in the cannula but the abdominal wall is insulated by the plastic anchor (Fig. 4.4).
2. Capacitive coupling also occurs when a conventionally insulated electrode is passed through a metal suction-irrigator. Approximately 70% of the current may be induced in the suction-irrigator.[12] This instrument combination is particularly dangerous when a plastic cannula is used, because all of the stray current may be transmitted through a narrow contact with the bowel. An all-metal cannula at the abdominal wall will "bleed off" the stray current through the wall. Standard electrodes should not be passed through metal suction irrigation devices.
3. Another significant capacitor is constructed when a surgical electrode is passed through the operating channel of an operating laparoscope.
4. Thin insulation increases capacitance. The extremely thin insulation of some instruments (particularly some ceramic coatings) decreases the effective separation of the electrode from the surrounding conductor and increases the capacitance effect. A partial thickness defect in the insulation of an electrode will increase the capacitively coupled current.

The potential for injury from capacitive coupled currents can be reduced with an understanding of the biophysics and good electrosurgical technique. The risks of capacitive coupling can be eliminated by the use of recently designed electrosurgical instruments (Electroscope), that collect the stray current, remove it from the surgical site, and monitor the total amount of current before delivering it to the return pad. This system confines capacitive coupling to the surgical instrument and monitoring circuit, thereby eliminating transmission to either the cannula or biologic tissues.

Direct Coupling

Direct coupling is the condition whereby the activated electrode touches other metal instruments (in particular, the laparoscope) within the abdomen, allowing the energy to be transferred unknowingly to tissue outside the view of the laparoscope (Fig. 4.5). All cannulas

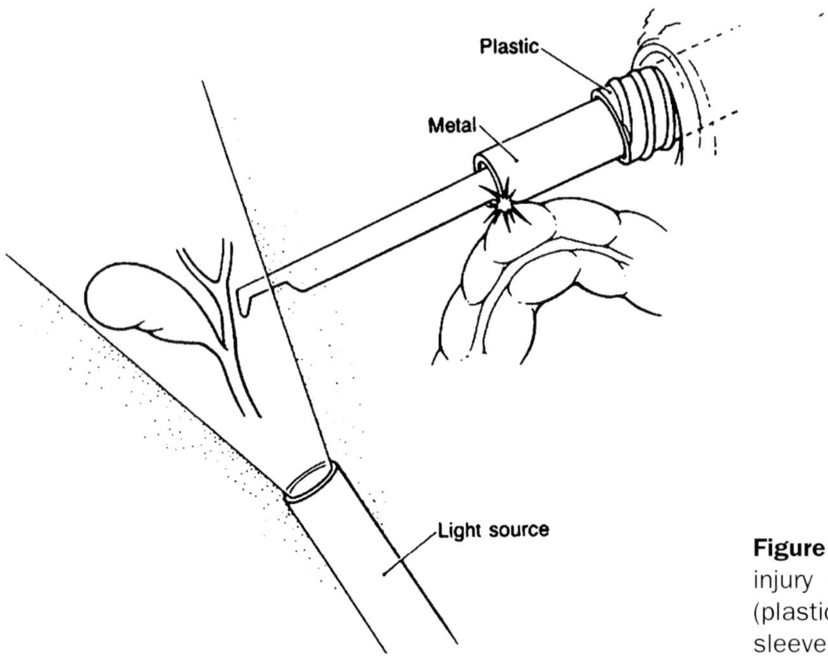

Figure 4.4. Capacitive coupling with bowel injury associated with a hybrid cannula (plastic anchor threads and a metal sleeve).

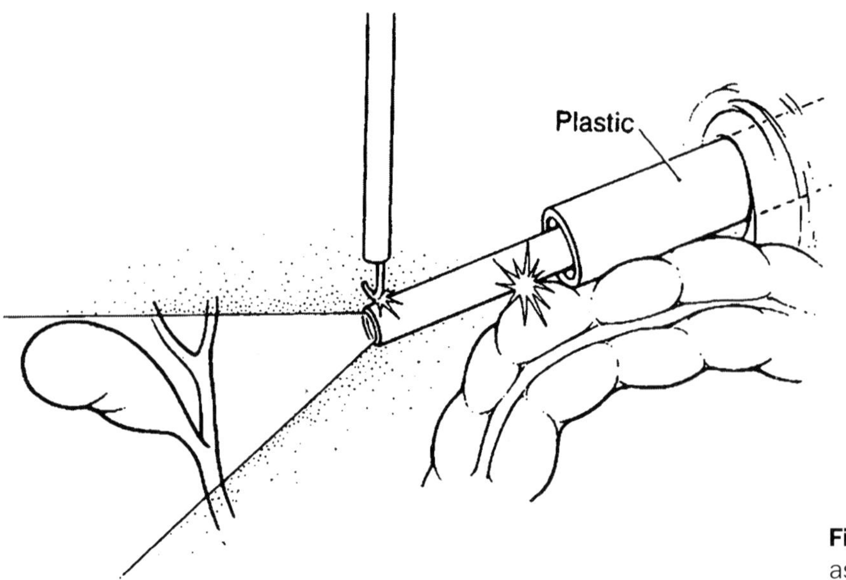

Figure 4.5. Direct coupling injury associated with plastic cannulas.

housing conductive instruments (laparoscope and metal graspers) should be introduced through metal cannulas.

SAFE USE OF MONOPOLAR ELECTROSURGERY: SUMMARY

In the relatively short history of laparoscopic surgery, many different energy sources have been used for tissue dissection. The laser was quickly introduced, but its use rapidly diminished because of its lack of efficacy and increased costs. Bipolar devices may have specific benefit in certain situations where desiccation alone is needed, but they are less efficacious than monopolar devices when an electrical cutting or fulguration effect is preferred. Additional energy sources relying on ultrasonic tissue manipulation have been advocated, but they increase costs and their efficacy for cholecystectomy is questionable; advocates describe a potential benefit with desiccation of moderate-size arterioles. At this point, the best energy source for both laparoscopy and laparotomy remains monopolar electrosurgery.

The fully developed art of electrosurgery is reflected by the surgeon's ability to manipulate fine electrodes and tissue to achieve a desired tissue effect with an appropriate wattage. The informed surgeon understands the relative advantages and disadvantages of both high- and low-voltage waveforms. If cutting alone is needed, a low-voltage, cut waveform is appropriate using a light, feathery motion in a noncontact mode. However, high voltage and high wattage are quite useful for deeper desiccation, especially for noncontact, superficial arc fulguration. Safety is enhanced with bursts of current rather than with continuous generator activation during laparoscopy.

The primary deficiency of laparoscopic mono-polar electrosurgery is not technological but rather is related to surgical education regarding the underlying biophysics. Injuries due to stray currents (insulation failure, capacitive coupling, and direct coupling) are most effectively eliminated with all-metal cannulas and actively monitored electrodes.

REFERENCES

1. Peterson HB, Ory HW, Greenspan JR, et al: Deaths associated with laparoscopic sterilization by uni-polar electrocoagulating devices. *Am J Obstet Gynecol* 139:141–143, 1978–1979.
2. Tucker RD, Fergusson S: Do surgical gloves protect staff during electrosurgical procedures? *Surgery* 110: 892–895, 1991.
3. Voyles CR, Tucker RD: Education and engineering solutions for potential problems with laparoscopic monopolar electrosurgery. *Am J Surg* 164:57–62, 1992.
4. ECRI Guidance Article: Monopolar electrosurgical safety during laparoscopy. *Health Devices* 24:6–22, 1995.
5. Martin DC, Soderstrom RM, Hulka JF, et al: *Electrosurgical Safety*. AAGL Technical Bulletin: American Association of Gynecologic Laparoscopy, 1995.
6. *Diathermy Injury during Laparoscopic Surgery*: Safety Action Bulletin. (94) 38, September 1994. (This bulletin from the United Kingdom is similar to FDA Alert).
7. Willson PD: A fatal complication of diathermy in laparoscopic surgery. *Minimally Invasive Therapy* 3:19–20, 1994.
8. Berry SM, Ose KJ, Bell RH, et al: Thermal injury of the posterior duodenum during laparoscopic cholecystectomy. *Surg Endosc* 8:197–200, 1994.
9. Levy BS, Soderstrom RM, Dail DH: Bowel injuries during laparoscopy: Gross anatomy and histology. *J Reprod Med* 30:168–172, 1985.
10. PIAA Laparoscopic Procedure Study: Physician Insurers Association of America, May 1994.
11. Tucker RD, Schmitt OH, Sievert CR, et al: Demodulated low frequency currents from electrosurgical procedures. *Surg Gynecol Obstet* 159:39–43, 1984.
12. Voyles CR, Tucker RD: Unrecognized hazards of surgical electrodes passed through metal suction irrigation devices. *Surg Endosc* 8:185–187, 1994.

chapter five

Laser Utilization in Minimally Invasive Surgery: Applications and Pitfalls

Raymond J. Lanzafame

The meteoric growth of laparoscopic cholecystectomy sparked a revolution in surgical thinking and application. Initially, surgeons had an intense interest in lasers and laser technology for use during laparoscopic cholecystectomies. However, the majority of them rapidly discarded the laser for electrosurgical devices and conventional instruments as they struggled to master new techniques and procedures with unfamiliar laparoscopes, video cameras, and skills they had never seen or used. While nearly 80% of all cholecystectomies performed in the United States in 1992 were performed laparoscopically, only 4% were performed with laser technology. The initial enthusiasm for the use of lasers in minimally invasive surgery can be traced to the work of Reddick, Schultz, Saye and McKernan. However, the advent of videoendoscopy, specific laparoscopic instrumentation for cholecystectomy and other procedures, and the development of multiple-load endostaplers has done much to simplify minimally invasive surgery for the skilled laparoscopist.

This chapter will review the array of laser technologies available for laparoscopic use and will discuss the relative merits and liabilities of each.

LASER VERSUS NONLASER USE

While the lay community remains enamored of the laser and is convinced that *laser* and *laparoscopy* are interchangeable terms, one must consider whether *any* laser adds anything to the laparoscopist's armamentarium. The surgical literature is replete with articles which purport to compare lasers to electrosurgical devices for use during laparoscopic cholecystectomy. The consensus is that electrosurgical devices are much more familiar, ubiquitous in the operating room, less expensive in terms of capital equipment purchases and *some* disposables, and faster, particularly since the surgeon is much more familiar with electrosurgical technology and its appropriate application.

There is little question that the appropriate use of lasers enhances patient comfort, reduces morbidity, and reduces the length of hospitalization when used for incisional (open) cholecystectomy and a number of other open procedures. The evidence is incontrovertible that laparoscopic cholecystectomy is a superior technique for cholecystectomy in the majority of cases. This is particularly true from the patient's perspective. However, it must be recognized that the use of the laparoscope, rather than a subcostal incision, is the main reason for the dramatic improvement in patient outcome.

The main advantage of electrosurgical devices are their ubiquity in the operating room and the fact that no additional training or safety considerations are needed. These factors, when coupled with the average surgeon's comfort with using them, make them the technology of choice for many surgeons. Both monopolar and bipolar instrumentation are available for laparoscopic use, and the majority of routine laparoscopic instrumentation is insulated to permit its use with electrosurgical devices. The main disadvantages of electrosurgical devices are due to the relative imprecision of energy delivery to the desired target. The buildup of char and debris on the electrode surface can result in the delivery of energy to areas adjacent to the desired target rather than to the target itself. In addition, debris can cause the electrode to adhere to the tissue or drag irregularly through it. Some manufacturers of disposable electrodes have attempted to solve this problem by coating the electrode with Teflon or other polymers and by using ceramic materials. However, the majority of laparoscopic instrumentation is untreated. Electrosurgical devices work poorly in the presence of blood, edema, and irrigating solutions. The majority of insulated laparoscopic hand instruments have relatively large exposed electrode surfaces (Figs. 5.1 and 5.2). A large electrode may result in damage to adjacent structures, particularly in close spaces. These issues, as well as the problem of capacitance coupling, are discussed in Chapter 4.

An array of laser technology is available for use during laparoscopy for incisional purposes. Currently, this includes the argon, CO_2, holmium, KTP, and Nd:YAG lasers. More recently, high-power diode laser technology has become available for use in soft tissue applications. It is likely that new instruments will be forthcoming. Laser technology is also available for lithotripsy. We will discuss each of these wavelengths and technologies in some detail below. Several points bear mention prior to the consideration of specific technologies.

Proponents of laser technology list the high degree of precision possible with these devices and the ability to control the tissue effect at the desired target as being the main advantages of these devices. Opponents often cite the expense of laser machinery and accessories, in addition to increased operative time, as the main disadvantages. Although these issues are often raised, few recognize that the cost of a technology is not necessarily correlated with its actual price and that the price has little to do with the charge or the reimbursement. It must be understood that the net global effect of a technology may be to lower the total cost of an illness when one considers factors such as the length of hospitalization, the degree and duration of disability, and the ability of the patient to return to normal productivity. Such a thesis is borne out by laparoscopic cholecystectomy: The cost of the technology necessary to perform the procedure is higher than that of its open counterpart, but the overall cost to industry, the primary payor for

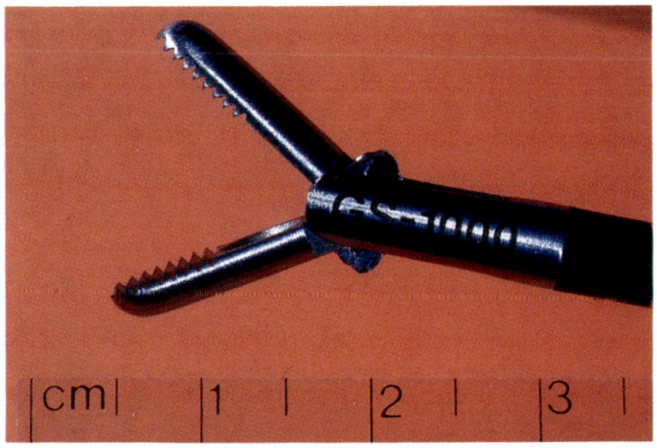

Figure 5.2. The length of exposed electrode is shown for a typical laparoscopic grasper. Note that the electrode is nearly 3 cm in length.

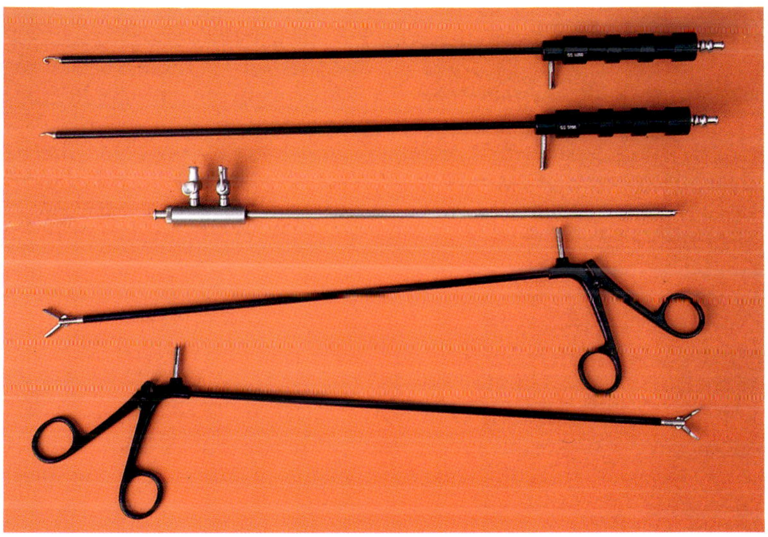

Figure 5.1. A typical array of insulated monopolar electrocautery capable instruments for laparoscopic procedures is shown.

health care, is lower due to the more rapid return to the workplace.

Similarly, when one considers the length of the procedure, it is important to note that speed improves *after* the surgeon becomes experienced and facile with the technique and the technology used to accomplish a procedure. It must also be recognized that a laser may be utilized for only a small portion of a procedure and that several other factors also determine the operative time.

The surgeon would do well to have a complete working understanding of lasers, their delivery systems, and their tissue effects *prior* to attempting to apply them to a laparoscopic or any other procedure. The surgeon should attend specific hands-on laser training programs if laser education and the opportunity to use these devices were not available during the residency training program or if the surgeon is not familiar with a particular device or delivery system. Clearly, the house officer is in an ideal position to acquire the intellectual and manual skills necessary to use lasers and other technologies properly if this opportunity is provided as a part of the residency training program. However, postgraduate continuing medical education programs can bridge the gap for those who did not have formal training elsewhere. It is then imperative that the surgeon continue to develop these newly acquired skills in an ongoing, graded fashion. This requires gradual incorporation of the use of laser technology into clinical practice by tackling the simpler procedures and tasks first, followed later by other, more difficult problems, once the surgeon has become comfortable with the technology and has acquired a working understanding of its limits and advantages. The surgeon must be aware that all lasers and delivery systems are not alike and that selection of the proper wavelength, the proper delivery system, and the proper laser parameters are central to achieving the desired clinical outcome given the appropriate technical expertise.

This point cannot be neglected by the surgeon. The selection of a laser device, delivery system, or any other instrument during the course of a procedure is critical to the conduct and outcome of that procedure. The surgeon must recognize that the selection of instrumentation for procedures involves a number of variables, as discussed above. However, it is clear that the preference of the surgeon is a major determinant in this process. Preference depends on availability, skill, judgment, experience, and the sense that a particular tool "feels right" or "works well" for a particular task in the hands of a particular surgeon. This is the clinical equivalent of the motto of the Stanley Tool Corporation: "The right tool for the right job." One need only examine the back table during an operative procedure to recognize that several alternatives exist for the surgeon's execution of a particular task.

We shall now examine the types of laser technology available for endoscopic use and discuss the applications and problems of each.

CO_2 LASER

CO_2 lasers have been used extensively for an array of gynecologic laparoscopic applications but have been rarely utilized for laparoscopic cholecystectomy and other minimally invasive surgical procedures. The energy of the CO_2 laser (wavelength = 10,600 nm) is in the far-infrared portion of the electromagnetic spectrum. This wavelength is intensely absorbed by cellular water. This property results in superficial injury to tissues and enables the sealing of blood vessels up to 0.5–1.0 mm in diameter, as well as lymphatics. The potential for inadvertent injury to deeper structures is minimal. When used at appropriate fluences in a cutting mode, the zone of necrosis is approximately 100–300 μm, which closely resembles the histology of an incision created by the scalpel. This wavelength is absorbed independently of the color of the tissue. Thus, the clinical effect seen in soft tissues is relative to their water content. Local infiltration of tissue with saline or anesthetic solutions will protect or insulate them from injury by the laser beam until the fluid has been vaporized. This laser is the most efficient modality available for ablation or vaporization of large volumes of tissue such as tumor nodules or endometriomas.

The CO_2 laser wavelength is carried via hollow tubes, waveguides, and mirrors. Conventional fiberoptics are not currently available for clinical use. The laparoscopic use of this wavelength is possible with the use of a focusing cube and an operative laparoscope or with a variety of waveguides designed for multipuncture laparoscopic applications. The focusing cube permits the use of the CO_2 laser free beam for cutting, vaporization, and coagulation of tissue. A variety of procedures such as myomectomy, partial oophorectomy, and even cholecystectomy have been performed successfully with this delivery system (Fig. 5.3). Cholecystectomy requires a McKernan-type approach. The successful use of this approach requires knowledge of and facility with the operative laparoscope and the surgeon's ability to visualize the desired target and maneuver a micromanipulator or joy stick. The surgeon can

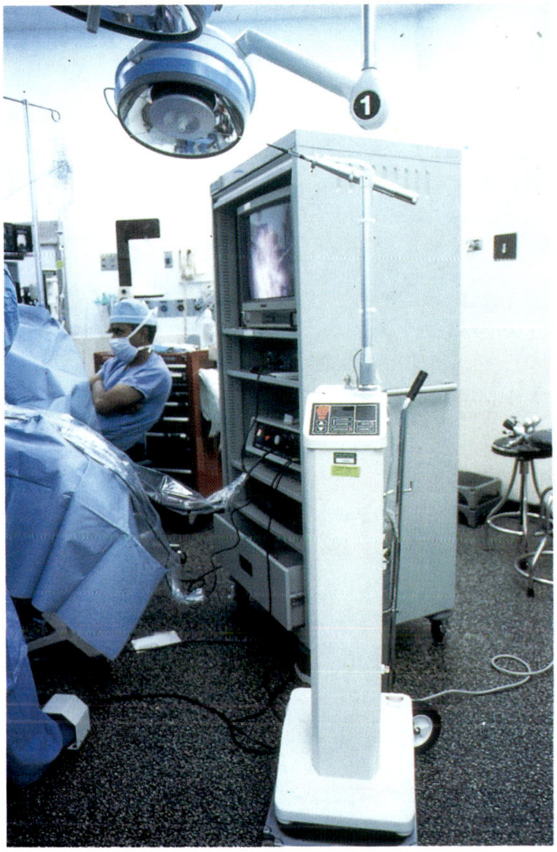

Figure 5.3. This figure demonstrates the use of a flexible waveguide with a 20 watt sealed tube CO_2 laser. A laparoscopic cholecystectomy is being performed.

alter the tissue effect by focusing or defocusing the laser beam, as well as by varying the laser wattage selected. Laser waveguides are hollow tubes with mirror-like surfaces which reflect the CO_2 wavelength. Waveguides are available in both rigid and flexible versions (Figs. 5.1–5.6) and can be used to achieve a spot size (i.e., burn or incision) which is in the range of 0.8–2.2 mm. As a general principle, the waveguide is used in a noncontact fashion, particularly since tissue contact can obstruct the waveguide and liquid can be drawn into it by capillary action. The result of these events is the irreversible destruction of the waveguide.

The successful use of this laser for dissection and hemostasis requires that the surgeon be expert with the laser, as this will affect the ability to dissect tissues and achieve an adequate degree of hemostasis. Both the focusing cube and waveguide systems require a direct line of sight or the use of angled mirrors, which further complicates the maneuverability of these devices—more so than that of fiber-capable lasers and conventional instruments. Both configurations require flowing gas to cool the system and prevent the vaporized tissue plume from being thrown into the device. The most frequently used purge gases are argon and CO_2. High CO_2 gas flow rates can actually absorb the laser energy and reduce its efficiency (i.e., the transmission of energy from the laser to the tissue). Therefore, lower flow rates (i.e., 1 L/min) are suggested. Some laser systems are equipped with a nitrogen purge gas system. The surgeon should *not* use nitrogen during laparoscopy, as its absorption from the peritoneum can produce "the bends."

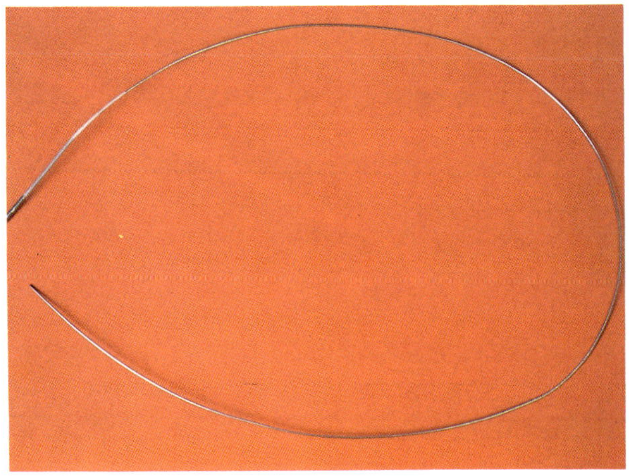

Figure 5.4. A metallic flexible waveguide for the CO_2 laser is shown.

The optimal use of the CO_2 laser for laparoscopic or open use is achieved when the beam is oriented perpendicular to the desired target. Hemostasis will be enhanced by tissue compression, the use of epinephrine-containing local anesthetic solutions, and the ability of the operator to recognize the presence of a vessel *prior* to its division. Under these conditions, the surgeon defocuses the laser (i.e., moves the handpiece, waveguide, or operating laparoscope farther away from the target) and then applies short bursts of energy to the vessel in the area to be divided (Fig. 5.7). This maneuver heats and coagulates the vessel, thereby enabling its bloodless division by the focused beam. The surgeon should use the highest power setting with which he or she is comfortable, as this will enable more efficient cutting, better hemostasis, and less thermal injury to the wound edges by minimizing conductive and radioactive heat loss into the wound. Intermittent evacuation of the vaporized tissue plume or the use of a recirculating filtration system ensures a clear field of

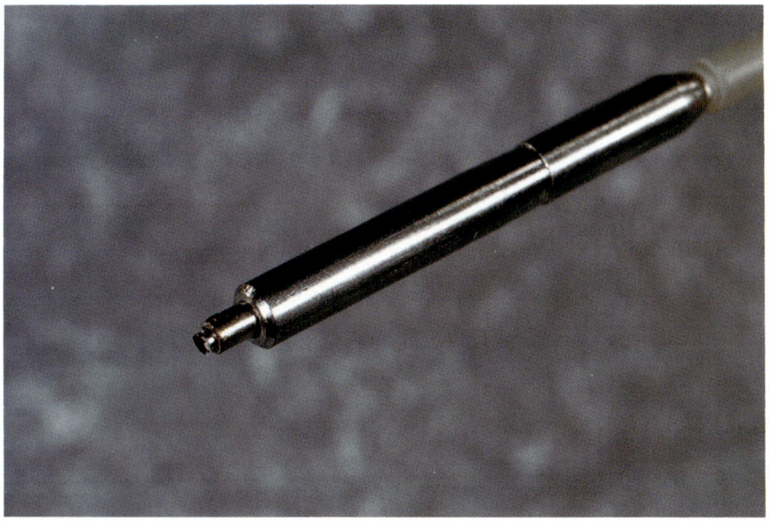

Figure 5.5. The CO_2 laser waveguide couples to the laser via a snap-in fitting (shown) which inserts into a coupling launch.

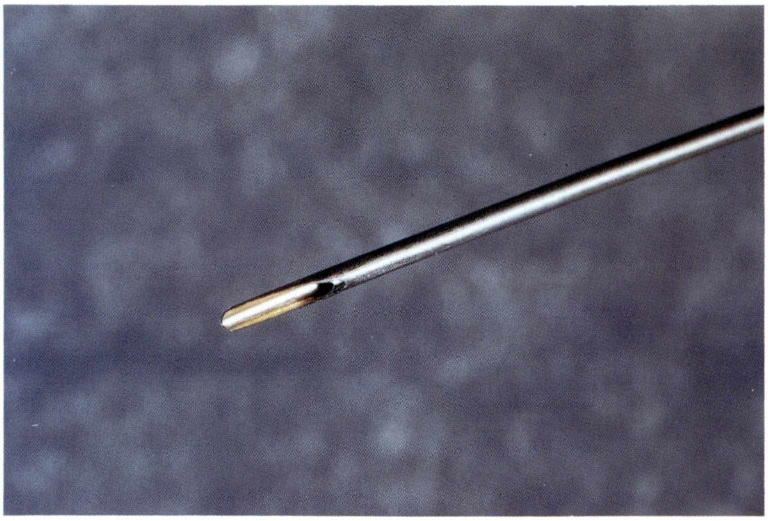

a

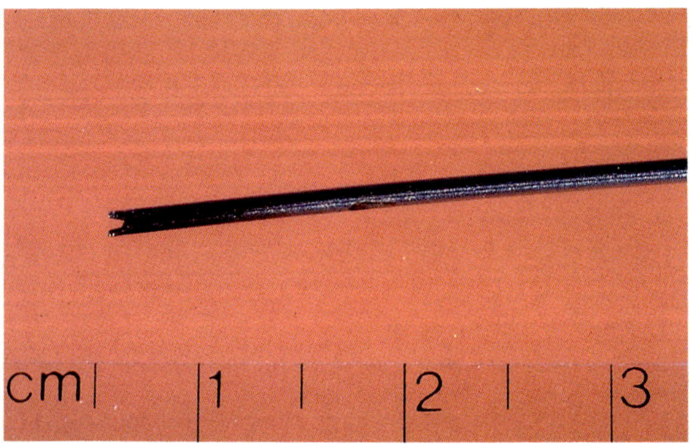

b

Figure 5.6. CO_2 laser waveguide tip configurations have been manufactured in a variety of styles. The fluted style is shown (a). The notched style is shown (b).

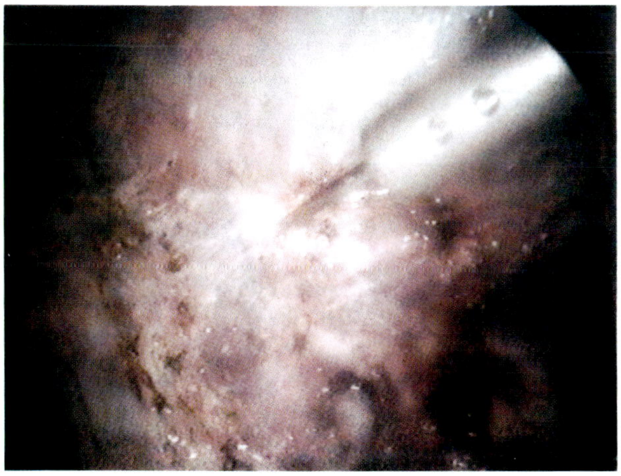

Figure 5.7. Intraoperative photograph depicting the use of the flexible CO_2 laser waveguide to dissect the gallbladder from the gallbladder bed. The waveguide is used in a non contact fashion and can be oriented either obliquely or perpendicularly relative to the plane of the dissection.

view and prevents the absorption of toxic products of combustion by the patient. This problem is identical in magnitude and toxicity to the absorption of the vaporized tissue plume created by any electrosurgical, thermal or laser source. Similarly, the "smoke" should not be vented into the operating room, as it should be considered hazardous for operating room personnel. (OSHA/NIOSH has written regulations which require that operating room staff be protected from this hazard, regardless of its source).

ARGON LASER

The argon laser has been used extensively for gynecologic laparoscopic procedures. This laser produces light in the visible portion of the spectrum. Although six lines (wavelengths) are produced, the majority of the laser output is in the blue-green spectrum (wavelengths = 488, 514 nm). This energy is intensely absorbed by hemoglobin and melanin, although other exogenous chromophores will also absorb these wavelengths efficiently. Visible light wavelengths can be passed through water, enabling the argon laser to be used in aqueous environments such as the bladder, during hysteroscopy, during arthroscopy, and in the presence of irrigating fluids. This property enables the surgeon to photocoagulate a bleeding area while irrigating the wound to locate the source of the bleeding.

Both free-beam and conventional fiberoptic applications are utilized during operative laparoscopy. A Microslad unit (micromanipulator) may be coupled with the operative laparoscope. A gimbaled mirror and joy stick allow the surgeon to maneuver the beam in the surgical field. The fiber can be used in both a contact and a noncontact mode.

Argon laser light penetrates and scatters in tissues. The resultant damage can be as much as 6 mm during free-beam applications. When used in an incisional mode, the speed of incision and the degree of hemostasis are adequate. Blood vessels on the order of 2 mm in diameter can be divided and coagulated with this wavelength. Although some authors have reported successful hemostasis of vessels as large as 3–4 mm in diameter, the possibility of delayed bleeding or rebleeding is real. Therefore, the surgeon would do well to use ligature and hemoclip methods for hemostasis in these instances. The cause of the delayed bleeding is necrosis of photocoagulated tissue and tissue slough. This condition also occurs after use of the Nd:YAG laser in a free-beam mode on similar tissues.

The contact or fiberoptic method is much more easily mastered than the free-beam approach since the surgeon has direct tactile feedback from the tissue. The speed of incision and the degree of hemostasis are adequate, and the more selective absorption of these wavelengths in hemoglobin enables the surgeon to photocoagulate vessels prior to their division by bringing the fiber away from the tissue surface. This maneuver is similar to that of defocusing the free beam. The defocused mode is used to vaporize endometriomas or photocoagulate vessels prior to their division. Some manufacturers produce a variety of sculpted fibers and metal-jacketed fiber delivery systems. These fibers are constructed to be more durable and perform more like a scalpel due to absorption of some of the laser energy in the fiber, which results in heating of the fiber. This produces an optically driven cautery effect. So-called bare or urologic fibers are easily used, and are cleaved and stripped as the fiber end degrades with use. Optimal cutting occurs by using the tip of the fiber either end-on or somewhat oblique to the plane of the dissection.

Since these wavelengths are color dependent, the surgeon should note that white or lightly colored tissues such as meniscus and tumor implants will not cut efficiently and will not be vaporized (ablated) unless they are first painted with India ink, indigo carmine dye, or another exogenous chromophore. A droplet of blood placed on the surface is sometimes effective for this purpose. Blackened or ebonized instruments and the use of optical backstops are required to prevent beam reflection and iatrogenic injury.

One of the main drawbacks to the laparoscopic use of the argon laser is the camera/eye safety filter. The eye and camera filters must block the six lines produced by the laser. These filters are usually a deep orange color and absorb 30–60% of the visible spectrum. As a result, the color balance of the image is distorted and the need for a high-power light source is critical to the surgeon's ability to visualize the operative field. Many laser systems have intermittent shutter mechanisms which place the filter in the visual field only while the laser is actually being fired. Nonetheless, the surgeon must be expert in the local anatomy and the details of the procedure prior to attempting to work with this laser.

ND:YAG LASER

The neodymium YAG laser produces near-infrared light at a wavelength of 1060 nm. This wavelength is carried via conventional fiberoptics and, as in visible-light lasers, the energy will be transmitted through water. The energy can be applied to tissues with a wide array of delivery systems, including cleaved bare fiber (i.e., urologic fiber), polished GI fiber, sapphire tip (i.e., the delivery device marketed as the SLT Contact Laser), and sculpted fiber (e.g., Surgimedics Microcontact tip and various other proprietary versions of this technology), as well as free beam via a micromanipulator or Microslad unit. The energy of the Nd:YAG laser is intensely absorbed in tissue protein and chromophores and is highly scattered in tissue. These properties result in deep penetration of the energy and much greater damage below the tissue than can be appreciated at the surface. This makes noncontact (i.e., GI fiber, free beam) and bare fiber applications of the Nd:YAG laser extremely dangerous unless the surgeon has a thorough understanding of the laser–tissue interaction and orients the beam in a direction which reduces the likelihood of damaging nearby structures. Recently, ADD fibers have been developed for use in photocoagulation of the prostate. These angled delivery devices project the beam at right angles to the long axis of the probe, allowing the prostatic tissue to be photocoagulated. These applications require knowledge of the anatomy and of tissue effects. The surgeon orients the laser output toward the 10:00 and 12:00 positions and fires the laser at a preset energy for a specified length of time based on the volume of tissue to be photocoagulated.

The Nd:YAG laser is a poor cutting instrument when it is used in a noncontact mode. The development of sapphire tips and sculpted fiber technologies facilitates use of this laser in contact with tissue. Free-beam applications can result in damage to as much as 2 cm of liver tissue and the photocoagulation of vessels up to 4 mm in diameter. However, the sapphire tip technology is a combination of thermal and optical interaction with tissue. Much of the Nd:YAG energy is absorbed by the sapphire or fiber tip and converted to heat (Figs. 5.8 and 5.9). The result is an optically driven cautery. The temperature of the tip can be tightly regulated for some applications. These instruments improve the cutting ability of the laser, and tissue damage and the extent of coagulation are reduced dramatically. The tissue effects of these devices are quite similar to those produced by electrosurgical devices. Since their main tissue interaction is thermal cautery, the rate of incision and the degree of hemostasis will be reduced when these devices are used in the presence of irrigating fluids or in the aqueous environment of the bladder or joint space. The surgeon must adjust the laser parameters accordingly to achieve the desired effect. Sapphire tips are fragile and are more expensive than other delivery systems. They remain hot for a short time after the laser has been turned off. This can cause damage or adherence to adjacent structures upon accidental contact. The sapphire tip may become disconnected from the fiber while operating and may be lost. When these devices are used in vascular and aqueous conditions such as in the bladder, prostate, or uterus, the fibers must *never* be cooled with air or gas, as embolism of gas has proven fatal. Fiber cooling with saline or irrigant is quite safe however.

Sculpted fibers and Microcontact tips (Fig. 5.10) have been developed with many of the same properties as the sapphire tip, but without the liability of the tip's remaining hot for any appreciable period of time after lasing has ceased and with less fragility of the tip. Some types of sculpted fibers transmit enough laser energy to permit the coagulation of bleeders by using the fiber in a noncontact mode. Sculpted fibers are a good compromise for many laparoscopic applications. However, many of the currently available fiber designs are much stiffer than conventional fibers, which makes them less pliable and more fragile than conventional silica-silica and quartz fibers.

Surgery with sapphire tips and sculpted fibers is facilitated by using them at an oblique angle relative to the plane of dissection. This technique enhances hemostasis by taking advantage of the heated mass of sapphire (or fiber tip), which coagulates the tissues prior

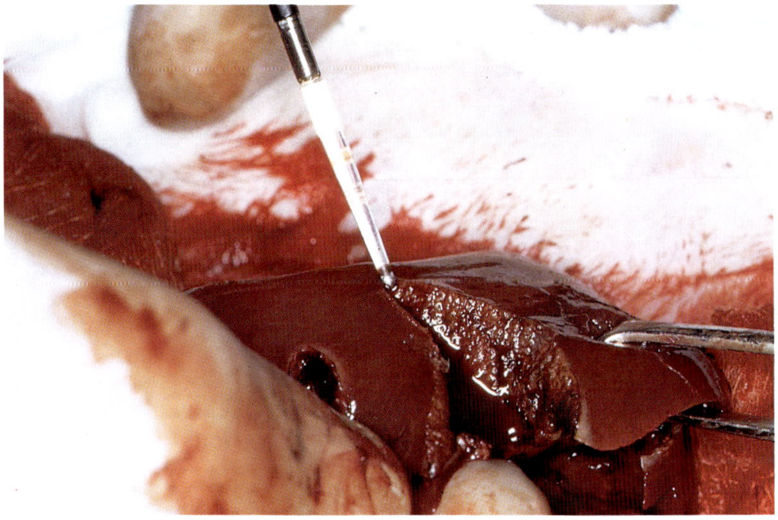

Figure 5.8. This figure demonstrates the use of a conical sapphire contact tip for hepatic division in an animal model. Note the oblique angle at which the tip is held relative to the plane of the dissection.

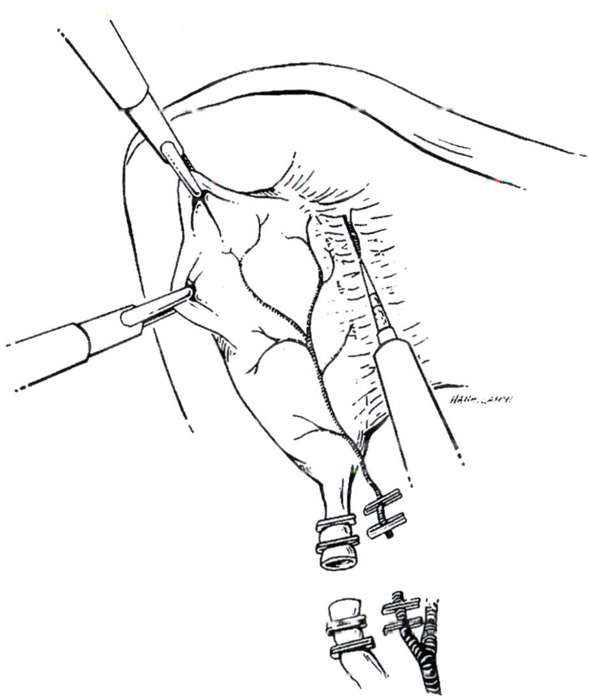

Figure 5.9. Schematic showing the use of a sapphire tip via a suction-irrigation cannula in order to dissect the gallbladder from the gallbladder bed.

to their division by the much hotter tip portion. Use of the bare fiber for dissection has been practiced safely by several European groups. However, the surgeon must have an intimate understanding of anatomy and should orient the fiber in a plane which is tangential to the line of incision to limit forward scattering of the energy into the tissues. The use of ebonized instruments and optical backstops is mandatory.

Hemostasis with the YAG laser is best accomplished by using the laser (fiber, beam) in a defocused mode and delivering short bursts of energy to the area and its immediate periphery. It is generally better to deliver a few pulses and then wait for a few minutes to observe the area rather than attempting to lase continuously. The latter practice will increase tissue damage unnecessarily and may result in vaporization of the clot and the resumption of bleeding.

The Nd:YAG laser has been used for the vaporization (ablation) of tumors. Typically, the surgeon will orient the beam parallel to the long axis of hollow viscera to avoid iatrogenic injury or perforation. Most techniques are performed in stages. The tumor is treated, allowed to slough, and then is treated as needed in subsequent sessions after debridement or natural sloughing of the photocoagulated tissue. The YAG wavelength is actually a poor ablating wavelength, particularly when compared to the CO_2, KTP, or holmium wavelengths, whose rates of ablation are significantly higher. Lightly colored tissues require substantially more energy to initiate tissue ablation. Ablation does not proceed until an area becomes desiccated and/or carbonized. The carbon particles absorb the laser energy and "catalyze" the ablation of the subjacent tissue. Painting the tissue with India ink, methylene blue, blood, or other chromophores makes the process much more efficient and safer by dramatically reducing the total amount of energy required to photoablate a given volume of tissue.

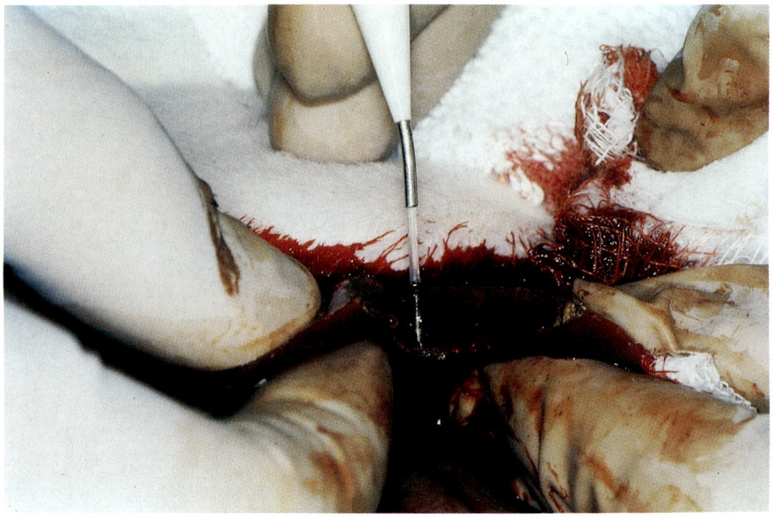

Figure 5.10. A sculpted fiber is shown in an open experimental hepatic division. Note that the fiber is angled obliquely relative to the plane of the incision.

KTP LASER

The KTP laser is a frequency-doubled YAG laser which produces pure lime green light at a wavelength of 532 nm. This wavelength is also available using crystals other than potassium-titanyl-phosphate. The Combo-laser version is produced by Laserscope (San Jose, CA) and is capable of delivering both the 532-nm KTP wavelength and the 1060-nm YAG wavelength. The surgeon can switch between these wavelengths, depending on the needs of the procedure. The KTP wavelength is intensely absorbed by hemoglobin and melanin. Its absorption by hemoglobin is quite efficient, as it is very close to the hemoglobin absorption peak at 540 nm. This wavelength is easily transmitted through water and is carried via conventional fiberoptics. Typically, a cleaved and stripped bare fiber is used with a suction-irrigation instrument (Figs. 5.11 and 5.12). Free-beam applications are possible with a micromanipulator (Microslad). The KTP laser is capable of incision, coagulation, and vaporization of tissue. Its wavelength is much more efficient than that of the argon laser for these functions and surpasses the YAG laser in its cutting and vaporization functions. These properties make this laser quite versatile for laparoscopic procedures. Vessels up to 2 mm in diameter are easily coagulated. The hemoglobin selectivity of this wavelength enables the surgeon to defocus the beam (move the fiber away from the tissue surface) and preferentially coagulate a vessel prior to its division. Bleeders such as those encountered in the gallbladder bed during cholecystectomy are dealt with by irrigating the area with saline and using the laser in a defocused mode, delivering short bursts of energy. Persistent bleeding can be dealt with by switching to the Nd:YAG laser output if a dual-wavelength laser is available. Like the argon and Nd:YAG lasers, the KTP laser requires eye safety and camera filters. Optical backstops, along with ebonized instruments, prevent damage from stray light or beam reflection hazards. Since the KTP laser produces a single visible light line, interference filters are available. These filters protect the camera and the eyes from injury by blocking the transmission of the 532- and 1060-nm wavelengths. This causes little if any color distortion. The charge coupled device camera and monitor are easily adjusted to compensate for the filtered color. As noted above, the tip of the fiber is the portion emitting the laser energy and is therefore the part which incises and/or coagulates the tissue. Therefore, the surgeon must position the fiber either perpendicularly or obliquely relative to the plane of dissection (Figs. 5.12–5.13).

HOLMIUM LASER

The holmium laser produces infrared light at a wavelength of 2100 nm. This wavelength is intensely absorbed by water. Unlike the CO_2 wavelength, the holmium laser wavelength can be carried via conventional fiberoptics. The fiber is usually encased in a metallic sheath for single-puncture use or in application with a suction-irrigation probe (Fig. 5.14). This delivery system is quite durable and tends to be self-

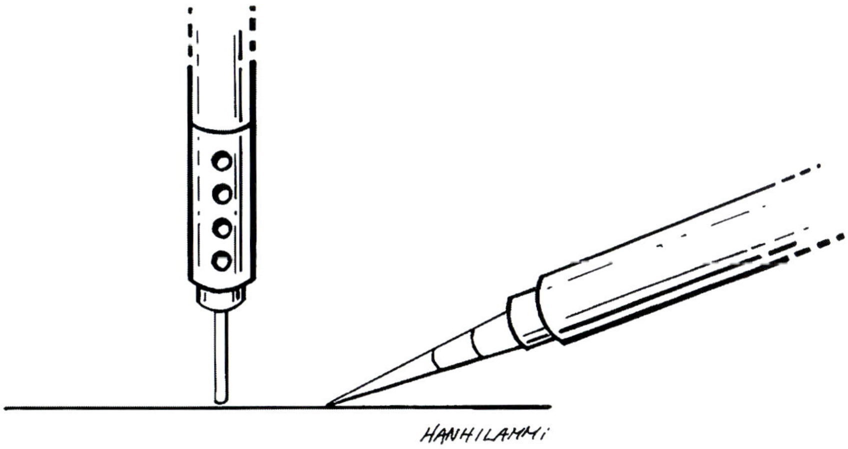

Figure 5.11. This schematic demonstrates the proper positioning of a bare fiber or waveguide for incision (left) and the proper positioning of a sapphire tip or sculpted fiber (right) relative to the tissue plane. KTP laser, bare fiber, and CO_2 waveguides are optimally placed perpendicular to the plane of incision whereas sapphire tips and sculpted fibers should be oriented obliquely and are dragged across the tissue.

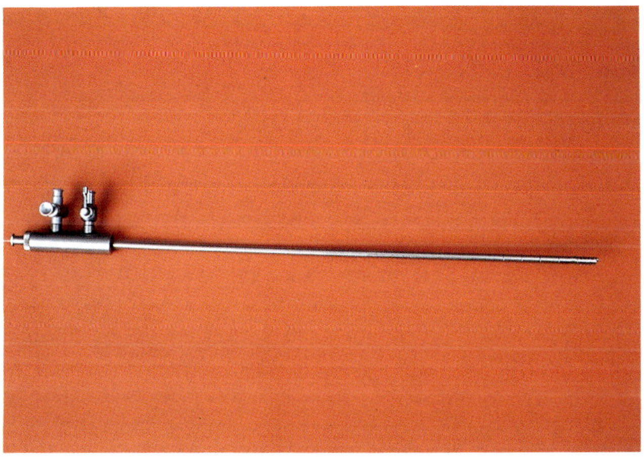

a

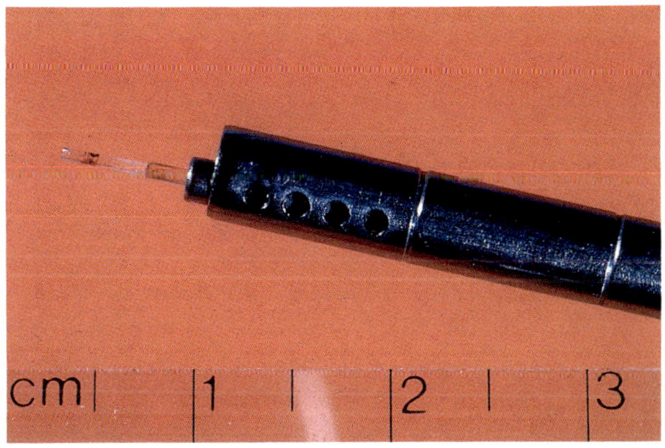

b

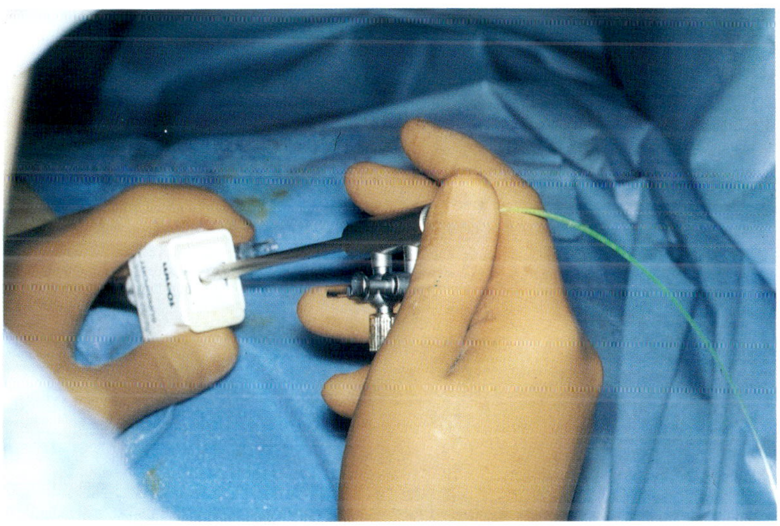

c

Figure 5.12. A bare, cleaved fiber is used for surgery with the KTP laser. The fiber is usually positioned through a suction irrigation instrument (a). The fiber should extend approximately 1–2 cm from the tip of the probe (b). The probe and fiber can be maneuvered easily during surgery (c).

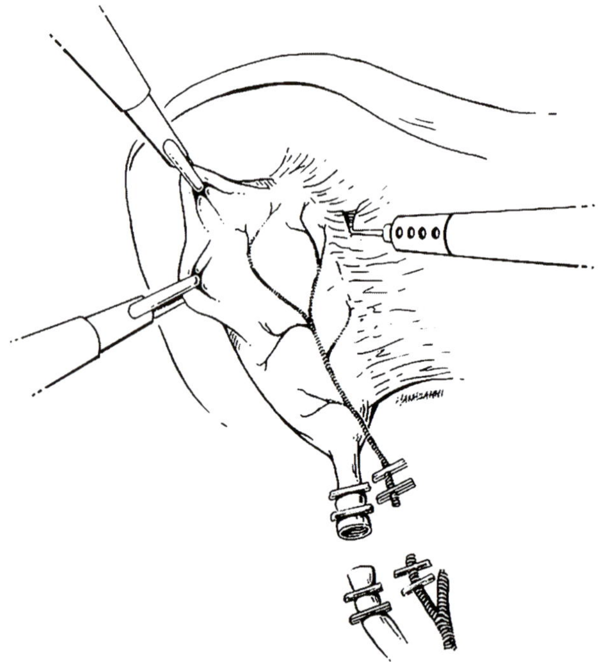

Figure 5.13. This schematic demonstrates the proper orientation of the bare fiber and suction-irrigator for use during the dissection of the gallbladder. The tip of the fiber is used and should be ideally positioned perpendicular to the plane of the incision.

cleaning. The highly efficient absorption of this wavelength by water permits cutting and ablation of bone and cartilage. Despite its water absorption, this laser can be used in an aqueous environment due to the development of a vapor bubble between the fiber and the tissue. This "Moses effect" transmits the laser energy to the tissue. Current systems can achieve outputs of 40 watts. The laser output is pulsed, and high fluences may produce significant splattering and sputtering of tissue from the target area. This can coat the laparoscope and obscure the view. This problem can be minimized by selecting an appropriate power output and repetition rate, as well as viewing the surgical site at a slightly greater distance than one would use with other modalities. A self-washing laparoscope is available.

The incisional and ablative speed of this laser is somewhat slower than that of many of the other wavelengths available for laparoscopic use. However, this problem is offset by the ease of use and durability of the fiberoptics. The zone of coagulation is similar to that seen with electrosurgical devices and sculpted fibers. This laser is the most efficient wavelength for meniscectomy and percutaneous laser disc decompression.

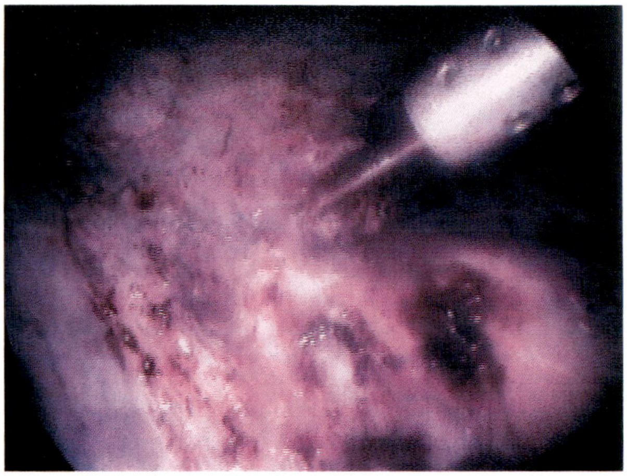

Figure 5.14. Intraoperative view of a holmium laser fiber being used to dissect the gallbladder. The fiber is passed through a suction-irrigation cannula.

DIODE LASER TECHNOLOGY

High-power diode laser systems are becoming available for clinical use. The advantages of these systems are their compact size, portability, and the potential for lower capital and maintenance costs. The Diomed laser (Diomed, Inc., The Woodlands, TX) is the first unit approved for several surgical uses. This laser produces near-infrared light at a wavelength of 805 nm. This wavelength is carried by conventional fiberoptics and is most frequently applied with sculpted fiber technology. The wound histology and the incisional speed of this device are quite similar to those of the Nd:YAG laser. It is likely that other diode arrays will become available in the future. Eye safety and intraoperative measures to prevent iatrogenic injury are similar to those described for the Nd:YAG laser. However, this wavelength scatters less in tissue; therefore, the depth of penetration of the free beam is shallower than that of the free-beam YAG.

LITHOTRIPSY DEVICES

The early years of laparoscopic cholecystectomy left surgeons with a limited number of options regarding management of the patient with choledocholithiasis. As surgeons became more expert in minimally invasive surgical techniques and as smaller-diameter fiberscopes and glidewires became available, it became possible to perform common duct exploration and stone extraction laparoscopically.

Stone extraction with baskets and forceps proceeds in a manner similar to that of open common duct exploration. However, these procedures can be difficult in the presence of large stones or stones which have become impacted. These patients can be managed successfully with a variety of lithotripsy techniques. Both laser- and nonlaser-based technologies have been applied. Electrohydraulic or spark-gap lithotripsy devices were created several years ago with the development of flexible choledochoscopy. These devices relied on a piezoelectric or spark-gap device implanted at the distal end of the catheter to generate shock waves which fragmented the calculus. These catheters were relatively inexpensive compared to other devices. However, they were rather large in diameter, which made them impractical for use with small-diameter, flexible fiber choledochosopes.

Laser-based lithotripsy devices are available for laparoscopic and ureteroscopic use. A variety of lasers have been tested, including pulsed dye, alexandrite, holmium, and excimer lasers. Of these, the pulsed dye and alexandrite lasers are available for clinical use at the present time. Both lasers generate photoacoustic shock waves at the surface of the calculus, which jackhammers and disintegrates the stone into small particles which can be flushed from the duct. A cleaved fiber is placed in contact with the stone, and a cavitation bubble develops as the laser is fired. Absorption of laser energy at the proper fluence and duty cycle causes the bubble to vibrate and fragment the stone. These devices are quite simple to use, as they can be applied under direct vision with a fiber scope, placed percutaneously, or threaded into the duct or ureter blindly. A characteristic cracking or snapping sound is audible as the stone is contacted and as fragmentation occurs. Matching of the wavelength to the stone material and the relatively low fluences required for this photoacoustic effort enable destruction of the calculus without damage to the tissues of the duct or ureter.

PRACTICAL TIPS FOR LASER USE

Throughout this chapter, we have considered the various laser technologies and delivery systems available for laparoscopic use. This section will discuss various practical tips to optimize the clinical results obtained with these devices.

It must again be emphasized that the surgeon should have an intimate understanding of the details of the procedure, as well as the laser technology and delivery systems selected for use. It is preferable to learn the procedure and become comfortable with it by using conventional devices *prior* to attempting to perform it with laser technologies. The surgeon should practice with laser devices as much as possible prior to using them clinically. A thorough understanding of tissue effects and the ability to assemble and troubleshoot the instrumentation are critical. It is helpful to work with the laser technology in a pelvic trainer and then gradually introduce it into clinical procedures.

Trocar placement should be well thought out and based on the needs of the procedure as well as the habitus of the patient. As a general principle, the operative port should be positioned such that the laser fiber (and other instruments) can easily reach the intended surgical site end on. This is particularly important for direct fiber systems such as bare fibers for KTP, holmium, or argon lasers or waveguides for CO_2 lasers. Sculpted fibers and contact tips (sapphire tips) cut and coagulate optimally when they can be dragged obliquely across the tissues rather than using them end on (Figs. 5.8, 5.9, 5.11). Therefore trocar placement may need to be modified for the specific laser and delivery system to be utilized.

The assistant surgeon should provide steady countertraction to distract the line of incision, facilitate exposure, and optimize the efficiency and efficacy of laser use. The tissues should be incised in fluid, complete strokes, as this too will increase the efficiency of the dissection and enable it to proceed with better hemostasis. Staccatto, repetitive passage of the laser fiber over the same area tends to produce a more irregular incision and frequently causes bleeding as vessels become injured at multiple points in the irregular wound. Typically, the fiber-capable lasers are applied by placing the fiber into a suction-irrigation cannula. The fiber should be positioned such that it is easily visualized and the proposed line of incision is not obstructed by the suction irrigator. An optimal distance is 1–2 cm for fiber extension from the end of the probe (Fig. 5.12). This permits visualization and maneuverability of the fiber at the surgical site without making the fiber too floppy as a result of having too much fiber protruding from the suction irrigator. It is also critical that the fiber be retracted completely within the instrument when the instrument is being removed or inserted into the abdomen (or another site). This maneuver prevents fiber breakage or iatrogenic injury. The foot pedal for the laser and the electrosurgical device should be within easy reach while the monitor is viewed and the instrumentation is manipulated. Ideally, the surgeon should have access to only one pedal at a time to prevent inadvertent triggering of the wrong device. Several devices are available which angulate the bare fiber, permitting the surgeon to optimize the position of the fiber relative to the topography of the dissection. Again, the fiber should be positioned to enhance visualization and minimize fiber breakage.

The surgeon should learn to apply a light touch when using laser fibers of all types. The rate of movement of the fiber should be deliberately slow enough to allow the tissue to be cut through completely prior to advancing the fiber. The fiber should not be visibly bowed, as this indicates undue pressure or too deep placement of the fiber into the wound. These conditions reduce efficiency and increase the likelihood of fiber breakage.

Sapphire tips and sculpted fibers should be used in a similar fashion to the method suggested for bare fibers. However, the tip or probe should be oriented more obliquely or tangential to the line of incision. This optimizes the coagulative effect of the laser and facilitates dissection. The surgeon should also recognize that no laser system is a panacea. He or she should be prepared to use other modalities to accomplish dissection or hemostasis if the laser is not successful.

SUMMARY

This chapter has discussed the tissue effects and delivery systems available for laser utilization during minimally invasive surgical procedures. These versatile devices have many justifiable uses during surgery. The surgeon should have a thorough understanding of the procedure to be performed, as well as familiarity with the laser device, its delivery systems, and safety considerations. Practice and continued use of these devices will lead to improved outcomes.

BIBLIOGRAPHY

Borderlon BM, Hobday KA, Hunter JG: Laser vs. electrosurgery in laparoscopic cholecystectomy. A prospective randomized trail. *Arch Surg* 128(2): 33–36, 1993.

Carroll B, Chandra M, Papaioannou T, et al: Biliary lithotripsy as an adjunct to laparoscopic common bile duct stone extraction. *Surg Endosc* 7(4):356– 359, 1993.

Corbitt JD Jr: Laparoscopic cholecystectomy: Laser versus electrosurgery. *Surg Laparosc Endosc* 1(4): 268–269, 1991.

Hershman MJ, Rosin RD: Laparoscopic laser cholecystectomy: Our first 200 patients. *Ann R Coll Surg Engl* 74(4): 242–247, 1992.

Hinshaw JR, Daykhovsky L, Glantz G, et al: Current controversies in laparoscopic cholecystectomy: A roundtable discussion. *J Laparoendosc Surg* 1(1): 17–29, 1990.

Hunter JG: Exposure, dissection, and laser versus electrosurgery in laparoscopic cholecystectomy. *Am J Surg* 165(4):492–496, 1993.

Lanzafame RJ: Applications of lasers in laparoscopic cholecystectomy. *J Laparoendosc Surg* 1(1):33–36, 1990.

Lanzafame RJ: Applications of laser in laparoscopic cholecystectomy: Technical considerations and future directions. *SPIE* 1421:189–196, 1991.

Lanzafame RJ, Brien T, Rogers DW, et al: Comparison of sapphire contact scalpels for surgery. *Lasers Surg Med* 2(Suppl):9, 1990.

Phillips E, Daykhovsky L, Carroll B, et al: Laparoscopic cholecystectomy: Instrumentation and technique. *J Laparoendosc Surg* 1(1):3–15, 1990.

Reddick EJ, Olsen DO: Laparoscopic laser cholecystectomy. A comparison with mini-lap cholecystectomy. *Surg Endosc* 3(3):131–133, 1989.

Reddick EJ, Baird D, Daniel J, et al: Laparoscopic laser cholecystectomy. *Ann Chir Gynaecol* 79(4):189–191, 1990.

Reddick EJ, Olsen D, Alexander W, et al: Laparoscopic laser cholecystectomy and choledocholithiasis. *Surg Endosc* 4(3):133–134, 1990.

Reddick EJ, Olsen D: Outpatient laparoscopic laser cholecystectomy. *Am J Surg* 160(5):485–487, 1990.

Schultz LS, Hickok DF, Garber JN, et al: The use of lasers in general surgery. A preliminary assessment. *Minn Med* 70(8):439–442, 1987.

Smith EB: Complications of laparoscopic cholecystectomy. *J Natl Med Assoc* 84(10):880–882, 1992.

Spaw AT, Reddick EJ, Olsen DO: Laparoscopic laser cholecystectomy: Analysis of 500 procedures. *Surg Laparosc Endosc* 1(1):2–7, 1991.

Steger AC, Moore KM, Hira N: Contact laser or conventional cholecystectomy: A controlled trial. *Br J Surg* 75(3): 223–225, 1988.

Unger SW, Edelman DS, Scott JS, et al: Laparoscopic treatment of acute cholecystitis. *Surg Laparosc Endosc* 1(1): 14–16, 1991.

Williams IM, Lewis DK, Shandall AA, et al: Laparoscopic cholecystectomy: Laser or electrosurgery. *J R Coll Surg Edinb* 39(6):348–349, 1994.

chapter six
Strategies to Control Basic Problems

Stacey L. Mazzacco
John V. White

INTRODUCTION

Diagnostic laparoscopy was first described by Kellog in 1902.[1] During the ensuing years, laparoscopy was most widely applied in the field of gynecology. With the popularization of laparoscopic cholecystectomy in the late 1980s came the achievement of reduced hospital stays, limited postoperative pain, early return to normal activity, and improved cosmesis.[2,3] As a result, myriad minimally invasive procedures have been developed to deal with a wide variety of surgical disease. The continuous development and improvement of technology and techniques have extended the limits of minimally invasive surgery. Operations thought to be impossible without large incisions, such as aneurysm resections and coronary artery bypass grafting, are rapidly succumbing to miniaturization. This explosion of minimally invasive techniques has been accompanied by the recognition of complications unique to this field. The comprehension of the prevention and management of several basic complications that may be encountered during a variety of procedures, such as hemorrhage, trocar hernias, pneumothorax, hypothermia, and carbon dioxide embolus, as well as the basic physiologic changes associated with laparoscopy, are essential for all laparoscopic surgeons. Complications unique to specific procedures will be discussed in subsequent chapters.

PHYSIOLOGIC ALTERATIONS ASSOCIATED WITH CO_2 PNEUMOPERITONEUM

Respiratory Changes

Normally, CO_2 is virtually ubiquitous within the body as an end product of aerobic metabolism. Produced within cells, CO_2 is released into the blood stream, where it is dissolved and transported to the lungs. The scant amount of CO_2 in inspired alveolar air generates a large chemical gradient driving the CO_2 from the blood into the lungs, so that it may be excreted during expiration.

CO_2 significantly influences respiratory function and is a profound stimulant of respiratory function in the nonexercising patient.[4] Increasing blood levels of CO_2 result in a significant increase in respiratory minute ventilation. Studies in which normal volunteers inhaled high concentrations of CO_2 (1–30%) have clearly demonstrated that there is an increase in minute ventilation with each increase in pCO_2 despite normal ranges of pO_2.[5] This increase in respiration is also associated with bronchodilation.

Mechanical effects of abdominal insufflation alter respiratory physiology. The changes induced include increased peak inspiratory pressures and decreased lung compliance, presumably related to decreased diaphragmatic excursion caused by intra-abdominal insufflation. Elevation of the diaphragm results in an increase in physiologic dead space, which is the volume of lung not available for gas exchange. These effects are augmented by the Trendelenberg position.[6,7] Peak inspiratory pressures are markedly increased as intra-abdominal pressures exceed 20 mmHg. Although usually tolerated well in otherwise healthy patients, these high peak inspiratory pressures can rupture bullae and induce pneumothorax in patients with chronic pulmonary disease.

Introduction of CO_2 into the blood, such as during peritoneal absorption of the gas during laparoscopy, transiently affects the bicarbonate blood buffer system. During normal metabolism, much of the CO_2 produced is converted to carbonic acid, which replenishes the blood buffer system by establishing an equilibrium with bicarbonate.[8] The H^+ ion is accepted by deoxygenated hemoglobin to maintain blood pH. The infusion of larger amounts of CO_2 into the blood will result in rapid production of carbonic acid and excessive H^+ ions which cannot be accepted by deoxygenated hemoglobin. The hydrogen ions become bound to bicarbonate, which results in a transient decrease in blood pH and a fall in the bicarbonate level. The body attempts to reduce the elevated level of pCO_2 by increasing the respiratory rate, which promotes clearance of CO_2 and the restoration of normal blood pH and bicarbonate levels. The accommodation of transient, rapid increases in blood levels of CO_2 is limited only by the ability of the lungs to increase minute ventilation and excrete the gas.

Systemic alterations associated with hypercarbia and acidosis include pulmonary hypertension, a condition poorly tolerated by patients with right heart failure or advanced cardiomyopathy, and, if the acidosis is severe, results in decreased myocardial contractility and lowered arrhythmia thresholds. Such arrhythmias may be refractory to medical therapy, resulting in circulatory collapse.[9,10] In addition to acidosis-induced arrhythmia, significant bradyarrhythmias may result from peritoneal stimulation combined with the parasympathetic potentiation by CO_2.

Insufflation of the abdomen with CO_2 frequently results in a transient increase in blood CO_2 level. Risk factors related to greater increases in $PaCO_2$ include the length of insufflation time, the presence of subcutaneous emphysema, and the use of extraperitoneal approaches. $PaCO_2$ can increase significantly within the first 15 min after CO_2 introduction into the peritoneum.[11]

During minimally invasive procedures, more than 60 L of CO_2 may be infused into the peritoneal cavity. A recent study documented the magnitude of the acid-base changes induced in 16 patients.[12] End-tidal CO_2 levels increased from 31.4 ± 0.7 to 42.1 ± 1.6 mmHg and pCO_2 levels increased from 33.3 ± 0.7 to 43.7 ± 1.2 mmHg. These increases were associated with a fall in blood pH from 7.43 ± 0.01 to 7.34 ± 0.01. The bicarbonate concentration did not change significantly. Despite these changes, there was no significant alteration in cardiac output. Increases in minute ventilation can rapidly return blood pCO_2 and blood pH to normal levels.

The clinical significance of CO_2 absorption from the peritoneum, then, is underscored by alterations in respiratory mechanics and CO_2 excretion. Prevention of significant alterations in blood pH and vascular tone depends on the ability of the patient to increase ventilation. Therefore, a thorough preoperative pulmonary evaluation, including pulmonary function testing and a room air arterial blood gas determination, would be wise in high-risk patients. End-tidal CO_2 should be monitored during the procedure to assess CO_2 excretion, however, $ETCO_2$ and $PaCO_2$ do not correlate well in patients with pulmonary disease, making periodic arterial blood gas determinations essential.[13] CO_2 may be stored in large quantities in muscle, bone, and visceral tissues during lengthy procedures.[14] As a result, CO_2 levels may remain elevated postoperatively as these storage deposits return to baseline. This concept must be kept in mind especially when evaluating patients with limited respiratory capacity who are experiencing difficulties in the recovery room after extubation. All patients experiencing respiratory difficulties in the immediately postoperative period should be treated with respiratory support aimed at increasing minute ventilation while the source of the pulmonary embarrassment is investigated.

The risk of respiratory compromise during minimally invasive surgery in patients with impaired pulmonary function has led to a search for alternative techniques of abdominal expansion, such as gasless laparoscopy, and alternative insufflation gases. Helium is an inert, nonexplosive gas which is rapidly and totally excreted from the arterial blood into alveoli.[15] Although helium is less soluble in blood and water than CO_2, it is more diffusible due to its low density, making the dissolution of small helium emboli similar to that of CO_2. Neither CO_2 nor helium emboli result in bronchoconstriction. Animal models have shown minimal increases in $PaCO_2$ when utilizing helium as the insufflating agent, a finding confirmed in human studies.[11,16] As such, future trends may be toward helium insufflation in patients with advanced pulmonary disease.

Cardiovascular and Hemodynamic Changes

Carbon dioxide also has a significant effect on local and systemic vascular tone (Table 6.1). Systemically, elevations in pCO_2 lead to an increase in pulse rate and cardiac output due to both a direct effect on the myocardium and the triggering of chemoreceptors near the aortic arch and the carotid bifurcations.[17] Locally, increases in pCO_2 cause vasodilation in most vascular beds.[18] The locally high CO_2 concentrations also enhance the release of hemoglobin-bound O_2 by red blood cells in the region.

The hemodynamic response to CO_2 infusion into the peritoneum is governed by the mechanical effects of increased intra-abdominal pressure, the cardiovascular stimulation related to CO_2 absorption, and the volume shifts imposed by patient position on the operating room table—for example, Trendelenberg versus reverse Trendelenberg. At low intra-abdominal pressures (5–10 mmHg) venous return may actually increase, with a concomitant increase in cardiac output.[19] This may be due to the venodilation which accompanies absorption of small amounts of CO_2. With pressure increases to 10–20 mmHg, which are commonly used during laparoscopy, inferior vena cava flow is decreased, thereby reducing preload and cardiac output.[6,20] These effects can be dramatic in the setting of intra-abdominal pressures of 20–40 mmHg, especially if the patient is hypovolemic, stressing the importance of patient hydration and close monitoring of intra-abdominal pressures.

Despite these changes in preload induced by increased intra-abdominal pressures, there is frequently little deterioration of cardiac output when CO_2 is the agent utilized to establish pneumoperitoneum. This is due to the central stimulatory effect of CO_2 on the sympathetic nervous system, resulting in augmented levels of circulating catecholamines, increased heart rate, contractility, and systemic vascular resistance.[6,21] In addition, the Trendelenberg position may augment venous return.[22] Given these compensations, there seems to be little change in cardiac output or blood pressure in young, healthy patients. The potential for complications in patients with cardiomyopathy or severe ischemic heart disease can easily be appreciated. In this subset of patients, thorough preoperative optimization of cardiac status is essential. Invasive pulmonary artery monitoring is also helpful intraoperatively to assess and monitor the physiologic alterations induced by the elevations in blood CO_2. Conversion to gasless laparoscopy or to an open procedure in those patients who experience irreversible hemodynamic compromise from the gas is prudent.

Another effect of decreased venous return induced by increased intra-abdominal pressure is venous stasis in the lower extremities. Animal studies have revealed a decrease in femoral venous flow rates associated with insufflation pressures of 10–20 mmHg.[23] This reduction in venous outflow from the lower extremity can be aggravated by the reverse Trendelenberg position. It is recognized (Virchow's triad) that venous stasis can increase the likelihood of deep venous thrombosis of the lower extremities. Therefore, in patients undergoing significant pelvic or prolonged abdominal procedures, deep venous thrombosis prophylaxis should be administered. The form of prophylaxis can be chosen to suit the patient's requirements. Graduated compression stockings, intermittent sequential pneumatic compression devices, and anticoagulants and antiplatelet medications can all be of use in selected patients. Those at highest risk, including patients over the age of 60, the obese, and those with cancer or a previous history of deep venous thrombosis, may require a combination of methods.

Table 6.1. Physiological Effects of Elevations of Blood Carbon Dioxide Levels

Systemic
Increased pulse rate
Increased stroke volume
Increased cardiac output
Bronchodilation
Increased respiratory rate
Transient mild acidemia
Local
Vasodilation
Enhanced oxyhemoglobin dissociation

OTHER BASIC PROBLEMS

Hemorrhage

Hemorrhage related to minimally invasive surgery can range from minor nuisance bleeding from a trocar site to life-threatening major vascular injury. Minor bleeding from a trocar site can usually be controlled with electrocautery. There are several newer models of trocars, including visualization and/or cautery to prevent trocar-related bleeding from the abdominal wall during insertion. These may be of benefit to some practitioners but are not necessary. Simple safety measures taken during trocar placement, such as the use of the modified open placement technique in patients who are large or who have had previous procedures, are generally sufficient to avoid bleeding from the trocar site. Nonetheless, all trocar sites should be laparoscopically inspected after the trocar is removed and the pneumoperitoneum is partially released (5 mmHg) to reveal any site of bleeding that may have been tamponaded during the procedure. If the patient is unresponsive to cautery, full-thickness fascial closure, either with conventional means or with newer devices designed specifically for this purpose, will usually be effective. Balloon tamponade utilizing a Foley catheter has also been used effectively. More troublesome trocar bleeding is seen with inadvertent inferior epigastric vessel injury within the rectus sheath. Knowledge of its anatomic course can help in planning torcar placement to avoid injury. Although trocar bleeding can sometimes be controlled by cauterizing the parietal peritoneum proximal and distal to the trocar site, ligation of the vessels either by fascial closure or wound exploration and direct visualization may be required.[24]

Although infrequent, major vessel injury can be a fatal complication of minimally invasive surgery, occurring with a reported incidence of 39 cases per 10,000 laparoscopies. The majority of these injuries occur during Veress needle or trocar insertion. The vessels most likely to be injured are the aorta, iliac artery, and iliac vein, although large mesenteric vessels may also be involved.[25,26] Vascular injuries can usually be avoided by careful placement of at least the first trocar using the open technique. Despite careful introduction of the trocars and instruments, vascular injury may occur. It is crucial that these injuries be quickly recognized and treated. Having a complete set of open surgical instruments in the operating room at all times will allow a prompt response in the case of inadvertent injury. A preset plan of maneuvers, such as pressure application with a blunt laparoscopic instrument accompanied by rapid conversion to an open procedure, is recommended.[27] Veress needle vascular injuries can be minimized by applying firm upward traction on the abdominal wall and inserting the needle at a 45° downward angle to the abdominal wall.[28] In addition, grasping the needle 2–3 cm from its tip will prevent too deep an insertion. Recognition of patients at high risk of injury, such as those with previous abdominal surgery, combined with careful attention to proper technique, will help guard against vascular misadventure. A thorough questioning with the patient to elicit a history of bleeding disorders is recommended prior to any surgical procedure.

In addition to access-related bleeding, major hemorrhage may occur, either by inadvertent injury to larger vessels or by slippage of previously placed clips or loops. Venous bleeding may not become evident until after the pneumoperitoneum is released, reversing its venous tamponade effect. The first symptoms of hemorrhage may not become apparent until the procedure is completed and the patient is in the recovery room. A sound knowledge of anatomy coupled with careful dissection techniques will allow proximal placement of double clips or loops prior to vessel division. There is no substitute for visualization while dissecting around or near major vascular structures. Blind application of clips in an effort to control hemorrhage within an inadequately dissected field is fraught with disaster. Familiarity with the use of preformed loops and sutures to gain vascular control is of obvious importance.[27] When dividing large vascular bundles, such as the renal artery and vein, it is wise to dissect and ligate each vessel separately to prevent acute bleeding and the possibility of delayed atrioventricular fistula formation.[29]

Bleeding from solid organs due to instrument injury or dissection is usually limited or easily controlled by gentle pressure. If the injury is unresponsive to these maneuvers, topical hemostats (Surgicel, Thrombin, Gelfoam, Avitene) may be applied. Laparoscopic injection of fibrin glue may be a future alternative as this medication becomes available.[30]

Trocar Hernias

Laparoscopic procedures generally employ trocars ranging from 5 to 15 mm in diameter. Although hernias have been reported to occur at 5-mm sites, the majority of cases occur after the use of 10-mm or larger trocars. The incidence of trocar hernia increases both with increasing trocar size, from 0.23% to 3.1% in one series, and with failure to close the fascia adequately.[31] These hernias may contain omentum or small bowel; Richter hernias are particularly common.[32,33] Patients may be asymptomatic or present with local pain or bowel obstruction.

Several factors are thought to predispose a patient to hernia formation. These include the presence of a preexisting umbilical hernia, coughing during reversal of anesthesia at the comple-tion of the procedure, poor relaxation when the sheaths are removed, failure to close trocar sites of 10 mm or more, and obesity, with the concomitant difficulty of adequately repairing trocar sites. To avoid incisional hernias, some laparoscopists avoid the umbilicus due to its inherent fascial weakness,[34] while others utilize a Z-path through the subcutaneous tissues or puncture off the midline to provide soft tissue support of fascial defects. Thorough evacuation of CO_2 before trocar removal, accompanied by shaking of the abdominal wall, will prevent the entrapment of omentum or bowel within the trocar site after removal. Maintaining the trocar valve in the open position and inserting a probe into the trocar during removal will facilitate the same goal. Perhaps most important is adequate closure of all 10 mm trocar sites. If the trocar was placed through the rectus sheath, confirming proper closure of the posterior sheath by laparoscopic inspection has been advocated. In fact, if possible, all fascial repairs should be inspected both digitally and laparoscopically to ensure integrity, especially in the obese patient. Newer instruments designed specifically for fascial closure will make this task easier and more efficient. Proper fascial closure will also help decrease the incidence of acute ascities leakage postoperatively.

Bowel Injury

Bowel injuries complicating minimally invasive surgery may have lethal consequences, especially if recognition and treatment are delayed. These injuries are usually penetrating and occur during the placement of the Veress needle or sharp trocars, with an overall incidence of 2.7 per 1000 procedures.[35] Patients who have had prior open abdominal surgery are at higher risk because of the increased likelihood of bowel adherence to the anterior abdominal wall. Proper techniques of both open and closed trocar placement help to minimize these injuries. When these injuries are recognized, immediate suture or staple repair should be undertaken.

Bowel injury can also be induced by injudicious grasping or retraction. Gentle retraction of the bowel with instruments designed for that purpose will minimize injury. Handling extremely friable, adherent bowel with laparoscopic instruments carries a high risk of bowel injury. Finally, in resecting inflamed bowel, staple lines should be placed across noninflamed sites to reduce the likelihood of subsequent leakage. If the bowel is too friable to handle with currently available techniques, conversion to an open procedure is warranted.[36]

Thermal bowel injury may result from improperly applied electrocautery or laser energy and can involve partial or full wall thickness. These injuries may be particularly problematic because they are often delayed. The mechanisms of cautery injury include misdirected cautery application and arcing of the electric current. In the first mechanism, a contact point proximal to the target may deliver some or all of the current force to an unseen segment of bowel. This was a common mechanism of injury with older laparoscopic electrocautery instruments, which had a long length of exposed metal proximal to the instrument tip. Frequently, the proximal portion of the exposed metal of the instrument was not visible during cautery application. This mechanism of injury can be avoided by full visualization of the noninsulated portion of the cautery instrument prior to the initiating current. The second major method of electrocautery injury, arcing of the current, most commonly occurs with higher levels of direct current. The current may travel to the closest organ during instrument movement. This mechanism of injury can be avoided by refraining from initiating current prior to fixation of the instrument on the target tissue. Laser injuries occur in much the same way as electrocautery injuries. Contact laser fibers can discharge energy at unintentional targets if energy delivery begins prior to contact with the target tissue. Free beam energy, such as from the CO_2 laser, will penetrate visible tissue and injure underlying, poorly visualized tissue. Laser use during minimally invasive surgery requires a clear understanding not only of laparoscopic tissue dissection but also of laser physics.

Bowel perforation due to a partial-thickness thermal injury or ischemic necrosis related to devascularization or mesenteric vein thrombosis may present in a delayed fashion.[37] The mortality associated with delayed recognition of intestinal perforation can be substantial,[38] mandating a high degree of suspicion in postoperative patients with pain out of proportion to their procedure. As a confounding variable, diffuse abdominal pain after minimally invasive surgery is not uncommon and may last for 12–36 hr.[39] Its causes include the formation of carbonic acid from CO_2 and peritoneal fluid which acts as a peritoneal irritant, as well as loss of the natural "suction" effect of the right diaphragm on the liver, resulting in undue traction on the peritoneum as it suspends the liver. Both of these effects can be reduced by thorough evacuation of CO_2 at the conclusion of the procedure.

Assurance of adequate pneumoperitoneum, use of atraumatic retraction, gastric decompression, and judicious use of the laser and cautery will help prevent bowel injury. If recognized intraoperatively, most bowel injuries can be repaired without conversion to an open procedure. If, however, the diagnosis is delayed, formal laparotomy to ensure clear identification of the injury, adequate repair, drainage, and irrigation should be considered, especially in patients with signs of diffuse peritoneal irritation and sepsis.

Subcutaneous Emphysema and Pneumothorax

Subcutaneous emphysema occurs in 0.43–2% of patients undergoing laparoscopy.[40] It is usually a benign complication of abdominal insufflation resulting from incorrect positioning of an insufflation needle or leakage around a trocar site.[41] Additional sources include malfunction of insufflators and excessive intra-abdominal pressure. Attempts to minimize this complication include assurance of proper Veress needle position aided by the "water test," use of newer trocars with an outer corkscrew-like outer coating, and placement of trocars through an angled plane to minimize trocar manipulation and enlargement of fascial defects.[42] The water test consists of placing 1 mL of sterile saline in the open end of the Veress needle. If the needle is in the peritoneal space, the saline will be rapidly drawn up; however, if it is in the higher-pressure environment of the preperitoneal space, the saline level will change minimally. Once insufflation commences, high pressures with a low delivered volume indicate improper positioning. Though the open technique of trocar placement often ensures correct insufflation position, if initial incisions are too large gas leakage may occur, with subsequent development of subcutaneous emphysema.

The presence of subcutaneous emphysema, especially around the head, neck, or chest, should alert the surgeon to the possibility of pneumothorax. Although rare, occurring in 0.03–0.08% of cases,[43] pneumothorax and pneumomediastinum can be fatal due to respiratory and cardiac insufficiency. Extraperitoneal and retroperitoneal dissection may allow gas to track cephalad along the great vessels, causing pneumomediastinum or pneumopericardium. This could result in a tamponade effect, which requires surgical decompression if cardiac embarrassment occurs.[24] Insufflation gas can rupture through the mediastinal pleura, causing a pneumothorax. Tension pneumothorax can be rapidly induced by gas leakage into the pleural cavity through previously unrecognized diaphragmatic defects, either congenital or traumatic, or by excessive dissection around the esophageal hiatus, such as during the performance of a Nissen fundoplication. Increased peak inspiratory pressures caused by pneumoperitoneum may rupture blebs in patients with underlying emphysematous pulmonary disease. Small pneumothoraces detected postoperatively on routine X-rays that are asymptomatic may be treated expectantly, but large pneumothoraces or those causing symptoms require tube thoracostomy. Sudden intraoperative hemodynamic embarrassment should alert the surgeon to the possibility of tension pneumothorax. Emergent needle decompression should be performed if breath sounds are not detectable on auscultation. The penumoperitoneum should also be evacuated if the source of the pneumothorax is gas leakage from the abdomen.

CO_2 Embolus

CO_2 embolism is another potentially fatal form of cardiopulmonary compromise which may complicate minimally invasive surgery. The incidence is quite low, occurring in 0.002–0.02% of cases.[43,44] The majority of cases occur during the first few minutes of the procedure and are usually related to Veress needle introduction into a major vein, including portal venous tributaries within the liver. Gas emboli cause symptoms of hypoxia/ hypercapnia and hypotension by blocking the right ventricular outflow tract and pulmonary arteries. Cyanosis and dysrhythmia may ensue, and the classic mill wheel murmer can be detected on physical exam. A sudden, large end-tidal CO_2 may reveal an incomplete flow obstruction, whereas a sudden, large decrease in exhaled CO_2 may indicate complete cessation of pulmonary blood flow.[45,46] These changes are often accompanied by an electrocardiographic tracing which reveals evidence of right heart strain or a widened QRS complex. Treatment begins with the rapid releases of pneumoperitoneum. The patient should be placed in a steep left lateral Trendelenberg position and ventilated with 100% oxygen via an endotracheal tube. Attempts to aspirate the gas from the right ventricle using a central venous catheter may be considered.

Hypothermia

During lengthy procedures, multiple factors contribute to the development of hypothermia, including anesthetic effects of impaired body temperature maintenance, skin exposure, use of large volumes of insufflating gas, and the administration of cold intravenous solutions. General anesthesia with neuromuscular blockade inhibits shivering, preventing the generation of muscular heat and peripheral vasoconstriction. Blood reaching the hypothalmus is at a lower temperature, and the mechanisms which normally regulate body temperature are impaired.[47] Prolonged laparoscopy has been associated with a 0.3°C heat loss per 40–50 L CO_2 delivered to the peritoneum, further compounding the above effects.[48]

If a procedure is anticipated to be lengthy, the patient's core temperature should be monitored, warming blankets applied, and IV solutions warmed. Minimizing procedure time and maintaining an operating room temperatures above 23°C are recommended.[49] Thermal losses during laparoscopy can be lessened by the use of warmed, humidified CO_2 to establish and maintain pneumoperitoneum. Although the majority of heat loss mechanisms are related specifically to anaesthesia, it is important to recognize the heat loss capacity of high-volume CO_2 use.

SUMMARY

Following widespread acceptance of laparoscopic cholecystectomy, the field of minimally invasive surgery grew rapidly as novel equipment and surgical approaches were developed. Although these procedures are generally considered low in morbidity and mortality, there are a number of associated complications and physiologic alterations. Knowledge of their occurrence, prevention, and treatment coupled with careful patient selection will maintain the high degree of safety associated with this field.

REFERENCES

1. Kelling G: Uber Oesophagoskopie, Gastroskopie, and Zolio Skopiel. *Münch Med Wochenschr*. 1902; 49:21–24.
2. Soper NJ, Barteau JA, Clayman RV, et al: Comparison of early post operative results for laparoscopic versus standard open cholecystectomy. *Surg Gynecol Obstet* 1992; 174:114–118.
3. Peters JH, Ellison EC, Innes JT, et al: Safety and efficacy of laparoscopic cholecystectomy: A prospective analysis of 100 initial patients. *Ann Surg* 1991; 213:3–12.
4. Lambertson CJ: Chemical control of respiration at rest. In: Mountcastle VB, ed. *Medical Physiology*. St. Louis, Mo: CV Mosby Co; 1980; 1774– 1827.
5. Lambertson CJ: Therapeutic cases: Oxygen, carbon dioxide, and helium. In: DiPalma JR, ed. *Drill's Pharmacology in Medicine*. 4th ed. New York: McGraw-Hill Book Co; 1971.
6. Richardson DW, Wasserman AJ, Patterson JL: General and regional circulatory responses to change in blood pH and carbon dioxide tension. *J Clin Invest* 1961; 40:294–302.
7. Monk TG, Weldon BC, Lemon D: Alterations in pulmonary function during laparoscopic surgery. *Anesth Analg* 1993; 76:S274.
8. Gamble JL Jr: Acid Base Physiology. Baltimore: The Johns Hopkins University Press; 1982.
9. Scott DB, Julian DG: Observations on cardiac arrhythmias during laparoscopy. *Br Med J* 1972; 1:411–413.
10. Harris MNE, Planteueim OM, Crowther A: Cardiac arrhythmias during anesthesia for laparoscopy. *Br J Anaesth* 1984; 56:1213–1217.
11. Leighton TA, Bongard FS, Liu SY, et al: Comparative cardiopulmonary effects of CO2 and helium pneumoperitoneum. *Surg Forum* 1991; 62:485– 487.
12. Liu SY, Leighton T, Davis I, et al: Perspective analysis of cardiopulmonary responses to laparoscopic cholecystectomy. *J Laparoendosc Surg* 1993; 1:241–246.
13. Wittgen CM, Andrus CH, Fitzgerald SD, et al: Analysis of hemodynamics and ventilation during laparoscopic cholecystectomy. *Arch Surg* 1991; 126:997–1001.
14. Nunn JF: Carbon dioxide. In: *Nunn's Applied Respiratory Physiology*, 3rd ed. London: Butterworth-Heinemann Ltd. 1987; pp 207–234.
15. Smith TC, Gross JB, Wolman H: The therapeutic gases. The pharmacologic basis of therapeutics, 5th ed. In: Goodman LS, Gilman A, eds. New York: Macmillan Publishing Co. 1975.
16. Bongard FS, Pianim NA, Leightion TA, et al: Helium insufflation for laparoscopic operation. *Surg Gyn Obstet* 1993; 177:140–146.
17. Marshall RJ, Sheperd JT: *Cardiac Function in Health and Disease*. Philadelphia: WB Saunders Co; 1968.
18. Milnor WR: Autonomic and peripheral control mechanisms. In: Mountcastle VB, ed. *Medical Physiology*, St. Louis, Mo: CV Mosby Co, 1980; 1047–1060.
19. Delman GR, Swapp GH, Smith I, et al: Cardiac output and arterial blood-gas tension during laparoscopy. *Brit J Anaesth* 1972; 44:1155.
20. McKenzie R, Wadha RK, Bedger RC: Non-invasive measurement of cardiac output during laparoscopy. *J Rep Med* 1980; 24:247–250.
21. Price HL: Effects of carbon dioxide on the cardiovascular system. *Anesthesiology* 1968; 21(6): 633–663.
22. Centili DR, Benjamin B, Darger SR, et al: Cardiopulmonary effects of the head down xxx position in elderly postoperative patients; A prospective study. *South Med J* 1988; 81:1258.

23. Jorgenson JO, Gillies RB, Lalak NJ, et al: Lower limb venous hemodynamics during laparoscopy: An animal study. *Surg Laparosc Endosc* 1994; 4:32–35.
24. Evans RM, Hulbert JC, Reddy PK: Complications of laparoscopy. *Seminars in Urology* 1992; 10: 164–168.
25. Peterson HB, Greenspan JR, Ory HW: Death following puncture of the aorta during laparoscopic sterilization. *Obstet Gynecol* 1982; 59:133.
26. Katz M, Beck P, Tancer ML: Major vessel injury during laparoscopy: Anatomy of two cases. *Am J Obstet Gynecol* 1979; 135:344.
27. Gill IS, Kavoussi LR, Clayman RH, et al: Complications of laparoscopic neplurectomy in 185 patients: A multi-institutional review. *J Urol* 1995; 154:479–483.
28. Palmer R: Safety in laparoscopy. *J Reprod Med* 1974; 13:1.
29. Kerbl K, Chandhoke PS, Clayman RV, et al: Ligation of the renal pedicle during laparoscopic nephrectomy: A comparison of staples, clips, and sutures. *J Laparoendosc Surg* 1993; 3:7.
30. Salvino CK, Esposito TJ, Smith DK, et al: Laparoscopic injection of glue to arrest intraparenchymal abdominal hemorrhage: An experimental study. *J Trauma* 1993; 35: 762–766.
31. Kadar N, Reich H, Liu CY, et al: Incisional hernias after major laparoscopic gynecologic procedures. *Am J Obstet Gynecol* 1993; 168:1493–1495.
32. Sauer M, Jarrett J: Small bowel obstruction following diagnostic laparoscopy. *Fertil Steril* 1984; 42: 635–654.
33. Kiiholma P, Makinena J: Incarcerated Richter's hernia after laparoscopy: A case report. *Eur J Obstet Gynecol Reprod Med* 1988; 28:75–77.
34. Hogdall C, Roosen J: Incarcerated hernia following laparoscopy. *Acta Obstet Gynaecol Scand* 1987; 66: 735–736.
35. Phillips J, Keith D, Hulka J, et al: Gynecologic laparoscopy in 1975. *J Reprod Med* 1976; 16: 105–117.
36. Connor TJ, Garcha TS, Ramshaw BJ, et al: Diagnostic laparoscopy for suspected appendicitis. *Am Surg* 1995; 61:187–189.
37. Reich H: Laparoscopic bowel injury. *Surg Laparosc Endosc* 1992; 2:74–78.
38. Wolfe BM, Gardiner BN, Leary BF, et al: Endoscopic cholecystectomy: An analysis of complications. *Arch Surg* 1991; 126:1192–1198.
39. Alexander JI, Hull MGR: Abdominal pain after laparoscopy: The value of a gna drain. *Br J Obstet Gynaccol* 1987; 94:267–269.
40. Kalhan SB, Reaney JA: Pneumomediastinum and subcutaneous emphysema during laparoscopy. *Cleve Clin J Med* 1990; 57:639–642.
41. Bard PA, Chen L: Subcutaneous emphysema associated with laparoscopy. *Anesth Analg* 1990; 71: 100–106.
42. Kent RB: Subcutaneous emphysema and hypercarbia following laparoscopic cholecystectomy. *Arch Surg* 1991; 126:1154–1156.
43. Bruhl W: Complications of laparoscopy and liver biopsey under vision: The results of a survey. *German Med Monthly* 1967; 12:31.
44. Loeffer FD, Pent D: Indications, contraindications, and complications of laparoscopy. *Obst Gynec Surg* 1975; 30:407.
45. Shulman D, Aronson HB: Capnography in the early diagnosis of carbon dioxide embolism during laparoscopy. *Canad Anaesth Soc J* 1984; 31:455.
46. Ostman PL, Pantl-Fisher FH, Faure BA, et al: Circulatory collapse during laparoscopy. *J Clin Anesth* 1990; 2:129.
47. Ott DE: Correction of laparoscopic insufflation hypothermia. *J Laparoendosc Surg* 1991; 1:183– 186.
48. Ott DE: Laparoscopic hypothermia. *J Laparoendosc Surg* 1991; 1:127–131.
49. Morris R, Wilkey R: The effects of ambient temperature on patient temperature during surgery not involving body cavities. *Anesthesiology* 1970; 32:102–1078.
50. Liu SY, Leighton TA, Bongard FS, et al: Cardiopulmonary effects of laparoscopic cholecystectomy. *J Laparoendoscopic Surg* 1991; 5:241–246.

section two

Techniques in Biliary Surgery

chapter seven

Techniques of Laparoscopic Cholecystectomy to Avoid Complications

Douglas O. Olsen

In 1882, Langenbuch performed one of the first cholecystectomies.[1] He was later quoted as saying, "The gallbladder should be removed not because it contains stones, but because it forms stones." The surgical removal of the gallbladder has thus become the gold standard in the management of biliary calculous disease. Although the procedure can be performed with minimal morbidity and mortality, physicians and patients have continued to seek alternatives to surgical treatment. With the introduction of laparoscopic cholecystectomy, patients were given the option of a treatment that managed their disease definitively without the morbidity of a surgical incision. This led to widespread acceptance of the procedure, which occurred so rapidly and with such explosive force that is has been compared to a revolution. This has stimulated a growth of new technologies that has been unprecedented in surgical history.

Despite the wide acceptance of laparoscopic cholecystectomy, significant complications continue to be reported.[2] Bile duct injury is perhaps the most devastating one and emphasizes the need to continue the refinement of the basic surgical technique. Complications with laparoscopic cholecystectomy can be divided into two groups: those related to laparoscopic access and those specifically related to removal of the gallbladder. Complications related to the access technique are common to all laparoscopic procedures and can be considered laparoscopic complications. Gaining safe access to the abdominal cavity is the key to safe laparoscopic surgery. The techniques of safe access are covered in Chapter 3 and will vary, depending on the surgeon's experience and the type of patient being treated. The complications of gallbladder removal are technique specific and are seen in both the open procedure and its laparoscopic counterpart. The incidence of complications is related to the surgical technique, and by adhering to certain basic principles of surgery, many of these complications can be avoided. These basic principles include the following:

1. Ensuring adequate exposure before proceeding with the operation.
2. Careful, meticulous dissection with maintenance of hemostasis—no blind clipping or cauterization of bleeding sites.
3. Positive identification of the anatomy before any structure is ligated or divided.

By observing these principles and by converting quickly to an open cholecystectomy when these principles cannot be adhered to, reported complications of laparoscopic cholecystectomy will be significantly reduced.

GAINING ADEQUATE EXPOSURE

It is hard to match the exposure that can be achieved with the laparoscopic approach, and this is perhaps the reason that laparoscopic cholecystectomy was accepted by physicians as quickly as it was by their patients. The exposure, however, still depends on certain techniques that will ensure the surgeon the best possible view.

Trocar Position

The first step in achieving adequate laparoscopic exposure is attaining proper trocar position. Once the initial umbilical trocar access is achieved, the placement of the accessory trocars can make a significant difference in the surgeon's ability to see the tissues and the area of dissection. The most critical of trocar position is the 10-mm operating port that is placed in the epigastrium. This trocar should be placed as high in the epigastrium as possible so that the angle between the instruments and the axis of the camera is at its maximum (Fig. 7.1). This will allow the surgeon to see the tips of the dissecting instruments and clip applier much more easily than if they are passed along the viewing axis. Caution must be used to ensure that the trocar is placed at or below the edge of the liver. Since the falciform ligament fixes the liver at this location, elevating the liver will not compensate for a trocar that is placed too high, as is the case with the lateral trocars. The two 5-mm trocars that are placed laterally are placed just below the costal margin, one along the midclavicular line and the other along the anterior axillary line (Fig. 7.2). Even when the liver extends below the costal margin, the edge of the liver is ultimately elevated, and with the high position of the 5-mm trocars, the surgeon has better leverage to manipulate the tissues for exposure. The placement of these lateral trocars is not as critical as placement of the epigastric trocar, but the increased ability to manipulate and elevate the tissues will still aid in gaining the best optimum exposure.

Table Positioning

Gravity is the surgeon's friend during laparoscopic surgery. With the pneumoperitoneum that is created, elevating the head of the table in a steep reverse Trendelenburg position allows the intestinal contents to slide down into the pelvic cavity (Fig. 7.3). Since the liver is attached to the diaphragm, the liver, along with the biliary structures, remains in the upper abdominal cavity. A slight rotation of the table to the left will further draw the organs away from the right upper quadrant. This rotation will also allow the surgeon to operate in a more comfortable position.

Exposing the Porta Hepatis

The ultimate ability to gain exposure with laparoscopic cholecystectomy lies in the ability of the surgeon to grasp the gallbladder and elevate the right lobe of the liver, exposing the gallbladder and the porta hepatis. A normal liver is folded back on itself within the space created by the pneumoperitoneum, giving an exposure which is literally a textbook view. This is achieved by grasping the fundus of the gallbladder with an atraumatic grasper placed through the lateral 5-mm trocar cannula and lifting and elevating the fundus over the liver edge (Fig. 7.4). Care must be taken to release any

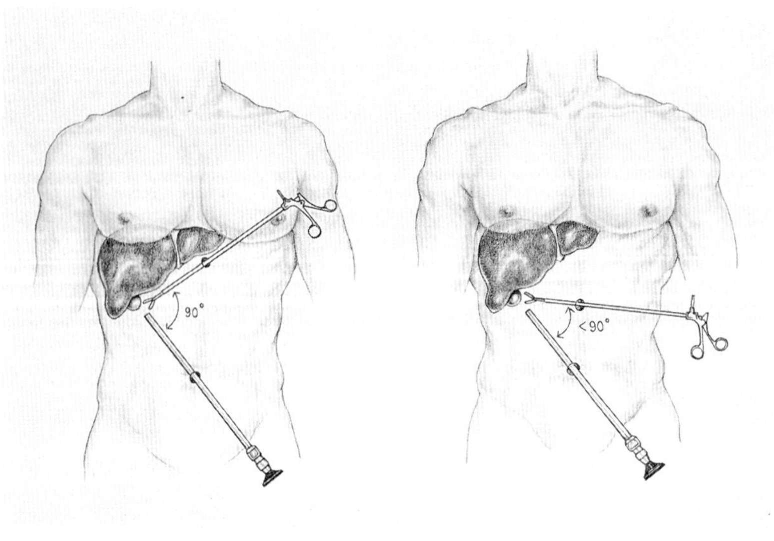

Figure 7.1. The epigastric trocar should be placed high to maximize the angle between the path of the trocar and the laparoscope at the umbilicus.

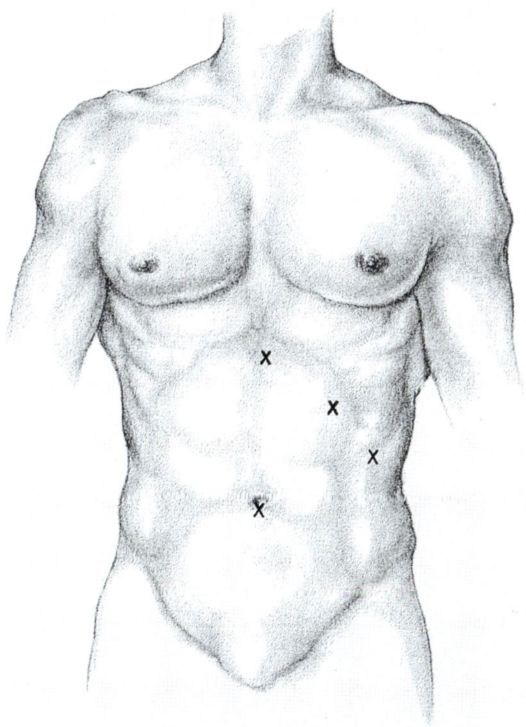

Figure 7.2. The usual positions for trocar placement.

adhesions to the gallbladder and/or liver that may prevent this elevation (Fig. 7.5). Often the elevation needs to be achieved in steps. As the adhesions are released, additional traction is applied to gain more and more elevation until maximum exposure has been achieved. This is best achieved by grasping the tip of the fundus. If the liver is thickened due to fatty infiltration, edema, or cirrhosis and effective folding over of the liver cannot be achieved, the surgeon must rely on simple lifting of the liver. This is best achieved by grasping the gallbladder in midbody and lifting it straight up toward the anterior abdominal wall, as opposed to up and toward the diaphragm (Fig. 7.6). The gallbladder is grasped further down the body if additional lift is required.

With proper lifting, exposure of the porta hepatis is completed by grasping Hartman's pouch and applying downward and lateral traction with an atraumatic grasper placed through the midclavicular 5 mm trocar cannula. This helps to reestablish the normal angle between the cystic duct and the common bile duct that is closed with the upward traction applied to the gallbladder (Fig. 7.7). This distorts the normal anatomic relationship between these two structures and can lead to confusion in the identification of the anatomy. By reestablishing a more normal angle between the cystic duct and the common bile duct, the surgeon will increase his or her ability to identify and correctly dissect out the neck of the gallbladder. Care must be taken to not grab the gallbladder too close to the neck. If this occurs, the surgeon can pull the structures in the he-

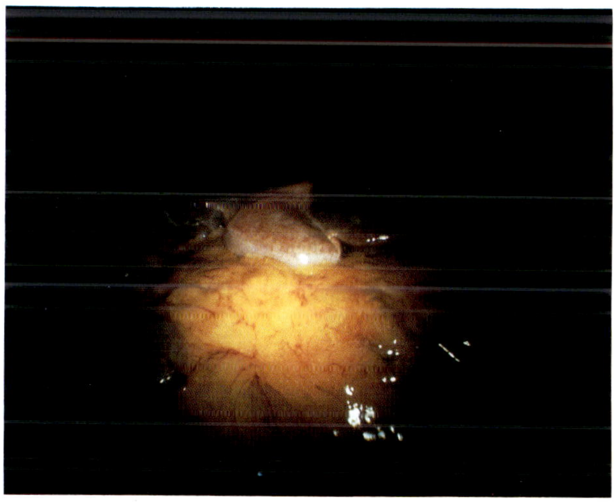

Figure 7.3a. View of a gallbladder with the patient in a neutral position.

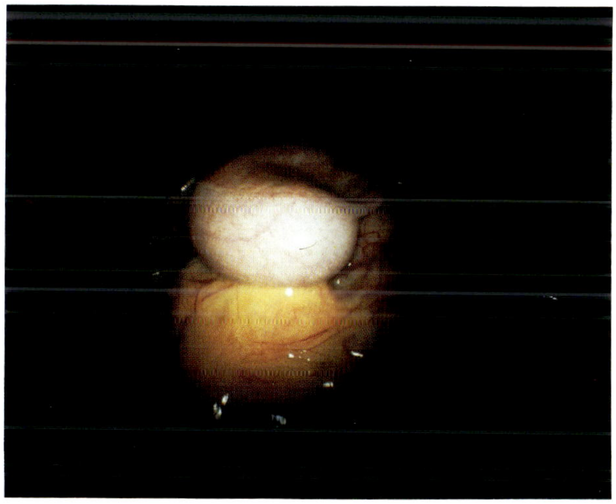

Figure 7.3b. View of the same gallbladder with the patient placed in the steep Trendelenburg position.

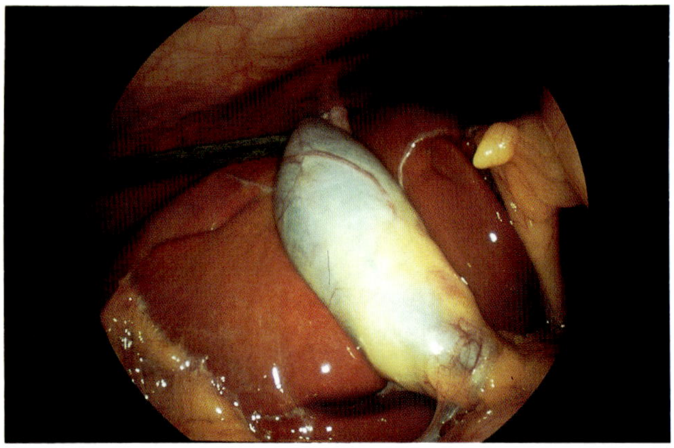

Figure 7.4. Exposure achieved by lifting the gallbladder up over the edge of the liver.

patoduodenal ligament into the operative field, leading to inadvertent dissection of the common bile duct (Fig. 7.8).

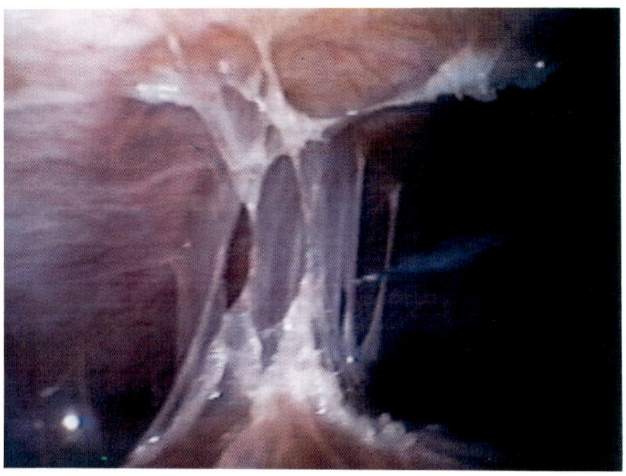

Figure 7.5. Adhesions over the dome of the liver can restrict the elevation of the liver and must be divided.

DIFFICULT EXPOSURE PROBLEMS

Although these exposure techniques should work for most normal gallbladders, there are certain difficult situations that pose unique problems which make it difficult to gain adequate exposure. If these difficulties cannot be overcome, the surgeon is faced with the prospect of converting the case to an open cholecystectomy to allow the procedure to be done safely. Difficult situations most commonly seen include the following:

1. The obese patient.
2. The large, redundant left lobe of the liver.
3. The acute gallbladder.

These situations create exposure difficulty due to excessive tissue that may obscure the surgeon's view. The obese patient has an excessively large, thick omentum.

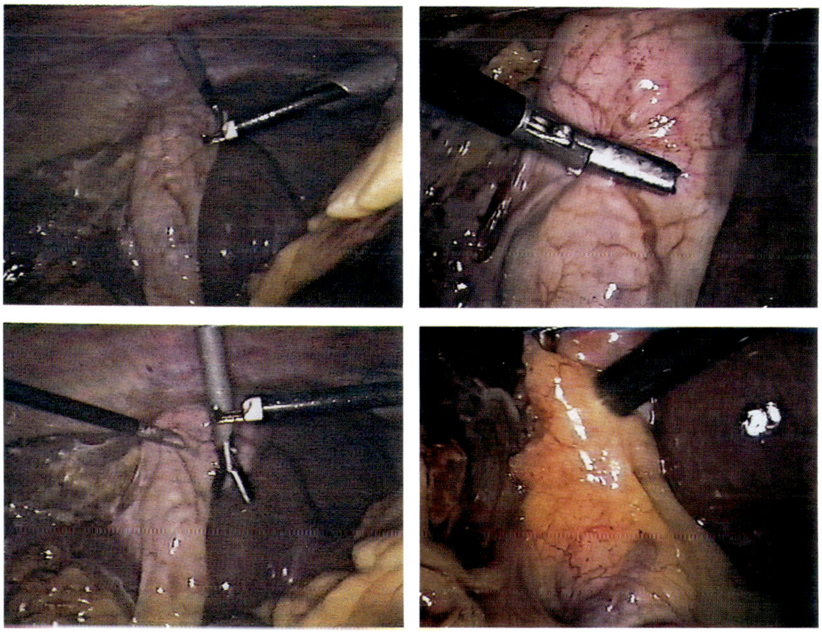

Figure 7.6. Sequence of photographs showing how "cheating" up on the gallbladder can help achieve the elevation needed to visualize the portal structures, as seen in the last picture.

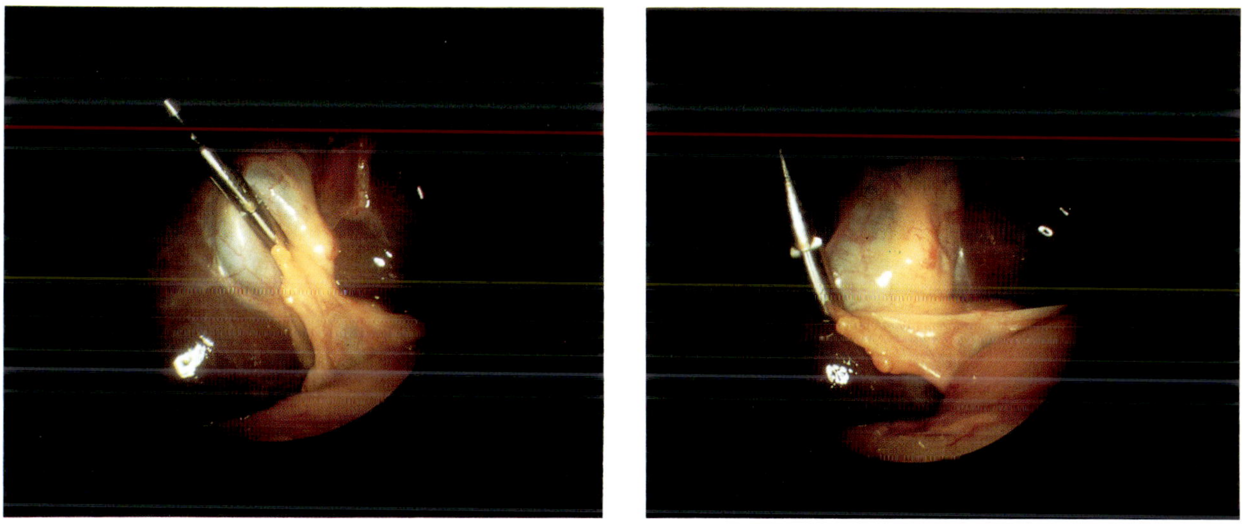

a b

Figure 7.7. The upward and medial traction on Hartman's pouch (a) tends to collapse the triangle of Calot, where downward and lateral traction (b) tends to open up the triangle of Calot.

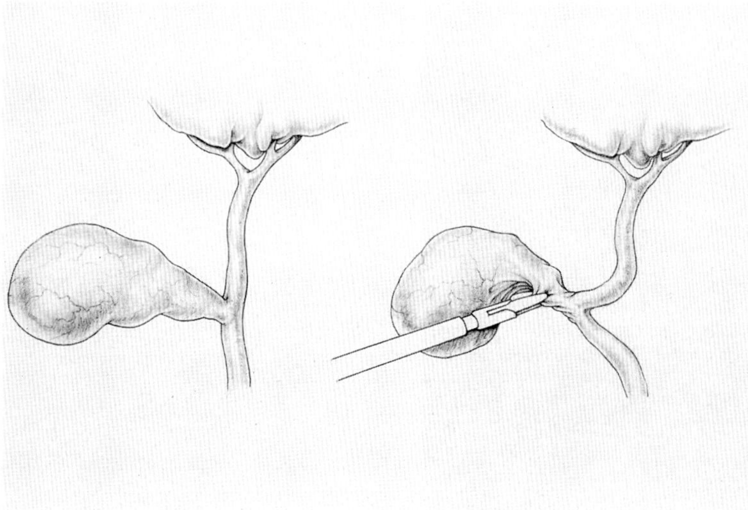

Figure 7.8. Example of how grasping too close to the neck of the gallbladder can cause tenting and possible misidentification of the common bile duct.

The patient with a large, floppy left liver lobe has a liver that continues to fall into the operative view despite normal retraction techniques. Alternatively, difficulty with exposure can occur from the inability to grasp and control the gallbladder in order to gain the upward lift needed for exposure, such as in the acute gallbladder. Additionally, even the smallest amount of bleeding that obscures the operative field can preclude the visualization necessary to carry out the laparoscopic procedure safely. Although the surgeon can usually prevent this type of bleeding through careful dissection, with an acute cholecystitis it is unavoidable.

The Obese Patient

The obese patient creates an exposure problem due to both the thickened liver that is more difficult to elevate and the increased amounts of intra-abdominal fat that thickens all of the abdominal organs and significantly increases the size of the omentum. In these patients, normal table positioning is not sufficient to gain exposure once the liver is elevated. As noted above with regard to the thickened liver, the gallbladder is grasped in midbody and lifted. To gain the proper view of the porta hepatis, the surgeon must either look over the thickened omentum, or displace it downward. With a straight-angled telescope (0 degrees), the thickened omentum increases the height of the horizon, precluding adequate vision (Fig. 7.9). By choosing an angled scope of 30–45 degrees, the surgeon can pass the scope over the horizon and look down to see the porta hepatis (Fig. 7.10). This alone is usually sufficient to give the surgeon adequate exposure.

An alternative to an angled scope, if one is not available, is to displace the tissue that is obscuring the horizon downward (Fig. 7.11). This can be achieved by inserting a fifth trocar in the left midabdomen for placement of a retracting instrument. The surgeon should choose an instrument that is very blunt and atraumatic, since the device will be outside the field of view during parts of the procedure. In especially difficult situations, both the angled telescope and the fifth trocar may be used.

The Large Left Lobe of the Liver

A particularly large, floppy left lobe of the liver is a unique problem that can often be seen in thin, older female patients. This floppiness of the liver causes difficulty. As the liver is elevated in the usual fashion, the left lobe, which is not directly attached to the right lobe, falls down into the operative view, obscuring vision (Fig. 7.12). Even if vision can be restored using an angled scope, the left lobe is usually still in the way of the operative port, preventing direct surgical access to the portal structures. The easiest and most direct way of regaining exposure is to use torque on the liver to rotate the left lobe out of the way. The proper torque is gained by elevating the fundus of the gallbladder upward and medially. This will usually produce a slight rotation of the liver on its axis and cause the left lobe to fall out of the way. If this is not successful, placing an additional 5 mm trocar in the left upper quadrant will allow the surgeon to retract the left lobe of the liver out of the way (Fig. 7.13).

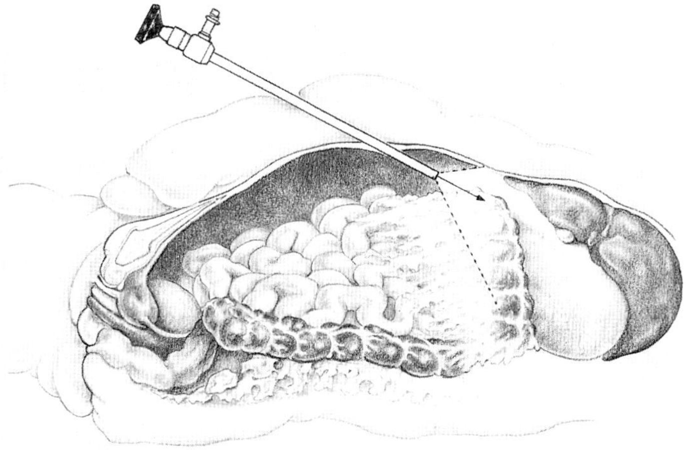

Figure 7.9. Thickened omentum or transverse colon can obscure the line of site if using a 0 degree telescope.

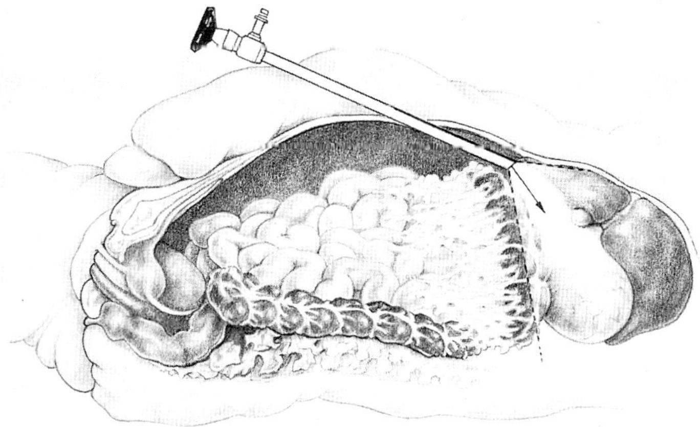

Figure 7.10. An angled scope allows the surgeon to get above the obscuring tissue and still visualize the portal area.

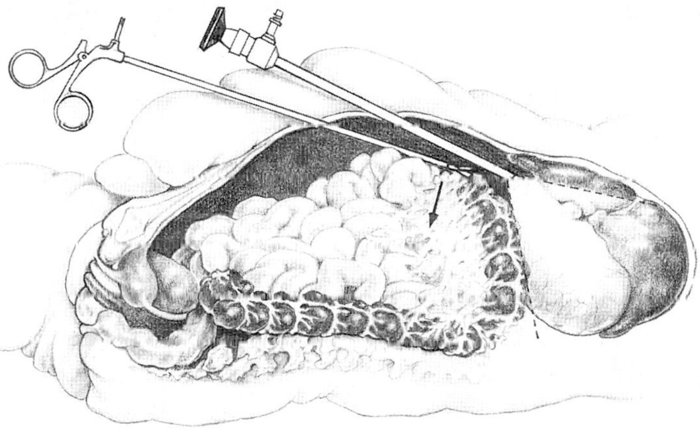

Figure 7.11. A fifth trocar can be placed to allow an additional instrument to be used to retract downward on the obscuring tissues.

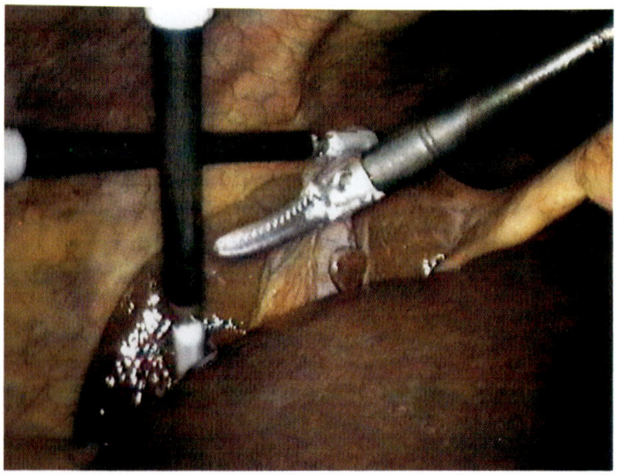

Figure 7.12. A floppy, enlarged left lobe of the liver can obscure the operative field.

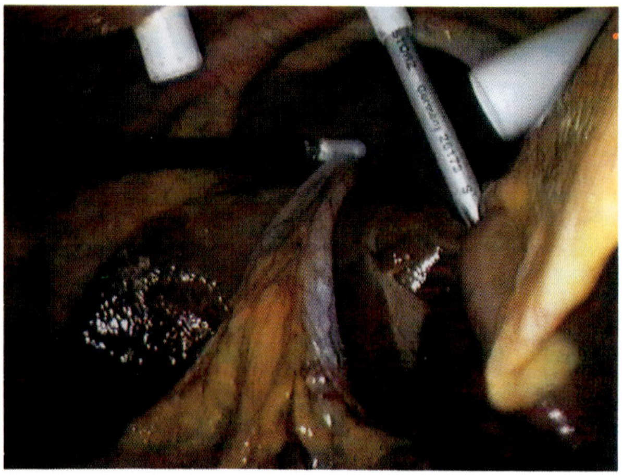

Figure 7.13. Same patient as in Figure 7.12. A fifth trocar has been placed to allow an additional instrument to be used to elevate the enlarged left lobe of the liver.

The Acute Gallbladder

The acute gallbladder possesses several challenges that make the performance of a laparoscopic cholecystectomy extremely difficult. The first is dealing with the thickened phlegmon that must be peeled off the acutely inflamed gallbladder. This is handled similarly to the thickened omentum in the obese patient. With the acute gallbladder, it is often necessary not only to use the angled scope but also to insert an additional 5-mm port for retraction.

Another problem is dealing with the tense, distended gallbladder that normally cannot be grasped with the standard laparoscopic graspers. As soon as the fundus of the gallbladder is exposed, the gallbladder should be decompressed. Although a needle is one method used to decompress the gallbladder, the acute gallbladder is often filled with thick, viscous bile that is hard to aspirate with a needle. To facilitate decompression, the midclavicular trocar can be inserted directly through the fundus under direct vision (Fig. 7.14). With the trocar inside the lumen of the gallbladder, a 5-mm suction-irrigator can be inserted and used not only to decompress the gallbladder but also to irrigate it clear so that any tears in the gallbladder will not result in the spill of contaminated bile as the organ is being removed. After the gallbladder is decompressed, the puncture hole is closed with a loop ligature. Even with the gallbladder decompressed, the standard laparoscopic graspers will have a difficult time holding on to the thickened gallbladder.

To facilitate elevation of the gallbladder, a 5-mm claw grasper can be inserted and utilized to grasp and elevate the gallbladder (Fig. 7.15). Although the gallbladder has been decompressed, care should still be used to avoid tearing it. The claw grasper is a very traumatic instrument and will most likely cause some tearing of the gallbladder. To minimize tearing, the surgeon should avoid repositioning the claw grasper and

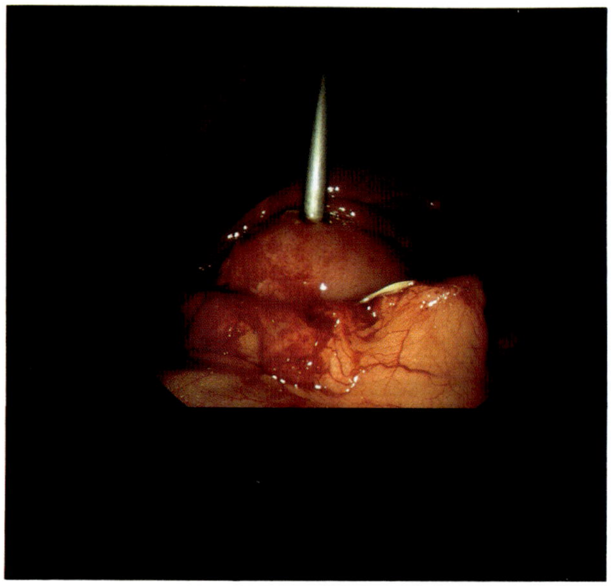

Figure 7.14. Decompression of an inflamed gallbladder using the midclavicular 5-mm trocar.

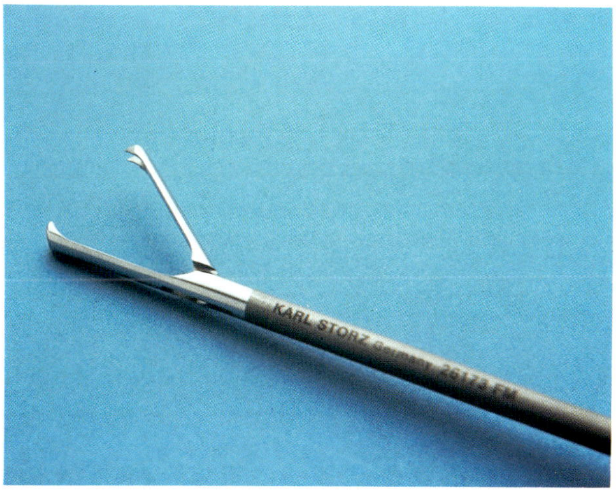

Figure 7.15. A 5-mm claw grasper allows positive grasping of even the most difficult gallbladder.

should make sure that a good healthy bite of tissue is achieved with its initial placement. With a good grasp on the gallbladder, exposure should be achieved in virtually every case.

The final problem with the acute gallbladder that challenges the laparoscopic surgeon is that of the constant oozing of blood from the dissection of inflamed tissue. This can obscure the plane of dissection quickly, making laparoscopic dissection impossible. To overcome this problem, the use of continuous irrigation will help wash away the blood, keeping the operative plane clear. By having proper lift on the gallbladder, the excess fluid will collect in the "gutter," and with occasional aspiration of this fluid, the surgeon can maintain a clean field. To prevent the blood from clotting and becoming difficult to aspirate, 5000 units of heparin should be added to each liter of irrigation fluid. This will keep the bloody pool fluid for easy aspiration. Once the cystic artery is ligated and the gallbladder is removed from the liver bed, all bleeding ceases. Any residual ooze should prompt the surgeon to place a drain.

IDENTIFICATION OF THE ANATOMY

Identification of the biliary anatomy is one of the most basic yet most important factors in performing a safe cholecystectomy. The majority of bile duct injuries are a direct result of misidentification of the biliary anatomy.[3,4] For this reason, the surgeon needs to be absolutely positive of his or her identification of the cystic duct before proceeding to ligate and divide that structure. Proper identification of the anatomy in a difficult case can be forbidding, but the surgeon has several options available to perform the task. Anatomic identification is not only the safest but also the most cost-effective means of verifying the anatomy. To achieve this goal, the surgeon must identify either the cystic duct common bile duct junction or the infundibulum of the gallbladder. The latter is used during a fundus first dissection practiced in open cholecystectomy. Because of the need to maintain the fundal attachments of the gallbladder to aid retraction of the liver during laparoscopic cholecystectomy, a classic fundus-first dissection is difficult with a laparoscopic approach. The same results can be achieved if the surgeon completely dissects out the neck and proximal body of the gallbladder. By clearly demonstrating the "funneling down" of the gallbladder to form the cystic duct, the surgeon has identified the infundibulum of the gallbladder and can be assured of the identification of the cystic duct. This dissection needs to be circumferential to ensure that the common bile duct has not been tented up into the operative field, with the common hepatic duct lying posterior (Fig. 7.16). With the infundibulum identified, the surgeon can safely proceed to cholangiography, or proceed to ligation of the duct if there are no indications for cholangiography.

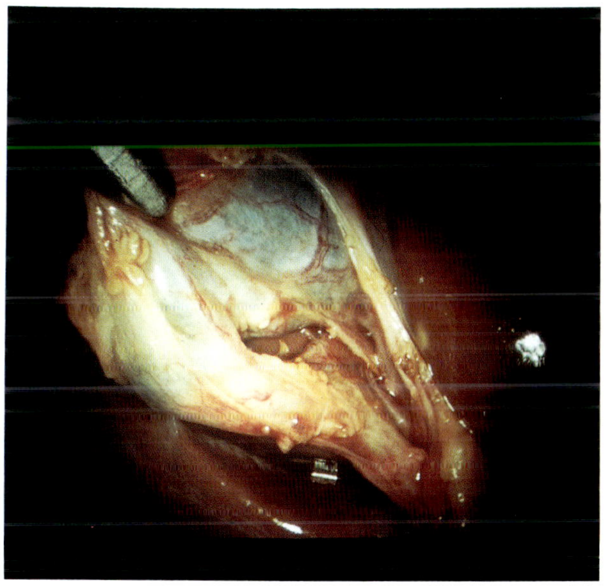

Figure 7.16. Complete dissection of the infundibulum and neck of the gallbladder must be achieved.

Routine cholangiography is of benefit and is covered elsewhere.

If the infundibulum cannot be clearly delineated due to inflammation or anatomy, the dissection is continued down the cystic duct, attempting to identify the cystic duct–common bile duct junction. To achieve this identification, the surgeon must be able to visualize the common hepatic duct, the cystic duct, and the common bile duct. Care must be taken to limit the dissection of the common bile duct or common hepatic duct to minimize possible ischemic injury to these structures, yet expose enough of the anatomy to assure positive identification (Fig. 7.17).

If the anatomy cannot be unequivocally identified by demonstrating the above-mentioned anatomic landmarks, the surgeon is obligated to perform a cholangiogram to verify the anatomy prior to ligating or dividing a ductal structure. If inflammation has totally obscured the anatomy, the patient is best served by either tube cholecystostomy or conversion to open cholecystectomy. There have been reports on partial cholecystectomies in which the anterior portion of the gallbladder is removed, leaving the posterior wall, but enough experience with this technique is not available to recommend it as an alternative in these difficult cases.

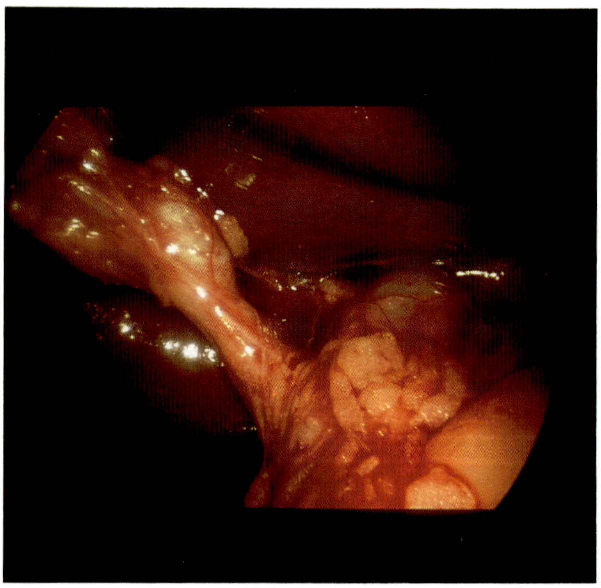

Figure 7.17. Enough dissection of the cystic duct and common bile duct must be achieved to allow absolute identification of the cystic duct.

DISSECTION AND HEMOSTASIS

Maintaining and ensuring adequate hemostasis is a basic principle of surgery. During open surgery, this principle requires a surgeon to proceed in an orderly fashion in exposing the anatomic area, ligating vessels as he or she continues and controlling active bleeding as it develops. With laparoscopic surgery the same principles hold true. The difference is that the surgeon is much less capable of controlling the bleeding. The concept of ligating vessels appropriately during dissection is easy enough to follow, and in fact is necessary because a clean operative field is of special importance during laparoscopic surgery. The difficulty occurs when bleeding starts after the tissue is divided. With laparoscopic surgery, the surgeon cannot simply apply pressure with a lap sponge or digital pressure. Suturing techniques are difficult, and even when they are mastered, they cannot be done quickly enough to control brisk bleeding. The only solution is to convert to an open procedure early enough to perform it in a controlled, orderly fashion before significant blood loss has taken place. This takes mature judgment on the part of the surgeon.

Dissection Techniques to Maintain Hemostasis

The key to hemostasis is to prevent any potential source of bleeding before it occurs. In laparoscopic cholecystectomy, the areas that create situations that prompt conversion to open cholecystectomy (excluding trocar injuries) include those in which a branch of the cystic artery is missed and cut across, bleeding from the liver bed occurs, or bleeding in the triangle of Calot develops. The last is avoided by staying lateral to the triangle of Calot until the cystic duct is clearly identified. Once the cystic duct is identified, the dissection is maintained right on the duct until a sufficient length of cystic duct has been dissected to verify the identification of the duct. Identification of the cystic artery is not attempted until after the cystic duct has been divided. This allows the surgeon to stay lateral of the triangle of Calot, avoiding the "depths" of the triangle. This approach will significantly minimize bleeding in the triangle of Calot. If a small amount of bleeding occurs during dissection, application of slight pressure with a

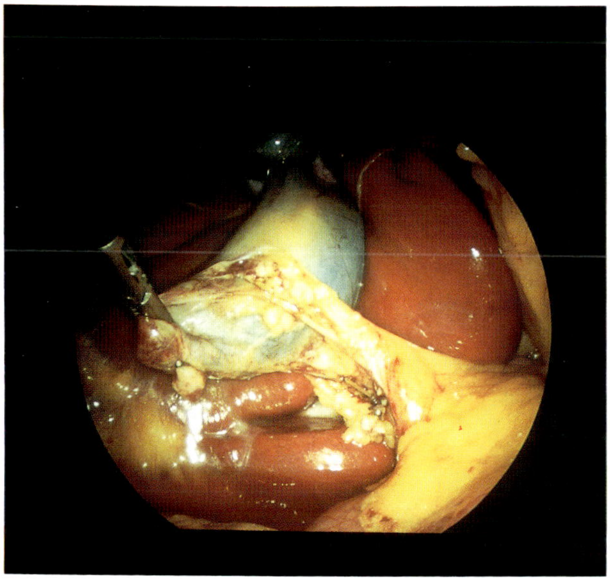

Figure 7.18. Exposure of the cystic artery is greatly enhanced by first dividing the cystic duct and retracting the neck laterally.

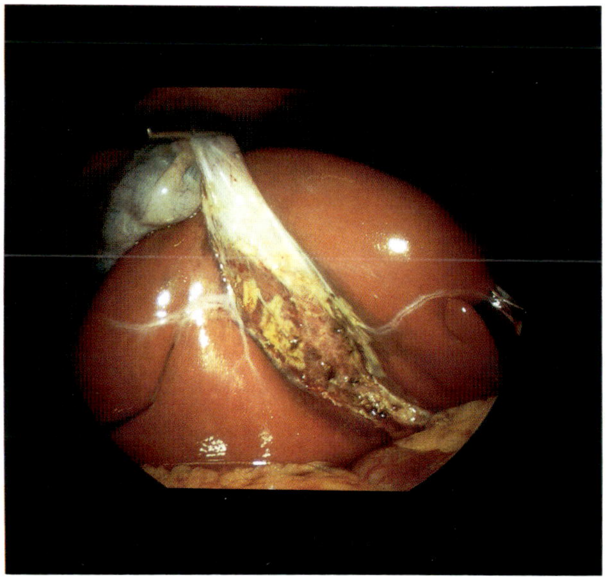

Figure 7.19. Before dividing the last attachments of the gallbladder, the liver bed should be carefully inspected.

grasper for several minutes will most often achieve hemostasis. Once the cystic duct has been identified and divided, the neck of the gallbladder can be elevated and retracted laterally to allow identification of the cystic artery high on the gallbladder, once again staying out of the depths of the triangle of Calot (Fig. 7.18).

A second bleed occurs when a posterior branch of the cystic artery is cut across while the surgeon is attempting to remove the gallbladder from the liver bed. The first step in avoiding this source of bleeding is to recognize the possibility of cutting this posterior branch and look for it prospectively. Blunt dissection at the neck of the gallbladder will most often allow recognition of this anatomic variant before the structure is divided without ligation. The surgeon should avoid cauterized division of tissues until the dissection has reached the liver bed.

The last major source of bleeding is within the liver bed. This usually occurs when the dissection enters the substance of the liver because the surgeon does not stay within the proper plane of dissection. The key to staying within the proper plane of dissection is to work on the lateral and medial serosal attachments of the gallbladder, working back and forth by flipping the gallbladder medially and laterally as the dissection continues. The dissection of the actual bed will follow automatically.

COMPLETING THE PROCEDURE

Before removing the last remaining attachments to the liver, the gallbladder should be used to elevate the liver to expose the porta hepatis and liver bed to check for hemostasis (Fig. 7.19). If there is a question about whether to drain or not to drain, the surgeon should place a drain and remove it in 12–24 hr if there is no significant drainage. If the gallbladder is perforated during its removal from the liver bed, the hole should be immediately closed to prevent further spillage and any spilled stones retrieved. The defect in the gallbladder is best closed using a loop ligature. Spilled bile should be aspirated and irrigated clear. With a gallbladder that has been violated or one that is acutely inflamed, the surgeon should place the specimen in a retrieval bag prior to removal (Fig. 7.20). After removing the gallbladder from the abdomen, the fascial defect at the umbilicus *must* be closed to prevent the complication of trocar site herniation.

By using careful technique and adhering to the basic principles of surgery, safe laparoscopic cholecystectomy can be achieved. The surgeon must not hesitate to convert to an open cholecystectomy if there is any doubt about maintaining exposure, gaining adequate hemostasis, or identifying the anatomy.

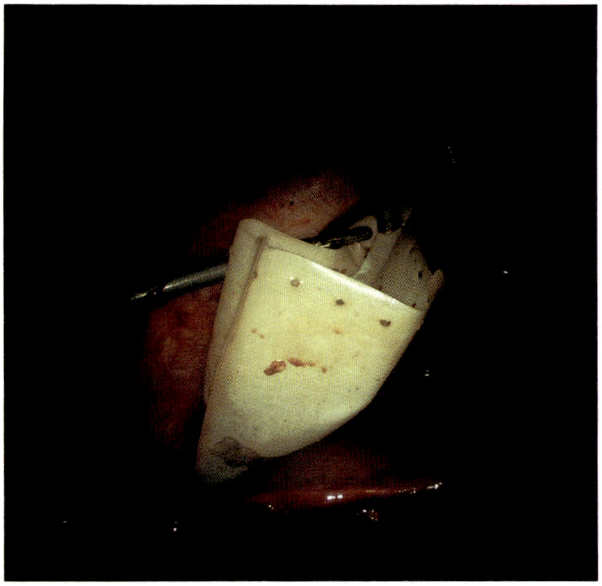

Figure 7.20. An inflamed or violated gallbladder should be placed in a specimen bag prior to removal from the abdominal cavity.

REFERENCES

1. Langenbuch C: Ein Fall von Exterpation der Gallenblase wegen chronischer Cholelithiasis: Heilung. *Klin Wochenschr* 19:725–727, 1882.
2. Deziel DJ, Millikan KW, Economou SG, et al: Complications of laparoscopic cholecystectomy: A national survey of 4,292 hospitals and an analysis of 77,604 cases. *Am J Surg* 165:9–14, 1993.
3. Davidof AM, Pappas TN, Murray EA, et al: Mechanisms of major biliary injury during laparoscopic cholecystectomy. *Ann Surg* 215:196–202, 1992.
4. Deziel DJ: Complications of cholecystectomy: Incidence, clinical manifestation and diagnosis. *Surg Clin North Am* 74(4):809–823, 1994.

chapter eight

Operative Cholangiography Techniques

Leonard S. Schultz

INTRODUCTION

The techniques for introduction of iodinated or radioactive contrast material into the biliary tract have varied over the years, but their purpose has remained the same: identification of anatomy to best plan for treatment options. Earlier methods, such as intravenous cholangiography and oral cholecystography, have largely been replaced by scans using radioactive material and ultrasonography of the biliary tree for preoperative investigations, while cholecystocholangiography and cystic duct cholangiography have become reliable intraoperative methods for verification of anatomic landmarks. Despite their usefulness, even these may soon be supplanted by laparoscopic ultrasonography. However, no matter what method the surgeon employs, the purpose remains the same: identification of anatomy to help prevent complications and/or incomplete surgery.

In an effort to determine the value of such intraoperative studies, certain questions have been asked to help define the controversy over whether intraoperative cholangiography should be done routinely or only in specific instances during laparoscopic cholecystectomy. Such questions include the following:

1. Does routine cholangiography decrease the incidence of complications?
2. Is its use cost effective?
3. Should cystic duct cholangiography or cholecystcholangiography be used as the standard approach, and, if so, at what time during the procedure?

Attempts to answer such questions have produced a surfeit of journal articles but very few, if any, definitive answers. These many opinions can be summarized as follows:

1. Variations in cystic duct anatomy are not uncommon,[1] and include low union of parallel or spiral cystic ducts[2] and congenitally short ducts of less than 2 cm,[3] which, if unrecognized at the time of laparoscopic cholecystectomy, can lead to a host of serious ductal injuries.[4]
2. Routine cholangiography is controversial,[5–8] but selective use is indicated in patients with abnormal liver function tests who have not been subjected to preoperative endoscopic retrograde cholangiopancreatography (ERCP) or in those with ill-defined operative anatomy.
3. Although not yet proven in a randomized prospective study, most experienced laparoscopic biliary surgeons practice and/or advocate routine use of intraoperative cholangiography to identify anatomy, possibly to prevent ductal injuries, and to gain facility with cystic duct manipulation in preparation for common bile duct stone extraction via the transcystic approach.[9–18] These opinions are based on the fact that classic indications for intraoperative cholangiography are lacking when the laparoscopic approach is used.
4. The ease of real-time C-arm fluoroscopic cholangiography keeps costs to a minimum, in contrast to the cost of a single common bile duct injury and/or lawsuit settlement that such a study could

have prevented, not to mention the cost in human terms.[15]

5. Although most authors use cystic duct cannulation, some favor injection of dilute dye directly into the gallbladder to prevent possible inadvertent placement of the catheter into the common bile duct,[19] to obtain an accurate anatomic representation of the biliary tree prior to surgical dissection, and to evaluate defects within the common bile duct.[20,21]

For any or all of these reasons, any student or practitioner of laparoscopic biliary surgery should learn the techniques of intraoperative cholangiography. Who would not want a precise, informative cholangiogram in cases of acute cholecystitis where ductal structures are subject to distortion by inflammatory edema?

CYSTIC DUCT CHOLANGIOGRAPHY

The standard method of intraoperative visualization of the biliary tract is with the use of dilute iodinated dye infused through a catheter placed within the cystic duct and secured with some method of fixation.[22–25] The examination is most commonly done with a single infusion of 7–10 cc of contrast into the biliary tract, with an x-ray taken just as the infusion is concluded. More recently, C-arm fluoroscopy has greatly facilitated this process and has added a measure of cost effectiveness.

To prevent false-positive results secondary to the infusion of air bubbles along with the dye, a segment of IV tubing is joined to a stopcock (through which air can be vented), and is then attached to the dye-filled syringe. The tubing then connects to the hub of the cystic duct catheter or to a metal needle with a flared tip. Prior to dye infusion, a second syringe partially filled with saline is also attached to the stopcock and used to aspirate any unwanted bile and/or air from the biliary tree, catheter, and dye syringe.

Although relatively easy to perform with the abdomen open, this test can be most challenging when done under fluoroscopic conditions. Here we must consider the best placement of the access device, the materials needed to guide the catheter into the cystic duct, and how to keep the catheter secured.

As with the open method, the cystic duct must first be dissected out. This means that unrealized aberrant anatomy could cause the common bile duct to be mistaken for the cystic duct, with resultant choledochotomy. Such an event would require immediate repair utilizing T-tube drainage, although primary closure could be done without decompression in a normal common bile duct. Assuming no untoward events, the infundibulum is retracted cephalad with a 5-mm grasper, and a hemostatic clip occludes the gallbladder–cystic duct junction. If available, a modified 5-mm metal sleeve with a Touhy-Borst pneumo-valve is used as an access device and is placed in the mid-right subcostal position. Just as easily, a 5-mm trocar may be substituted (Fig. 8.1). Once placed, a microscissors is used to cut a hole in the cystic duct (Fig. 8.2); a catheter is threaded through the valve and, if semirigid, can be passed into the cystic duct (Fig. 8.3). If the catheter is not stiff, then a dilator sheath is advanced

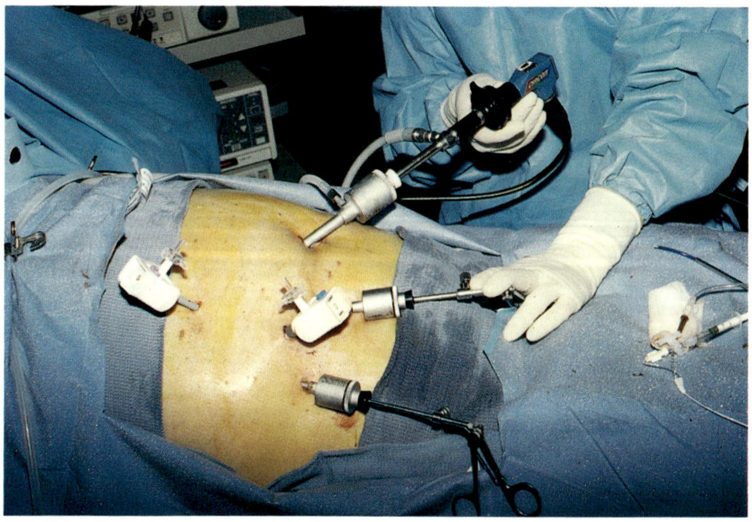

Figure 8.1. The 5-mm trocar for cystic duct catheter access is positioned midway below the right costal margin. It is cephalad to the other closely grouped trocars.

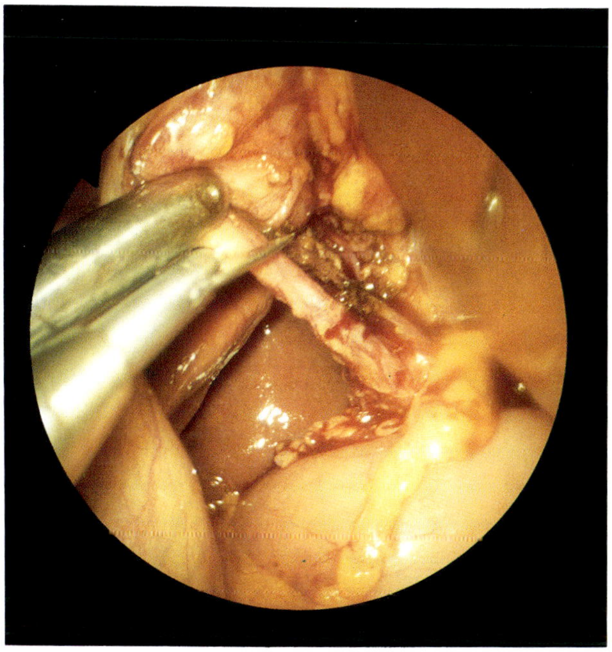

Figure 8.2. Just to the right of the grasper, a microscissors is about to cut an opening in the cystic duct.

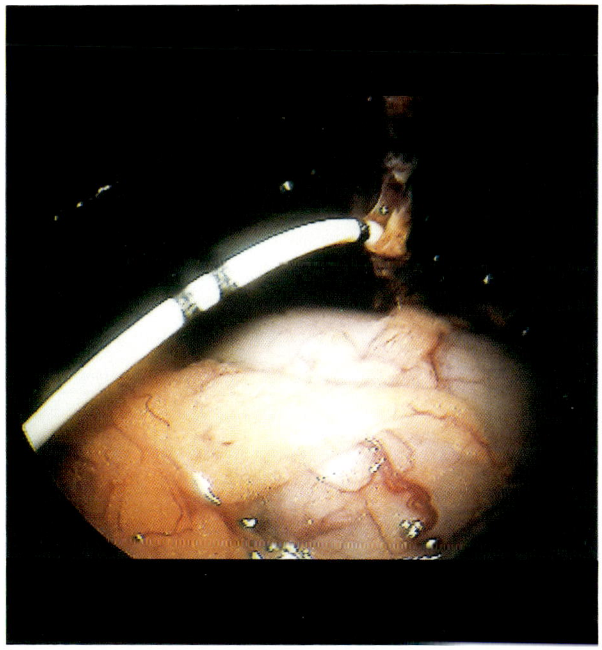

Figure 8.3. A firm catheter has been threaded into the cystic duct but has not yet been secured.

down the metal sleeve and into the cystic duct. This is tricky to use at first, and vigorous dilation of the duct is to be avoided. In fact, only gentle pressure on the hollow dilator should be used as it is passed into the duct. Once in place, the catheter can be passed down the lumen of the sheath, advanced into the cystic duct (Fig. 8.4), and secured with either balloon inflation or a hemostatic clip. If cystic ductal dilation is needed for common bile duct exploration, it can be achieved better with guidewire and balloon technique than with plastic dilators (see Chapter 9). If a clip is used to secure the catheter, I suggest using a single-clip applier to do this so that you can feel the pressure exerted on the clip thereby preventing occlusive compression of the catheter (Fig. 8.5). If a softer catheter is used, an attached balloon near the tip will usually suffice as an anchor following its inflation. Unfortunately, if the catheter tip ends up in the common bile duct, balloon inflation can cause obstruction and confuse the interpretation of the cholangiogram.[26]

Once the catheter is in place, the same dye and equipment described previously can be used to complete the cholangiogram (Fig. 8.6). At this point, a few additional comments are needed. Remember to withdraw the laparoscope into the umbilical trocar without removing it. This maneuver will prevent the tip of the

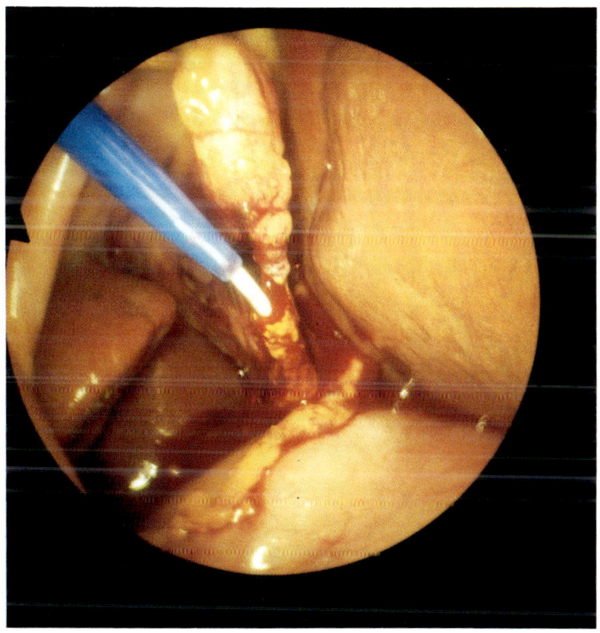

Figure 8.4. The blue dilator sheath, which has already widened the cystic duct, has been pulled back to serve as a guide for the cholangiogram catheter.

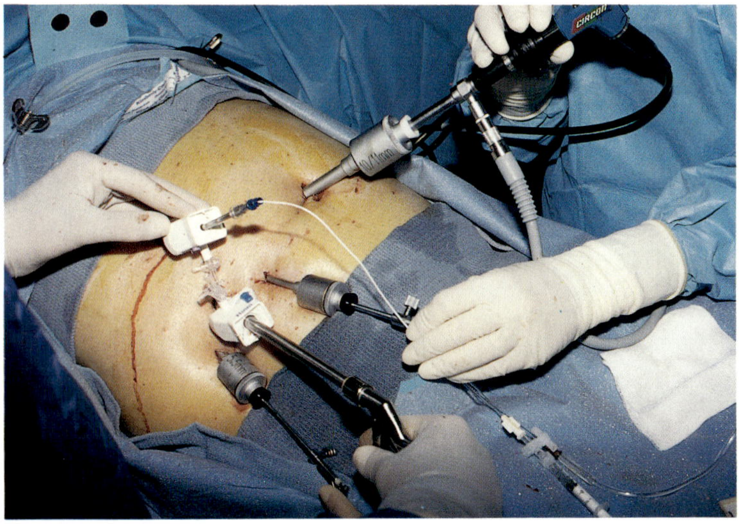

Figure 8.5. The surgeon's right hand is using a single clip applier (second instrument from the left) to secure a clip on the cholangiogram catheter.

laparoscope from obscuring the distal common bile duct on the x-ray. Further, the patient should be in a neutral position on the table to ensure proper dispersal of dye following its infusion. Once the x-ray is taken, leave everything in place until the x-ray is returned to the operating room for interpretation. Only after you verify that the cholangiogram is successful should the catheter be removed. Once it is withdrawn, two or three clips are placed on the cystic duct between the small incision and the cystic duct–common bile duct junction. Leave the metallic access sleeve in place until the end of the case to prevent loss of pneumoperitoneum.

CHOLECYSTOCHOLANGIOGRAPHY

As an alternative to this classic method, one may wish to use cholecystocholangiography since it provides immediate visualization of the cystic duct's entry into the ductal system, as well as an assessment of any common bile duct abnormalities (Fig. 8.7).

Prior to installation of dye, the fundus of the gallbladder is grasped with a bitoothed biopsy forceps which has been placed through a 5-mm trocar positioned approximately 3–5 cm caudad of the right costal margin along the anterior axillary line (Fig. 8.8). The

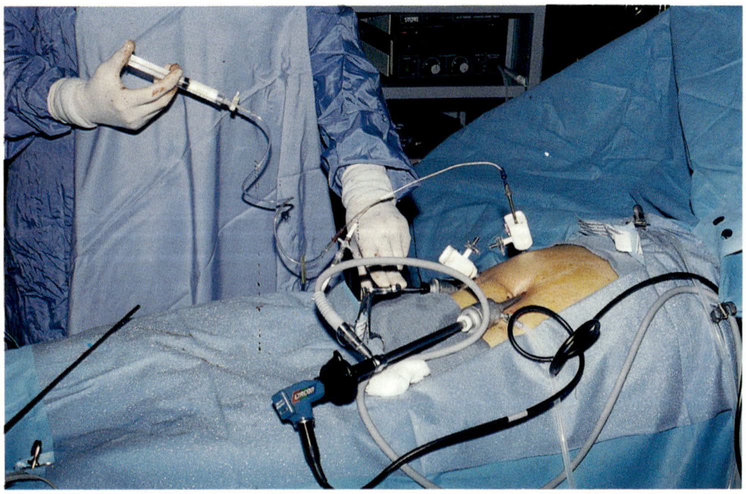

Figure 8.6. The laparoscope has been pulled back into the trocar sleeve, the surgeon stands behind a draped lead shield protector, and the dye is being infused for a cystic duct cholangiogram.

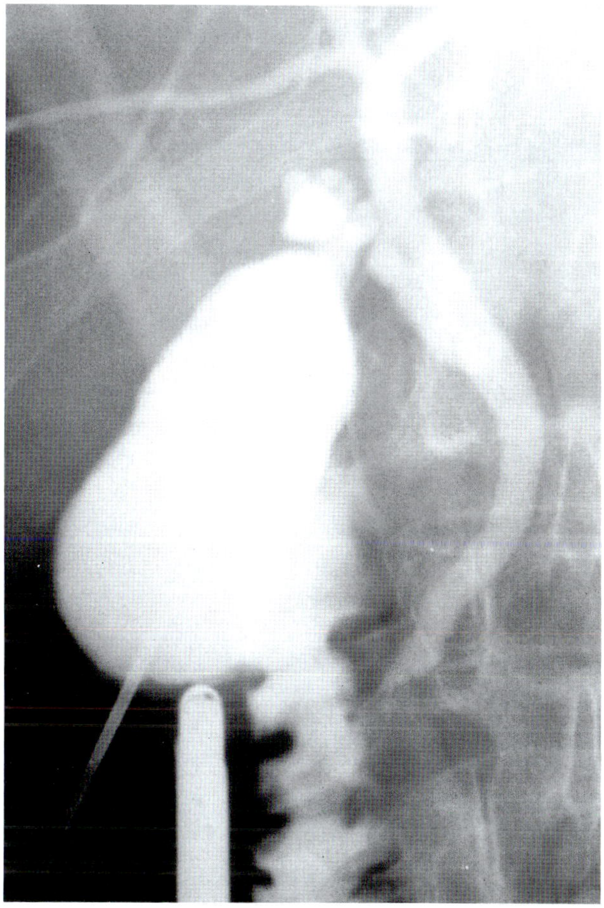

Figure 8.7. The cholecystocholangiogram demonstrates all pertinent parts of the biliary tree before dissection is begun.

forceps exerts upward traction toward the anterior abdominal wall. Viewed externally, there is an angle between the rib margin and the longitudinal axis of the instrument, and it is through this angle that a 17-gauge pericardial needle is passed percutaneously into the gallbladder (Fig. 8.9). Its internal course is monitored laparoscopically, with the needle positioned so that its tip enters the gallbladder about 1–2 cm from the end of the fundus and is directed toward the infundibulum (Fig. 8.10a,b). In most cases, one can see the needle within the gallbladder by pushing the hub of the needle cephalad, resulting in caudad displacement of the tip against the anterior wall of the gallbladder.

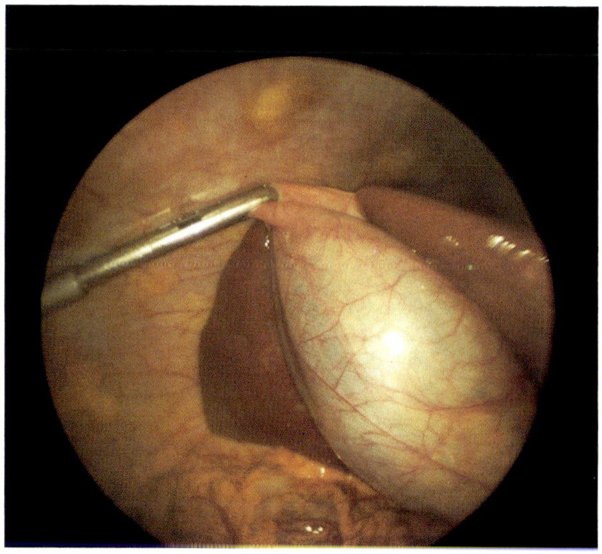

Figure 8.8. Upward retraction makes the bile-filled gallbladder, an easy target for the needle.

Once the needle is in place, bile is aspirated directly through it into a syringe and discarded (Fig. 8.11). One end of the IV tubing is connected to the hub of the needle and the other end is connected to the stopcock. Two other syringes, one partially filled with saline for flushing and/or aspiration and one containing 60 cc of dilute dye, also connect to the stopcock. After the line is cleared of air, the x-ray unit is positioned over the abdomen, the table assessed for neutral position, the x-ray plate checked for proper location, a protective shield placed in front of the surgeon, and infusion of 50 cc of dye is begun (Fig. 8.12). During this time, the patient's respirations are halted and the x-ray is taken immediately upon conclusion of dye infusion (Fig. 8.13). X-ray plates are exchanged while a very slow, continuous infusion is maintained. When the second dose of the remaining 10 cc of dye is delivered, the second of two x-rays is taken.

While waiting for the return of the processed x-rays, any residual dye is aspirated (Fig. 8.14). Once the x-rays are viewed and considered satisfactory, the needle is removed from the decompressed gallbladder and the operation proceeds.

The x-rays are viewed for evaluation of the cystic duct anatomy and for any common bile duct defects and/or drainage abnormalities. This road map can prove invaluable in alerting the surgeon to unusual configurations, such as entry of the cystic duct into the

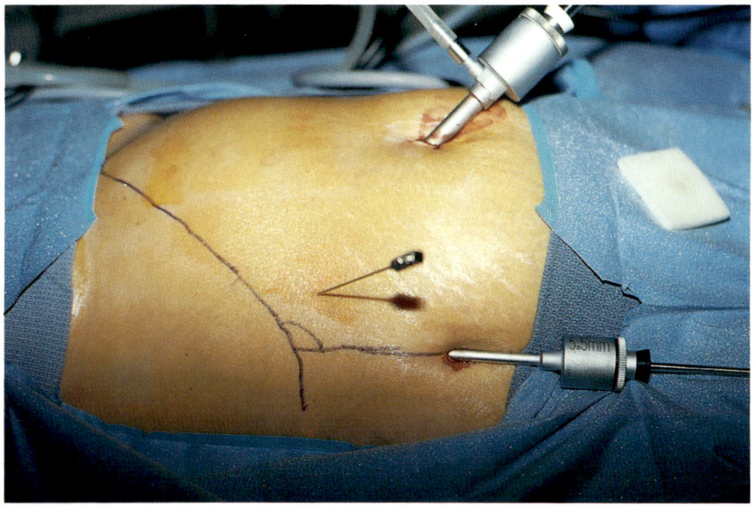

Figure 8.9. Pen marks define the angle made by the right rib margin and the direction of the grasper.

a

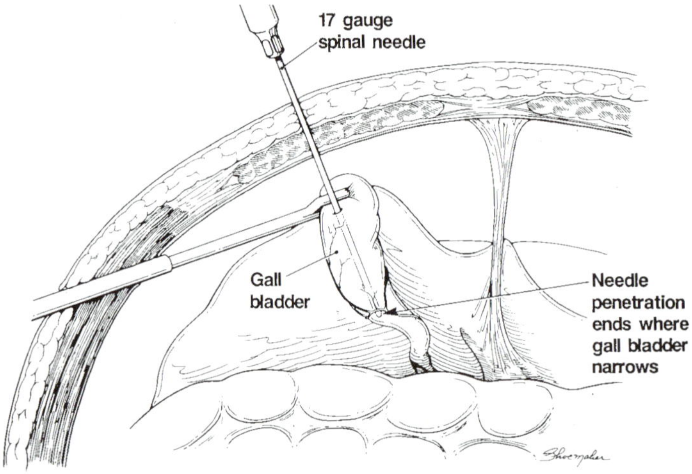

b

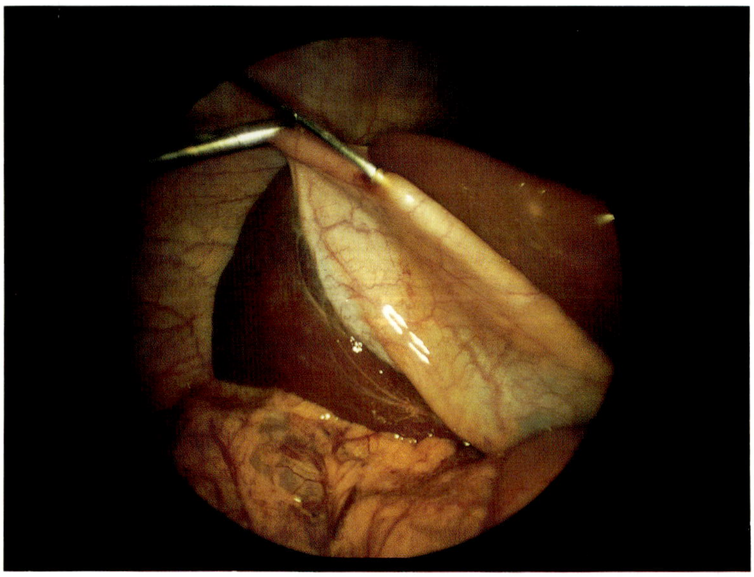

Figure 8.10. (a) The laparoscope's view of the needle as it passes into the gallbladder. (b) Internal view of the gallbladder during aspiration of bile.

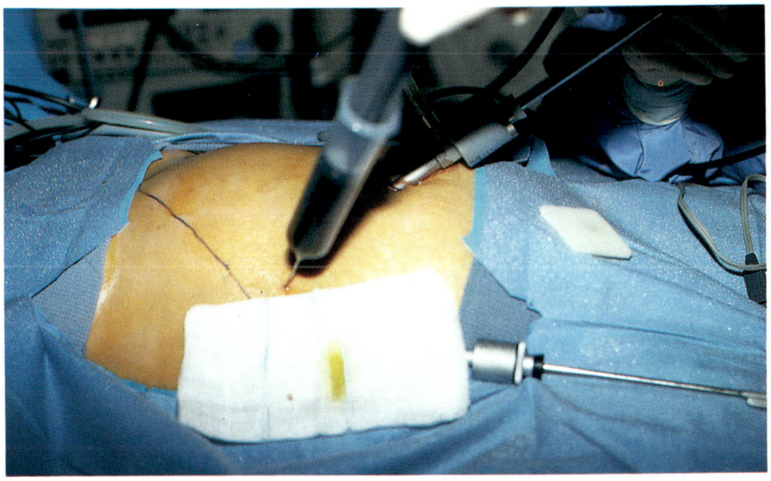

Figure 8.11. The volume of aspirated bile is about 30 cc. If it is too viscid to aspirate, it is left and the same amount of dye is infused, regardless of the amount of bile left within the gallbladder.

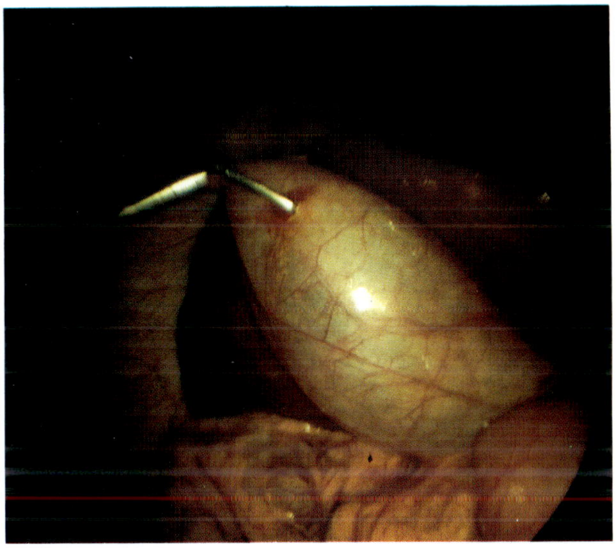

Figure 8.12. Despite the tenseness of the dye-filled gallbladder, little escapes from the site of needle puncture.

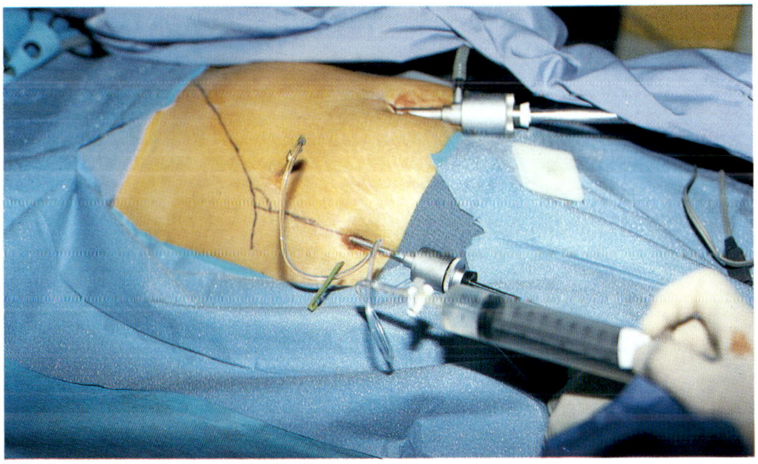

Figure 8.13. A total of 50 cc of dye has been infused and the first x-ray has been taken. While the film is changed, the remaining 10 cc of dye is continuously and slowly infused until the second x-ray has been taken. By that time, all the dye should have been instilled.

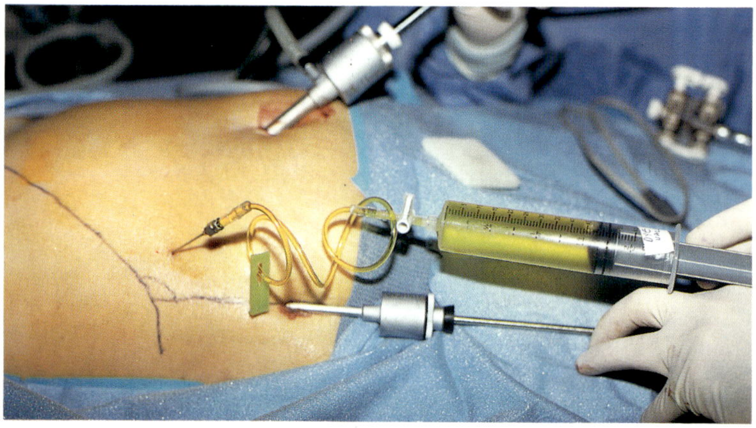

Figure 8.14. Bile and excess dye are aspirated to provide as much decompression of the gallbladder as possible to facilitate later extraction from the abdomen.

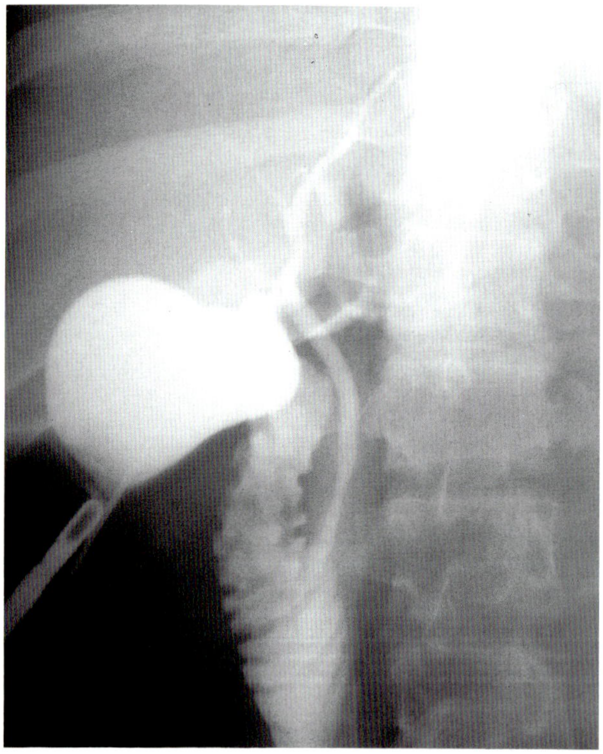

Figure 8.15. What surgeon would not want to be forewarned that, in this case, the cystic duct enters the right hepatic duct adjacent to the bifurcation?

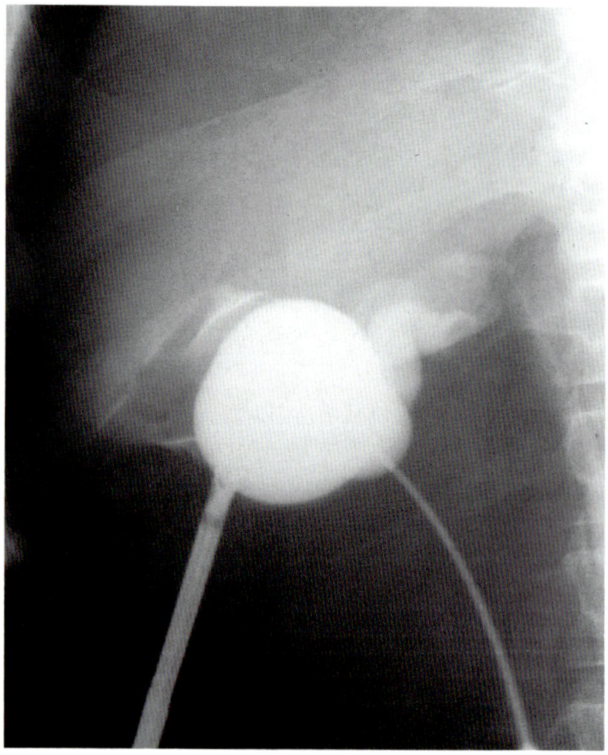

Figure 8.16. Visualization of acute inflammation or tense distention of the gallbladder and/or white bile indicates the futility of cholecystocholangiography.

right hepatic duct (Fig. 8.15) or low entrance into the common bile duct. One must be reminded that obtaining a complete cholangiogram is not enough; to gain benefit from the process, one must look carefully at the x-ray and use it to help guide further dissection. Our initial results with this method were reported in 1991.[27] Despite hundreds of x-rays done since that time, the data remain consistent. Visualization of the biliary ductal system is satisfactory in 90% of cases, technical failures exist in 1%, and x rays are not indicated in 8–9% because of acute cholecystitis secondary to cystic duct obstruction, where passage of dye into the common bile duct is not expected (Fig. 8.16). It is in these latter cases that one must rely on cystic duct cholangiograms for verification of anatomy. Leakage of minimal amounts of bile and dye at the site of entry of the needle has not precipitated infections, since our incidence of postoperative subhepatic infection is 0.5%.

SUMMARY

Despite the enthusiasm for and success of cholecystocholangiography in our hands, there have been and will continue to be cases where cystic duct cholangiography is advantageous. Both methods must be part of the laparoscopist's skills, especially those that pursue common bile duct exploration.

The question of the cost effectiveness of such procedures should not be dealt with in a global statistical manner. Instead, one must be willing to support whatever information is needed for a surgeon to consistently provide successful laparoscopic cholecystectomy. If intraoperative cholangiography furthers that goal, then it should be an integral part of that operation.

REFERENCES

1. Benson EA, Page RE: A practical reappraisal of the anatomy of the extrahepatic bile ducts and arteries. *Br J Surg* 63:853–860, 1976.
2. Adams DB: The importance of extrahepatic biliary anatomy in preventing complications at laparoscopic cholecystectomy. *Surg Clin North Am* 73:861–871, 1993.
3. Hollinshead W: *Anatomy for Surgeons. Vol 2: The Thorax, Abdomen and Pelvis.* New York, Harper & Row, 1971, pp 314–374.
4. Hunter JG: Avoidance of bile duct injury during laparoscopic cholecystectomy. *Am J Surg* 162:71–76, 1991.
5. Mansberger JA, Davis JB, Scarborough MD, et al: Selective intraoperative cholangiography. A case for its use on an anatomic basis. *Am Surg* 54:31–33, 1988.
6. Hauer-Jensen M, Karesen R, Nygaard K, et al: Prospective randomized study of routine intraoperative cholangiography during open cholecystectomy. Long-term follow-up and multivariate analysis of predictors of choledocholithiasis. *Surgery* 113:318–323, 1993.
7. Clair DG, Carr-Locke DL, Becker JM, et al: Routine cholangiography is not warranted during laparoscopic cholecystectomy. *Arch Surg* 128:551–555, 1993.
8. Clair DG, Brooks DC: Laparoscopic cholangiography. The case for a selective approach. *Surg Clin North Am* 74:961–966, 1994.
9. Phillips EA, Berci G, Carroll B, et al: The importance of intraoperative cholangiography during laparoscopic cholecystectomy. *Am Surg* 56:792–795, 1990.
10. Berci G, Sackier JM, Paz-Partlow M. Routine or selected intraoperative cholangiography during laparoscopic cholecystectomy? *Am J Surg* 161: 355–360, 1991.
11. Sackier JM, Berci G, Phillips E, et al: The role of cholangiography in laparoscopic cholecystectomy. *Arch Surg* 126:1021–1026, 1991.
12. Flowers JL, Zucker KA, Graham SM, et al: Laparoscopic cholecystectomy. Results and indications. *Ann Surg* 215: 209–215, 1991.
13. Lillemoe KD, Yeo CJ, Talamini MA, et al: Selective cholangiography. Current role in laparoscopic cholecystectomy. *Ann Surg* 215:669–676, 1992.
14. Berci G: Biliary ductal anatomy and anomalies. The role of intraoperative cholangiography during laparoscopic cholecystectomy. *Surg Clin North Am* 72:1069–1075, 1992.
15. Phillips EA: Routine versus selective intraoperative cholangiography. *Am J Surg* 165:505–507, 1993.
16. Nathanson LK, Pietrabissa A: Intraoperative cholangiography during laparoscopic cholecystectomy. *Surg Endosc* 8:302–305, 1994.
17. Traverso LW, Hauptmann EM, Lynge DC: Routine intraoperative cholangiography and its contribution to the selective cholangiographer. *Am J Surg* 167:464–468, 1994.
18. Soper NJ, Brunt LM: The case for routine operative cholangiography during laparoscopic cholecystectomy. *Surg Clin North Am* 74:953–959, 1994.
19. Hawasli A: Does routine cystic duct cholangiography during laparoscopic cholecystectomy prevent CBD injury? *Surg Laparosc Endosc* 3:290–295, 1993.
20. Kuster GGR, Gilroy S, Graefen M: Intraoperative chol-

angiography for laparoscopic cholecystectomy. *Surg Gynecol Obstet* 176:411–417, 1993.

21. Glattli A, Metzger A, Klaiber C, et al: Cholecystocholangiography during vs. cystic duct cholangiography during laparoscopic cholecystectomy. *Surg Endosc* 8:299–301, 1994.
22. Fligelstone LJ, Foster ME, Hay D: Laparoscopic operative cholangiography: A simple, successful cost-effective method. *Ann R Coll Surg Eng* 74: 252–253, 1992.
23. Hunter DC, Jeffs N, Mee WM: Easy technique for cholangiography during laparoscopic cholecystectomy. *Br J Surg* 80:211, 1993.
24. Evans RJ, Shirley AJ: A technique for cholangiography during laparoscopic cholecystectomy. *Aust NZ J Surg* 63:975–976, 1993.
25. Willekes CL, Edoga JK, Castronuovo JJ, et al: Technical elements of successful laparoscopic cholangiography as defined by radiologic criteria. *Arch Surg* 130:398–400, 1995.
26. Velanovick V, Kaufmann C: Two pitfalls of laparoscopic balloon cholangiography. Recognition and correction. *Am Surg* 5:290–292, 1993.
27. Pietrafitta JJ, Schultz LS, Graber JN, et al: Cholecystocholangiography during laparoscopic cholecystectomy: Cholecystocholangiography or cystic duct cholangiography. *J Laparoendosc Surg* 1:197– 206, 1991.

chapter nine

Managing Common Duct Stones, Common Duct Injuries, and Bile Leaks

Jeffrey M. Marks
Jeffrey Ponsky

INTRODUCTION

Since the first laparoscopic cholecystectomy (LC) by Mouret in 1987, LC has rapidly become the standard treatment for symptomatic cholecystolithiasis. With the rapid adoption of the highly popular minimally invasive surgery so attractive to patients, providers, and physicians, there soon developed the realization that the problems and complications attending these methods were not entirely the same as those commonly seen with traditional open procedures. At the forefront of these new complications was the increased incidence of biliary tract problems including leaks, strictures, and extrahepatic bile duct injuries. Recent advances in laparoscopic techniques have also provided new alternatives in the management of choledocholithiasis. It is appropriate to examine the emerging techniques for management of choledocholithiasis, as well as the approach to the prevention, diagnosis, and therapy of problems attendant on laparoscopic biliary tract surgery.

Management of Common Bile Duct Stones

With the rapid development of multiple therapeutic options, the optimal management of common bile duct stones (CBDS) is a heavily debated topic among endoscopic surgeons. The incidence of choledocholithiasis is directly related to age, and occult CBDS are found in 4–10% of all cases.[1–3] Preoperative suspicion of choledocholithiasis is based on clinical, laboratory, and radiologic examinations. Numerous studies have attempted to identify the preoperative markers most predictive of CBDS. A history of gallstone pancreatitis, jaundice, or a dilated common bile duct (CBD) on ultrasound may all suggest CBDS. The only findings shown to correlate with the actual occurrence of CBDS, however, are a persistent elevated conjugated bilirubin level and choledocholithiasis identified on ultrasound exam.[4–6] Pancreatitis, transaminase elevation, and CBD enlargement are less predictive of CBDS.[4–7]

When the preoperative suspicion of CBDS exists, the choice of therapy will depend on the experience and resources available to the endoscopic surgeon. Previously, open common bile duct exploration (OCBDE) was the only tool utilized by the biliary surgeon. Now choledocholithiasis can be managed in a minimally invasive fashion, with excellent results, utilizing both endoscopic and laparoscopic techniques.

Endoscopic Management of CBDS

For the diagnosis and treatment of suspected CBDS, endoscopic retrograde cholangiopancreatography (ERCP) can be performed preoperatively or postoperatively and has been utilized most recently intraoperatively in conjunction with laparoscopic techniques. The endoscopic management of CBDS almost always requires electrosurgical division of the ampullary sphincter. The overall risks and complications associated with ERCP and sphincterotomy are well documented (Table 9.1). The overall success rate of ERCP

Table 9.1. Complications of Endoscopic Sphincterotomy

Pancreatitis	1.0–3.0%
Bleeding	1.0–4.0%
Cholangitis	1.0–2.0%
Perforation	0.4–1.0%
Stone impaction	<0.2%
Death	<1%

with the clearance of all CBDS is documented to be 85–90%.[4,8–16] The actual rate of successful CBD clearance is very much dependent on the skill of the endoscopist and the size of the stone.[8,17] Preoperative ERCP offers the advantage of assessment and potential clearance of the duct prior to LC, reducing operative time and difficulty during surgery. Also, if unsuccessful, the surgeon will have to rely on laparoscopic or open techniques to remove CBDS. Once identified, CBDS are removed utilizing balloons, baskets, or mechanical lithotripsy devices[18] (Figs. 9.1, 9.2). More difficult CBDS may require pulsed dye laser therapy or electrohydraulic lithotripsy (EHL). EHL utilizes high-pressure shock waves and can be safely delivered under cholangioscopic guidance[19] (Fig. 9.3). Pulse dye laser lithotripsy has also proven effective, fragmenting all stones in patients with CBDS in a series by Ponchon et al.[20] In addition, ultrasonic lithotripsy and extracorporeal shock wave lithotripsy have been used to achieve stone fragmentation with varying success.[21,22] In patients with CBDS lager than 3 cm, or in those who have multiple CBDS, endoscopic clearance may not be possible and surgical CBD exploration or choledochoenterostomy may be required. If a cholangiogram has been performed with unsuccessful decompression or clearance of the CBD, a biliary stent or nasobiliary tube is recommended to decrease the incidence of cholangitis. Biliary stenting can also be utilized permanently in patients with significant choledocholithiasis who are poor surgical candidates (Fig. 9.4). Stent changes are usually required every 3–6 months to prevent stent occlusion and resultant cholangitis.

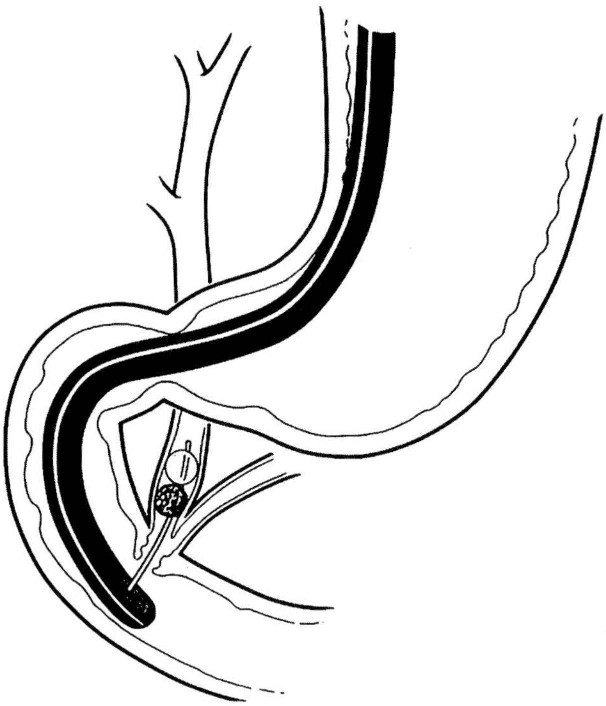

Figure 9.1. After endoscopic sphincterotomy, a biliary balloon is passed beyond the common bile duct stone, inflated, and then withdrawn to extract the stone. (From Ponsky JL: *Atlas of Surgical Endoscopy.* St Louis CV Mosby, Year Book Medical, 1992. Reprinted with permission.)

Intraoperative ERCP

The combination of laparoscopic and endoscopic tools has been attempted by several investigators. Previously, intraoperative ERCP had been utilized as a diagnostic tool in the management of patients with pancreatic trauma. Now antegrade and retrograde approaches to the papilla can be successfully performed at the time of laparoscopic cholecystectomy. Deslandres et al. reported four cases of choledocholithiasis managed with endoscopic sphincterotomy and laparoscopic cholecystectomy performed in one session.[23] A transcystic catheter is passed into the duodenum to identify the papilla for the endoscopist. A sphincterotomy is then performed in a retrograde fashion using a dyathermic needle knife sphincterotome. CBDS were removed successfully in all cases with an endoscopic Dormia stone retrieval basket. Cited advantages to this combined procedure include a single anesthetic, no need for T-tubes, and decreased total fluoroscopic exposure.[23] Another potential advantage of this approach is the ability to clear CBDS without cystic duct dilation or choledochotomy, which are commonly required for transcystic or laparoscopic CBD exploration. We have modified this approach by utilizing a wire-guided retrograde technique. A long (480-cm) wire is passed

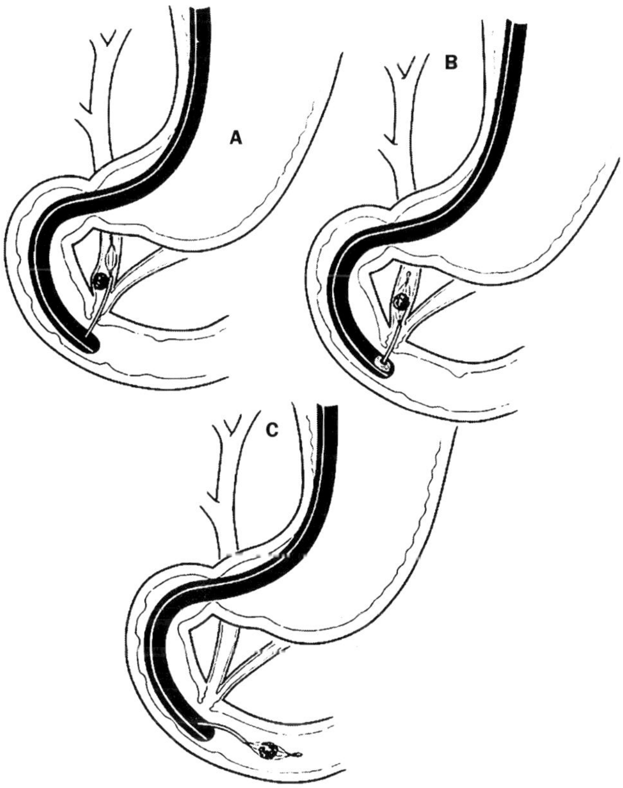

Figure 9.2. (a–c) A Dormia stone-retrieval basket is used to extract a CBDS following an endoscopic sphincterotomy. After removal, the stone is allowed to pass through the gastrointestinal tract. (From Ponsky JL: *Atlas of Surgical Endoscopy.* St Louis, CV Mosby, Year Book Medical, 1992. Reprinted with permission.)

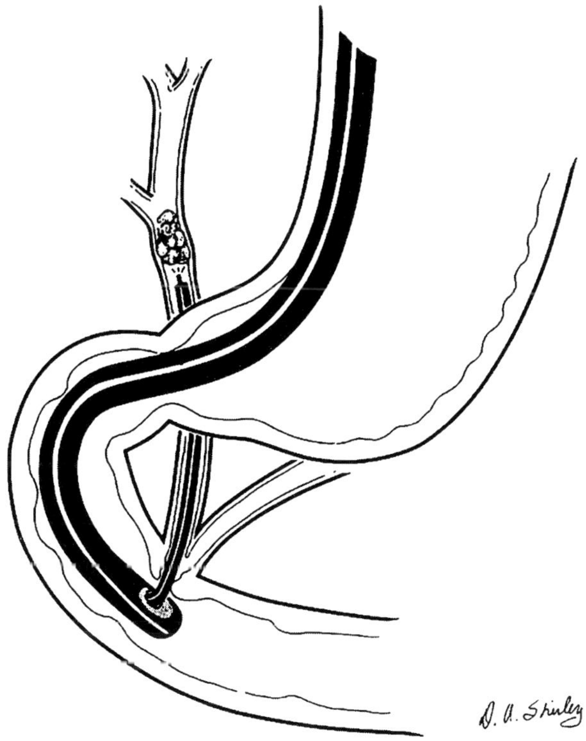

Figure 9.3. A small cholangioscope passed into the CBD allows safe delivery of EHL or pulse dye laser lithotripsy. (From Ponsky JL: *Atlas of Surgical Endoscopy.* St Louis, CV Mosby, Year Book Medical, 1992. Reprinted with permission.)

transcystically into the duodenum and, after the duodenoscope is positioned, the wire is grasped with an endoscopic snare. A double-channel sphincterotome is then passed over the wire to perform a sphincterotomy, and endoscopic biliary balloons are passed retrograde to complete the clearance of the CBD (Fig. 9.5).

An antegrade approach to the papilla, combining endoscopic and laparoscopic techniques, has also been described by DePaula et al.[24] At the time of laparoscopic cholecystectomy, a double-channel endoscopic sphincterotome is passed transcystically or via a choledochotomy. Under endoscopic guidance the sphincterotome is placed across the papilla and a sphincterotomy is performed[24] (Fig. 9.6). DePaula et al. were successful in all 22 cases attempted, with this maneuver adding a mean of 17 minutes to the overall surgical procedure. Two patients had elevated postoperative amylase levels without clinical pancreatitis, and one patient had a 6% drop in hematocrit but did not require transfusion. None of the patients had evidence of retained CBDS at follow-up periods ranging from 1 to 18 months. Intraoperative ERCP utilizing antegrade or retrograde approaches provides a safe, effective alternative in the management of CBDS.

Laparoscopic Management of CBDS

Many surgeons prefer to address CBDS at the time of LC rather than utilizing preoperative or postoperative ERCP. Intraoperative cholangiograms (IOC) are vital

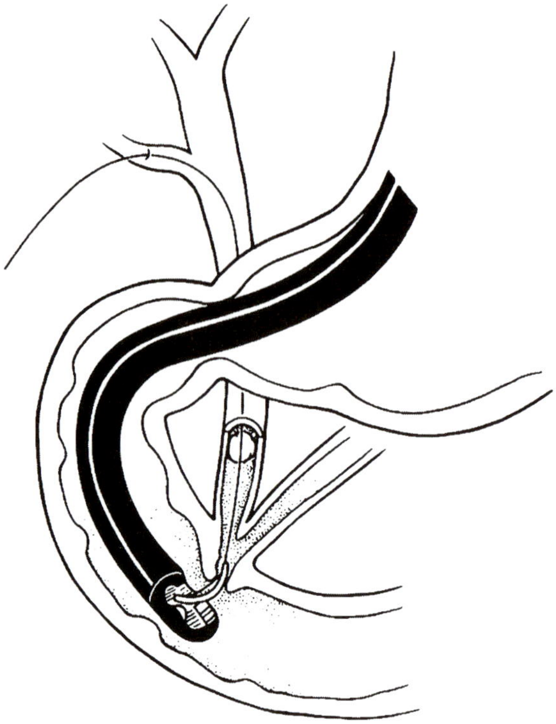

Figure 9.4. A combined laparoscopic and endoscopic technique for management of CBDS, utilizing a wire-guided retrograde technique.

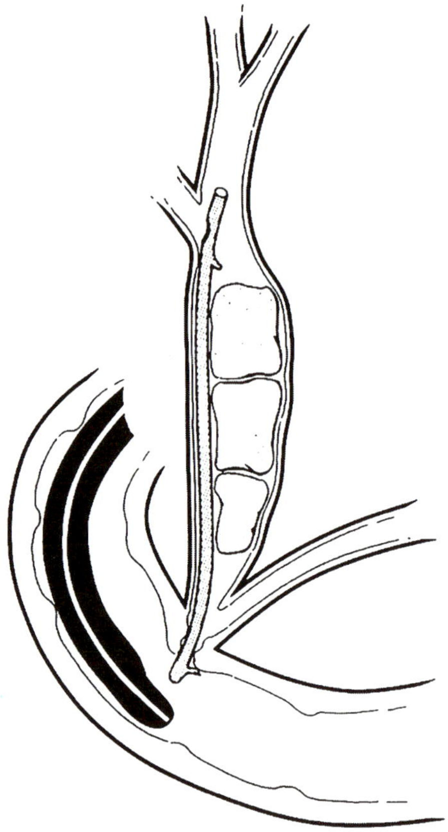

Figure 9.5. A straight biliary endoprosthesis passed alongside multiple CBDS allows temporary biliary decompression. (From Ponsky JL: *Atlas of Surgical Endoscopy*. St Louis, CV Mosby, Year Book Medical, 1992. Reprinted with permission.)

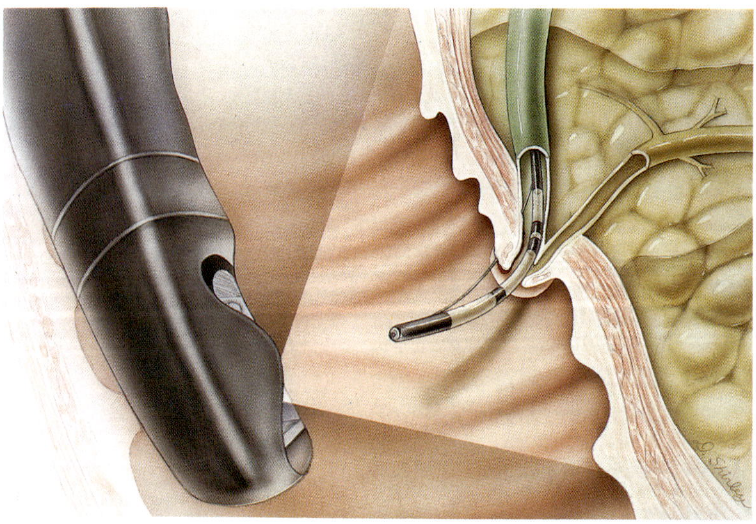

Figure 9.6. An antegrade sphincterotomy performed under endoscopic guidance at the time of laparoscopic cholecystectomy.

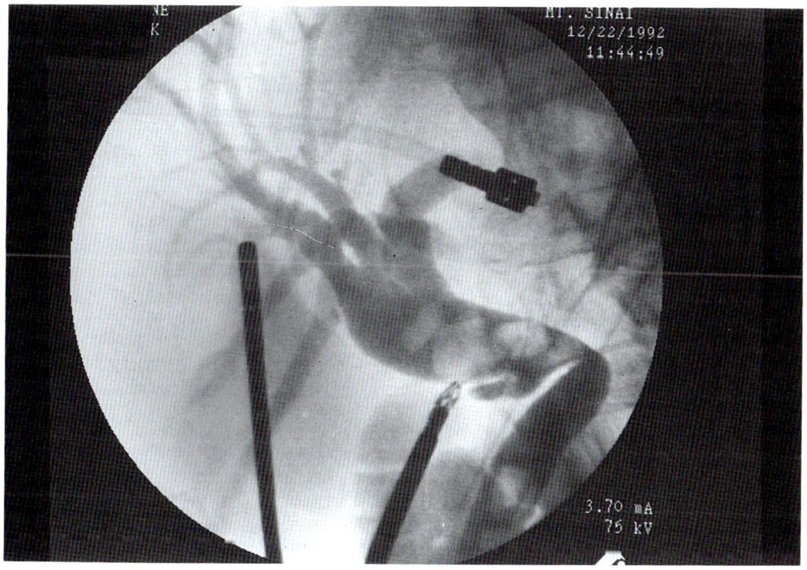

Figure 9.7. Multiple CBDS identified on an intraoperative cholangiogram.

not only to define anatomy but also to identify occult CBDS (Fig. 9.7). The availability of real-time fluoroscopy is of paramount importance in the laparoscopic management of CBDS. The size of the stones, the diameter of the CBD, and the skill of the surgeon are important factors in choosing the appropriate laparoscopic technique to clear the CBD. Small stones (less than 3 mm) will most likely pass spontaneously or can be flushed through the ampulla at the time of surgery. Sphincter of Oddi relaxation can be achieved to aid in clearance of the duct after a 1 mg IV dose of Glucagon. Ampullary dilation has also been attempted with balloons to allow for flushing of small CBDS (Fig. 9.8). When stones cannot be simply flushed through the ampulla, the surgeon must decide to either proceed to more advanced laparoscopic techniques, perform an OCBDE, or electively treat the patient endoscopically if the patient becomes symptomatic postoperatively. The skill of the surgeon, as well as the availability of an experienced endoscopist, will help guide this decision. In situations where an experienced endoscopist if not available, surgeons who do not possess the laparo-

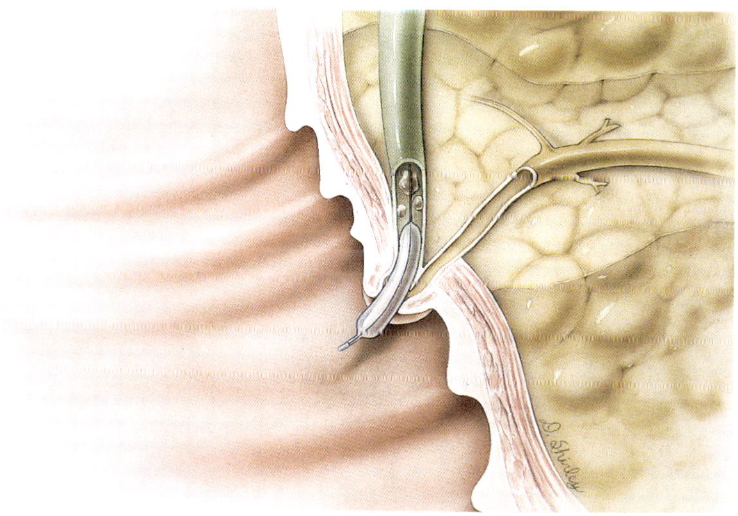

Figure 9.8. Ampullary dilation is performed with a biliary balloon passed transcystically under fluoroscopic guidance.

scopic skills and/or necessary instrumentation to perform transcystic common bile duct exploration (TCBDE) should proceed to OCBDE. It is never considered a complication to convert a laparoscopic case to an open surgery, and a good surgeon should know his or her own limitations.

For those surgeons who lack the laparoscopic skills, or who do not possess the necessary tools (i.e., flexible choledochoscopes, intraoperative fluoroscopy) but do have an experienced endoscopist available, we recommend leaving access to the biliary tree at the time of surgery if CBD stones are left behind. A catheter can be placed into the cystic duct, secured with endoscopic clips or pretied loops, and brought out of one of the trocar sites (Fig. 9.9). It is also appropriate to leave a closed suction drain adjacent to the catheter in the subhepatic region. At the time of ERCP postoperatively, a guidewire can be advanced through the catheter into the duodenum to help the endoscopist identify the papilla. Next, a double-channel papillatome is passed over this guidewire to perform a sphincterotomy and achieve endoscopic clearance of the CBD. The transcystic catheter is then managed like a T-tube and can be removed after 10–14 days.

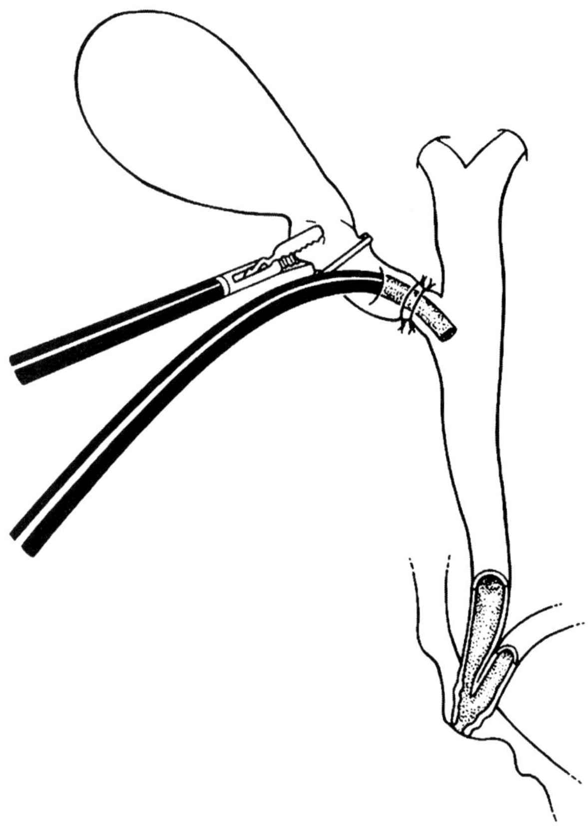

Figure 9.9. A catheter placed in the cystic duct and secured with pretied ligatures maintains access to the biliary tree to assist postoperative endoscopic management of CBDS.

Transcystic Common Bile Duct Exploration

After the identification of CBDS on intraoperative cholangiography, surgeons with advanced laparoscopic skills can proceed to a TCBDE. Excellent results have been reported using transcystic approaches to CBDS, with successful clearance in up to 90% of cases.[25,26] As described in the previous section, flushing of small stones should be attempted initially. Sphincter relaxation with intravenous Glucagon or balloon dilation of the ampulla have been described to aid in this procedure. These techniques, however, have been associated with postoperative pancreatitis. If they are unsuccessful, the surgeon must next evaluate the anatomic configuration of the biliary system and the size of the cystic duct. Fewer than one-third of patients will have the commonly described biliary anatomy with a lateral insertion of the cystic duct into the CBD (Fig. 9.10a–d). A long common septum or a distal insertion of the cystic duct will make transcystic exploration difficult. Even with caudad traction on the cystic duct to straighten the natural angulation at the cystic duct–common duct junction, access into the hepatic ducts can sometimes be impossible (Fig. 9.11). If the diameter of the cystic duct is less than 3 mm, cystic duct dilation with hydrostatic balloons or dilators passed over a wire is commonly required to allow passage of a choledochoscope or removal of snared CBDS. Care must be taken during this procedure to prevent avulsion or tearing of the cystic duct (Fig. 9.12). Also, injury to the CBD must be carefully avoided during dilation. Passage of ureteral dilators over a wire and under fluoroscopic visualization will decrease the chance of injury to the back wall of the CBD. The length of the cystic duct is also important. If the duct is long and tortuous, as seen on the IOC, entry into the duct closer to its insertion into the CBD can facilitate TCBDE. In patients with intrahepatic stones or biliary anatomy not amenable to TCBDE, laparoscopic choledochotomy, antegrade sphincterotomy, or postoperative endoscopy may be necessary.[25]

The first therapeutic maneuver of TCBDE utilizes Dormia stone retrieval baskets and balloons (Fig. 9.13). Some investigators perform this first procedure

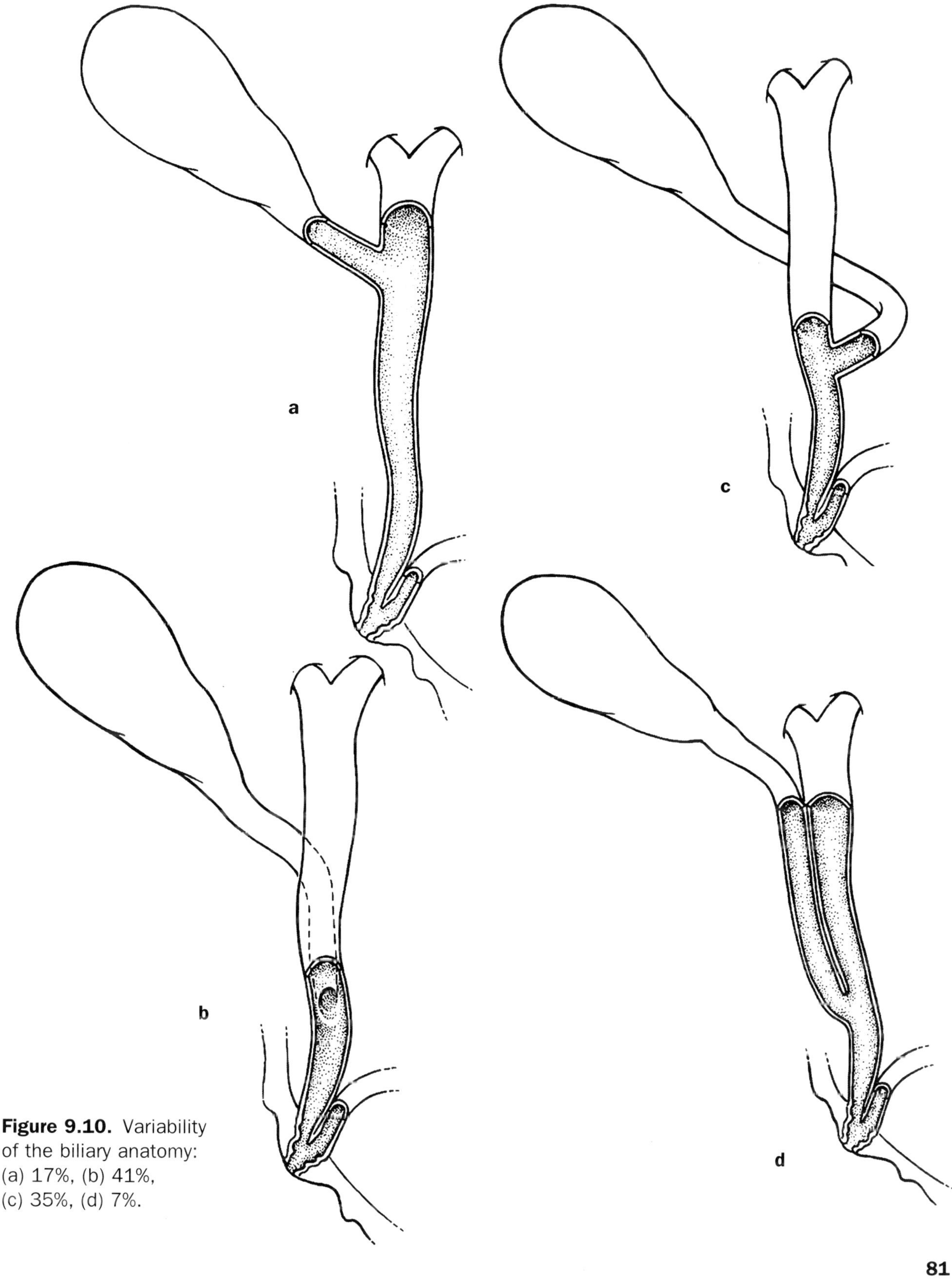

Figure 9.10. Variability of the biliary anatomy: (a) 17%, (b) 41%, (c) 35%, (d) 7%.

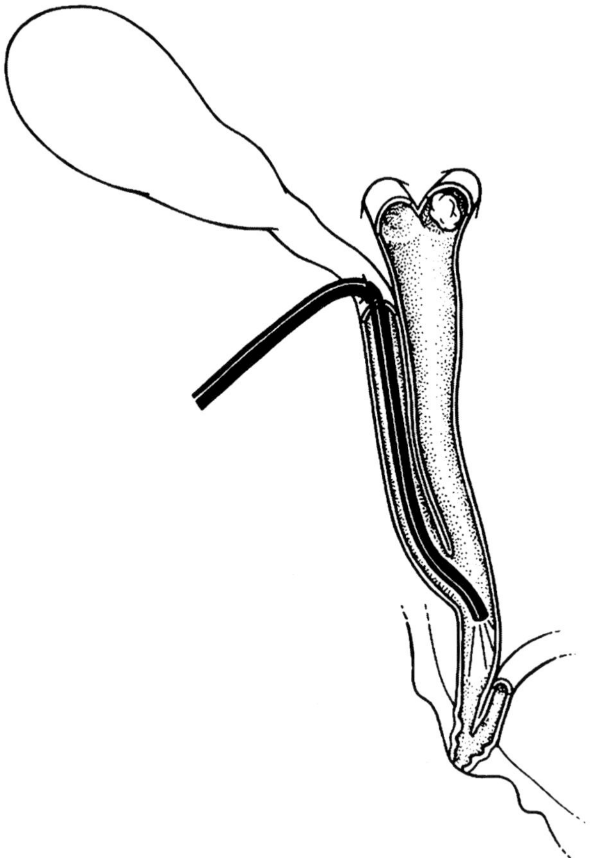

Figure 9.11. Transcystic removal of hepatic duct stones may be impossible in patients with distal insertion of the cystic duct or in those with a long common septum.

blindly. However, in our experience, fluoroscopic guidance increases the effectiveness of this procedure and shortens the operation. If the stones are not easily extracted, transcystic choledochoscopy should be considered. Flexible fiberoptic scopes with bidirectional maneuverability and a single working channel have been designed for this procedure. They are small (less than 3 mm) and can be attached to a camera system to allow for videoscopic viewing. Some video endoscopic programs allow both the laparoscopic and cholangioscopic images to be displayed on the same video screen. During TCBDE, access to the CBD is maintained with a guidewire or an introducer sheath placed into or near the cystic duct opening (Fig. 9.14). As in other cholangioscopic procedures, infusion of saline allows for optimal visualization. After identification of a CBDS, a Dormia basket or four-wire stone basket is used to snare the CBDS. The basket is passed beyond the stone initially and then opened prior to its withdrawal. This will capture the stone and allow it to be crushed or removed. Cholangioscopic and fluoroscopic visualization is helpful in guiding successful stone entrapment. Obviously, multiple stones will require repeat passes of the scope and basket. For CBDS that are very large or impacted, alternative procedures such as EHL or pulse dye laser therapy may be required.[27,28] Endoscopic guidance during these procedures will decrease the chance of injury to the walls of the CBD. Perforations can occur if energy from these sources is incorrectly aimed. Following TCBDE, it is recommended to ligate the cystic duct with either a pretied loop ligature or an intracorporeal suture. Manipulation of stones in the distal duct, as well as transphincteric maneuvers to eliminate CBDS, can lead to edema at the ampulla, resulting in increased biliary pressure. Clip dislodgement and resultant cystic duct leaks can be related to this process, as well as to direct tissue edema at the site of cystic duct dilation.

Laparoscopic Common Bile Duct Exploration Via Choledochotomy

Several factors will occasionally preclude TCBDE and require proceeding to a laparoscopic common bile duct exploration (LCBDE) via a choledochotomy. In a series by Carroll and Phillips, 10% of patients with CBDS managed laparoscopically required LCBDE.[25] DePaula et al. also reported excellent success with TCBDE. Conversion to LCBDE was necessary in only 6.2% of their patients.[29] The major indications for LCBDE include large stones in a dilated CBD, intrahepatic or common hepatic duct stones not accessible by transcystic approaches, or a cystic duct not amenable anatomically to transcystic maneuvers. LCBDE is most safely and easily performed in patients with CBD in excess of 15 mm. As in open surgery, the laparoscopic approach to CBD stones, LCBDE, utilizes a choledochotomy, followed by choledochoscopy with extraction of stones, and finally placement of a T-tube.

The choledochotomy initially should be small, and excessive cleaning of the bile duct should be avoided to prevent vascular compromise and resultant strictures. The incision can be placed transversely or longitudinally and is best performed at the level of the cystic duct–common bile duct junction. A fifth laparoscopic port in the left upper quadrant is usually required for

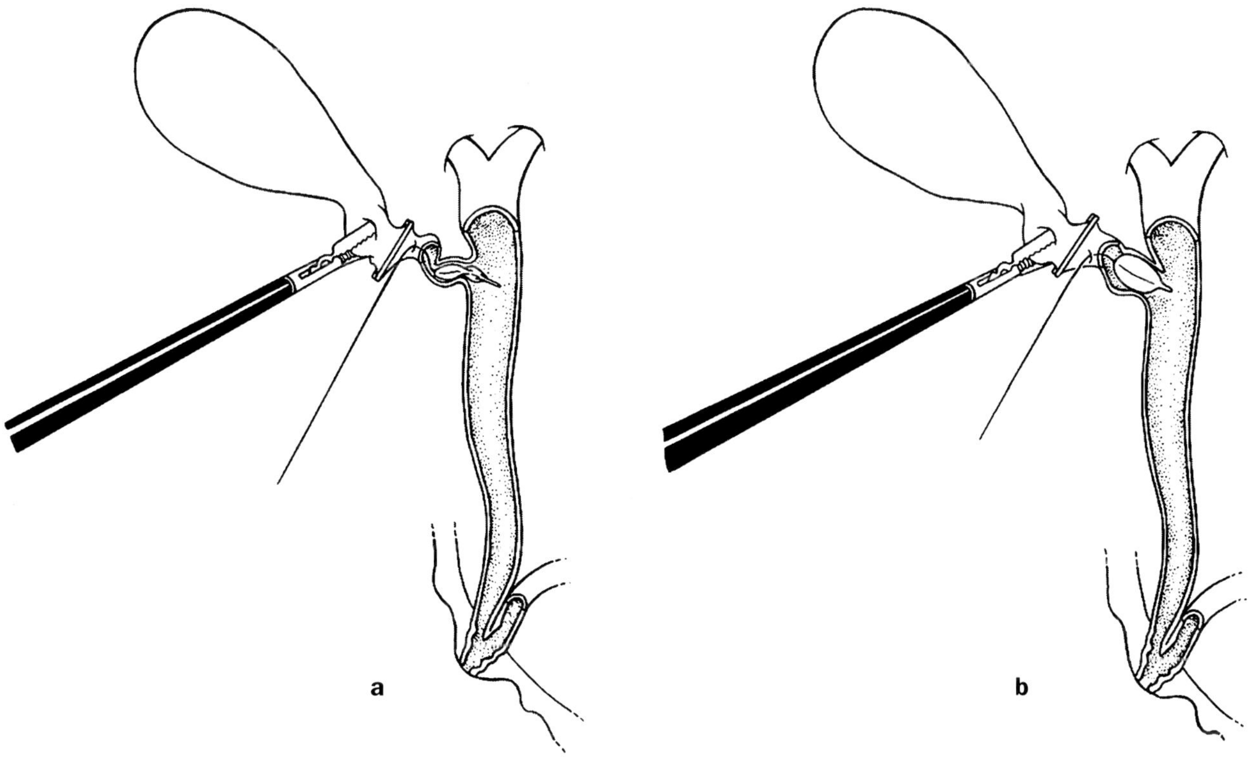

Figure 9.12. (a,b) Balloon dilation of the cystic duct is often necessary prior to transcystic CBD exploration.

exposure, as well as for suturing of the CBD. The gallbladder is not removed, and the cystic duct is not transsected until completion of CBD exploration. Retraction of the gallbladder fundus and infundibulum is done via the right inferior and epigastric ports, respectively. The right subcostal port will be used for delivery of balloons, baskets, and the choledochoscope. The additional left upper quadrant port, which will be used for suturing the CBD after completion of the CBD exploration, can also be utilized for exposing the choledochotomy.

As in routine open CBD exploration, biliary balloons, baskets and red rubber catheters to flush the CBDs are first utilized. These maneuvers are performed both proximally and distally until all stones are believed to be cleared. Next, a standard flexible choledochoscope is passed into the CBD while instilling saline irrigation to improve visualization.

Passage into the duodenum as well as the hepatic radicals can easily be performed. If no further CBD stones are identified, a T-tube of appropriate size is then placed completely into the peritoneal cavity. The arms of the T-tube are inserted and the choledochotomy is closed, using intracorporeal or extracorporeal suturing techniques (Figs. 9.15 and 9.16). To prevent accidental removal of the T-tube, it is not brought through the abdominal wall until the gallbladder has been completely dissected and removed. A T-tube cholangiogram should be performed in the operating room to rule out retained CBDS or leaks at the choledochotomy. A short, straight course for the T-tube will best enable the radiologist to perform percutaneous extraction of any retained CBD stones. A closed suction drain is also placed near the choledochotomy. The T-tube and drain are managed as in open CBD exploration. Strictures, leaks, pancreatitis, and retained CBDS are the major complications of laparoscopic CBD exploration via choledochotomy. As in any laparoscopic technique, conversion to open CBD exploration should not be considered a complication of the procedure. Open CBD exploration should be performed when the biliary anatomy is unclear when excessive

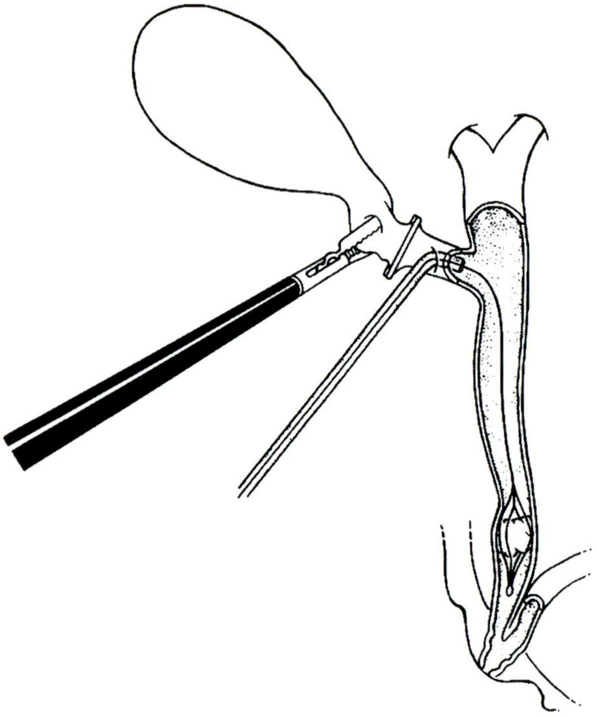

Figure 9.13. Transcystic CBD exploration using a Dormia stone-retrieval basket is aided by placing an introducer sheath into the cystic duct to maintain access to the biliary tree.

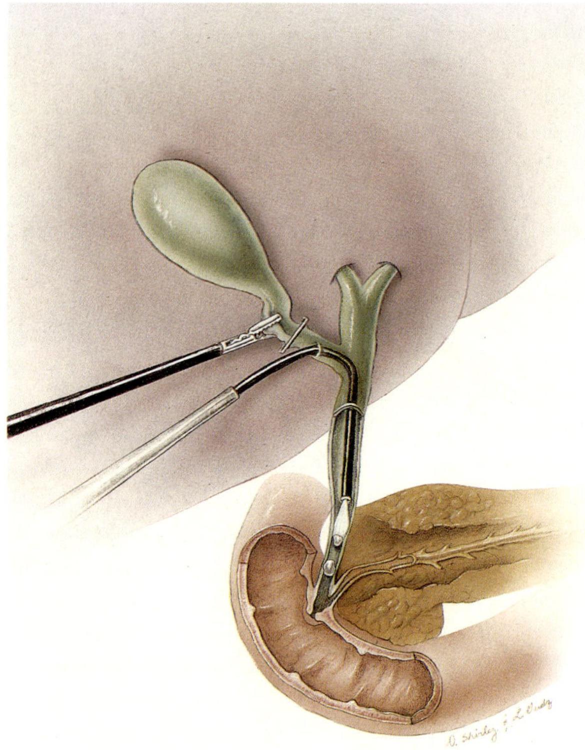

Figure 9.14. Access to the CBD during transcystic choledochoscopy is maintained with an introducer sheath placed into or near the cystic duct opening. (From Marks JM, Ponsky JL: Recent advances in choledochoscopy. In *Contemporary Surgery.* Bobitt Publishing, 1994, p 45. Reprinted with permission.)

bleeding occurs, when large stones are discovered which cannot be removed, or when a choledochoenterostomy is indicated.

Bile Duct Injuries, Strictures, and Leaks

LC has become the standard approach for patients with symptomatic cholelithiasis. Inherent in the advancement of any new procedure is the identification of new complications and problems. In the case of LC, bile duct injuries, strictures, and leaks have been at the forefront. Bile duct injuries associated with LC have been reported to occur in 0.5–2.7% of cases in the United States and in 0.25–3% in Europe.[30–36] The incidence of bile duct injuries during open cholecystectomy has been shown previously to range from 0.2% to 0.5%.[37] Lack of tactile sensation, inexperience of the surgeon, and reluctance to convert to an open procedure have all been identified as reasons for this increased rate of bile duct complications.[38,39] Another issue of debate in the discussion of bile duct injuries is whether the use of routine intraoperative cholangiography could have an impact on the rate of complications. Several authors have reported that routine cholangiography does not alter the risk of CBD injury, and that meticulous dissection at the infundibulum–cystic duct junction and delineation of the anatomy are the key to avoiding injuries.[40,41] However, review of several series of patients who sustained CBD injuries in the absence of IOC reveals that cholangiography may not have prevented these complications but at least may have allowed earlier identification and pri-

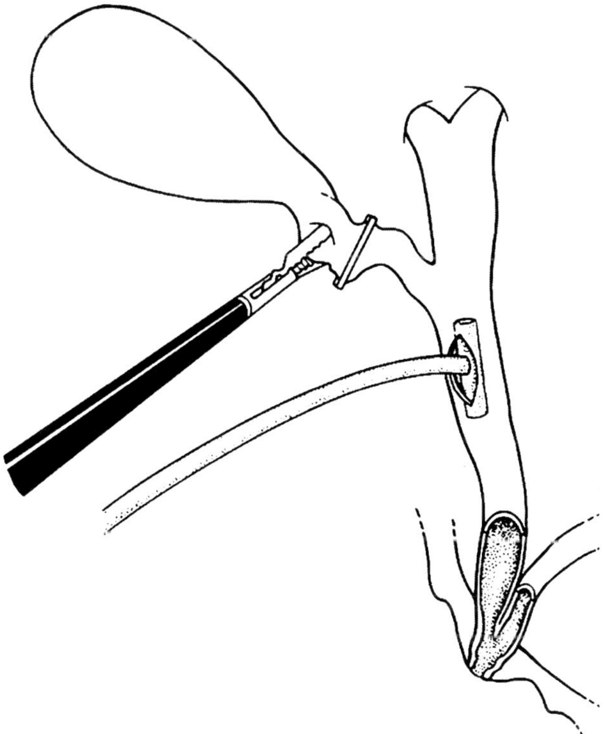

Figure 9.15. After completion of a laparoscopic CBD exploration, a T-tube is placed in the small choledochotomy which has been made near the cystic duct–CBD junction.

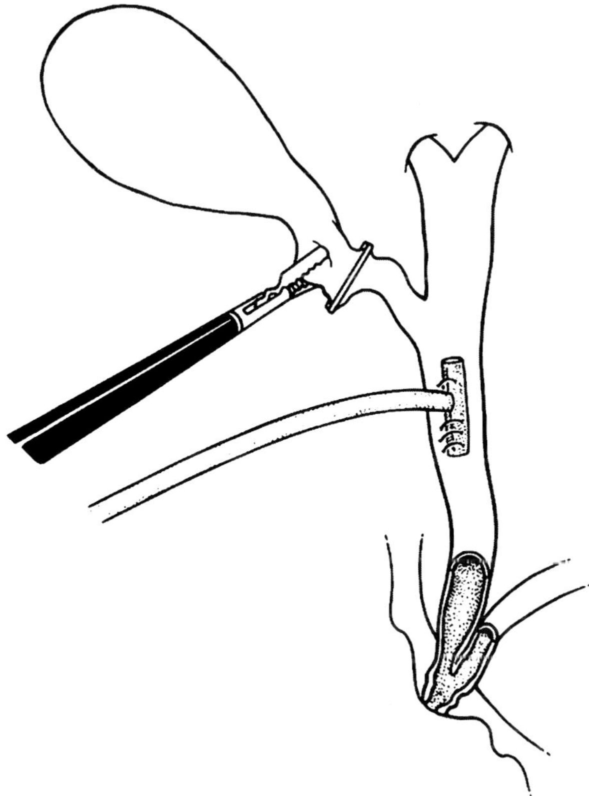

Figure 9.16. Closure of the choledochotomy around the T-tube can be done with intracorporeal or extracorporeal suture techniques.

mary repair. Also, correct interpretation of the cholangiograms that were performed would have helped identify ductal injuries in 64% of the cases.[42–45] Intraoperative cholangiography may never be proven to decrease the rate of bile duct injuries. However, it may allow earlier intraoperative recognition and may reduce the severity of injury.[46–48] Immediate recognition of a bile duct injury affords the best chance for primary repair and may decrease postoperative and long-term complications.[49,50]

A broad range of bile duct injuries have been described, including strictures, leaks, and actual bile duct transsections or resections. If not identified immediately at the time of surgery, bile duct injuries can produce dramatic early postoperative morbidity or may present up to several months after the initial surgery.[51] A high index of suspicion for bile leak or injury should be present for any patient who does not have an uncomplicated postoperative recovery following laparoscopic cholecystectomy.[52] Patients with nausea, anorexia, abdominal pain, or malaise should be suspected of having a complication.[52]

Biliary Leaks

Biliary leaks with resultant bile peritonitis or biloma formation usually present with persistent abdominal pain, distention, malaise, and shoulder pain secondary to diaphragmatic irritation. Bile duct leaks may produce these symptoms anywhere from 2 days to 2 weeks following surgery.[51–54] There are multiple sites in the hepatobiliary system where bile leakage may occur, as well as multiple etiologies. Also, bile duct leaks can occur in conjunction with a bile duct injury or transsection, and bile peritonitis rather than jaundice may be the initial presenting symptom.

There are varied opinions as to the appropriate diagnostic workup of a patient with suspected bile duct leak. Some investigators believe that immediate ERCP without other diagnostic imaging studies is the most beneficial and cost-effective plan.[54] In support of this opinion is the fact that clinically irrelevant fluid collections in the gallbladder bed are commonly seen radiographically on ultrasound and computed tomography scans after LC.[55] Also, ERCP will provide information on the existence and site of the biliary leak, will diagnose other associated hepatobiliary injuries or retained CBDS, and may offer immediate therapy in a number of situations (Fig. 9.17). Ultrasound, computed tomography, and nuclear scans are obviously less specific and will not delineate the source and etiology of the bile leak.

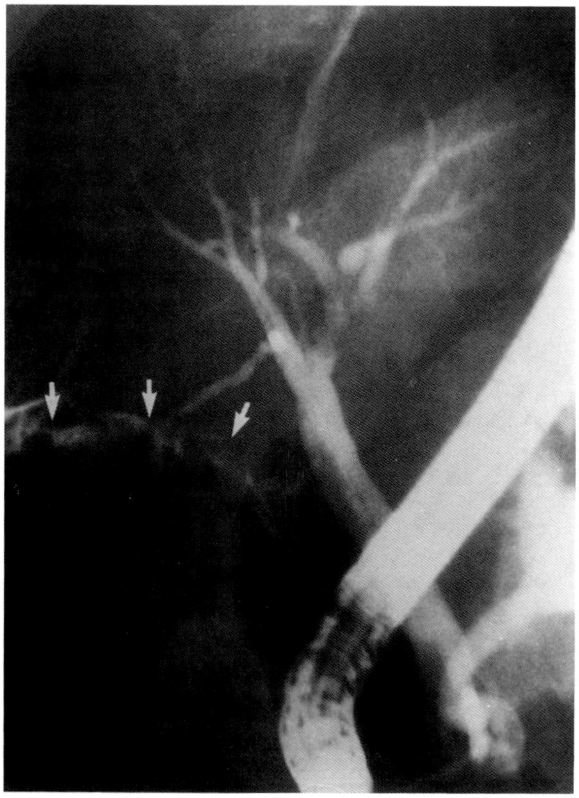

Figure 9.17. Postoperative ERCP revealing a biliary leak from a cystohepatic duct. (From Jenkins MA, Ponsky JL, Lehman GA, et al: Treatment of bile leaks from the cystohepatic ducts after laparoscopic cholecystectomy. In *Surgical Endoscopy,* vol. 8. New York, Springer-Verlag, 1994. Reprinted with permission.)

There are also cited advantages to performing radiographic imaging studies prior to ERCP. Ultrasound and computed tomography can be used for therapeutic percutaneous catheter placement to drain resultant bilomas and allow for resolution of bile peritonitis.[51] Pigtail catheters, placed under radiographic guidance, can be introduced for drainage of bile collections in both the abdomen and pelvis, with excellent symptomatic relief of abdominal pain. A controlled biliary fistula is created and a formal therapeutic endoscopic or surgical procedure, if required, can be performed electively. In addition, nuclear scans can be used initially to identify bile extravasation, as well as the continuity of bile flow into the duodenum (Fig. 9.18). ERCP or percutaneous transhepatic cholangiography (PTC) would then be indicated if the nuclear scan reveals any abnormalities.

After a postoperative biliary leak has been confirmed by radiographic or endoscopic studies, the appropriate management includes biliary diversion and resolution of bile peritonitis. The source of the biliary fistula, as well as the presence or absence of bile duct continuity, will dictate the appropriate management. In patients with a patent bile duct system and an uncomplicated biliary fistula, endoscopic decompression utilizing a sphincterotomy and/or a biliary endoprosthesis provides adequate treatment[54,56–59] (Fig. 9.19a,b). This includes patients with biliary leaks from cystohepatic ducts (ducts of Lushka) or cystic duct stumps, without associated bile duct strictures or injuries.[60,61] Short-term stent placement (4–6 weeks) is recommended, as well as percutaneous drainage of associated bilomas.[54,56] Biliary fistulas secondary to bile duct lacerations or thermal injuries will have a higher risk of strictures and are less likely to be successfully treated with minimally invasive maneuvers.[53] Overall, the long-term complication rates of endoscopically treated biliary leaks secondary to laparoscopic cholecystectomy are not yet known. Short-term results thus far, however, appear promising.[51,54,56]

Biliary Strictures

Postoperative biliary strictures associated with LC have been attributed to thermal and ischemic injuries, as well as impingement on the CBD secondary to inappropriate clip placement. Thermal injuries are related to extensive electrocauterization or laser dissection and can present up to 6 months after LC.[51,56] The type of instrument used for dissection (laser vs. electrocautery) has not been shown to significantly change

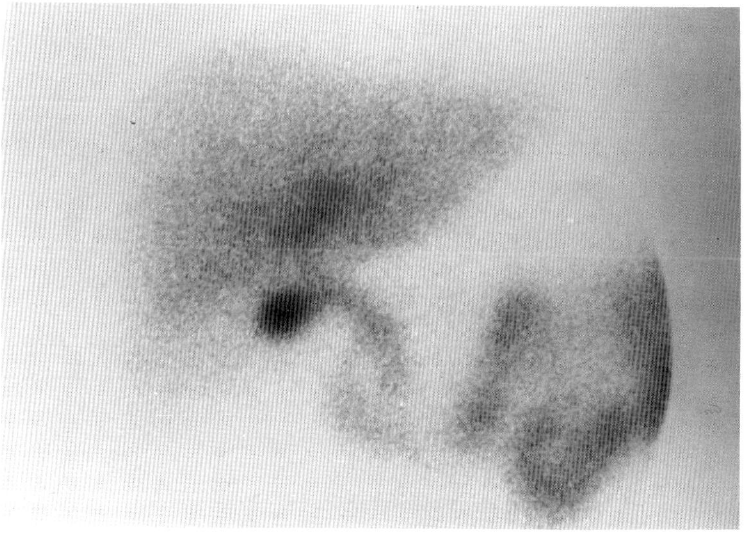

Figure 9.18. A HIDA scan after laparoscopic cholecystectomy revealing a leak from the cystic duct.

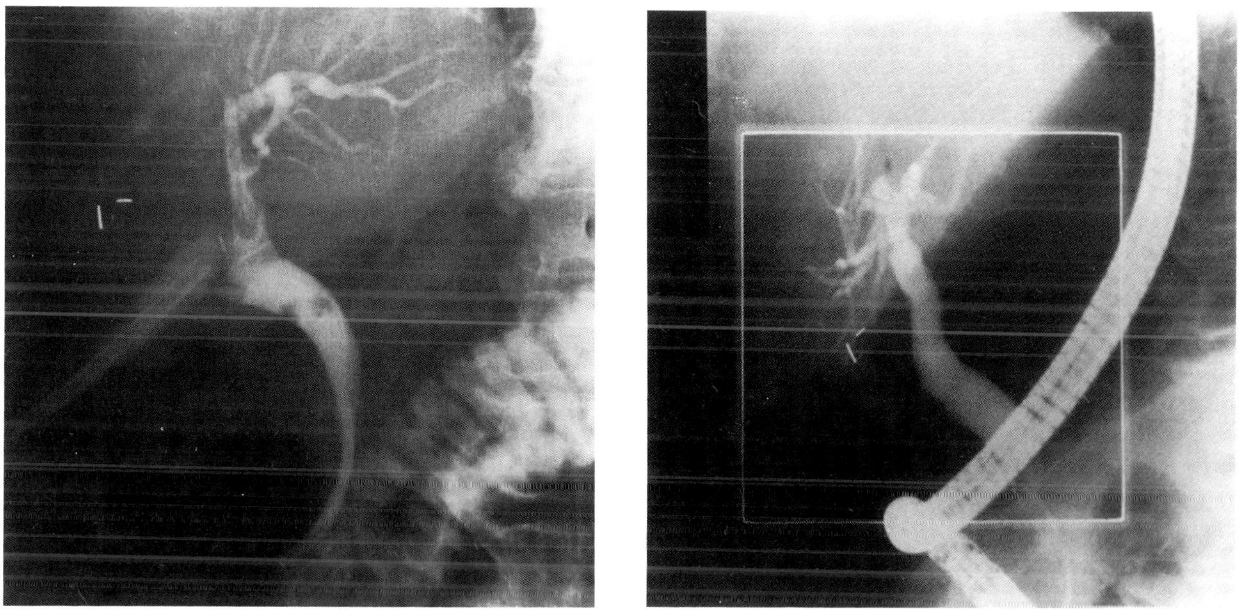

a b

Figure 9.19. (a) A postoperative ERCP revealing a leak from the region of the cystic duct. An endoscopic stent has been placed. (b) Follow-up ERCP 6 weeks following stent placement reveals complete resolution of the bile leak, and the stent was removed. (From Ponsky JL: Management of complications of laparoscopic cholecystectomy. In *Endoscopy* vol. 24. Thieme Medical, 1992. Reprinted with permission.)

the risk of thermal-induced injuries.[44,51] Also, the site of injury is variable, with strictures occurring in the hilum as well as in the mid-CBD region. Ischemic injuries are also responsible for postoperative strictures and are probably due to extensive dissection and "cleaning" of the cystic duct–common bile duct junction. This type of injury was seen during the era of open surgery when surgeons attempted to leave a short cystic duct stump and performed extensive cleaning of the cystic duct–common bile duct region. Impingement on the CBD, due to inappropriate clip placement, is a source of biliary strictures which appears to be unique to LC (Fig. 9.20). The two previously described injuries, thermal and ischemic were documented prior to the laparoscopic era. Due to inadequate exposure, poor hemostasis, or an unidentified short cystic duct, biliary strictures have become more common since the advancement of laparoscopic techniques.[49,51,56]

Biliary strictures can present with painless jaundice, fatigue, or delayed bile leak and bile peritonitis.[51,53,56] Patients with biliary strictures after LC can also have retained bile duct stones.[56] Once suspected, imaging of the biliary tree is required. ERCP, PTC, or both may be necessary to obtain access across some biliary strictures. Nonoperative management of biliary strictures has been described by many authors.[51,56,58,59,62,63] Current management includes periodic balloon dilation and endoprosthesis placement for 6–12 months[56,64,65] (Fig. 9.21a–d). Subsequent dilations and stent changes are required every 3–6 months until no evidence of stricture re-formation is seen on follow-up ERCP. Patients are then followed with periodic liver function studies, and repeat ERCP is performed for any laboratory changes suggesting recurrent stenosis. As with biliary leaks, the long-term complication rates of patients with endoscopically treated biliary strictures after laparoscopic cholecystectomy are not yet known. Although the initial results are encouraging, the follow-up period is still too short to determine if a high percentage of these patients will develop recurrent stenosis requiring long-term stenting or surgical repair. Patients with recurrent symptoms or those in whom stent placement is unsatisfactory will require surgical intervention. The surgical procedure most appropriate is Roux-en-Y hepaticojejunostomy. Primary direct repair of postoperative strictures or simple placement of T-tubes is associated with a high failure rate and a high incidence of recurrent stenosis.[53,66]

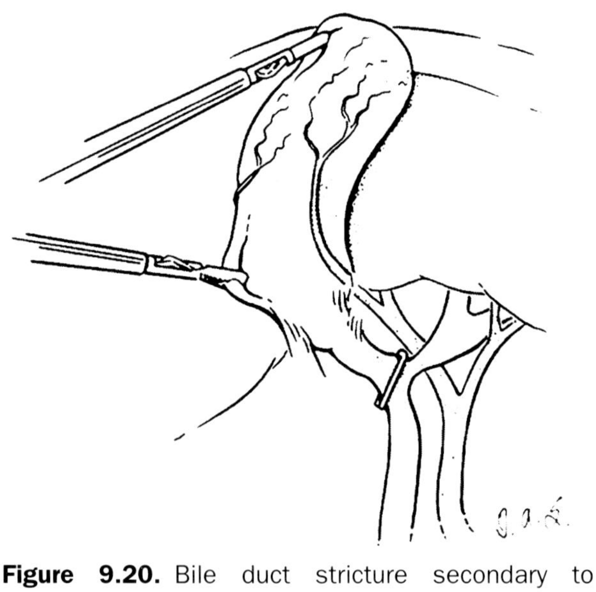

Figure 9.20. Bile duct stricture secondary to impingement of the CBD by inappropriate clip placement (From Ponksy JL: Management of complications of laparoscopic cholecystectomy. In *Endoscopy,* vol. 24. Thieme Medical, 1992. Reprinted with permission.)

CBD Injuries

Actual injuries to the hepatobiliary tree can be divided into lacerations, transsections, and resections. Therefore, these injuries will present in association with bile leaks and/or biliary strictures. As stated previously, any patient who does not have an uncomplicated postoperative course after LC should be investigated for a bile duct injury.[49,52,56] Endoscopic and/or radiographic imaging (ERCP, PTC) are the diagnostic tools of choice to delineate the abnormality in the hepatobiliary anatomy. Lacerations and transsections of the hepatobiliary tree occur when exposure is poor, secondary to bleeding and/or extensive inflammation, or when aberrant biliary anatomy is unrecognized.[49,51,67,68] They may also occur in apparently easy cases when identification of ductal anatomy is inadequate. These injuries may be associated with excessive dissection with scissors or electrocautery instruments, inadvertent or uncalculated clip placement, inappropriate identification of biliary strictures, and/or inexperience of the laparoscopic surgeon.[38,39,44,53,66,69] Early identification of "clean-cut" injuries at the time of the original surgery may allow primary repair or reanastomosis.[48,49,70] We believe, as do many authors, that while IOC may not avert all injuries of the bile duct, it may prevent simple

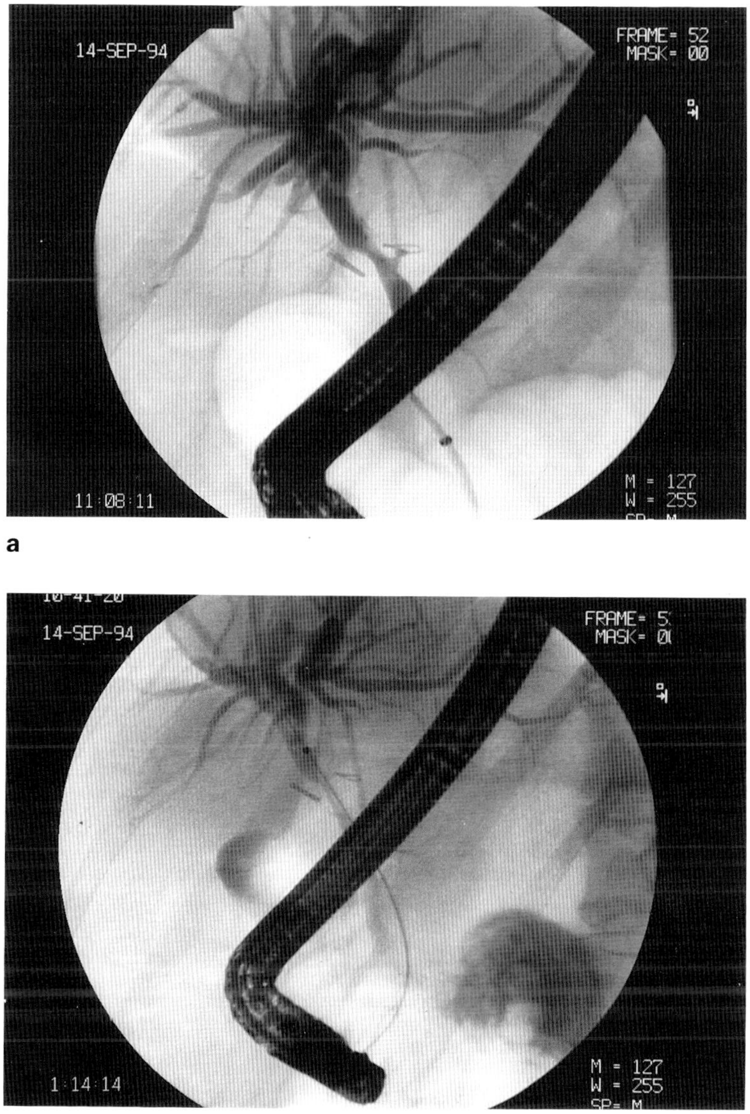

Figure 9.21. (a) A bile duct stricture at the level of the cystic duct after laparoscopic cholecystectomy. (b) A hydrostatic balloon is placed across the stricture.

injuries from becoming transsections or resections of biliary structures.[48,51] Unfortunately, no prospective studies have been done to show that IOC will aid the surgeon in avoiding bile duct injuries.

In patients with a short cystic duct or extensive inflammation between the gallbladder and the CBD or common hepatic duct, severe injuries can occur if the surgeon is not careful (Fig. 9.22a). Resections of segments of the bile duct will take place when the CBD is mistaken for the distal cystic duct (Fig. 9.22b). Usually the surgeon will have to divide two "structures" in addition to the cystic duct to remove the gallbladder (Fig. 9.22c). Caudal and lateral traction on the gallbladder will open Calot's triangle and help differentiation of the cystic and common bile ducts. Also, compulsive dissection of the lateral aspect of the gallbladder will help identify the infundibulum–cystic duct junction[40,71,72] (Fig. 9.23). Transsections of the bile

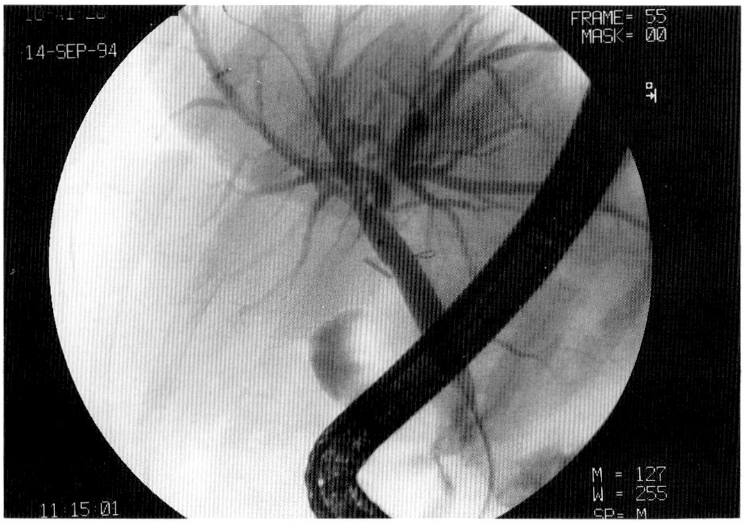

c

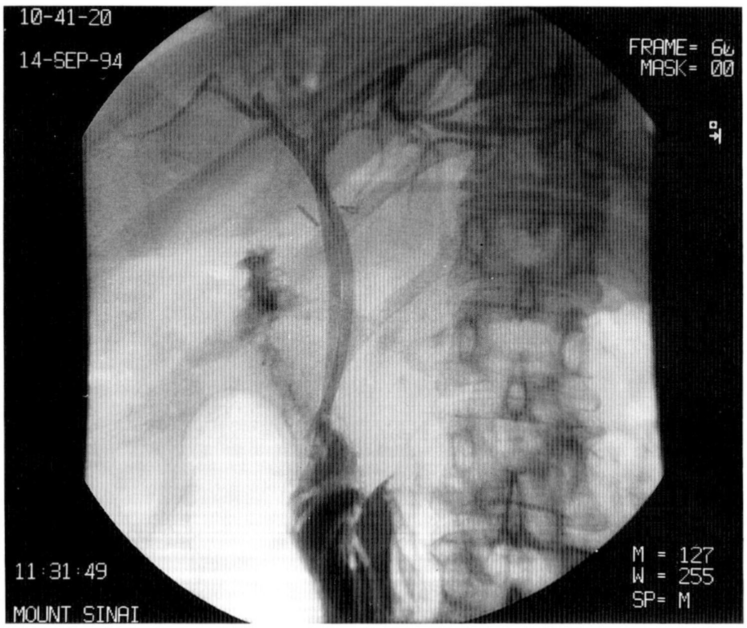

d

Figure 9.21. (c) Dilation is performed until waist ablation of the balloon is seen at the level of the stricture. (d) Following balloon dilation, double stenting is performed to help prevent recurrent stricture formation.

duct which go unrecognized, and injuries which result in loss or destruction of tissue of the hepatobiliary tree, will require Roux-en-Y-hepaticojejunostomy.[19,51,53,66] Attempting to reanastomose the bile duct after a resection injury will lead to increased tension and ischemia at the suture line, with resultant stricture formation. Delayed repair is associated with increased morbidity and will make surgical repair even more difficult due to the inflammatory reaction secondary to bile peritonitis. Prior to a secondary or delayed hepatobiliary reconstructive surgery, diversion of bile leakage and resolution of biliary sepsis is recommended. This may require temporary endoscopic or transhepatic biliary decompression, as well as percutaneous pigtail catheter placement for creation of a controlled biliary fistula. Referral to a tertiary care center with radiologic, endoscopic, and surgical specialists experienced in the management of complex biliary injuries is recommended.

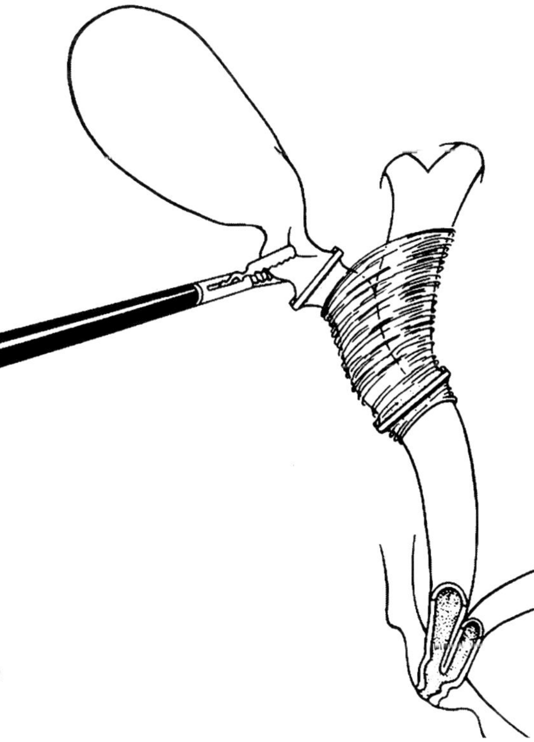

b

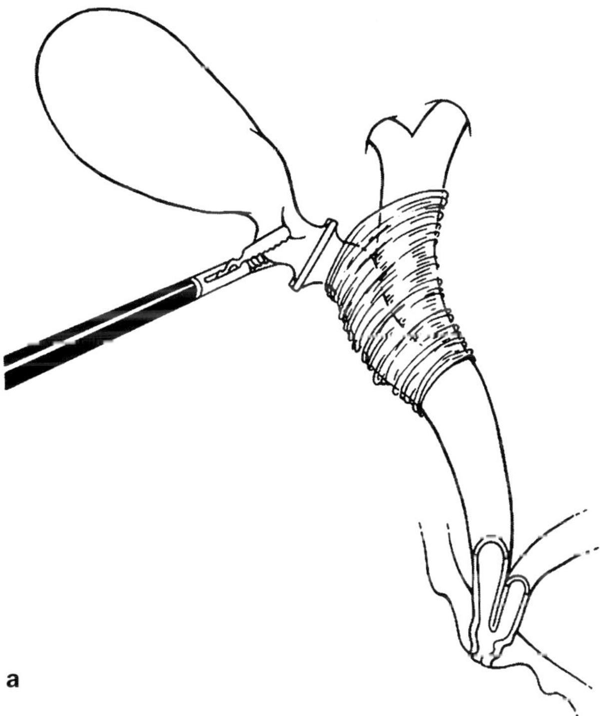

a

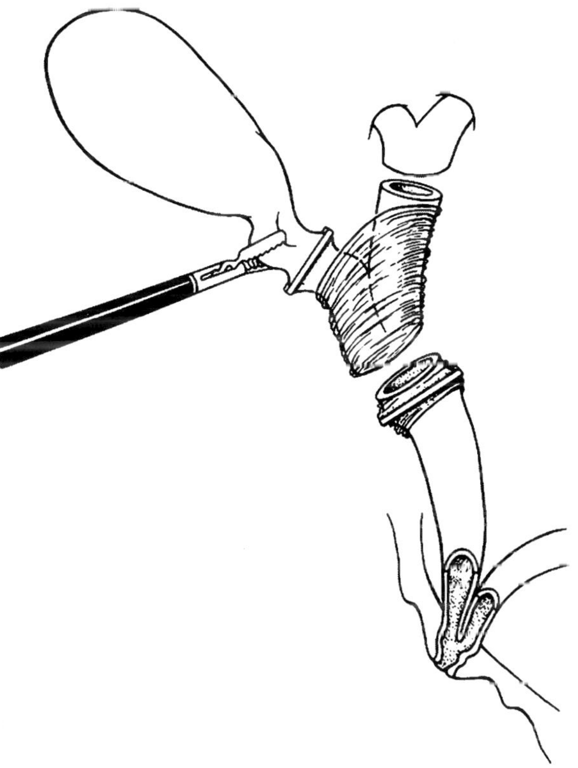

c

Figure 9.22. (a) Adhesions between the cystic duct and CBD or common hepatic duct can predispose patients to bile duct injuries. (b) The CBD can be mistaken for the distal cystic duct in patients with extensive adhesions. (c) Resection of a segment of the biliary tree will then occur with this type of injury.

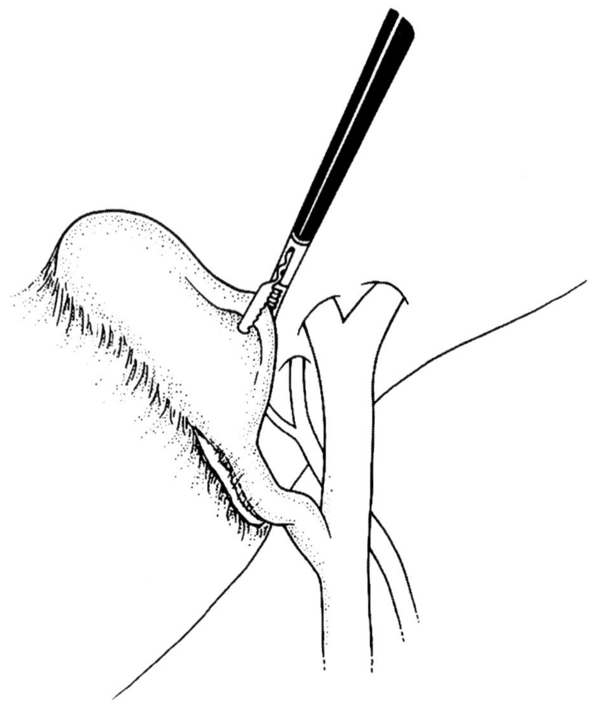

Figure 9.23. Compulsive dissection of the lateral aspect of the gallbladder helps to identify the infundibulum–cystic duct junction.

REFERENCES

1. Panton ONM, Nagy AG, Scudamore CH, et al: Laparoscopic cholecystectomy: A continuing plea for routine cholangiography. *Surg Laparosc Endosc* 5:43–49, 1995.
2. Allen B, Shapiro H, Way LW: Management of recurrent and residual common duct stones. *Am J Surg* 142:41, 1981.
3. McSherry CK, Glenn F: The incidence and causes of death following surgery for non-malignant biliary tract disease. *Ann Surg* 191:271, 1980.
4. Graham SM, Flowers JL, Scott TR, et al: Laparoscopic cholecystectomy and common bile duct stones. *Ann Surg* 218:61–67, 1993.
5. Arregui ME, Davis CJ, Arkush AM, et al: Laparoscopic cholecystectomy combined with endoscopic sphincterotomy and stone extraction or laparoscopic choledochoscopy and electrohydraulic lithotripsy for management of cholelithiasis and choledocholithiasis. *Surg Endosc* 6:10–15, 1992.
6. Franceschi D, Brandt C, Margolin D, et al: The management of common bile duct stones in patients undergoing laparoscopic cholecystectomy. *Am Surg* 59:525–532, 1993.
7. Vanneman W, Kingsbury R, Duberman E, et al: When is ERCP indicated before laparoscopic cholecystectomy? *Gastroenterol Endosc* 38:265, 1993.
8. Silvis SE: Current status of endoscopic sphincterotomy (editorial). *Am J Gastroenterol* 79:731, 1984.
9. Cotton PB: Nonoperative removal of bile duct stones by duodenoscopic sphincterotomy. *Br J Surg* 67:1–5, 1980.
10. Kawai K, Nakajima M: Present status and complications of EST in Japan. *Endoscopy* 15:169–172, 1983.
11. Escourrou J, Cordova J, Lazorthes F, et al: Early and late complications after endoscopic sphincterotomy for biliary lithiasis with and without the gallbladder in situ. *Gut* 25:598–602, 1984.
12. Leese T, Neoptolemos JP, Carr-Locke DL: Successes, failure, early complications and their management following endoscopic sphincterotomy: Results in 394 consecutive patients from a single center. *Br J Surg* 72:215–219, 1985.
13. Ikeda S, Tanaka M, Matsumoto S, et al: Endoscopic sphincterotomy: Long-term results in 408 patients with complete follow-up. *Endoscopy* 20:13–17, 1988.
14. Cotton PB, Vallon AC: British experience with duodenoscopic sphincterotomy for removal of bile duct stones. *Br J Surg* 68:373–375, 1981.
15. Lambert ME, Betts CD, Hill J, et al: Endoscopic sphincterotomy: The whole truth. *Br J Surg* 78:743–746, 1991.
16. Frazee RC, Roberts J, Symmonds R, et al: Combined laparoscopic and endoscopic management of cholelithiasis and choledocholithiasis. *Am J Surg* 166:702–706, 1993.
17. Geenan JE, Vennes JA, Silvis SE: Resume of a seminar on endoscopic retrograde sphincterotomy. *Gastroenterol Endosc* 27:31, 1981.
18. Demling L, Seuberth K, Reiman JF: A mechanical lithotripter. *Endoscopy* 14:100, 1982.
19. Leung JW, Chung SS: Electrohydraulic lithotripsy with peroral choledochoscopy. *Br Med J* 299: 595–597, 1989.
20. Ponchon T, Gagnon P, Valette PJ, et al: Pulsed dye laser lithotripsy of bile duct stones. *Gastroenterology* 100: 1730–1736, 1991.
21. Sauerbruch T, Delius M, Paumgartner G, et al: Fragmentation of gallstones by extracorporeal shockwaves. *N Engl J Med* 314:818, 1986.
22. Noar M, Grimm H, Sollano J, et al: Extracorporeal shock wave lithotripsy (ESWL) of endoscopically nonextractable bile duct stones (abstract). *Gastroenterol Endosc* 34:208, 1988.
23. Deslandres E, Gagner M, Pomp A, et al: Intraoperative endoscopic sphincterotomy for common bile duct stones during laparoscopic cholecystectomy. *Gastroenterol Endosc* 39:54–58, 1993.

24. DePaula A, Hashiba K, Bafutto M, et al: Laparoscopic antegrade sphincterotomy. *Surg Laparosc Endosc* 3:157–160, 1993.
25. Carroll BJ, Phillips EH: Laparoscopic removal of common duct stones. *Gastroenterol Endosc Clin North Am* 3:239–246, 1993.
26. Cotton PB, Vennes J, Geenen JE, et al: Endoscopic sphincterotomy complications and their management: An attempt at consensus. *Gastroenterol Endosc* 37:383–386, 1991.
27. Phillips EH, Carroll BJ, Pearlstein AR: Laparoscopic choledochoscopy and extraction of common bile duct stones. *World J Surg* 27:22–28, 1993.
28. Picus D, Weyman PJ, Marx MV: Role of percutaneous intracorporeal lithotripsy in the treatment of biliary tract calculi. *Radiology* 170:989–993, 1989.
29. DePaula AL, Hashiba K, Bafutto M: Laparoscopic management of choledocholithiasis. *Surg Endosc* 8:1399–1403, 1994.
30. Kalk H, Bruhl W: *Leitfaden der Laproskopie*. Stuttgart, Thieme, 1951.
31. Kelling G: Zur Goelioskopie. *Arch Klin Chir* 126: 226–229, 1923.
32. Lingeman E, Newman DM: *Shock Wave Lithotripsy*. New York, Plenum Press, 1988.
33. Moosa AR, Mayer AD, Stabile B: Iatrogenic injuries to the bile duct. *Arch Surg* 125:1028–1030, 1990.
34. Morgenstern L, Berci G, Wong L: Twelve hundred consecutive cholecystectomies before the laparoscopic era: Morbidity, mortality and general observations. *Arch Surg* 127:400–403, 1992.
35. O'Donnell LDJ, Heaton KW: Postdissolution gallstone recurrence: A lifetime sentence to the rock pile or not? *Gut* 29:655, 1988.
36. Perissat J, Collet D, Belliard R: Gallstones: Laparoscopic treatment. *Surg Endosc* 4:1–5, 1990.
37. Phillips E, Berci G, Carroll B, et al: The value of operative cholangiography during laparoscopic cholecystectomy. *Am Surg* in press.
38. Scott TR, Zucker KA, Bailey RW: Laparoscopic cholecystectomy: A review of 12,937 patients. *Surg Laparosc Endosc* 2:191–198, 1992.
39. Orlando R, Russell JC, Lynch J, et al: Laparoscopic chole cystectomy: A statewide experience. *Arch Surg* 128:494–499, 1993.
40. Clair DG, Carr-Locke DL, Becker JM, et al: Routine cholangiography is not warranted during laparoscopic cholecystectomy. *Cholangiogr Laparosc Cholecyst* 128: 551–555, 1993.
41. Barkun JS, Fried GM, Barkun AN, et al: Cholecystectomy without operative cholangiography. *Ann Surg* 218:371–379, 1993.
42. Davidoff AM, Pappas TN, Murray EA, et al: Mechanisms of major biliary injury during laparoscopic cholecystectomy. *Ann Surg* 215:196–202, 1992.
43. Moosa AR, Easter DW, van Sonnenberg E, et al: Laparoscopic injuries to the bile duct: A cause for concern. *Ann Surg* 215:203–208, 1992.
44. Rossi RL, Schirmer WJ, Braasch WJ, et al: Laparoscopic bile duct injuries: Risk factors, recognition, and repair. *Arch Surg* 127:596–602, 1992.
45. Soper NJ, Flye MW, Brunt LM, et al: Diagnosis and management of biliary complications of laparoscopic cholecystectomy. *Am J Surg* 165:663–669, 1993.
46. Soper NJ, Brunt LM: The case for routine operative cholangiography during laparoscopic cholecystectomy. *Surg Clin North Am* 74(4):953–959, 1994.
47. Phillips EH: Routine versus selected intraoperative cholangiography. *Am J Surg* 165:505–507, 1993.
48. Cantwell DV: Routine cholangiography during laparoscopic cholesystectomy. *Arch Surg* 127: 483–484, 1991.
49. Rantis PC, Greenlee HB, Pickleman J, et al: Laparoscopic cholecystectomy bile duct injuries: More than meets the eye. *Am Surg* 59:533–540, 1993.
50. Way LW, Bernhoft RA, Thomas MJ: Biliary stricture. *Surg Clin North Am* 61:963–972, 1981.
51. Bezzi M, Silecchia G, Orsi F, et al: Complications after laparoscopic cholecystectomy. *Surg Endosc* 9:29–36, 1995.
52. Morgenstern L, Berci G, Pasternak EH: Bile leakage after biliary tract surgery: A laparoscopic perspective. *Surg Endosc* 7:432–438, 1993.
53. Huang S-M, Wu C-W, Hong H-T, et al: Bile duct injury and bile leakage in laparoscopic cholecystectomy. *Br J Surg* 80:1590–1592, 1993.
54. Davids PHP, Ringers EAJ, deWit L Th, et al: Bile duct injury after laparoscopic cholecystectomy: The value of endoscopic retrograde cholangiopancreatography. *Gut* 34:1250–1254, 1993.
55. Kang EH, Middleton WD, Balfe DM, et al: Laparoscopic cholecystectomy: Sonographic evaluation. *Radiology* 181:439–442, 1991.
56. Manoukian AV, Schmaiz MJ, Geenan JE, et al: Endoscopic treatment of problems encountered after cholecystectomy. *Gastroenterol Endosc* 39: 9–14, 1993.
57. Ponchon T, Gallez J-F, Valette P-J, et al: Endoscopic treatment of biliary tract fistulas. *Gastroenterol Endosc* 35:490–498, 1989.
58. Kozarek RA, Ganan R, Baerg R, et al: Bile leak after laparoscopic cholecystectomy: Diagnostic and therapeutic application of ERCP. *Arch Intern Med* 151:1040–1042, 1992.
59. O'Rahilly S, Duignan VP, Lennon JR, et al: Successful treatment of a postoperative external biliary fistula by endoscopic papillotomy. *Endoscopy* 15:68–69, 1983.

60. Dubois F, Icard P, Berthelot G, et al: Coelioscopic cholecystectomy: Preliminary report of 36 cases. *Ann Surg* 211:60–62, 1990.
61. Peters JH, Gibbus GD, Innes JT, et al: Complications of laparoscopic cholecystectomy. *Surgery* 110:769–778, 1991.
62. Gibson RN, Adam A, Yeung E, et al: Percutaneous techniques in benign hilar and intrahepatic strictures. *J Intervent Radiol* 3:125–130,
63. Rossi P, Salvatori FM, Bezzi M, et al: Percutaneous management of benign biliary strictures with balloon dilation and self-expanding metallic stents. *Cardiovasc Intervent Radiol* 13:231–239,
64. Geenen DJ, Geenen JE, Hogan WJ, et al: Endoscopic therapy of benign bile duct strictures. *Gastroenterol Endosc* 35:367–371, 1989.
65. Davids PHD, Rauws EAJ, Coene PPLO, et al: Endoscopic stenting for postoperative biliary strictures. *Gastroenterol Endosc* 38:12–18, 1992.
66. Davidoff AM, Pappas TN, Murray EA, et al: Mechanisms of major biliary injury during laparoscopic cholecystectomy. *Ann Surg* 215:196–202, 1992.
67. Reddick EJ, Olson D, Spaw A, et al: Safe performance of difficult laparoscopic cholecystectomies. *Am J Surg* 161: 377–381, 1991.
68. Flowers JL, Bailey RW, Scovill WA, et al: The Baltimore experience with laparoscopic management of acute cholecystitis. *Am J Surg* 161:388–392, 1991.
69. Flowers JL, Zucker KA, Graham SM, et al: Laparoscopic cholangiography results and indications. *Ann Surg* 215: 209–216, 1992.
70. Blumgart LH: Benign biliary strictures. In Blumgart LH (ed): *Surgery of the Liver and Biliary Tract.* Edinburgh, Churchill Livingstone, 1988, pp 721–752.
71. Lillemoe KD, Yeo CJ, Talamini MA, et al: Selective cholangiography: Current role in laparoscopic cholecystectomy. *Ann Surg* 215:669–676, 1992.
72. Soper NJ, Dunnegan DL: Routine versus selective intraoperative cholangiography during laparoscopic cholecystectomy. *World J Surg* 16:1133–1140, 1992.

chapter ten

Laparoscopic Cholecystectomy During Pregnancy

Jeffrey B. Comitalo

Numerous gastrointestinal surgical conditions such as acute appendicitis, biliary tract disease, pancreatitis, inflammatory bowel disease, and bowel obstruction can affect the pregnant patient. While many of these gastrointestinal conditions can be successfully managed medically, delay of surgery in certain conditions (e.g., acute appendicitis, acute cholecystitis) can lead to serious complications in the mother or the fetus. Approximately 1 of 500 to 1000 pregnant women will require laparotomy for a nonobstetric condition. The most common indications for laparotomy in the pregnant patient are acute appendicitis, adnexal masses, and symptomatic biliary tract disease.

Cholecystectomy is one of the most commonly preformed abdominal operations in the United States. The incidence of cholelithiasis in the United States is estimated to be 10% of the population.[1] Of these patients, 1–2% per year will require biliary tract surgery due to symptoms or complications secondary to cholelithiasis. Biliary tract disease is the second most common gastrointestinal disorder requiring laparotomy in the pregnant patient. Asymptomatic cholelithiasis is seen in 2.5–3.5% of all pregnant patients.[2,3] The incidence of symptomatic biliary tract disease is estimated at 0.05–0.1% in this population. Because cholelithiasis is so common, the general surgeon must be familiar with the presentation, diagnosis, and treatment of symptomatic biliary tract disease in the pregnant patient.

GALLBLADDER PHYSIOLOGY DURING PREGNANCY

Over 80% of gallstones contain cholesterol, and its oversaturation in bile is thought to play a major role in the formation of gallstones. Although the etiology of cholesterol gallstones is multifactorial, pregnancy may lead to the formation of gallstones or increased symptoms from previously formed gallstones due to several physiologic changes that occur in the gallbladder during pregnancy. In the first trimester, gallbladder function differs little from that in the nongravid patient. Beginning in the second trimester, gallbladder volume during fasting is double that of the nonpregnant patient. The rate of gallbladder emptying slows, and the maximum percentage emptied (ejection fraction) is decreased. The last two changes are also seen in first-trimester patients, but to a lesser degree. Finally, the residual gallbladder volume after maximum emptying is increased.[4]

Changes in gallbladder physiology may occur as a result of the unique hormonal environment associated with pregnancy. Progesterone is known to be a smooth muscle relaxant, and serum levels increase significantly after the 11th week. Progesterone also impairs the gall bladder's response to exogenously administered cholecystokinin in the animal model, but this has not been tested in humans.[5] Decreased tone, increased relaxation of the gallbladder, or a reduced response to cholecystokinin may account for the increased gallbladder volume seen after the first trimester. Decreased water absorption by the gallbladder may also cause increased fasting volumes. This is thought to be due to the effect of estrogens on the sodium-potassium ATPase pump, which plays an integral role in the reabsorption of water from the gallbladder.[4]

These findings suggest that pregnancy increases the risk of gallstone formation. Increased fasting volumes and incomplete emptying of the gallbladder may lead to stasis (an etiologic factor in the formation of cholesterol stones) or promote the formation of biliary sludge, a possible precursor of cholesterol stones. Immediately postpartum, up to 25% of women have biliary sludge on ultrasound, but only 4% have persistent sludge 1 year later.[6]

BILIARY COLIC AND ACUTE CHOLECYSTITIS

Diagnosis

The clinical features of biliary colic and acute cholecystitis in the pregnant patient differ little from those in the nongravid patient. As many as 50% of patients have a history of biliary colic prior to pregnancy.[7] Midepigastric or right upper quadrant (RUQ) pain is the most characteristic feature of biliary colic and is seen in 60–90% of these patients.[7,8] Over 95% of patients with acute cholecystitis will have this finding.[9] Other symptoms such as nausea, vomiting, and fatty food intolerance are seen in 30–50% of cases are therefore less helpful in establishing the diagnosis.

The most common physical examination finding is RUQ tenderness. Murphy's sign (inability of the patient to take a deep inspiration when the RUQ is deep palpated below the hepatic margin), a common finding in patients with acute cholecystitis, may be seen less commonly in the pregnant woman.[10] Systemic symptoms such as fever and tachycardia may also be present. Laboratory values tend to be nonspecific and include leukocytosis and elevation of the alkaline phosphatase level. Pregnancy normally causes an increase in the alkaline phosphatase level. Elevated serum bilirubin or amylase levels raise the possibility of choledocholithiasis or pancreatitis, though cholecystitis or choledocholithiasis accounts for only a minority of pregnant patients who are jaundiced (5%).

When considering the diagnosis of acute cholecystitis, the differential includes several diagnoses unique to the pregnant patient, including acute fatty liver of pregnancy, severe preeclampsia, and HEELP syndrome (*HE*molysis, *E*levated *L*iver enzymes, and *L*ow *P*latelets)[11] Also, acute appendicitis must always be considered in the pregnant patient with right-sided abdominal pain. It is the most common condition requiring laparotomy in the pregnant patient, and the appendix is often displaced into the RUQ in the latter part of pregnancy.

Ultrasonography is the radiologic procedure of choice for determining the presence of gallstones in the pregnant patient. It is a noninvasive test, has a high degree of sensitivity in diagnosing cholelithiasis (greater than 95%), and involves no ionizing radiation. The pancreas, intrahepatic duct, and extrahepatic duct may also be visualized in many cases. Ideally, the patient should be in a fasting state prior to the exam to allow greater distension of the gallbladder and therefore better visualization. Radioisotope scanning is not recommended unless the diagnosis remains in doubt.

Medical Management

Traditionally, the management of recurrent biliary colic and acute cholecystitis has been medical. There are numerous examples in the literature favoring nonoperative management of symptomatic biliary tract disease due to the possibly increased risk of spontaneous abortion and preterm labor associated with surgery.[8-10] Anesthetic agents may also pose a risk to the fetus, especially in the first trimester. Resolution of the pregnancy without surgical intervention is the ultimate goal of medical management of biliary tract disease during pregnancy.

Medical management consists of bed rest, analgesics, intravenous fluids, elimination of oral intake, and nasogastric suction (in the presence of severe emesis). Antibiotics are usually reserved for patients with evidence of sepsis. The use of broad-spectrum antibiotics during short-term attacks to prevent acute cholecystitis have been advocated by some.[8] Using these methods, up to 84% of patients can be successfully managed without surgical intervention in the initial episode.[9,12] These patients are then followed closely during the remainder of their pregnancy, and cholecystectomy is performed in the postpartum period. Advocates of medical management state that the "surgical strategy for acute biliary tract disease in pregnancy includes recognition of pregnancy, diagnosis using ultrasonography, avoidance of medications that cross the placenta, treatment of hyperamylasemia by medical regimens, and *delay of surgical therapy* (italics added) until delivery unless therapeutic abortion is desired by the mother."[8]

Surgical Management

Surgical treatment of symptomatic biliary tract disease in the pregnant patient has, until recently, been confined to those patients who fail medical management. Failure of medical therapy has been defined as three or more episodes of biliary colic in one trimester, persistent or worsening clinical symptoms beyond the fourth hospital day, suspected perforation, severe toxicity, significant obstructive jaundice, or uncertainty about the diagnosis.[9,10] This method of management differs significantly from that of the nongravid patient in that early surgical intervention is usually advocated over medical management with delayed cholecystectomy when severe biliary colic, acute cholecystitis, or gallstone pancreatitis is present.[13]

Open cholecystectomy

Advances in perioperative fetal monitoring and anesthetic care have allowed surgeons to consider a more aggressive approach to the treatment of symptomatic cholelithiasis in the pregnant patient. Numerous articles published over the last decade advocate just such an approach. Dixon et al.,[14] in their review of 44 patients, found that of the 26 patients managed medically, 58% (15 patients) experienced recurrent episodes of biliary colic and 27% (7 patients) were hospitalized several times. Two patients required total parenteral nutrition due to intractable symptoms, and three patients suffered spontaneous abortions after the biliary symptoms began (7, 12, and 14 weeks). Of the 18 operative patients, 3 had surgery in the first trimester and *elective* abortion was performed in all 3. Fourteen patients were operated on in the second trimester and one in the third, with no significant maternal morbidity, preterm labor, or spontaneous abortion noted.

Swisher et al.[12] found similar results: a 69% relapse rate in those patients treated medically, 90% of whom required rehospitalization. Medical management failed in 44% of patients with acute cholecystitis. Relapse prior to delivery was noted in 60% of patients with gallstone pancreatitis and in 71% of those with biliary colic. Relapse rates following initial successful medical therapy of symptomatic biliary tract disease depend on the trimester of presentation. A rate of 92% was noted in the first trimester, 64% in the second, and 44% in the third. In the patients treated surgically (all open), no maternal or fetal morbidity was noted, though there was a 13% incidence of postoperative uterine contractions (treated successfully with tocolytic agents).

Reluctance to perform cholecystectomy during pregnancy is largely based on the reported high incidence of premature labor or spontaneous abortion. This avoidance of elective biliary tract surgery in the pregnant patient may no longer be warranted. In a review article by McKeller,[15] the rate of spontaneous abortion after cholecystectomy was found to be the highest in the first trimester, at 12%, followed by 5.6% in the second trimester and 0% in the third. The rate of premature labor was highest in the third trimester, and tocolytic agents were successfully employed to prevent premature delivery. Several of the articles cited by McKeller are over 20 years old. A review of the recent literature shows that the rates of fetal complications after cholecystectomy (including open and laparoscopic cases) to be even lower (Table 10.1).

Based on the numerous recent studies of biliary tract disease during pregnancy, cholecystectomy in the pregnant patient appears to be a safe and reasonable alternative to medical management for cases of acute cholecystitis, gallstone pancreatitis, or recurrent episodes of biliary colic. The benefits of early cholecystectomy compared to medical management include rapid eradication of the disease and a reduction in hospital costs from recurrent admissions. The optimal time to perform the operation is in the second trimester, as organogenesis is complete and there is a low incidence of spontaneous abortion and premature labor. First- and third-trimester patients should be treated conservatively and offered cholecystectomy in the second trimester or postpartum period, respectively. Regardless of the trimester, if surgery is thought to be indicated, delay should be avoided, as it can only place the mother and fetus at greater risk for postoperative problems.

Laparoscopic cholecystectomy

Laparoscopic cholecystectomy was first performed in the United States in 1988[16] and has since become the procedure of choice when cholecystectomy is indicated. It has the advantages over open cholecystectomy of a reduced hospital stay, rapid convalescence, and less postoperative pain and immobility. Although most patients are candidates for the laparoscopic approach, several contraindications do exist. Absolute contraindications most often cited include severe cardiac disease (class IV), chronic obstructive pulmonary disease with hypercarbia, inability to tolerate general anesthesia, presence of an abdominal wall stoma, and peritonitis with bowel distention. Relative contraindications include severe bleeding disorders, morbid obesity, portal hypertension, and diaphragmatic hernia.[17] Preg-

Table 10.1. Outcome of Pregnancy After Cholecystectomy (Open and Laparoscopic)

Study	No. of Patients	Trimester I	Trimester II	Trimester III	Spontaneous Abortion	Premature Labor	Elective Abortion
Landers[9]	9	3	3	3	1*	2†	2
Swisher[12]	16	3	12	1	0	2‡	0
Dixon[14]	16	3	12	1	0	1‡	3
McKellar[15]	9	2	4	3	0	0	0
Laparoscopic Cases (Table 10.2)[19–39]	46	4	38	4	0	2‡	0
Total	96	15	69	12	1 (1.05%)	7 (7.36%)	5 (5.26%)

* Occurred in the first trimester.

† Resulted in preterm delivery in both patients.

‡ Occurred in the third trimester; successfully treated with tocolytic agents.

nancy was once thought to be an absolute contraindication to laparoscopic cholecystectomy,[18] but several recent reports in the literature demonstrate that it can be performed safely.

The first laparoscopic cholecystectomy during pregnancy was reported in June 1991 by Arvidsson and Gerdin.[19] Two other case reports followed later in 1991.[20,21] Numerous series and case reports have since been published[22–39] To date, a total of 46 pregnant patients undergoing laparoscopic cholecystectomy have been reported in the literature (Table 10.2). The majority of patients were in the second trimester. The most common indication for surgery was severe biliary colic (37 patients), followed by acute cholecystitis (6 patients) and recurrent gallstone pancreatitis (3 patients). An open technique to gain initial access to the peritoneal cavity was utilized in 31 patients. Intraoperative cholangiograms were performed in 15 patients. Spontaneous abortion was not seen in any patient postoperatively, and no maternal morbidity was noted. Premature labor was noted in two patients postoperatively.[38] Both were in the third trimester, and the uterine contractions were eliminated with tocolytic agents. Despite the numerous cases presented here, a significant number of laparoscopic cholecystectomies have been performed in pregnant patients but have not been reported in the literature.[40]

Arguments against the use of laparoscopic cholecystectomy in the pregnant patient are based on the unknown effects of the CO_2 pneumoperitoneum on fetal physiology. Insufflation of CO_2 into the peritoneal cavity can cause changes due to increased absorption of CO_2 and increased intra-abdominal pressure. The acid-base changes induced by CO_2 pneumoperitoneum have been studied. While changes in the pH, end-tidal CO_2 value, and $PaCO_2$ value were noted, these changes were not significant in patients without cardiopulmonary disease.[41] In the animal model (pregnant ewe), CO_2 pneumoperitoneum (20 mmhG) was noted to cause a decrease in maternal perfusion pressure and maternal placental blood flow and an increase in placental vascular resistance. Despite these changes, the fetal placental perfusion pressure and blood flow, pH, and blood gas tensions were unaffected by insufflation or desufflation.[42] Though these results cannot be generalized to the pregnant human, no fetal complications have been reported after laparoscopic cholecystectomy. Further study is needed to better define the physiologic changes of CO_2 pneumoperitoneum on the human fetus.

Numerous cardiovascular changes are seen in patients undergoing laparoscopic cholecystectomy. These changes include a decrease in cardiac index and stroke volume of up to 30% and increases in mean arterial pressure of 15–28% and the calculated peripheral resistance index of 79%.[43] Increased intra-abdominal pressure, anesthesia, and the reverse Trendelenberg position are all thought to contribute to these hemodynamic changes.[44,45] While cardiac disease is rarely seen in the pregnant patient (approximately 1%),[46] if it is present, specialized hemodynamic monitoring may be required.

Although there are little data on the physiologic changes in the fetus induced by laparoscopy, other laparoscopic procedures have been performed in the pregnant patient, with similarly good results. Ovarian

Table 10.2. Laparoscopic Cholecystectomy During Pregnancy

Study	No. of Patients	Trimester I	Trimester II	Trimester III	Initial Access Hasson	Initial Access Veress	IOC	Spontaneous Abortion	Premature Labor
Arvidsson[19]	1		1		1		0*	0	0
Pucci[20]	1			1		1	0*	0	0
Weber[21]	1		1		1		0*	0	0
Soper[22]	5		5		5		0	0	0
Morrell[23]	5		5		5		5	0	0
Adamson[24]	2		2			2	0	0	0
Bennett[25]	1		1			1	0	0	0
Elerding[26]	5	1	3	1	5		5	0	0
Fabiani[27]	1		1			1	0	0	0
Hart[28]	3	1	2		3		1	0	0
Jackson[29]	1		1		1		0*	0	0
Rusher[30]	1		1			1	0*	0	0
Schorr[31]	2		2		2		0	0	0
Chandra[32]	1	1				1	1	0	0
Comitalo[33]	4		4		4		2	0	0
Constantino[34]	2		2			2	0*	0	0
Csaba[35]	1		1			1	0	0	0
Shaked[36]	1	1				1	0*	0	0
Wilson[37]	2		2		2		0	0	0
Lanzafame[38]	5		3	2	1	4	0	0	2†
Panton[39]	1		1		1		1	0	2†
Total	46	4	38	4	31(67%)	15(33%)	15(33%)	0	2(4.4%)

* If not specifically stated, cholangiogram was assumed not to have been performed.
† Successfully treated with tocolytic agents.

cystectomy,[47] diagnosis and treatment of ovarian torsion,[48,49] and appendectomy[50] have been performed laparoscopically during pregnancy, with minimal morbidity to the mother or fetus. Laparoscopic cholecystectomy has been shown to be as safe and effective as open cholecystectomy for symptomatic gallstone disease. Given the numerous advantages of the laparoscopic approach, this may be the procedure of choice when cholecystectomy is indicated in the gravid patient.

GALLSTONE PANCREATITIS AND CHOLEDOCHOLITHIASIS

Gallstone pancreatitis may also occur during pregnancy, though it is less common than biliary colic (incidence of 0.05%). Management is similar to that in nongravid patients. Early cholecystectomy is advocated to prevent recurrent attacks of pancreatitis, which may occur in up to 72% of patients. The rate of relapse appears to be highest when the first episode occurs in the first trimester. Surgical treatment depends on the trimester of the patient. First-trimester patients should be managed medically until the second trimester, when elective cholecystectomy can be performed. Third-trimester patients are managed in a similar fashion, and cholecystectomy is performed in the postpartum period. Second-trimester patients are operated on when the acute pancreatitis subsides.[51,52] This surgical strategy will result in fewer episodes of recurrent gallstone pancreatitis and does not appear to cause increased maternal/fetal morbidity or mortality when compared to medical management.

In patient who present with cholangitis, severe pancreatitis which does not quickly resolve or with ultrasonically demonstrated choledocholithiasis, endoscopic retrograde cholangiopancre-atography (ERCP) may be required. Preoperative ERCP need not be performed in all patients with gallstone pancreatitis, as a minority of these patients (38% in nongravid patients) will be found to have common duct stones.[53] Also, as surgical techniques improve, laparoscopic clearance of the common duct will become more common. ERCP has been performed in the pregnant patient with favorable results.[33,54] Lead shielding of the pelvis and conservative use of fluoroscopy will minimize radiation exposure to the fetus.

TECHNICAL CONSIDERATIONS

While the basic technique of laparoscopic cholecystectomy in the pregnant patient is unchanged from that in the nongravid patient, several technical changes should be employed to lower the risk of perioperative complications. Technical points to be discussed include the timing of surgery, perioperative fetal monitoring, the use of prophylactic tocolytics, methods of peritoneal access, prophylaxis against deep venous thrombosis, and intraoperative cholangiography in the pregnant patient.

The first consideration should be the timing of the surgery. As stated previously, numerous reports have shown that cholecystectomy in the second trimester has a low incidence of premature labor and spontaneous abortion. This is also the ideal time to perform laparoscopic cholecystectomy, as the uterus is not yet large enough to obscure the operative field. Although laparoscopic cholecystectomy has been performed during pregnancy as late as 31 weeks of gestation,[20] increased difficulty due to the enlarged uterus will be encountered during the middle to late third trimester. These patients may not be candidates for the laparoscopic approach if cholecystectomy is indicated. For patients undergoing cholecystectomy in the late second or early third trimester, the site of trocar placement may need to be modified to avoid difficulties in visualization secondary to the enlarged uterus (Fig. 10.1). Though one report recommends restricting the operation to first-trimester patients to prevent uterine injury,[36] most authors recommend cholecystectomy (laparoscopic or open) during the second trimester for the aforementioned reasons.

Perioperative monitoring of the fetus is strongly recommended when cholecystectomy is to be performed. Several methods are available, including pre- and postoperative monitoring of fetal heart tones and continu-

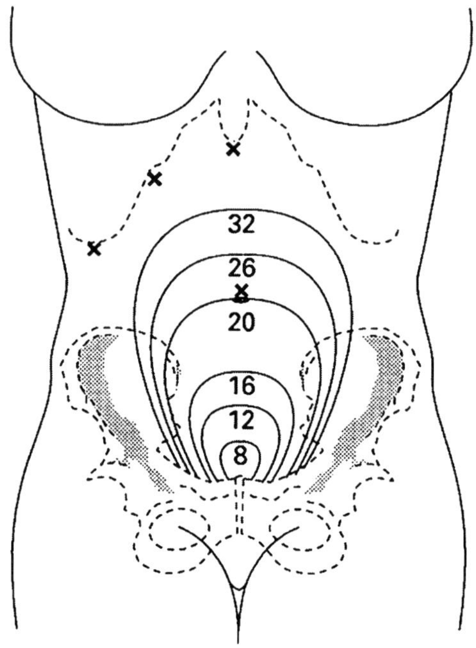

Figure 10.1. Uterine size from 8 to 32 weeks. "X" represents standard port placement for laparoscopic cholecystectomy.

ous intraoperative monitoring using an transabdominal monitor or an intravaginal ultrasound. Hart et al.[28] state that intraoperative monitoring "allows appropriate corrective steps to be taken in the event of a complication" and recommend the transvaginal route as the most efficient method. If fetal distress is encountered intraoperatively (assuming intraoperative fetal monitoring), rapid release of the pneumoperitoneum is suggested. Conversion to an open procedure should be considered.

The use of perioperative tocolytics to prevent preterm labor is controversial. Several studies have shown no decrease in preterm labor when prophylactic tocolytics were used.[55,56] Close surveillance for preterm labor is recommended for the first week postoperatively, as delayed uterine irritability may be seen during this time period.[55] While the use of prophylactic tocolytic agents has been reported in pregnant patients undergoing laparoscopic cholecystectomy,[22,38] the only clear indication for their use is when postoperative premature labor develops.

Initial access to the peritoneal cavity can be obtained using either a closed or an open technique. While both methods have been used in the pregnant patient, the open technique seems to be preferred (see Table 10.2). The only advantage of closed laparoscopy is rapid access to the peritoneal cavity. There are numerous disadvantages, including the possibility of uterine injury in the pregnant patient following blind insertion of the Veress needle and initial trocar. Other complications associated with the closed technique include intestinal perforation and vascular injury. The open technique using the Hasson trocar should eliminate these complications, as there is no initial blind puncture. The length of the procedure is not significantly changed and may in fact be shortened when using the open technique.[57] The potential for causing a serious complication if the closed technique is used, though rare, must be considered. It is therefore recommended that the open technique be used to gain access when performing laparoscopic surgery in the pregnant patient. If a Veress needle is used, an alternate site should be used for insertion, such as the RUQ or epigastrium.

Prophylaxis against deep venous thrombosis (DVT) during laparoscopic cholecystectomy is generally recommended. Although there has been no study comparing the incidence of DVT in open and laparoscopic cholecystectomy, the risk may be increased due to the patient's positioning and increased intra-abdominal pressure seen with laparoscopic procedures. Abdominal insufflation has been shown to increase femoral venous pressure, slow peak blood velocity, increase femoral vein diameter, and reduce or eliminate pulsatility of the common femoral vein.[58,59] Insufflation pressures as low as 12 mmHg were noted to cause significant venous stasis. From these studies, it appears that significant venous stasis, a well-recognized risk factor for developing DVT, occurs during prolonged laparoscopic procedures.

The pregnant patient undergoing laparoscopic surgery is not at increased risk for developing DVT not only from venous stasis but from the pregnant state as well. Although there is no change in the standard coagulation function tests, pregnancy is generally thought to be a hypercoagulable state. The risk of thromboembolic disease is increased by a factor of 1.5 to 2 during pregnancy compared to the nongravid patient.[60] Venous stasis (induced by the gravid uterus), vascular injury (secondary to labor and delivery), and activation of blood coagulation may predispose the pregnant patient to venous thromboembolic disease.[61] Because of the venous stasis seen with laparoscopy and the hypercoagulable state associated with pregnancy, some form of DVT prophylaxis is required when laparoscopic surgery is performed in the gravid patient. Several methods are available, including pneumatic compression stockings and heparin (heparin does not cross the placenta and should not produce any fetal complications). Although pneumatic compression devices can produce pulsatile venous blood flow, there is little change in venous blood flow velocity.[58] Further studies are needed to determine the best method of DVT prophylaxis during laparoscopic surgery.

The need for intraoperative cholangiography (IOC) during laparoscopic cholecystectomy remains controversial. It is not within the scope of this chapter to discuss the pros and cons of routine versus selective cholangiography; rather, our purpose is to consider if it can be performed safely during laparoscopic cholecystectomy in the pregnant patient. IOC has been performed in the pregnant patient with no apparent ill effects (see Table 10.1). According to the American College of Radiology, no single diagnostic procedure results in a radiation dose significant enough to affect the well-being of the developing fetus.[62] A plain radiograph of the abdomen is preferable to fluoroscopy when IOC is to be performed due to the lower radiation exposure with the former. A lead apron placed over the patient's lower abdomen should effectively shield the fetus from any significant radiation exposure.

The technical considerations when laparoscopic cholecystectomy is to be performed in the pregnant patient are presented in Table 10.3. Several authors recommend maintaining the intra-abdominal pressure below 12 mmHg.[22,23] Though there is no scientific evidence that the standard pressure of 15 mmHg is harmful, a lower intra-abdominal pressure may produce less venous stasis. Also, in patients undergoing surgery in the late second third trimester, the operating room table should be rotated to displace the uterus from the vena cava so that venous return is unimpaired. This would seem to be a prudent maneuver given the venous stasis seen during laparoscopic procedures.

Table 10.3. Technical Considerations for Laparoscopic Cholecystectomy in the Pregnant Patient

DVT prophylaxis
Open laparoscopy
Rotate patient to displace gravid uterus from vena cava
Maintain intraabdominal pressure at 10–12 mmHg
Shield pelvis when performing IOC
Perioperative fetal monitoring
No clear role for prophylactic tocolytics

SUMMARY

Historically, surgeons have been reluctant to operate on the pregnant patient with symptomatic biliary tract disease for fear of inducing premature labor or spontaneous abortion. However, numerous articles over the past decade have shown that cholecystectomy, both open and laparoscopic, can be performed safely in this group of patients with minimal maternal or fetal morbidity. Symptomatic cholelithiasis during pregnancy is no longer an absolute contraindication for laparoscopic cholecystectomy, according to a recent National Institute of Health consensus conference on gallstones and laparoscopic cholecystectomy.[63] Although further study is required to clarify the effects of CO_2 pneumoperitoneum on the fetus, given the numerous advantages of laparoscopic cholecystectomy over open cholecystectomy, the laparoscopic approach may be the procedure of choice when cholecystectomy is indicated in the gravid patient.

REFERENCES

1. Saunders KD, Cates JA, Roslyn JJ: Pathogenesis of gallstones. *Surg Clin North Am* 70:1197–1216, 1990.
2. Chesson RR, Gallup DG, Gibbs RL, et al: Ultrasonic diagnosis of asymptomatic cholelithiasis in pregnancy. *J Reprod Med* 30:920–922, 1985.
3. Stauffer RA, Adams A, Wygal J, et al: Gallbladder disease in pregnancy. *Am J Obstet Gynecol* 144:661–664, 1982.
4. Braverman DZ, Johnson ML, Kern F: effects of pregnancy and contraceptive steroids on gallbladder function. *N Engl J Med* 302:362–364, 1980.
5. Smith JJ, Pomaranc MM, Ivy AC: The influence of pregnancy and sex hormones on gallbladder motility in the guinea pig. *Am J Physiol* 132:129–140, 1941.
6. Cunningham FG: Gastrointestinal disorders. In Cunningham FG, MacDonald PC, Gant NF, et al (eds): *Williams Obstetrics*, ed 19, Suppl 7. Norwalk, CT, Appleton & Lange, 1993, p 11.
7. Hill LM, Johnson CE, Lee RA: Cholecystectomy in pregnancy. *Obstet Gynecol* 46:291–293, 1975.
8. Hiatt JR, Hiatt JCG, Williams RA, et al: Biliary disease in pregnancy: Strategy for surgical management. *Am J Surg* 151:263–265, 1986.
9. Landers D, Carmona R, Crombleholme W, et al: Acute cholecystitis in pregnancy. *Obstet Gynecol* 69:131–133, 1987.
10. Simon JA: Biliary tract disease and related surgical disorders during pregnancy. *Clin Obstet Gynecol* 26:810–821, 1983.
11. Sharp HT: Gastrointestinal surgical conditions during pregnancy. *Clin Obstet Gynecol* 37:306–315, 1994.
12. Swisher SG, Schmit PJ, Hunt KK, et al: Biliary disease during pregnancy. *Am J Surg* 168:576–581, 1994.
13. Morgenstern L, Sackier JM: Acute and chronic cholecystitis. In Cameron JL (ed): *Current Surgical Therapy*, ed 4. St Louis, Mosby Year Book, 1992, p 340.
14. Dixon NP, Faddis DM, Silberman H: Aggressive management of cholecystitis during pregnancy. *Am J Surg* 154: 292–294, 1987.
15. McKellar DP, Anderson CT, Boynton CJ, et al: Cholecystectomy during pregnancy without fetal loss. *Surg Gynecol Obstet* 174:465–468, 1992.
16. Reddick EA, Olsen DO: Laparoscopic laser cholecystectomy: A comparison with mini-lap cholecystectomy. *Surg Endosc* 3:131–133, 1989.
17. Cappuccino H, Cargill S, Nguyen T: Laparoscopic cholecystectomy: 563 cases at a community teaching hospital and a review of 12,201 cases in the literature. *Surg Laparosc Endosc* 4:213–221, 1994.
18. Gadacz TR, Talamini MA: Traditional versus laparoscopic cholecystectomy. *Am J Surg* 161:336–338, 1991.
19. Arvidsson D, Gerdin E: Laparoscopic cholecystectomy during pregnancy. *Surg Laparosc Endosc* 1:193–194, 1991.
20. Pucci RO, Seed RW: Case report of laparoscopic cholecystectomy in the third trimester of pregnancy. *Am J Obstet Gynecol* 165:401–402, 1991.
21. Weber AM, Bloom GP, Allan TR, et al: Laparoscopic cholecystectomy during pregnancy. *Obstet Gynecol* 78: 958–959, 1991.
22. Soper NJ, Hunter JG, Petrie RH: Laparoscopic cholecystectomy during pregnancy. *Surg Endosc* 6:115–117, 1992.
23. Morell DG, Mullins JR, Harrison PB: Laparoscopic cholecystectomy during pregnancy in symptomatic patients. *Surgery* 112:856–859, 1992.
24. Adamsen S, Jacobsen B, Bentzon N: Laparoscopic cholecystectomy during pregnancy. [Danish] *Ugeskrift for Laeger* 155:2215–2216, 1993.
25. Bennett TL, Estes N: Laparoscopic cholecystectomy in the second trimester of pregnancy: A case report. *J Reprod Med* 38:833–834, 1993.
26. Elerding S: Laparoscopic cholecystectomy in pregnancy. *Am J Surg* 165:625–627, 1993.
27. Fabiani P, Bongain A, Persch M, et al: Endoscopic surgery during pregnancy: a case report of cholecystectomy. [French] *J Gynecol Obstet Biol Reprod* 22:317–319, 1993.
28. Hart RO, Tamadon A, Fitzgibbons RJ, et al: Open laparo-

scopic cholecystectomy in pregnancy. *Surg Laparosc Endosc* 3:13–16, 1993.

29. Jackson SJ, Sigman HH: Laparoscopic cholecystectomy in pregnancy. *J Laparoendosc Surg* 3:35–39, 1993.
30. Rusher AH, Fields B, Henson K: Laparoscopic cholecystectomy in pregnancy: Contraindicated or indicated. *J Ark Med Soc* 89:383–384, 1993.
31. Schorr RT: Laparoscopic cholecystectomy and pregnancy. *J Laparoendosc Surg* 3:291–293, 1993.
32. Chandra M, Shapiro SJ, Gordon LA: Laparoscopic cholecystectomy in the first trimester of pregnancy. *Surg Laparosc Endosc* 4:68–69, 1994.
33. Comitalo JB, Lynch D: Laparoscopic cholecystectomy in the pregnant patient. *Surg Laparosc Endosc* 4:268–271, 1994.
34. Constantino GN, Vincent GJ, Mukalian GG, et al: Laparoscopic cholecystectomy in pregnancy. *J Laparoendosc Surg* 4:161–164, 1994.
35. Csaba J, Orban I: Laparoscopic cholecystectomy during the 25th week of pregnancy. [Hungarian] *Orvosi Hetilap* 135:1421–1422, 1994.
36. Shaked G, Twena M, Charuzi I: Laparoscopic cholecystectomy for empyema of gallbladder during pregnancy. *Surg Laparosc Endosc* 4:65–67, 1994.
37. Wilson RB, McKenzie RJ, Fisher JW: Laparoscopic cholecystectomy in pregnancy: Two case reports. *Aust NZ J Surg* 64:647–649, 1994.
38. Lanzafame RJ: Laparoscopic cholecystectomy in pregnancy. *Surgery* 118:627–633, 1995.
39. Panton ONM, Nagy AG, Scudamore CH, et al: Laparoscopic cholecystectomy, a continuing plea for routine cholangiography. *Surg Laparosc Endosc* 5:43–49, 1995.
40. Reedy MB: Laparoscopy during pregnancy. *SLS Report*, 3:3, 1994.
41. Wittgen CM, Andrus CH, Fitzgerald SD, et al: Analysis of hemodynamic and ventilatory effects of laparoscopic cholecystectomy. *Arch Surg* 126:997–1001, 1991.
42. Barnard JM, Chaffin D, Droste S, et al: Fetal response to carbon dioxide pneumoperitoneum in the pregnant ewe. *Obstet Gynecol* 85:669–674, 1995.
43. Westerband A, Van De Water JM, Amzallag M, et al: Cardiovascular changes during laparoscopic cholecystectomy. *Surg Gynecol Obstet* 175:535–538, 1992.
44. Noirot D, Legrand JM, Lamy M: Hemodynamic changes during pneumoperitoneum for laparoscopic cholecystectomy. *Anesthesiology* 77:A69, 1992.
45. Mclaughlin JG, Bonnell BW, Scheeres DE, et al: The adverse hemodynamic effects related to laparoscopic cholecystectomy. *Anesthesiology* 77:A70, 1992.
46. Cunningham FG, MacDonald PC, Gant NF, et al (eds): *Williams Obstetrics*, ed 19. Norwalk, CT, Appleton & Lange, 1993, p 1083.
47. Nezhat F, Nezhat C, Silfen SL, et al: Laparoscopic ovarian cystectomy during pregnancy. *J Laparoendosc Surg* 1:161–164, 1991.
48. Wittich AC, Lockrow EG: Laparoscopic management of adnexal torsion in early pregnancy: A case report. *Milit Med* 159:254–255, 1994.
49. Shalev E, Peleg D: Laparoscopic treatment of adnexal torsion. *Surg Gynecol Obstet* 176:448–450, 1993.
50. Schreiber JH: Results of outpatient laparoscopic appendectomy in women. *Endoscopy* 26:292–298, 1994.
51. Swisher SG, Hunt KK, Schmit PJ, et al: Management of pancreatitis complicating pregnancy. *Am Surg* 60:759–762, 1994.
52. Block P, Kelly TR: Management of gallstone pancreatitis during pregnancy and the postpartum period. *Surg Gynecol Obstet* 168:426–428, 1989.
53. Soper NJ, Brunt M, Callery MP, et al: Role of laparoscopic cholecystectomy in the management of acute gallstone pancreatitis. *Am J Surg* 167:42–51, 1994.
54. Baillie J, Cairns SR, Cotton PB: Endoscopic management of choledocholithiasis during pregnancy. *Surg Gynecol Obstet* 171:1–4, 1990.
55. Kort B, Katz VL, Watson WJ: The effect of nonobstetric operation during pregnancy. *Surg Gynecol Obstet* 177:371–376, 1993.
56. Hunt MG, Martin JN, Martin RW, et al: Perinatal aspects of abdominal surgery for nonobstetric disease. *Am J Perinatol* 6:412–417, 1989.
57. Sigman HH, Fried GM, Garzon J, et al: Risks of blind versus open approach to celiotomy for laparoscopic surgery. *Surg Laparosc Endosc* 3:296–299, 1993.
58. Beebe DS, McNevin MP, Crain JM, et al: Evidence of venous stasis after abdominal insufflation for laparoscopic cholecystectomy. *Surg Gynecol Obstet* 176:443–447, 1993.
59. Jorgensen JO, Lalak NJ, North L, et al: Venous stasis during laparoscopic cholecystectomy. *Surg Laparosc Endosc* 4:128–133, 1994.
60. Martin C, Varner MW: Physiologic changes in pregnancy: Surgical implications. *Clin Obstet Gynecol* 37:241–255, 1994.
61. LeClerc JR, Hirsh J: Venous thromboembolic disorders. In Burrow GN, Ferris TF (eds). *Medical Complications During Pregnancy*, ed 3. Philadelphia, Saunders, 1988, pp 204–206.
62. Cunningham FG, MacDonald PC, Gant NF, et al (eds): *Williams Obstetrics*, ed 19. Norwalk, CT, Appleton & Lange, 1993, p 984.
63. NIH Consensus Conference: Gallstones and laparoscopic cholecystectomy. *JAMA* 269:1018– 1024,1993.

section three

Hernias and Pelvic Surgery

chapter eleven

Anatomy of the Anterior Abdominal Wall and Deep Inguinal Region from the Laparoscopic Surgeon's Perspective

Thomas H. Quinn
Ardith Ryberg
Riccardo Annibali
Robert J. Fitzgibbons, Jr.

The advent of laparoscopy has introduced an element of remoteness to surgical practice. Surgeons can no longer rely on the sensitivity of fingertips or direct visualization of the operative field for sensory cues. Palpation of structures is distanced by intervening instrumentation. Magnified laparoscopic images fill video screens during laparoscopy in lieu of direct visual input. The techniques advocated during the rapid development of laparoscopic hernia repair in the last decade have been analyzed by Salerno, Fitzgibbons, Camps, and their colleagues.[1–3] It is clear that the constant evolution of this new procedure mandates a thorough knowledge of the anatomy of this region. Minimally invasive surgery cannot be equated with minimum risk unless the perspective of the basic anatomy encountered in laparoscopic herniorrhaphy is mastered.

The vantage point used for laparoscopic procedures, including inguinal herniorrhaphy, is quite different from that used in conventional surgery or in basic anatomic study of the region. The anatomy of the inguinal region, as perceived from indirect visual information during laparoscopy, may be somewhat disorienting to one who is accustomed only to conventional repairs. The surgeon who has mastered the anatomy of the region significantly reduces the possibility of unforseen complications.

This chapter provides a thorough analysis of the surgical anatomy of the anterior abdominal wall and the deep inguinal region as it is encountered in laparoscopic herniorrhaphy. Emphasis is placed on those structures that may be used as landmarks and on structures most often inadvertently damaged during inguinal hernia repair.

INTERIOR ASPECT OF THE ANTERIOR ABDOMINAL WALL

The Peritoneal (Umbilical) Folds or Ligaments, Their Contents, and the Peritoneal Fossae

The traditional method of describing the anatomy of the abdominal wall and inguinal region in anatomy and surgery texts is a progression through the superficial layers of abdominal fascia and musculature proceeding to the deeper structures. The laparoscopic surgeon, however, must first concentrate on the interior of the anterior abdominal wall and the deep inguinal region. For this reason, our description begins with the peritoneal surface of the anterior abdominal wall.

The peritoneum of the anterior abdominal wall consists of a monolayer of mesothelial cells supported by a thin sheet of connective tissue. It is replete with blood vessels and nerves derived during development from the somatopleure and is therefore sensitive to mechanical, thermal, and chemical stimuli.[4] The principal anatomic landmarks of the anterior abdominal wall when the abdominal cavity is insufflated with CO_2 are the parietal peritoneal folds or ligaments (Fig. 11.1). The current nomenclature pertaining to these folds is, respectively, *median, medial*, and *lateral peritoneal folds*.[5]

The median fold is formed by the presence of the urachus, the fibrous remnant of the fetal allantois. This structure may be very conspicuous or nearly hidden from view. The urachus is attached inferiorly to the fundus of the bladder. The urachus may be partially patent in some individuals, forming an open connection with the bladder and, in rare instances, the umbilicus.[6,7]

The obliterated portion of the umbilical artery is found in the peritoneum, forming the medial umbilical folds, while the lateral umbilical folds cover the inferior epigastric vessels. The peritoneum is reflected further from the anterior abdominal wall by the bladder. A transverse vesical fold of peritoneum is sometimes present spanning the area between the deep inguinal rings.

The peritoneal folds and the bladder serve as the structural boundaries of shallow depressions called the *peritoneal fossae* (see Fig. 11.1). The supravesical fossa is superior to the bladder. Its borders are the median and medial umbilical ligaments. The median fossa is the site of egress of a direct inguinal hernia; it covers the inguinal (Hesselbach's) triangle. It is bounded by the medial and lateral umbilical ligaments. The lateral fossa, in which the deep inguinal ring is located, is the site of an indirect inguinal hernia. The lateral umbilical ligament covering the inferior epigastric vessels and the lateral border of the rectus abdominis form the distinct medial border of the fossa. The lateral border usually is not distinct when the abdominal wall is distended during laparoscopy.

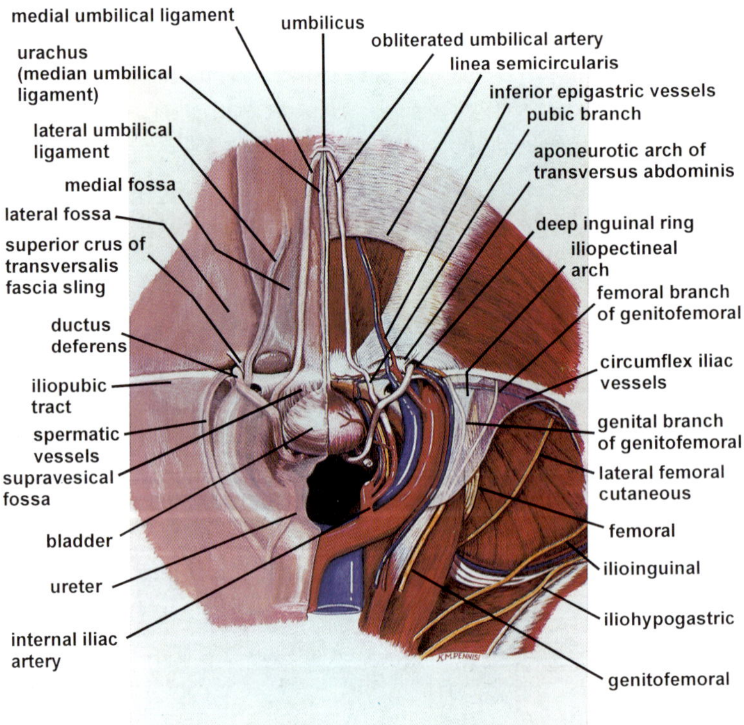

Figure 11.1. The anterior abdominal wall and deep inguinal region. The intact peritoneum, peritoneal folds, and fossae are shown on the left.

The Transversalis Fascia and the Preperitoneal Space

In order to carry out the transabdominal preperitoneal (TAPP) hernia repair now favored by many surgeons, the peritoneum is carefully opened from the anterior superior iliac spine to the medial umbilical ligament.[2] The preperitoneal structures may then be dissected.

The preperitoneal space is readily dissected, but its contents are complex and the subject of considerable contention. The debate centers on the first substantial layer of fibrous tissue encountered after the peritoneum is incised and reflected; should this layer be designated the *posterior lamina of the transversalis fascia* or the *preperitoneal fascia*? Cooper originally named and described the transversalis fascia, stating that it is a bilaminar structure.[8,9] Until recently, however, most authors have stated that there is only one layer of transversalis fascia.[10–12] Read recently reintroduced Cooper's original description of the transversalis fascia as a bilaminar structure.[13] He posed the following question: "is the transversalis fascia a single layer enveloping the abdomen, separate from the extraperitoneal fat in which the epigastric vasculature courses, or does it have a posterior lamina as described by Cooper, on which, as Mackay found, the blood supply to the recti passes?"[14]

In our experience, there is, in fact, a relatively dense second layer of tissue present just anterior (superficial) to and contiguous with the peritoneum. Our observations in the dissection laboratory and during the laparoscopic TAPP procedure, when only the peritoneal layer is incised, lend support to Read's concept of a substantial posterior lamina deep to the inferior epigastric vessels and attached to the pubic ramus inferiorly.[13] It is this layer that is often referred to as the *preperitoneal fascia*.[10,12,15–17] Throughout the remainder of this chapter, it will be called the *posterior lamina of the transversalis fascia*.

The plane created by blunt dissection between the peritoneum and the posterior lamina, if carried inferomedially, leads toward the urachus (median umbilical ligament) and the bladder and should therefore be avoided during hernia repair.[18] The posterior lamina, when opened, allows access to the preperitoneal fat and the epigastric vessels contained within it. Lateral dissection carried out in this plane proceeds unhindered until the linea semilunaris is encountered. Here fibers of the transversalis fascia fuse with anastomotic rectus sheath fibers, preventing further lateral progress into the retroperitoneal fat. The space encompassed by the layers of the transversalis fascia is further delimited as follows: (1) medially by intermeshing of posterior lamina fibers with the linea alba, (2) superiorly by the fusion of the lamina near the linea semicircularis (line of Douglas), and (3) inferiorly by its insertion on the superior ramus of the pubis.[18] The preperitoneal space thus formed is filled with a pyramid-shaped layer of fat, with its apex often nearly at the level of the umbilicus.

The concept of a bilaminar transversalis fascia is supported by Lytle, who described the deep inguinal ring as being formed by the transversalis fascia sling or "monk's hood" (Fig. 11.2). This sling is composed of a superior and an inferior crus.[19–22] The thicker medial aspect of the structure is formed by a redundant portion of the transversalis fascia created by the passage of the testicle during development. The crura of the deep ring are pulled upward and laterally when the abdominal muscles, especially the transversus abdominis, contract. This motion helps to create a valvular mechanism that normally prevents indirect hernia formation.[21,22] Our dissections indicate that the deep ring may incorporate tissue from both layers of the transversalis fascia, with the majority of the medial fibers arising from the anterior lamina of the transversalis fascia proper. The deep ring from which the internal spermatic fascia arises also transmits the ductus deferens, the testicular artery, the pampiniform plexus veins, and the genital branch of the genitofemoral nerve (Figs. 11.1, 11.2, and 11.3).

The anterior lamina of the transversalis fascia is generally accepted as the transversalis fascia proper. This layer of fascia is a portion of the endoabdominal fascia which covers separate muscles and aponeuroses or becomes attached to the periosteum of bony structures; it generally creates an envelope investing the entire abdomen.[12,23,21] The anterior lamina of the transversalis fascia covers the deep surface of the transversus abdominis and its aponeurosis, and is continuous with the fascia covering the psoas major and minor, the iliacus, and the obturator muscles.

Transversalis Fascia Analogues

The various condensations of the transversalis fascia have been called the *transversalis fascia analogues*.[25] One of these, the transversalis fascia sling, was previously discussed. Other transversalis fascia analogues important to the surgeon include the iliopubic tract, the pectineal (Cooper's) ligament, and the iliopectineal arch (Figs. 11.1 and 11.4). These analogues are among the most important structures to be considered since they provide vital landmarks and, in some cases, a firm substrate into which staples can be placed.

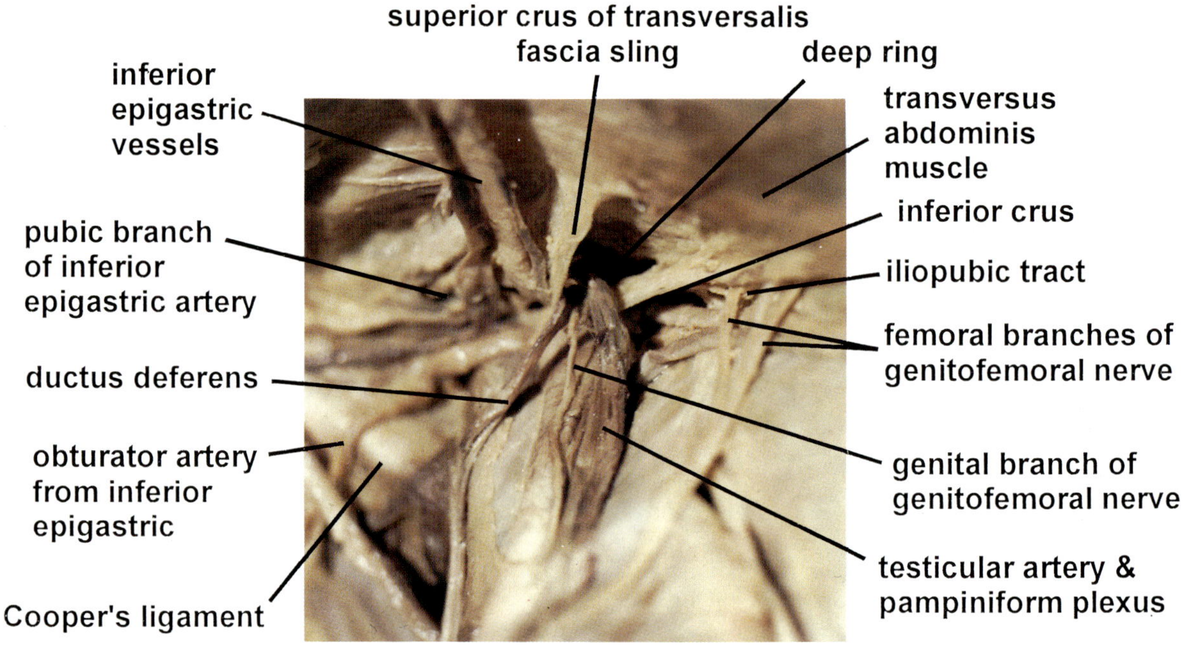

Figure 11.2. The deep inguinal ring and the structures it transmits. This is an enlarged view of the right deep inguinal ring of the dissection shown in Figure 11.3.

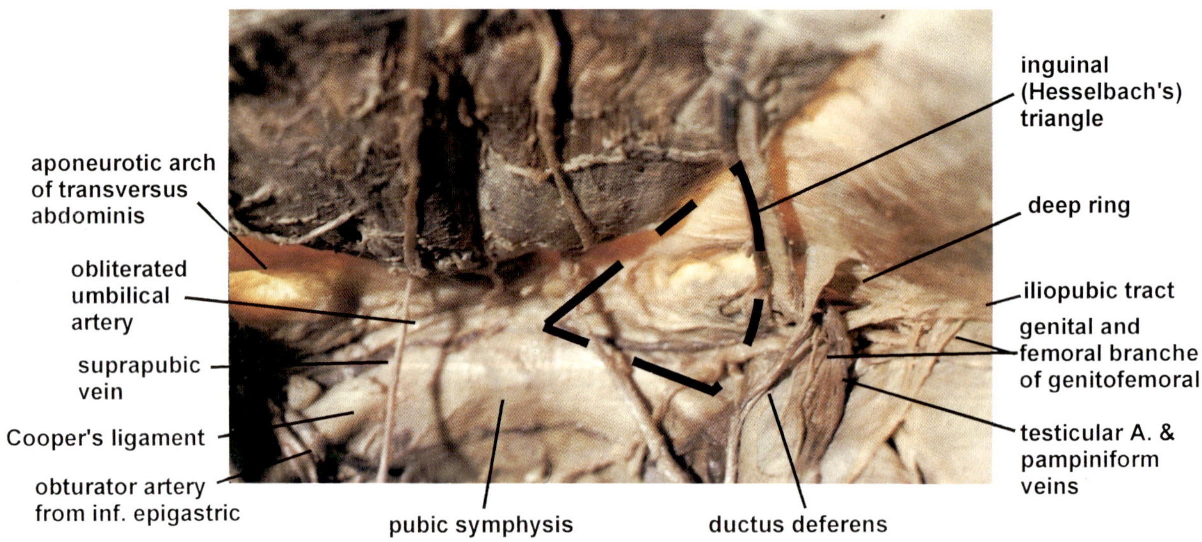

Figure 11.3. A transilluminated dissection of the deep anterior abdominal wall and inguinal region with the bladder and urachus removed. The supra- and retropubic vasculature can be seen.

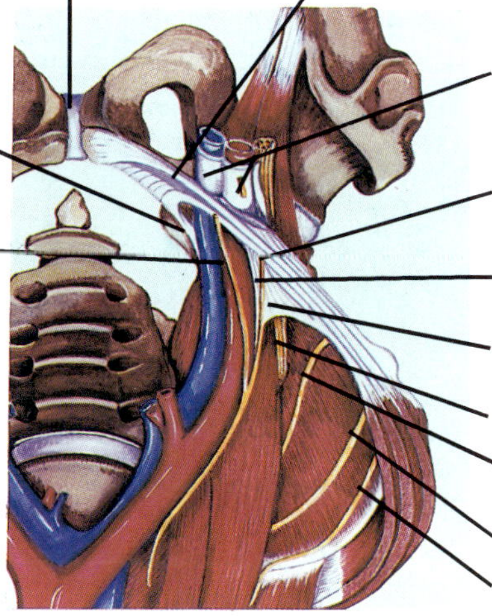

Figure 11.4. A view of the pelvis and inguinal region from the laparoscopic surgeon's perspective. Note the proximity of the branches of the lumbar plexus to the iliopubic ligament.

The *iliopubic tract* (Figs. 11.1, 11.2, and 11.4) is described as an aponeurotic band forming the inferior margin of the transversus abdominis lamina.[26] This portion of the transversalis fascia arises from the medial iliac crest and parallels the inguinal ligament in its course toward the pubis. It forms the inferior border of the deep inguinal ring and a portion of the anterior and medial femoral sheaths before insertion on the pubic tubercle and the medial part of Cooper's ligament. The iliopubic tract also forms the posterior wall of the inguinal canal and fuses with the inguinal ligament to form the floor of the canal. Although the importance of this structure to the surgeon is often debated, Gilroy et al. have recently shown that it contains both collagenous and elastic fibers and is a substantial structure in 42% of the specimens studied.[27] Condon observed that the iliopubic tract is often a substantial band useful in inguinal hernia repair.[28] Its usefulness may differ according to whether a conventional or laparoscopic approach is used. This possibility should be realized when the literature states that a structure is unsuitable for use in hernia repair.[29] Although the iliopubic tract is not always exposed during the course of a radical preperitoneal dissection for the TAPP procedure, its approximate location must be appreciated by the surgeon. Staples should be placed above the iliopubic tract (Figs. 11.1, 11,2, and 11.4) to avoid serious complications when stapling lateral to the testicular (internal spermatic) artery and pampiniform plexus (Fig. 11.2).

The pectineal (Cooper's) ligament (Fig. 11.1) is the combination of tough fibrous and periosteal tissue covering the superior pubic ramus.[30] Its medial aspect is blended with the lacunar ligament composed of reflected fibers of the inguinal ligament. The pectineal ligament is a substantial structure important not only as an easily distinguished landmark, but also as a sturdy anchoring surface when placing staples or sutures during hernia repair.[18,31,32]

The iliopectineal arch (Fig. 11.1) is a condensation of the transversalis fascia which commences at the medial border of the iliacus muscle and is continuous with the iliac fascia. The arch inserts medially at the iliopectineal eminence. Some of the muscular or aponeurotic fibers of all layers of the lateral abdominal wall originate from this arch.[22,28] The iliopectineal arch also separates the vascular compartment containing the femoral vessels from the neuromuscular compartment containing the iliopsoas muscle, as well as the femoral and lateral femoral cutaneous nerves. The proximal portion of the lateral femoral sheath is formed by the inferior most portion of the arch.

The Transversus Abdominis Muscle

The deepest muscle of the abdominal wall arises from the 6th to the 12th ribs, the lumbodorsal fascia, the iliopubic tract, and the iliopectineal arch. The muscle terminates in a relatively thick aponeurosis which forms a portion of the rectus abdominis sheath. The medial extent of the muscle fibers of the transversus abdominis varies. Thus, the aponeurosis covers more of the anterior abdominal wall than the muscular portion.[10,33,34] The inferior portion of the aponeurosis forms the aponeurotic arch (Figs. 11.1 and 11.3), which inserts on the pubic tubercle medially. This arch, along with the superior crus, forms the superior border of the deep inguinal ring. The height of the arch from the inguinal ligament determines the effectiveness of the transversus abdominis in providing a shutter mechanism which brings the arch closer to the inguinal ligament during abdominal muscle contraction.[22,35,36] The transversus abdominis in some individuals does not contribute any tissue to the lower abdominal wall in the region of the inguinal (Hesselbach's) triangle. Internal support is provided only by the transversalis fascia and the peritoneum.

The Inguinal (Hesselbach's) Triangle

The inguinal triangle (Fig. 11.3), as originally described by Hesselbach, is an area of the abdominal wall bounded superolaterally by the inferior epigastric vessels, medially by the rectus muscle, and inferiorly by the pectineal (Cooper's) ligament.[37,38] The inguinal ligament, however, provides the base of the triangle in most subsequent descriptions since it is visible in conventional herniorrhaphy.[39,40] We have retained the original description since it is visible and most useful to the surgeon approaching the area laparoscopically. Transillumination of the inguinal triangle (Fig. 11.3) demonstrates that the weakest (most translucent) area is bordered superiorly by the aponeurotic arch of the transversus abdominis in most cases. The remainder of the triangle internally is covered only by transversalis fascia and peritoneum. The aponeurotic portions of the external and internal abdominal oblique muscles primarily pass anterior to the rectus abdominis muscle at the linea semicircularis.[41] The inguinal triangle is located anteroinferiorly to the supravesical and medial umbilical fossae, the sites of direct inguinal herniation.

VASCULATURE OF THE ANTERIOR ABDOMINAL WALL AND DEEP INGUINAL REGION

Since many major vessels traverse the surgical field in a laparoscopic herniorrhaphy, a firm understanding of the location of these vessels is imperative. Although the inferior epigastric vessels and the umbilical arteries have been briefly considered in relation to the umbilical folds, some additional points concerning these arteries warrant discussion. The obliterated portion of the umbilical artery is seen as a distinct cord in the medial umbilical folds. The degree of obliteration of this branch of the internal iliac artery varies, and the lumen of the vessel may extend into the medial fold. A variable number of superficial vesical arteries arise from the patent portion of this artery.[42] The inferior epigastric vessels (Figs. 11.1, 11.2, and 11.3) may be easily seen through the peritoneum. The inferior epigastric artery normally arises from the external iliac artery at the level of the inguinal ligament. The inferior epigastric veins run in the manner of the vasa vasorum on either side of the artery; they are tributaries of the external iliac vein. The origin of the inferior epigastric artery is variable; it may, on rare occasions, arise from an unusually high (proximal) portion of the external iliac or from the femoral, obturator, or profunda femoris arteries.[43,44] The inferior epigastric vessels pierce the posterior lamina of the transversalis fascia and ascend in the preperitoneal fat for a short distance to enter the posterior rectus sheath at the linea semicircularis. The subsequent course and ramifications of the terminal branches of the inferior epigastric artery have been well documented by Milloy et al.[45]

Two small but important branches of the inferior epigastric artery are the cremasteric (formerly the external spermatic) artery and the pubic branch. The cremasteric artery courses along the medial aspect of the deep inguinal ring and pierces the external spermatic fascia to join the spermatic cord. The usually minute pubic branch of the inferior epigastric artery initially follows the iliopubic tract, then turns inferiorly to cross the pectineal ligament. It often anastomoses with the obturator artery (Figs. 11.1, 11.2, and 11.3).

The pubic branch of the inferior epigastric artery, when enlarged, is often either an accessory obturator artery or is the replacement of the more usual obturator branch from the internal iliac artery (Fig. 11.3). Pick et al. and Delitzin found that the obturator artery is a branch of the inferior epigastric in 27% of 640 dissections; it is a direct branch of the internal iliac artery or its other branches in the vast majority of specimens.[46,47] The course of the obturator artery from an inferior epigastric origin to the obturator foramen carries the artery across the pectineal ligament, where it may be inadvertently stapled during mesh fixation.[22]

The deep circumflex iliac artery arises from the distal external iliac artery just lateral to the origin of the inferior epigastric. The deep circumflex artery and vein run laterally between the iliopubic tract and the iliopectineal arch before piercing the transversalis fascia. Their initial course places them in contiguity with one of the ligamentous structures most often used to anchor surgical mesh in this area: the iliopubic tract.[22]

The veins of the preperitoneal space and deep inguinal region are considerably larger and more easily visualized than their accompanying arteries. The veins of this area (Fig. 11.3) have recently been described in some detail by Bendavid.[48] He indicated that anastomotic venous loops occur not only in the retropubic area between the obturator and retropubic veins, but also between the iliopubic vein and the so-called rectusial veins which drain a portion of the rectus abdominis muscle (Fig. 11.3). Familiarity with these vessels is necessary if serious hematomas in this area are to be avoided.

CONSTITUENTS OF THE SPERMATIC CORD

The component structures of the spermatic cord as they relate to laparoscopic surgery are best appreciated by first analyzing their course and relations just prior to entry into the deep inguinal ring (Figs. 11.1, 11.2, 11.3, and 11.5). The ductus (vas) deferens, testicular artery, pampiniform veins, and genital branch of the genitofemoral nerve converge at the deep ring. All are encountered and easily visualized during laparoscopic inguinal hernia repair. The tunica vaginalis, an important component of the enclosed spermatic cord structures, will be considered in this section due to its role in the development of inguinal hernias. The structures comprising the deep ring should also be reviewed at this point (Fig. 11.2).

The Ductus (Vas) Deferens

The ductus deferens (Figs. 11.1, 11.2, and 11.3) is intraoperatively observed as it exits the deep inguinal ring and turns medially rather sharply around the inferior epigastric vessels. Although it is covered by the peritoneum, it can be easily seen as it courses first across the external iliac vessels, the obliterated umbilical and superior vesical arteries, and the obturator nerve and artery. The ductus deferens receives its blood supply from the superior vesical arteries, which eventually anastomose with the testicular artery.

The Testicular Artery and Pampiniform Plexus

The testicular artery is an elongated branch of the abdominal aorta. It descends with the testicle during development, arising immediately inferior to the renal arteries but superior to the inferior mesenteric artery. The testicular artery is entwined by the pampiniform plexus of veins (Fig. 11.5). Because of its thin structure, the testicular artery must be manipulated carefully to avoid vascular compromise during reduction of a hernial sac.

The Genitofemoral Nerve

The genital branch of the genitofemoral nerve (Figs. 11.1 to 11.5) is usually a constituent of the cord which passes through the deep inguinal ring. However, the genitofemoral nerve is considered the most variable

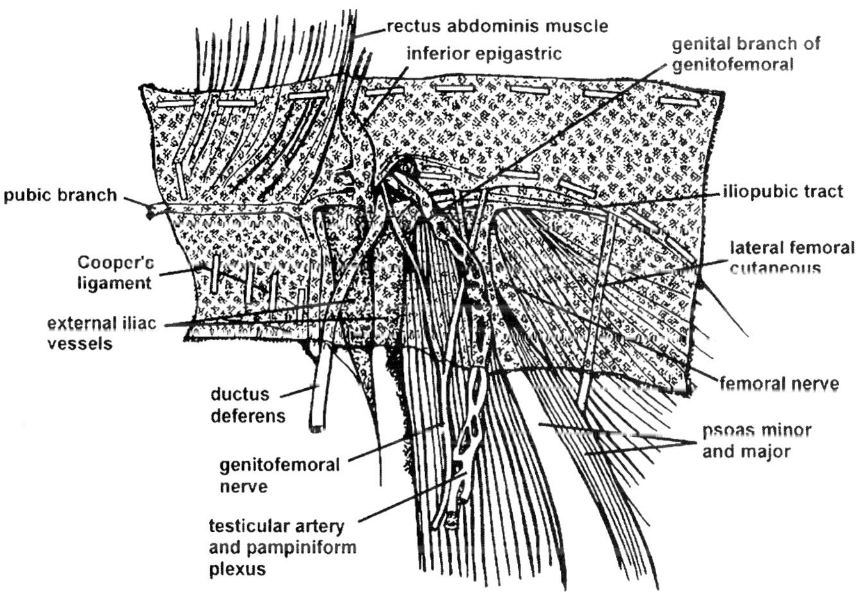

Figure 11.5. Drawing of the dissection seen in Figure 11.3. Mesh has been secured to Cooper's ligament; the posterior rectus abdominis muscle and the adjacent area along a horizontal line; and the area immediately superior to the iliopubic tract. Staples are placed lateral to the testicular artery and pampiniform plexus and above the iliopubic tract to avoid injury to nerves and vessels.

branch of the lumbar plexus. Occasionally it divides within the psoas muscle and emerges as two trunks. The genital branch may be located superior to the deep ring or it may be absent. If the nerve is not present, it may be replaced by a branch of the ilioinguinal nerve.[49,50]

Coverings of the Spermatic Cord

The cord is ensheathed by three layers (Fig. 11.6) which are acquired as the testicle descends through the layers of the abdominal wall. The innermost layer, the internal spermatic fascia, is derived from the transversalis fascia. The middle, or cremasteric, layer originates from the internal abdominal oblique muscle and provides the cremaster muscle fibers. The intermediate inguinal ring proposed by Yeager (Fig. 11.6) is the source of these fibers.[51] Finally, the external spermatic fascia is derived from the external abdominal oblique.

The Tunica Vaginalis

The tunica vaginalis is present in the spermatic cord, but in most cases its upper portion, which was in communication with the peritoneal cavity during fetal development, closes during the first year of life. It should be appreciated that the testicle does not descend into the tunica vaginalis but rather invaginates it posteriorly. Thus, the testicle is covered only anteriorly by an invaginated sac consisting of a visceral layer and a parietal layer of the tunica vaginalis. When the tunica vaginalis remains patent, intestinal loops may be forced into the canal, resulting in congenital inguinal hernia.

NERVES OF THE LUMBAR PLEXUS ENCOUNTERED DURING LAPAROSCOPIC HERNIA REPAIR

The results of a recent multicenter trial of laparoscopic herniorrhaphy indicate that a thorough knowledge of the anatomy of the nerve supply to the lower abdominal wall, groin, and thigh is indispensable if persistent postoperative pain due to improper staple placement is to be minimized.[3] It is now evident that staples placed inferior to the iliopubic tract and lateral to the femoral vessels may result in damage to the nerves of the lumbar plexus.[20,22,52] The placement of staples and mesh, as indicated in Figure 11.5, avoids neural and vascular damage while taking advantage of the strong fibers of Cooper's pectineal ligament and the iliopubic tract.

The innervation of the lower abdominal wall and the majority of the inguinal region is derived from the lumbar plexus. The nerve roots of the plexus, in turn, arise from the 12th thoracic nerve and from lumbar nerves 1 through 4. The branches of the five major nerves inner-

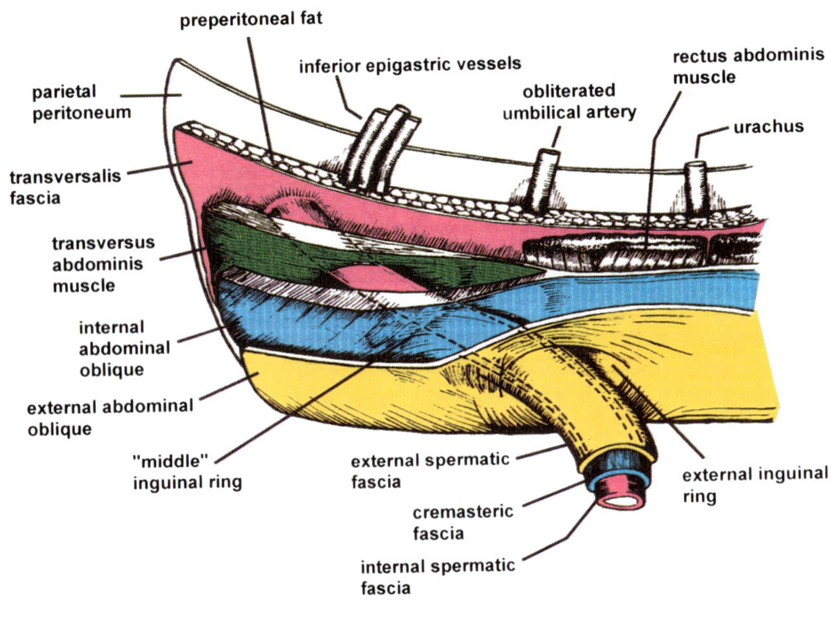

Figure 11.6. The middle inguinal ring and the coverings of the spermatic cord. (After Ref. 51.)

vating the area involved in hernia repair can normally be visualized through the peritoneum (Figs. 11.1, 11.3, and 11.4) as they course toward the anterior abdominal wall, groin, and thigh. Their cutaneous components innervate the areas indicated in Figure 11.7. All of the branches of the lumbar plexus are variable in terms of origin, interconnections with adjacent nerves, and intermuscular course. The five branches of the lumbar plexus in which we are particularly interested are related to the psoas major muscle. The most anterior of these nerves, and the one most often encountered directly during laparoscopy, is the genitofemoral nerve (Figs. 11.1 to 11.5).

The genitofemoral nerve is located retroperitonealy, most often as a single trunk (80%) emerging from the anterior portion of the psoas muscle. This nerve is considered by many, however, to be the most variable nerve in the plexus.[50,53] Its component genital and femoral branches may arise separately (20%) within the psoas muscle. The more medial of the two branches, the genital branch, enters the deep inguinal ring and traverses the inguinal canal. It is the motor nerve to the cremaster muscle and provides sensory innervation to part of the scrotum and penis. The femoral portion of the genitofemoral nerve usually bifurcates before crossing the deep circumflex iliac vessels and passing under the iliopubic tract. The normal cutaneous distribution of the femoral branch of the genitofemoral nerve is to the femoral triangle and the anteromedial surface of the upper thigh (Fig. 11.7). This distribution may be more extensive, covering up to two-thirds of the thigh.[49]

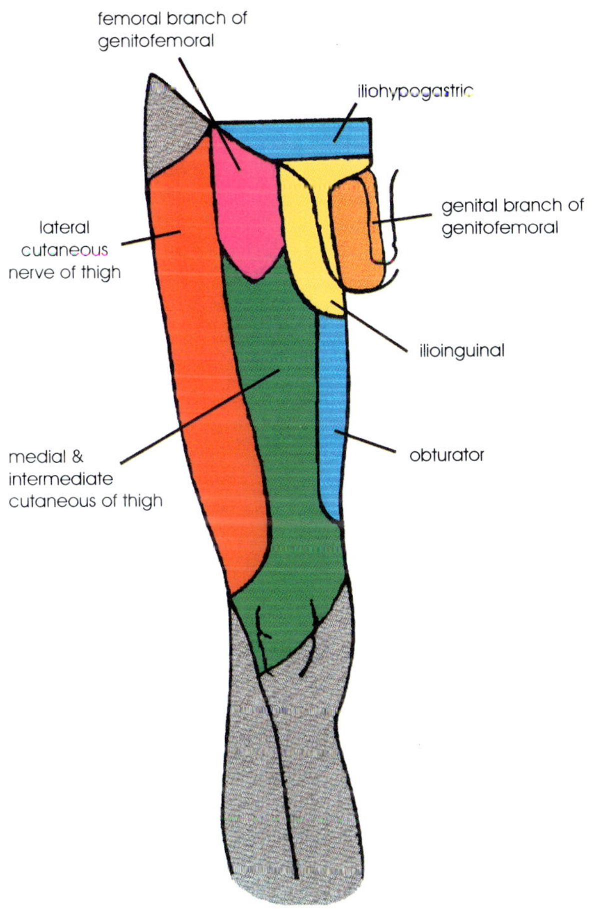

Figure 11.7. The cutaneous innervation of the thigh, inguinal region, and genitalia by branches of the lumbar plexus.

The iliohypogastric and the ilioinguinal nerves (Fig. 11.1) usually arise from the first lumbar nerve as a trunk. After initially diverging, they may subsequently have interconnections. The iliohypogastric is visible at the lateral aspect of the psoas major, crosses posteriorly along the inferior pole of the kidney and the quadratus lumborum muscle, and pierces the transversus abdominis muscle. The ilial branch is given off almost immediately and courses posteriorly to innervate anterolateral gluteal skin. The hypogastric branch is the main continuation of the nerve. After passing between the transversus abdominis and the internal abdominal oblique, it pierces the external abdominal oblique aponeurosis just above the external inguinal ring. The hypogastric branch innervates the suprapubic skin (Fig. 11.7). The interconnection and cutaneous terminations of both the ilioinguinal and iliohypogastric nerves have been analyzed in depth by Jamieson et al. and will not be considered here.[50]

The ilioinguinal nerve (Fig. 11.1) becomes visible just inferior to the iliohypogastric nerve. It pierces the transversus abdominis and internal abdominal oblique muscles. It then courses through the inguinal canal, emerges, and supplies the skin over the proximal portion of the penis and the upper medial thigh (Fig. 11.7).

The lateral femoral cutaneous nerve (Figs. 11.1, 11.4, and 11.5) is a large branch from the second and third lumbar nerves. After crossing the iliac fossa under cover of the iliac fascia, the nerve passes below the iliopubic tract and pierces the inguinal ligament to enter the thigh. The area innervated by the lateral femoral cutaneous is shown in Figure 11.7.

The femoral nerve (Figs. 11.1, 11.4, and 11.5) is usually covered by the lateral border of the psoas major muscle. It is not routinely exposed during laparoscopic herniorrhaphy and is generally considered to be at minimal risk for injury. Nevertheless, surgeons must be mindful of its location since damage to the nerve due to deeply placed, improperly positioned staples has been reported.[22] The femoral nerve runs under cover of the iliopectineal arch to the inguinal ligament and crosses beneath it. It then passes into the thigh, where it innervates the quadriceps muscle and the sartorius, as well as the overlying skin (Fig. 11.7).

CONCLUSION

The preface to Zimmerman and Anson's *Anatomy and Surgery of Hernia* concludes, in part, with the sentence "It is a salutary experience to find that investigation in gross anatomy unfailingly contributes to surgical precision."[54] The results of a recent multicenter trial of laparoscopic inguinal herniorrhaphy indicate that complications related to herniorrhaphy itself (e.g., transient leg or groin pain, seroma, hematoma, and transient testicular or spermatic cord problems) dramatically decreased as surgeons became more familiar with both the techniques and the anatomic viewpoint encountered in laparoscopic inguinal hernia repairs.[3] It is clear that a thorough review of the anatomy of the inguinal region from the laparoscopic perspective will help to ensure the effectiveness and safety of this alternative to conventional inguinal hernia repair.

REFERENCES

1. Salerno GM, Fitzgibbons RJ Jr, Filipi CJ, et al: Laparoscopic inguinal hernia repair. In Zucker KA (ed): *Surgical Laparoscopy*. St Louis, Quality Medical, 1991, pp 221–293.
2. Filipi CJ, Fitzgibbons RJ Jr, Salerno GM, et al: Laparoscopic herniorrhaphy. *Surg Clin North Am* 72:1109–1123, 1992.
3. Fitzgibbons RJ Jr, Camps J, Cornet DA, et al: Laparoscopic inguinal herniorrhaphy. Results of a multicenter trial. *Ann Surg* 221:3–13, 1995.
4. Williams PL, Warwick R, Dyson M, et al (eds): *Gray's Anatomy*, ed 37. Edinburgh, Churchill Livingstone, 1989, pp 1346–1347.
5. *Nomina Anatomica*: Authorized by the Twelfth International Congress of Anatomists in London. Edinburgh, Churchill Livingstone, 1989, p A51.
6. Begg RC: The urachus: Its anatomy, histology and development. *J Anat* 64:170–183, 1930.
7. Douglass M: Urachal cysts and fistulae. *Am J Surg* 22:557–560, 1933.
8. Cooper AP: *The Anatomy and Surgical Treatment of Inguinal and Congenital Hernia*. London, Longman, 1804.
9. Cooper AP: *The Anatomy and Surgical Treatment of Crural and Umbilical Hernia*. London, Longman, 1807, pp 3–4.
10. Anson BJ, Morgan EH, McVay CB: Surgical anatomy of the inguinal region based upon a study of 500 body-halves. *Surg Gynecol Obstet* 111: 707–725, 1960.
11. Lampe EW: Experiences with preperitoneal hernioplasty. In Nyhus LM, Condon RE (eds): *Hernia*, ed 3. Philadelphia, Lippincott, 1989, pp 242–247.
12. Skandalakis JE, Colborn GL, Gray SW, et al: The surgical anatomy of the inguinal area: part I. *Contemp Surg* 38:20–34, 1991.
13. Read RC: Cooper's posterior lamina of transversalis fascia. *Surg Gynecol Obstet* 174:426–433, 1992.
14. Cleland J, MacKay JY, Young BJ: The relations of the aponeurosis of the transversalis and internal oblique muscles to the deep epigastric artery and to the inguinal canal. In *Memoirs and Memoranda in Anatomy*, Vol. I London, Williams and Norgate, 1889, pp
15. Fowler R: Special comment: The preperitoneal fascia. In Nyhus LM, Condon RE (eds): *Hernia*, ed 2. Philadelphia, Lippincott, 1978, pp 64–67.
16. Condon RE: The anatomy of the inguinal region and its relation to groin hernia. In Nyhus LM, Condon RE (eds): *Hernia*, ed 3. Philadelphia, Lippincott, 1989, p 42.
17. Zimmerman LM, Anson BJ: *Anatomy and Surgery of Hernia*. Baltimore, Williams & Wilkins, 1953, p 71.
18. Arregui ME, Davis CJ, Yucel O, et al: Laparoscopic mesh repair of inguinal hernia using a preperitoneal approach: A preliminary report. *Surg Laparosc Endosc* 2:53–58, 1992.
19. Lytle W: The internal inguinal ring. *Br J Surg* 32: 441–446, 1945.
20. Quinn TH, Annibali R, Dalley AF, et al: Dissection of the anterior abdominal wall and deep inguinal region from a laparoscopic perspective. *Clin Anat* in press.
21. Annibali R, Quinn TH, Fitzgibbons RJ Jr: Surgical anatomy of the inguinal region and lower abdominal wall: The laparoscopic perspective. In Bendavid R (ed): *Prostheses and Abdominal Wall Hernias*. Austin, TX, Landes Medical, pp 82–103.
22. Skandalakis JE, Colborn G, Gray S, et al: The surgical anatomy of the inguinal area part II. *Contemp Surg* 38:28–38, 1991.
23. Hollingshead WH: *Anatomy for Surgeons*, Vol. 2: *The Thorax, Abdomen and Pelvis*. New York, Hoeber-Harper, 1961, pp 248–249.

24. Williams PL, Warwick R, Dyson M, et al (eds): *Gray's Anatomy*, ed 37. Edinburgh, Churchill Livingstone, 1989, p 603.
25. Nyhus LM, Condon RE, Harkins HN: Clinical experience with preperitoneal hernia repair for all types of hernia repair of the groin: With particular reference to the importance of the transversalis fascia analogs. *Am J Surg* 100:234–244, 1960.
26. Lichtenstein I, Shulman A, Amid P, et al: The pathophysiology of recurrent hernia. *Contemp Surg* 35:13–18, 1992.
27. Gilroy AM, Marks SC Jr, Quinfang L, et al: Anatomical characteristics of the iliopubic tract: Implications for repair of inguinal hernias. *Clin Anat* 5:255–263, 1992.
28. Condon RE: The anatomy of the inguinal region and its relation to groin hernia. In Nyhus LM, Condon RE (eds): *Hernia*, ed 3. Philadelphia, Lippincott, 1989, p 34.
29. McVay CB: The anatomic basis for inguinal and femoral hernioplasty. *Surg Gynecol Obstet* 139: 931–945, 1974.
30. Nyhus LM, Bombeck CT: Hernias. In Sabiston DC (ed): *Textbook of Surgery*, ed 13. Philadelphia, Saunders, 1986, pp 1231–1252.
31. Arregui ME: Preperitoneal repair of direct inguinal hernia with mesh. Presented at Advanced Laparoscopic Surgery: The International Experience, Indianapolis, May 20–22, 1991.
32. Rutledge RH: Cooper's ligament repairs for adult groin hernias. *Surgery* 87:601–610, 1980.
33. Anson BJ: *An Atlas of Human Anatomy*. Philadelphia, Saunders, 1950, p 421.
34. Chandler SB, Schadewald M: Studies on the inguinal region: I. The conjoined aponeurosis versus the conjoined tendon. *Anat Rec* 89:339–343, 1944.
35. Askar OM: Surgical anatomy of the aponeurotic expansions of the anterior abdominal wall. *Ann R Coll Surg Engl* 59:313–321, 1977.
36. Griffith CA: The Marcy repair of indirect inguinal hernia: 1870 to present. In Nyhus LM, Condon RE (eds): *Hernia*, ed 3. Philadelphia, Lippincott, 1989, pp 106–118.
37. Hesselbach FC: *Neuste anatomisch-pathologisch Untersuchungen ueber den Ursprung und das Fortschreiten der Leisten und Schenkelbruche*. Wurzburg, J Stahel, 1814.
38. Chandler SB: Studies on the inguinal region II. The anatomy of the inguinal (Hesselbach) triangle. *Ann Surg* 124:156–160, 1946.
39. Ponka JL: Surgical management of large bilateral sliding inguinal hernias. *Am J Surg* 112:52–57, 1966.
40. Anson BJ, McVay CB: The anatomy of inguinal hernia. *Surg Gynecol Obstet* 66:186–191, 1938.
41. Rizk NN: A new description of the anterior abdominal wall in man and mammals. *J Anat* 131:373–385, 1980.
42. Lipshutz B: A composite study of the hypogastric artery and its branches. *Ann Surg* 67:584–608, 1918.
43. Poynter CWM: Congenital anomalies of the arteries and veins of the human body with bibliography. *The University Studies of the University of Nebraska, Lincoln*. 16:229–345, 1916.
44. Hochstetter A von: Eine Schleife der Arteria epigastrica inferior in Canalis inguinalis. *Anat Anz* 109:221–224, 1961.
45. Milloy FJ, Anson BJ, McAffee DK: The rectus abdominis muscle and the epigastric arteries. *Surg Gynecol Obstet* 110:293–302, 1960.
46. Pick J, Anson BJ, Ashley FL: The origin of the obturator artery. A study of 640 body halves. *Am J Anat* 70: 317–344, 1942.
47. Delitzin S: Uber eine complicierte Anomalie in Gebiete der Arteria obturatoria und epigastrica inferior. *Arch Anat Physiol Wissensch Med*, 413–422, 1896.
48. Bendavid R: The space of Bogros and the deep inguinal venous circulation. *Surg Gynecol Obstet* 174:355–358, 1992.
49. Urbanowicz Z: External structure of the genitofemoral nerve in postfetal life in man. *Folia Morphol* 34:425–434, 1975.
50. Jamieson EB, Swigart La VL, Anson BJ: Points of parietal perforation of the ilioinguinal and iliohypogastric nerves in relation to optimal sites for local anesthesia. *Q Bull Northw Univ Med School* 26:34–35, 1952.
51. Yeager VL: Intermediate inguinal ring. *Clin Anat* 5:289–295, 1992.
52. Bendavid R: "Disejaculation": An unusual complication of inguinal herniorrhaphy. *Postgrad Gen Surg* 4:139–141, 1992.
53. Eckmann I: Ein Beitrag zur kenntnis des terminalen Verlaufs des N. ilioinguinalis. *Anat Anz* 140:15–30, 1976.
54. Zimmerman LM, Anson BJ: Preface to *Anatomy and Surgery of Hernia*. Baltimore, Williams & Wilkins, 1953.

chapter twelve

Complications in Transabdominal Preperitoneal Herniorrhaphy and How to Prevent Them

Michael S. Kavic

INTRODUCTION

The inguinal region is a portion of the abdominal wall not completely buttressed by a musculotendinous barrier. Because of this anatomic oversight, groin herniation is one of the more common problems to afflict mankind. More than 650,000 inguinal hernia operations are performed each year in the United States.[1]

The groin contains a potential space, a myopectineal orifice, through which the hernia traverses. Even experienced general surgeons may be unaware of the pivotal significance of this area. Specifically, the inguinal myopectineal orifice is bounded superiorly by the transversus abdominis and internal oblique muscles. Medially, the orifice is bounded by the rectus muscle; inferiorly and laterally, by the pubis and iliopsoas muscles. The myopectineal portal is spanned and divided by the inguinal ligament.[2]

Normally, the inguinal region is protected by a musculotendinous barrier that prevents intra-abdominal contents from exiting the abdominal cavity. The barrier is not static but rather functions as a shutter which is activated under certain physiologic conditions.

During physical work or straining, contraction of the transversus abdominis and internal oblique muscles cause a shutter-like approximation of these structures to the inguinal ligament.[3,4] The approximation of a strong musculotendinous layer to the inguinal ligament in a shutter-like fashion, buttresses the relatively thin transversalis fascia covering the inguinal myopectineal orifice. The shutter's exceptional strength prevents herniation through the direct and indirect inguinal rings.

Laparoscopic transabdominal access offers an unparalleled view of the inguinal wall. Structural relationships not well visualized during open hernia repair are clearly demonstrated during laparoscopic dissection. Rather than focus individually on direct or indirect inguinal defects, the entire myopectineal orifice should be reconstituted for an adequate repair of groin hernia. It is fundamental to the repair of inguinal hernia that the functional effect of the shutter mechanism be reproduced.[5]

TECHNIQUE

The laparoscopic transabdominal preperitoneal repair of inguinal hernia involves the use of a prosthetic material that serves as a preperitoneal aponeurotic-like buttress. The screen is positioned to extend from the transversus abdominis muscle and tendon superiorly to Cooper's ligament and the iliopubic tract inferiorly. There is no attempt to restore normal anatomy or to close the hernia defect under tension. Rather, by mimicking the effect of the inguinal shutter, a tension-free repair of hernia defects in the myopectineal orifice is achieved. Anything less than coverage of the myopectineal orifice is probably an inadequate repair, and anything more is superfluous.

COMPLICATIONS

It is important to recall the complications of open hernia repair when considering the complications of laparoscopic hernioplasty. The incidence of hernia recurrence after open repair has been well documented. Typically, it ranges from 10% for the Bassini procedure to 1.5% for the Shouldice method.[6,7]

Other significant complications of open repair include, but are not limited to, hematoma, wound infection, seroma, neuroma, epididymitis, orchitis, and bowel, vascular, and urinary bladder injuries.[8]

Complications associated with the laparoscopic transabdominal preperitoneal repair of inguinal hernia include misadventures related to laparoscopic access, problems with the use of large-bore cannulas, and complications arising from dissection and reconstitution of the inguinal myopectineal orifice.

Current technology limits the use of local and regional anesthesia for laparoscopic surgery. The laparoscopic transabdominal approach to hernia repair almost always requires general anesthesia. Complications related to general anesthesia are largely associated with the general health of the patient and the presence of comorbid factors. These anesthetic factors are reviewed elsewhere and lie outside the scope of this chapter.[9]

COMPLICATIONS ASSOCIATED WITH LAPAROSCOPIC ACCESS

The performance of laparoscopic access involves risks inherent in traversing the abdominal wall. These risks include skin infection, subcutaneous emphysema, hemorrhage, bowel perforation, and gas embolism.

Skin-level infection can be a complication of laparoscopic access which may be prevented with adequate preparation. Vigorous cleansing of the umbilicus should be performed with a cotton tip applicator and surgical scrub (Fig. 12.1).

Abdominal wall and omental emphysema result from incorrect placement of the Veress needle. Omental emphysema may obscure the operative field (Fig. 12.2), but visualization can be im-proved by table repositioning and the use of ancillary cannulas. Genital emphysema (Fig. 12.3) is common in males with indirect inguinal hernia and results from insufflation of the hernia defect with abdominal CO_2 gas. CO_2 is rapidly absorbed, and subcutaneous emphysema is transient, typically with no clinical sequelae. Genital emphysema usually resolves by the time the patient is discharged from the recovery area.

The frequency of troublesome abdominal wall bleeding is directly related to the presence of subcutaneous blood vessels and the use of large-bore cannulas. Laparoscopic illumination of the abdominal wall during trocar insertion can define larger vessels so that they may be avoided (Fig. 12.4). Generally, the use of large-bore cannulas is associated with a higher risk of incidental lateral abdominal wall bleeding than smaller ones. To minimize this risk, 5-mm cannulas are used in the right and left abdominal quadrant sites (Fig. 12.5). Incidental bleeding from the 5-mm peritoneal defect can usually be controlled with an electrosurgical device (Fig. 12.6).

Intra-abdominal vessels or intestine may be lacerated by trocars and cannulas. To reduce the risk of injury to

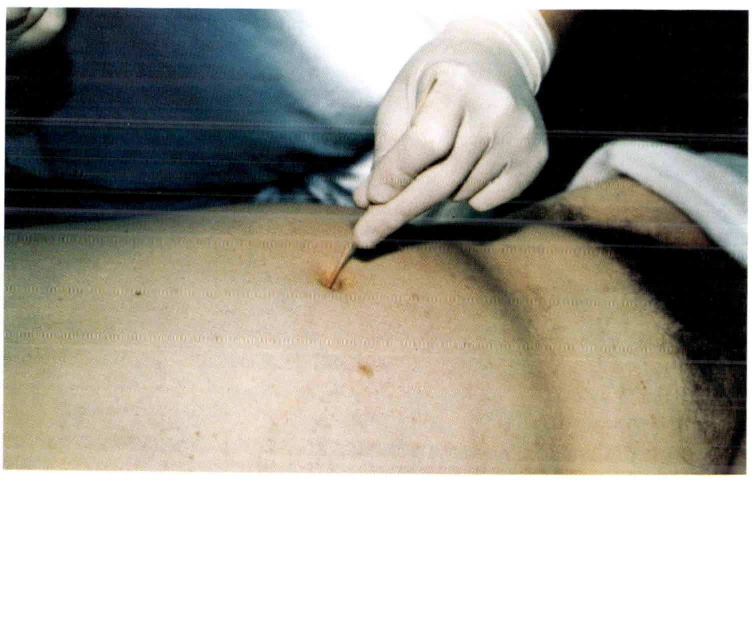

Figure 12.1. Umbilical preparation.

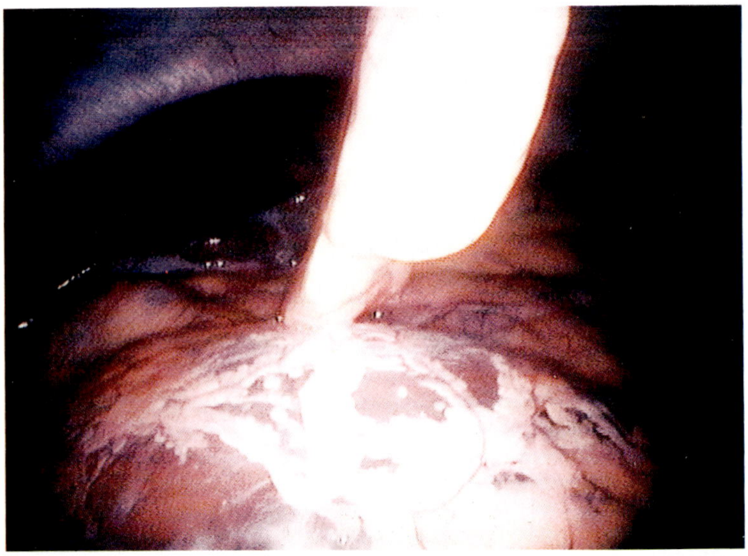

Figure 12.2. Omental emphysema.

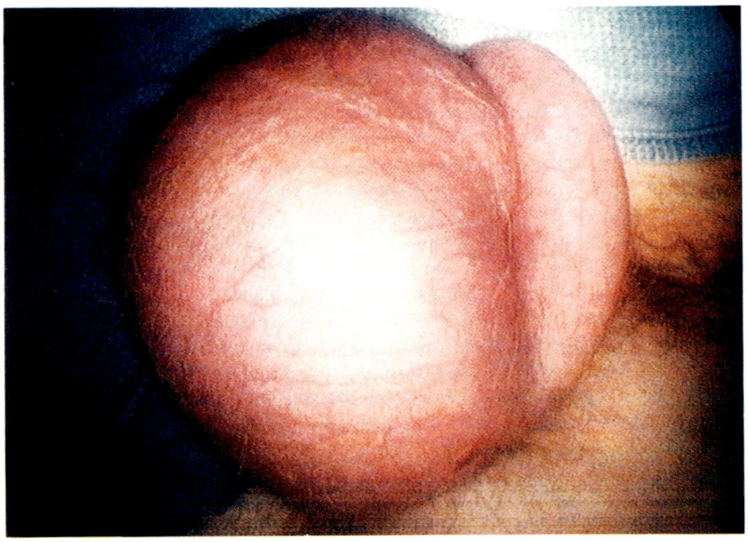

Figure 12.3. Genital emphysema.

the aorta and inferior vena cava during trocar insertion, it is necessary to direct the umbilical trocar toward the pelvis while the patient is maintained in the Trendelenberg position. Extension of the operator's third finger along the shaft of the cannula (Fig. 12.7) will help limit trocar incursion and the possibility of inadvertent abdominal injury. Preoperative administration of purgatives will decrease bowel size and reduce the possibility of iatrogenic harm.

Gas embolism, an uncommon complication, is caused by the introduction of a large amount of gas into a major vessel. Embolization may lead to right ventricular outflow obstruction. If this complication is encountered, the patient should be placed in the left lateral position, with a steep Trendelenberg posture to help decrease right outflow tract obstruction.[10] Careful attention to trocar placement, with avoidance of direct vascular injury, will avoid this potentially serious problem.

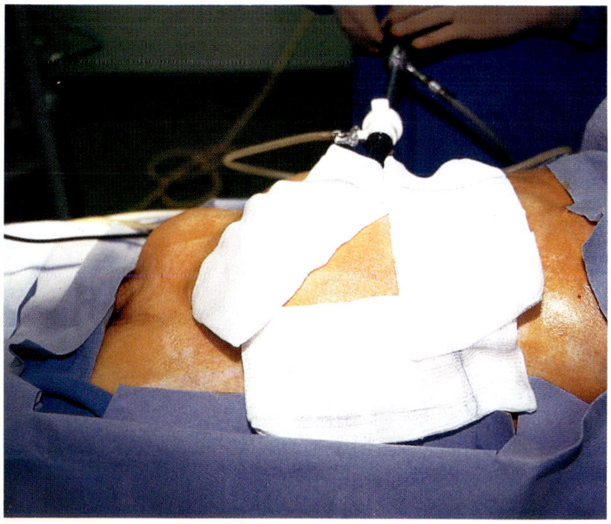

Figure 12.4. Laparoscopic illumination.

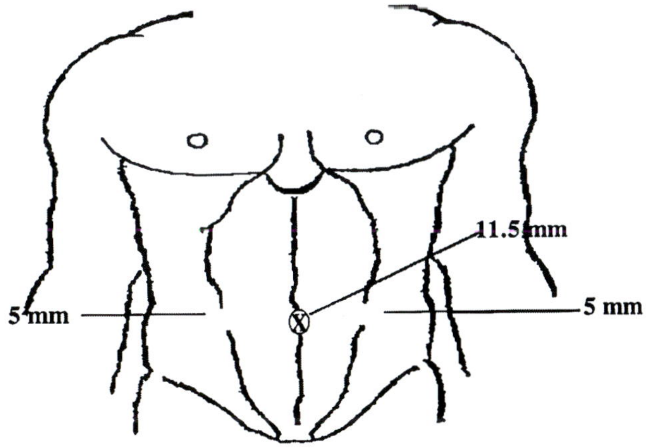

Figure 12.5. Trocar sites.

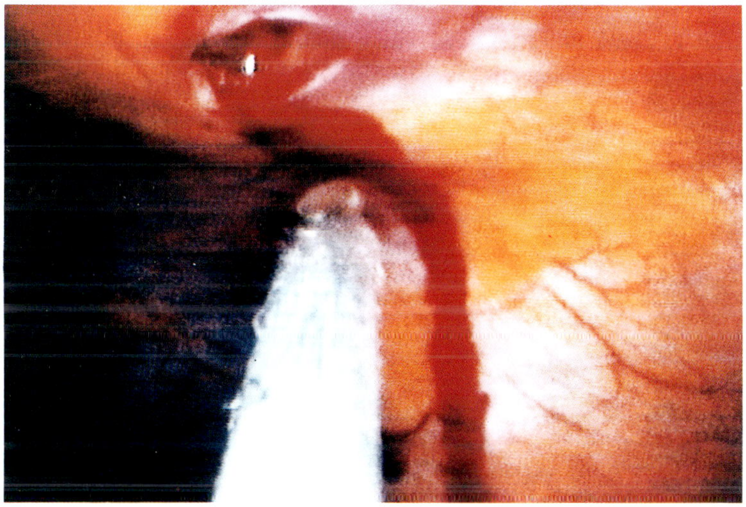

Figure 12.6. Electrocoagulation of trocar site bleeding.

COMPLICATIONS ASSOCIATED WITH LARGE-BORE CANNULAS

Large-bore cannulas used for passage of the laparoscope and endohernia stapler can be responsible for major injuries, including hemorrhage and abdominal wall hernia.

Hemorrhage at smaller cannula ports can usually be controlled with an electrosurgical unit. More vigorous bleeding from large cannula sites should be secured with extracorporeal suture utilizing a device such as Semms Notfall Nadel (Fig. 12.8) or a fascial suture device (Fig. 12.9; Excel-DR, Advanced Surgical).

Large-bore cannulas cause a substantial fascial defect, which may predispose to herniation of bowel or

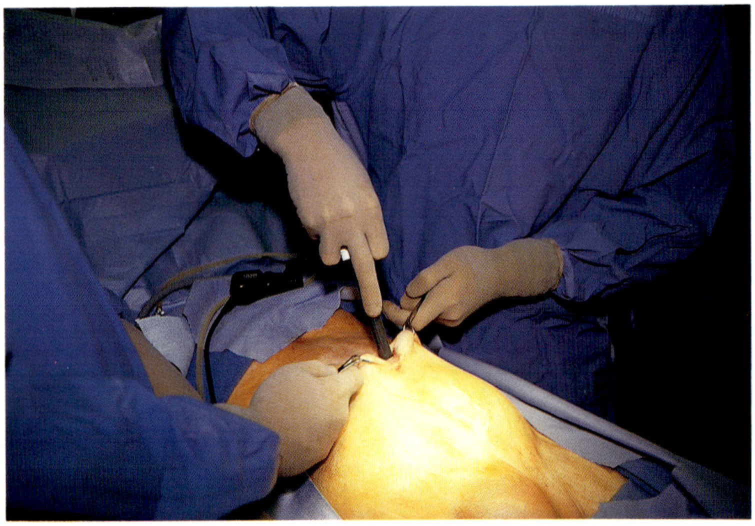

Figure 12.7. Limiting trocar incursion.

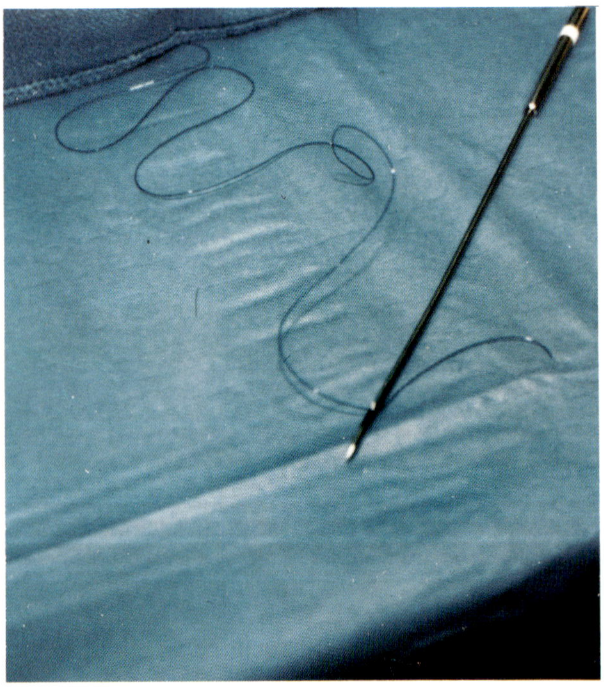

Figure 12.8. Semm's Notfall Nadel.

omentum. Incarceration and strangulation of bowel can occur if these cannula sites are not completely closed.[11] This complication can be lessened by careful suture closure of the fascial defect and the use of smaller cannulas. Limiting lateral wall cannulas to 5 mm will decrease the risk of trocar site hernia, as these smaller defects are not as prone to herniation.

Large (11.5-mm) cannulas are confined to the umbilical position. This central port allows passage of the 10-mm 0 degree laparoscope and the 12-mm endohernia stapler. Control of bleeding and the prevention of herniation at this site are facilitated by grasping the umbilical fascia with Köcher clamps and closing the defect with strong, absorbable suture. Closure of the umbilical fascia can be ensured by visualizing the abdominal aspect of the defect during closure with a 5-mm laparoscope passed through one of the lateral ports.

The possibility of incidental bleeding from lateral cannula sites is reduced if laparoscopic illumination of the abdominal wall is utilized during insertion of these 5-mm trocars. Laparoscopic light can define subcutaneous vessels so that they may be avoided. Subcutaneous suture is usually all that is required to close 5 mm sites and secure hemostasis.

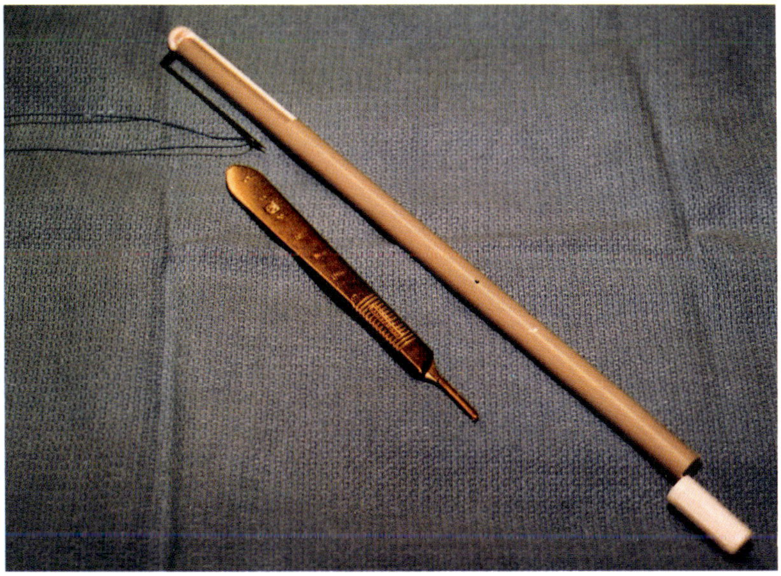

Figure 12.9. Excel (Advanced Surgical).

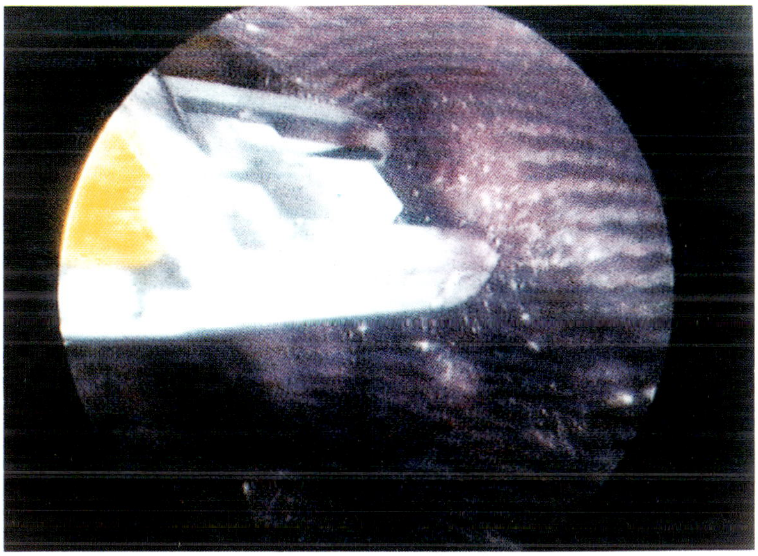

Figure 12.10. En face stapling.

Five-millimeter cannulas do not permit stapling from these ports. Current endohernia staplers are larger than 11 mm and require passage through a large (umbilical) cannula. Origin has recently introduced a 5 mm hernia screw for mesh fixation. However, traditional staples or suture closure are still required for closure of the peritoneum. A laterally-sited 5-mm laparoscope is employed to visualize the operative field during prosthetic screen stapling, which is accomplished by way of the umbilical port. The central position of the endohernia stapler, however, allows repair of either right- or left-sided inguinal hernia defects with a near en face attitude of the stapler (Fig. 12.10).

COMPLICATIONS ASSOCIATED WITH DISSECTION AND PREPARATION OF THE MYOPECTINEAL ORIFICE

Bleeding in the preperitoneal space can occur during laparoscopic dissection. This event may result in ecchymosis, seroma, or hematoma formation and occurs in approximately 3% of transabdominal repairs.[11] Preperitoneal seroma formation has been found to be slightly higher during the totally extraperitoneal repair, as blood sequestered in this space cannot readily drain into the peritoneal cavity.[11] Superficial preperitoneal bleeding can be reduced by dissecting just superior to the peritoneum. The transversalis fascia may be bilamellar, and dissection well above the peritoneum may violate this structure, leading to excessive bleeding (Fig. 12.11).

Small preperitoneal vessels can be secured with an electrosurgical device or endoclips. Hemorrhage from larger preperitoneal vessels, including the inferior epigastric vessels, may require control using intracorporeal or extracorporeal suture techniques. External suture may be passed with an instrument such as Semms Notfall Nadel. Intracorporeal suture may be tied with an intracorporeal or extracorporeal knot technique.

Closure of the peritoneal incision is most secure when suture approximation is used. This may be accomplished with interrupted figure of eight suture tied extracorporeally (Fig. 12.12a,b) or with running continuous suture (Fig. 12.13).

The introduction of suture with an attached needle is performed by grasping the suture proximal to the needle. The needle is allowed to follow the grasper as it is passed through the cannula and into the abdominal cavity. Laparoscopic graspers are used to pass suture, as they are relatively atraumatic. Specialized endoscopic needle drivers are typically fitted with aggressive jaws and may cut through suture during insertion.

Continuous suture closure of the peritoneal incision is usually started laterally (Fig. 12.14a). The stitch is secured by passing the needle through a previously tied loop of the tail (Fig. 12.14b). The suture is then run medially, closing the peritoneal defect, and "locked" into place with an endoclip (Fig. 12.14c). The risk of iatrogenic (needle) injury to the inferior epigastric vessels is lessened by traction on the peritoneal margins as the needle and suture are passed through these structures.

Specialized laparoscopic needle drivers such as R. Wolfe's advanced needle holder simplify suturing and enable the laparoscopic surgeon to perform this com-

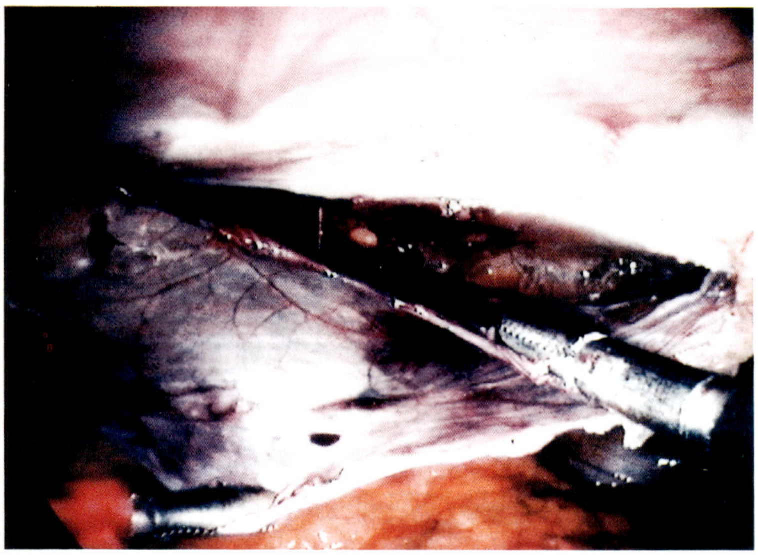

Figure 12.11. Transversalis fascia.

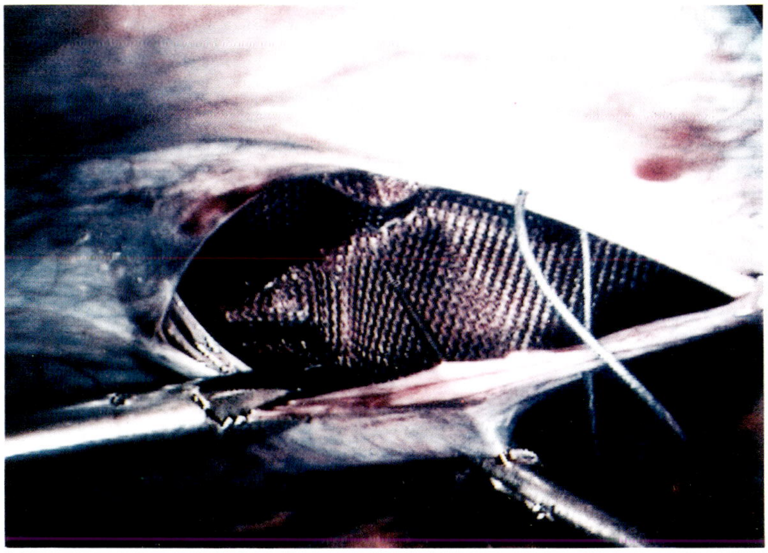

a

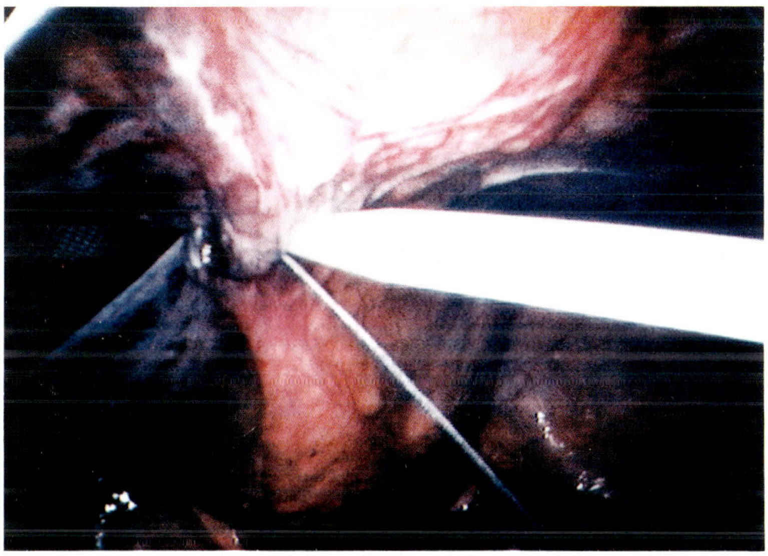

b

Figure 12.12. (a) Figure of eight suture. (b) Extracorporeal knot tie.

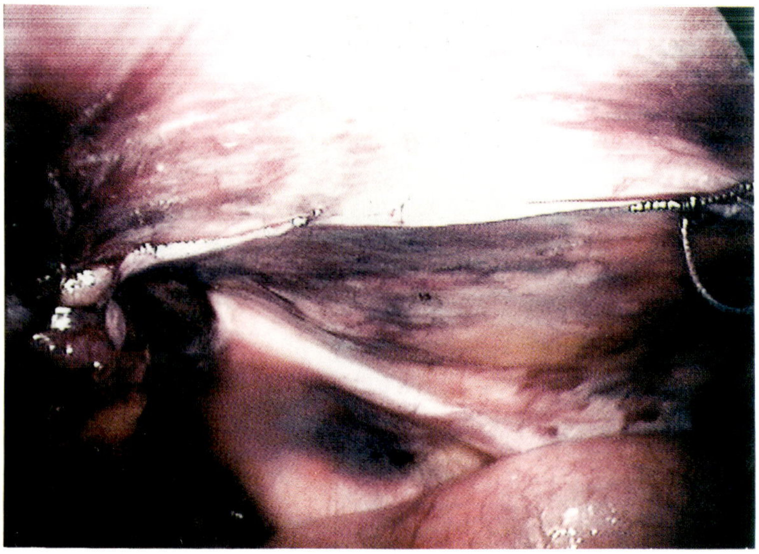

Figure 12.13. Completed preperitoneal closure with continuous suture.

mon surgical procedure com-fortably. Reusable laparoscopic instruments and inexpensive suture are cost-effective tools in the minimally invasive surgical armamentarium.

Complications associated with the use of prosthetic screens are principally technical in nature. In practice, the screen may be too small or improperly fixed. Small screens that are improperly fixed tend to migrate into the inguinal canal (Fig. 12.15). Adequate overlap of the myopectineal orifice is ensured with a large screen or the use of several screens. A double buttress technique, overlapping one screen with another, may be required to cover the hernia defects adequately.[12] Dependable fixation to Cooper's ligament, the symphysis pubis, and rectus sheath, and superiorly to the transversus abdominis muscle and tendon, is currently best accomplished with an endohernia stapler.

The "triangle of doom" has been well publicized in laparoscopic hernia repair literature and perhaps overdramatized.[13] This triangle is analogous to the triangle of Calot, and is no more or less dangerous to the trained general surgeon. Both triangles contain major blood vessels and important structures easily compromised by the inattentive. Surgery, however, can be safely performed in both areas with adequate knowledge, training, and caution. Major vascular injury has been remarkably uncommon during the initial experience with laparoscopic hernia repair. In a large, multi-institutional study, only one vascular injury was reported in a series of 3,229 laparoscopic hernioplasties performed on 2229 patients.[11] This is an incidence of 0.06% and may be compared to the incidence of vascular injury during open repair of 0.35–1.6%.[11]

Persistent anterior thigh paresthesia is a complication of laparoscopic hernioplasty and has been reported in 1.4–1.6% of transabdominal repairs.[5,11] Neuralgias occurred most frequently early in the laparoscopic hernia study and involved incomplete appreciation of genitofemoral and lateral femoral cutaneous nerve anatomy (Fig. 12.16). Branches of the genitofemoral nerve pass underneath and in close proximity to the inferior border of the iliopubic tract.

Stapling near or below the inferior margin of the iliopubic tract risks injury to the lumboinguinal branches of the genitofemoral nerve. More laterally, staples may impale branches of the lateral femoral cutaneous nerve. If stapling is required in the iliopubic tract, the possibility of nerve injury is reduced by vertically aligning and placing the staple **superior** to the inferior margin of the iliopubic tract. Only one or two staples are required to tack the prosthetic screen in this area.

A prosthetic screen will not lie flat in the inguinal region, as Cooper's ligament, the external iliac vessels, iliopubic tract, transversus abdominis muscle, and rectus sheath lie on different levels and different planes. The screen should drape about the external iliac vessels and spermatic cord, for these structures should be triangulated and not strangulated[14] (Fig. 12.17).

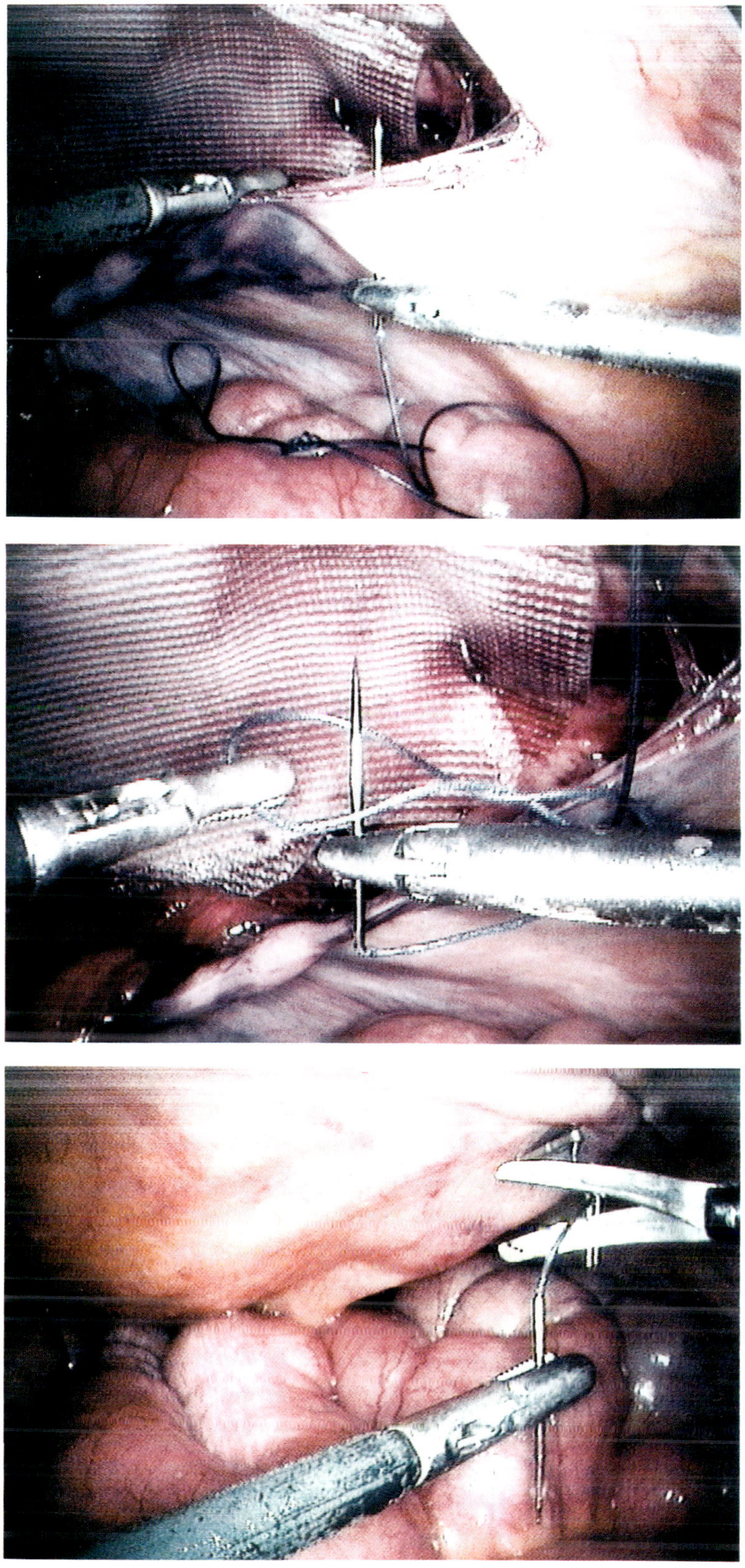

a

b

c

Figure 12.14. (a) Initial suture: continuous closure. (b) Pretied loop. (c) Continuous suture locked with an endoclip.

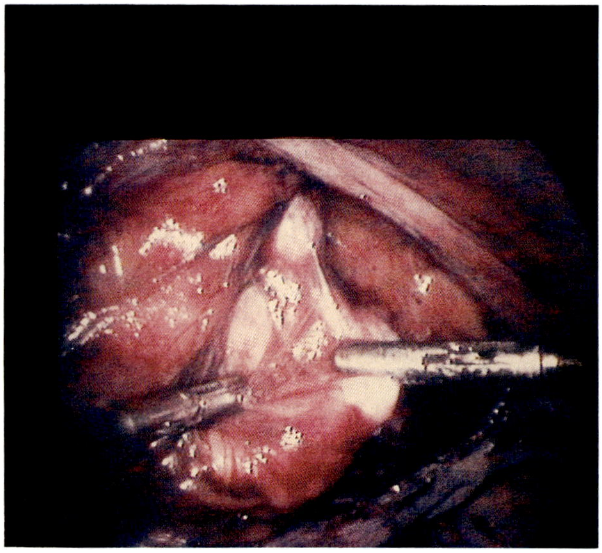

Figure 12.15. Migrated screen.

Bowel obstruction has been reported in 0.2% of laparoscopic transabdominal preperitoneal hernia repairs.[11] This complication has occurred when bowel has been trapped in incompletely closed trocar defects and inadequately stapled peritoneal closures. Close attention to peritoneal and fascial closure with suture will eliminate this problem.

Bowel injury has also occurred with the injudicious use of electrosurgery. To create a physical effect, monopolar electrical current must complete a circuit by passing through the patient's body and return to the grounding pad. If resistance to the flow of electrical current is encountered while completing a circuit, alternate current pathways are possible. Unintended alternate site electrical burns and injuries may result (Fig. 12.18). Careful use of monopolar electrosurgery, with short bursts of energy and low voltage, will diminish the possibility of alternate site pathway injury. The use of bipolar electrical devices will eliminate it.

Mortality has been rare in cases of laparoscopic hernia repair and essentially involved patients with significant comorbid factors. In a series of 3245 patients who underwent laparoscopic hernioplasty, two deaths were reported. One death was due to myocardial infarction, the other to hepatic failure.[11,15] Most other series have reported no mortality.[5,16]

Recurrence is the principal yardstick by which herniorrhaphy is evaluated. It is accepted that 5- and 10-year data are necessary to evaluate the true incidence of herniorrhaphy recurrence.[6] However, any recurrence after 2 or more years is probably not the result of surgical error but rather is due to tissue attenuation.[17] A large combined series of laparoscopic transabdominal preperitoneal hernia repairs has shown a recurrence rate of 1%.[11] It is noteworthy that these data also include recurrences experienced during the gene-

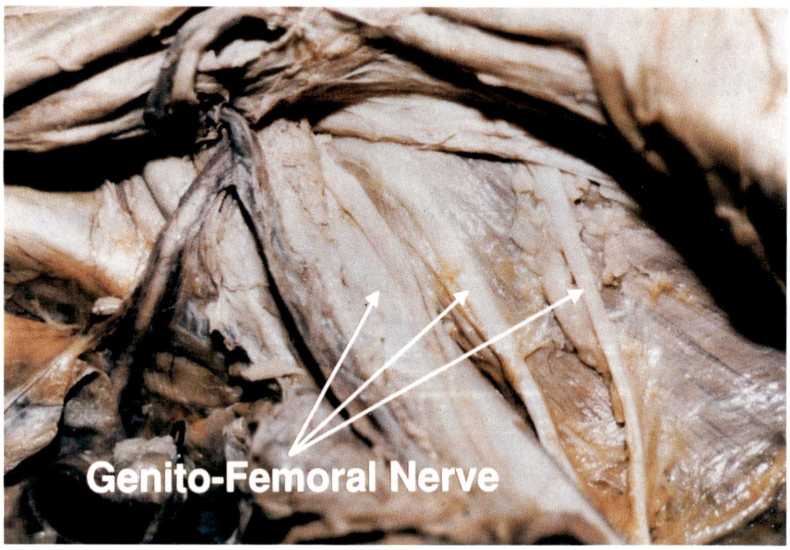

Figure 12.16. Genitofemoral nerve.

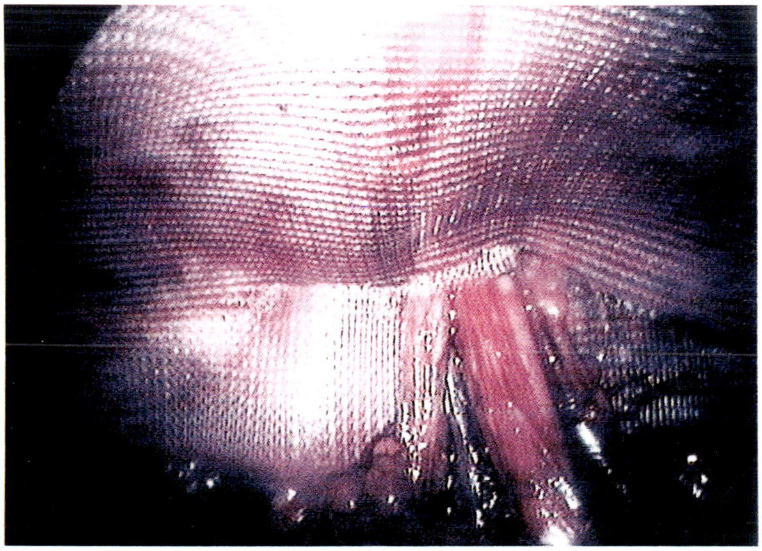

Figure 12.17. Proper screen position is shown.

sis of laparoscopic hernioplasty and reflect negotiation of the surgical/technical learning curve.

The issue of laparoscopic hernia recurrence seems to be essentially a technical one related to the size of the prosthetic screen and its method of fixation. An excellent way to ensure coverage of the myopectineal orifice is to affix larger (7 × 12 cm or more) screens with staples, taking care to overlap the prosthesis beyond the defect. This screen, or screens, should drape about the external iliac vessels and spermatic cord and not compromise them.

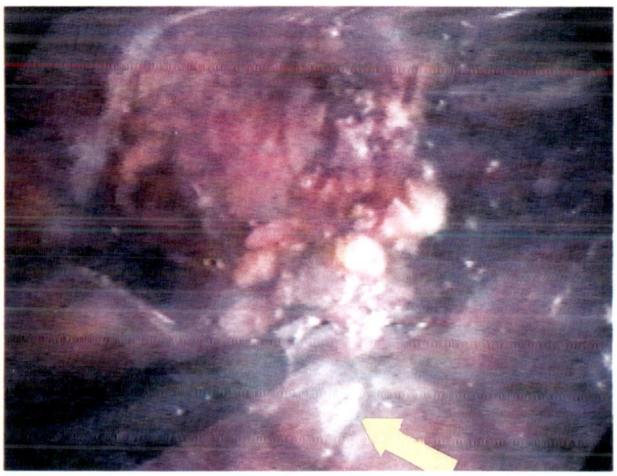

Figure 12.18. Alternate-site electrical burn.

Endohernia stapling devices are the most effective means to secure the prosthetic screen. Caution must be taken to avoid stapling near the inferior edge of the iliopubic tract so that branches of the genitofemoral nerve are not injured. Additionally, care must be taken not to staple the pudendal branch of the inferior epigastric artery as it courses near or on Cooper's ligament (Fig. 12.19). Coagulation of this vessel prior to screen positioning and staple fixation will reduce the risk of staple-induced bleeding. Bleeding after staple placement (Fig. 12.20) may be controlled with tamponade utilizing Codman surgical patties (Codman & Shurtleff, Inc., a Johnson & Johnson company) or rolled 4 × 4 gauze.[18] If this maneuver is unsuccessful, coagulation with an electrosurgical device may be used to secure hemostasis.

Inguinal hernia recurrence following laparoscopic hernioplasty compares favorably to recurrence rates after open methods of herniorrhaphy. Recurrence following the Bassini method is approximately 10%.[6] Lichtenstein has reported an 0.7% recurrence rate and Shouldice a 1.5% inguinal hernia recurrence rate.[7,19]

It is too early in the study of laparoscopic hernia repair to draw conclusions about its ultimate worth. There is evidence that patients with unilateral laparoscopic hernia repair have less morbidity than those who undergo open repair.[20] Also, there seems to be general agreement that the laparoscopic approach is desirable in patients with recurrence after open repair and in those with bilateral inguinal hernia.

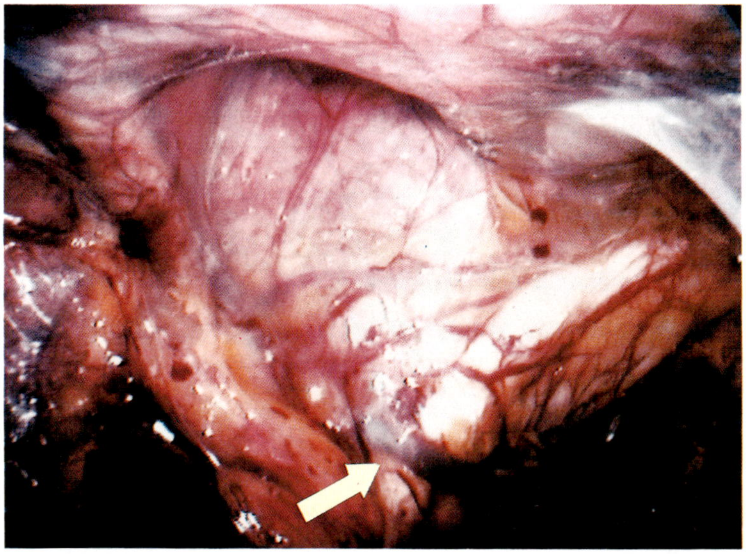

Figure 12.19. Pudendal branch inferior epigastric artery (arrow).

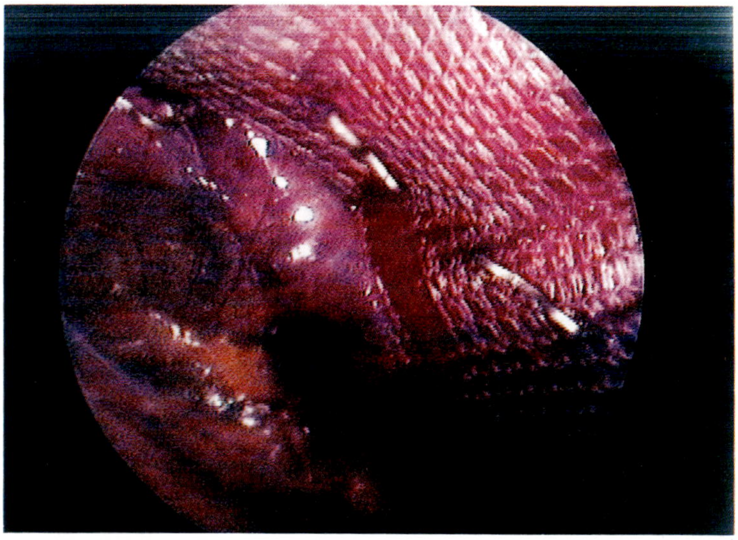

Figure 12.20. Staple site bleeding.

CONCLUSIONS

The application of laparoscopic technique to common surgical problems such as inguinal hernia is an exciting trend in general surgery. Initial results indicate decreased pain and rapid return to full activity. The severity of complications associated with laparoscopic hernia repair appears to be similar to that of open repair. The long-term benefit of laparoscopic hernioplasty, however, awaits a balance analysis of a large number of cases for a minimum of 5 years.

REFERENCES

1. Rutkow IM, Robbins AM: Demographic classificatory and socioeconomic aspects of hernia repair in the United States. *Surg Clin North Am* 73:3413–3426, 1993.

2. Fruchaud H: *Anatomie Chirurgicale des Hernies de l'Aine*. Paris, G Doin, 1956.
3. Keith A: The origin and nature of hernia. *Br J Surg* 11:455–475, 1923.
4. Hammond TE: Etiology of indirect inguinal hernia. *Lancet* 204:1206–1208, 1923.
5. Kavic MS: Laparoscopic hernia repair: Three year experience. *Surg Endosc* 9:12–15, 1995.
6. Heydron W: Abdominal Hernia. In James E, Corry R, Perry J (eds): *Principles of Basic Surgical Practice*. Philadelphia, Hanley & Belfus, 1987, pp 346–352.
7. Welsh D, Alexander AJ: The shouldice repair. *Surg Clin North Am* 73:451–470, 1993.
8. Nyhus LM, Condon RE: *Hernia*, ed 2. Philadelphia, Lippincott, 1978, pp 264–275.
9. Amado W: Anesthesia for hernia surgery. *Surg Clin North Am* 73:427–450, 1993.
10. Berci G, Cuschieri A: *Practical Laparoscopy*. London, Bailliere & Tindall, 1993, p 170.
11. Phillips EH, Arregui M, Carroll BJ: Incidence of complications following laparoscopic hernioplasty. *Surg Endosc* 9:16–21, 1995.
12. Felix E, Michas C: Double-buttress laparoscopic herniorrhaphy. *J Laparoendosc Surg* 3:1–17, 1993.
13. Spaw AT, Ennis BW, Spaw LPL Laparoscopic hernia repair: The anatomic basis. *J Laparoendosc Surg* 1:269–277, 1991.
14. Kavic MS: Laparoscopic hernia repair. *Surg Endosc* 7:163–167, 1993.
15. Fitzgibbons RJ, Carps J, Cornet D, et al: Laparoscopic inguinal herniorrhaphy: Results of a multicenter trial. *Ann Surg* 221:3–13, 1995.
16. Tucker JG, Wilson RA, Ramshaw BJ, et al: Laparoscopic herniorrhaphy: Technical concerns in prevention of complications and early recurrence. *Am Surg* 61:36–39, 1995.
17. Lichenstein IL: *Hernia Repair Without Disability*, ed 2. St. Louis, Ishiyaku Euroamerica, 1986, p 76.
18. Miguel PR, Figueirdo FA, Moreira da Rosa AL, et al: Use of gauze cylinders in laparoscopic cholecystectomy: A technical alternative. *Surg Laparosc Endosc*, 4:73–75, 1994.
19. Lichenstein IL: *Hernia Repair Without Disability*, ed 2. St Louis, Ishiyaku Euroamerica, 1986, p 212.
20. Payne JH Jr, Grininger LM, Izawa MT, et al: Laparoscopic or open inguinal herniorrhaphy? A randomized prospective trial. *Arch Surg* 129:973–981, 1994.

chapter thirteen

Complications of Laparoscopic Herniorrhaphy

John D. Corbitt, Jr.

INTRODUCTION

Following the surgical approach to hernia repair described in 1884 by Bassini, there have been many attempts to improve the technique of this tension-producing repair which placed tissue in opposition, creating a high recurrence rate.[1] The tension-free repair described by Lichtenstein et al.[1] and the extraperitoneal approach described by Stoppa, Nyhus and colleagues[2,3] produced excellent results and significantly lowered the recurrence rate. These transabdominal approaches require an abdominal wall incision to accomplish the repair. This incision traverses normal tissue to repair the defect. The pathology of the hernia usually lies on the posterior abdominal wall and has nothing to do with the cord itself. Therefore, it seems unnecessary to violate normal anatomic structures to repair the defect. In considering other laparoscopic procedures, it was not unreasonable to consider a laparoscopic approach to herniorrhaphy which would avoid destruction or manipulation of these uninvolved anatomic structures.

In 1989 early clinical attempts at laparoscopic herniorrhaphy were developed by Leonard Schultz[4] using a plug and patch technique to repair the hernia. John Corbitt[5] modified that repair using a plug and patch with high ligation of the sac. Early in both series, a large recurrence rate was noted as a major complication, necessitating both surgeons to modify the repair independently, resulting in the transabdominal preperitoneal approach to laparoscopic herniorrhaphy.[6-13]

Other attempts at hernia repair were initially proposed by Ralph Ger,[14] who performed a herniaplasty using Michelle clips on 13 patients undergoing exploratory laparotomy for other procedures. The 13th patient was repaired with a special instrument produced by Ger (the herniastat). Ger's early recurrences of 5 out of 33 repairs were attributed to smaller staple size, staple placed too far apart, and mechanical failure of the herniastat itself.[15]

The onlay or intraperitoneal method originally described by Giovanni Salerno, Robert Fitzgibbons, and Charles Filipi[16] resulted in a high recurrence rate in direct hernia repair and was modified to repair only indirect space hernias. Fitzgibbons et al. repair direct space hernias using a transabdominal preperitoneal method. Complications with intra-abdominal adhesions led these surgeons to discontinue the onlay method.[17] Another proponent of the onlay patch, Albert Spaw (personal communication), has modified his procedure to expose the medial portion of the preperitoneal area rather than attaching the mesh directly to the peritoneum in the area of Cooper's ligament.

Similarly, Frederick Toy and Ray Smoot[18,19] have modified the use of a small patch tacked directly to the peritoneum after reduction of the sac and high ligation. The sac is no longer reduced by most surgeons but rather left in place, and a larger piece of mesh is now being used by Toy, Smoot, and others. Toy and Smoot have also found it necessary to expose the area of the pubic tubercle, Cooper's ligament, and the inguinal ligament as it attached to the pubic tubercle, thus modifying their original description of the onlay technique. The extraperitoneal approach, which places a large piece of mesh in the same area as the preperitoneal approach, has been described extensively by Ed Phillips and Brendan Carol[20] and Barry McKernan and Henry Laws.[21,22] It would appear that the general trend of laparoscopic herniorrhaphy is toward the use of a large prosthesis placed over the entire inguinal floor, covering both the direct and indirect spaces. This large prosthesis is attached directly (preperitoneal and extraperitoneal repairs) or indirectly (onlay repairs) to the deep fascia, inguinal ligament, Cooper's ligament, and pubis. Although complications will be discussed for all of these repairs, the major emphasis will be placed on the preperitoneal and extraperitoneal repairs.

RECURRENCES

The plug, patch, and high ligation of the sac method of hernia repair had a recurrence rate in excess of 30% (Schultz and Corbitt)[11,12,23,24] after a 2-year follow-up. The recurrence rate of hernia was the major complication at that time. It was evident that a large piece of mesh covering both the direct and indirect spaces should be used and must be fixed using either sutures or staples, hence the development of the transabdominal preperitoneal repair (TAPP) and the extraperitoneal repair by multiple authors.[9,13,20–22] The onlay approach produced early recurrences in the direct space, causing authors such as Fitzgibbons to convert to the transabdominal preperitoneal approach for this type of hernia. Other proponents of the onlay repair have modified their repair to increase the size of the patch and anchor it to exposed or unexposed deep fascial structures. If a large recurrence rate is to be avoided, certain principles must be adhered to. Most important is the use of a large piece of mesh to cover the entire floor, as described by Rene Stoppa, Lloyd Nyhus, and Robert Condon[2,3] in the open approach to preperitoneal herniorrhaphy. This large piece of mesh should extend beyond the hernia defect by at least 2 to 3 cm to allow fibrous ingrowth to complete the repair in the early postoperative period.

Proponents of the onlay technique proposed anchoring the mesh to the deep structures such as the fascia, inguinal ligament, Cooper's ligament or the rim of the hernia defect itself.[17-19] These surgeons began exposing more of these fascial structures as time progressed in the development of hernia surgery. If these preperitoneal structures were exposed, early recurrence rates after 18 months were reported to be as low as 3% in a series of approximately 1000 patients, as reported at the Minimally Invasive Surgery and New Technology Congress in Luxembourg by Fitzgibbons.[25] As has been pointed out by Schultz (personal communication) and Corbitt, it is not sufficient to repair only the obvious hernia noted during laparoscopic examination; both the direct and indirect spaces must be repaired. This important observation was noted when repairing recurrences in the early plug and patch technique.[11,13,23,24] If an indirect hernia has been repaired, the recurrence may occur in the direct space or vice versa. It is also not sufficient to place the mesh behind the peritoneum without anchoring it firmly to the fascial structures to prevent migration of the mesh in the early postoperative period. Other observations of early recurrences confirmed that occasionally the patch had slipped to the side of the defect, allowing recurrence in this area. Therefore, to prevent recurrences, it is important to use a large prosthesis covering both the direct and indirect spaces, anchoring it to the fascial structures.

Finally, it should be noted that repair depends on fibrous ingrowth into the prosthesis. Anchoring the mesh in place holds the mesh until this ingrowth occurs. In this author's opinion, at present a polypropylene mesh works best, allowing early fibrous ingrowth securing the mesh in approximately 7 days; however, all polypropylene meshes should be covered with peritoneum to prevent complications, as will be discussed elsewhere. Under development is a mesh allowing ingrowth on one side and minimal cellular ingrowth or tissue attachment on the other side, which may eliminate the necessity to cover the mesh with peritoneum (Gore-Tex DualMesh).

LAPAROSCOPIC COMPLICATIONS

Laparoscopic complications, as well as the complications associated with the specific surgical procedure of herniorrhaphy, must be taken into consideration when evaluating the patient for hernia repair. The major indication for laparoscopic herniorrhaphy is bilateral or recurrent hernia. Specifically indicated for laparoscopic repair is the bilateral hernia because of decreased pain associated with the repair. Laparoscopic repair of the recurrent hernia affords the ability to repair the recurrence in an area of relatively undisturbed anatomy.

Prior to performing laparoscopic herniorrhaphy, the patient must be made aware not only of the complications peculiar to the procedure itself but also of those associated with general laparoscopy. Understanding these complications and the risk of general anesthesia will determine whether the patient is a candidate for laparoscopic herniorrhaphy. The size or type of hernia is of little significance since most hernias may be repaired laparoscopically.

There are many excellent groin approaches to hernia repair, as opposed to gallbladder surgery. Therefore, previous abdominal surgery with the inherent risks of bowel injury, vascular injury, and so on associated with laparoscopy must be a significant consideration in hernia surgery. However, if the incisions are limited to the area above the umbilicus, an extraperitoneal approach is an excellent choice. If the patient has a left inguinal hernia and a right lower quadrant appendectomy scar, the extraperitoneal repair is the procedure of choice.

MIGRATION OF MESH

Mesh that has not been firmly fixed to the pelvis may migrate. This migration of mesh away from the hernia site accounts for recurrences, as has been mentioned in the section on "Recurrences." Migration of the mesh also accounts for the presence of palpable, painful mesh in the inguinal canal. This is most commonly seen with the plug and patch method when the plug migrated distally down the canal and, on occasion, into the scrotal area. These repairs are still being made despite early large recurrence rates. This complication is prevented by securing the mesh to the fascia and Cooper's ligament using either staples or sutures. If the mesh is palpable in the canal or scrotum, the patient may become extremely dissatisfied. In general with current hernia repairs, the only possible situation in which this could occur is in the repair of a femoral hernia where a plug may still be used. Repair of the direct or indirect space hernia does not require the application of a plug. Free, large, unfixed mesh repairs are currently being evaluated. The larger hernias may have a high recurrence rate because of displacement of the mesh.

INTERFERENCE OF THE PROSTHESIS WITH THE ILIAC AND/OR SPERMATIC VESSELS

It is possible that a portion of prosthetic mesh placed on the floor of the inguinal canal could interfere later with the iliac or testicular vessels. This complication has not been observed to date in laparoscopic herniorrhaphy, nor has it been observed in similar repairs through open incisions by Stoppa, Condon, and Nyhus. It is, therefore, believed that this is a theoretical rather than a real complication. Mesh is not placed directly over these structures; instead, a layer of areolar tissue usually exists between the mesh and these important structures. This probably accounts for the protection of these structures from the prosthesis. Division of major vessels has not been reported.

Future vascular surgery requiring aortofemoral bypass has not been a problem following laparoscopic herniorrhaphy. A tunnel can always be made lateral to the graft or behind it.

BLADDER INJURY

Dissection of the pelvis through the laparoscope requires knowledge of the local anatomy. The dissection is usually performed anteriorly and lateral to the bladder. However, the possibility of bladder injury exists if dissection is carried too far medially. Generally, the umbilical ligament should be the medial boundary of the major portion of the dissection in laparoscopic herniorrhaphy. There has been one reported case in which the patient developed urinary symptoms postoperatively. Cystoscopy revealed a piece of mesh entering the bladder; it was removed without difficulty, and the patient became asymptomatic. The details of the cause of this injury are unknown; however, it is believed that the mesh was probably placed in the bladder at the time of herniorrhaphy rather than eroding into the bladder. There have been no other cases of erosion into the bladder postoperatively.

Large, direct hernias may contain bladder. During dissection, the muscular portion of the bladder is easily recognized and injury avoided. Blunt dissection of the fatty tissue in this area will help avoid this injury.

HYDROCELE

The majority of surgeons are now leaving the distal indirect sac in place, especially in the larger scrotal-type hernias, to prevent injury to the cord structures. The sac is amputated at the neck and allowed to remain in place. In open cases, long-term follow-up on this amputation procedure has not revealed the formation of hydroceles. Seroma or hematoma formation in the sac postoperatively may occur. This resolves in approximately 3 months. (All hematomas or seromas should be left in place and aspiration avoided unless absolutely necessary.) Experimental work by Ralph Ger, who performed herniaplasty with closure of the internal ring, has also supported the fact that the sac will be obliterated in approximately 6 weeks. During Ger's experiments, beagle dogs were used and sacrificed at varying intervals to establish hydrocele formation. Significant hydroceles were not seen in any of these animals, and the sac was noted to fibrose after several weeks.

If the patient is examined in the first postoperative week and there is an apparent hydrocele formation which is asymptomatic, nothing further need be done. If there is a question of a failed herniorrhaphy (early recurrence), ultrasound may be used to determine the exact diagnosis.

URINARY RETENTION

As with any type of surgery, and in particular with hernia surgery, the patient is at risk for postoperative urinary retention. This problem is not peculiar to laparoscopic herniorrhaphy and has not been seen to increase when the procedure is performed laparoscopically. Proper preoperative evaluation of the prostate will help prevent postoperative urinary retention; however, this is not infallible. Patients operated on on an outpatient basis do much better than those who are hospitalized. Fewer than 1% of these patients have difficulty, whereas over 20% of hospitalized patients are suggested to need catheterization by the nurse in charge.

HEMATOMAS

Scrotal hematomas and ecchymosis have been observed, as with open surgery. The hematomas resolve and usually are asymptomatic. The majority of them occur if the distal sac has been dissected from the scrotum. For this reason, it is recommended that the distal sac be left in place. More commonly, ecchymosis is seen because of dissection in the pelvic floor and free communication in the preperitoneal space between the soft tissue, scrotum, and direct area of repair. At present, a preoperative long-acting antibiotic is given because of the use of prosthetic material. This antibiotic probably helps prevent infection in the hematoma.

If the patient is seen in the office during the first postoperative week and the inguinal canal is examined, a bulge may be found in the canal. This is also thought to be a hematoma in the local area and/or a reaction to the mesh. This bulge will not respond to a Valsalva maneuver and is clearly not a recurrence. If the patient is followed for 3 months, the bulge will be found to resolve spontaneously. Hematomas between the peritoneum and the abdominal wall in preperitoneal and extraperitoneal repairs are not important.

Ecchymoses of the abdominal wall, as with all herniorrhaphies, have been observed, but usually to a lesser degree than with a trans-groin approach. They are not significant.

PARESTHESIA

The most common paresthesia observed in laparoscopic herniorrhaphy is that involving the lateral femoral cutaneous nerve of the thigh, which produces hypesthesia and/or paresthesia along the lateral aspect of the upper thigh. The lateral femoral cutaneous nerve of the thigh courses 1–2 cm medial to the anterior superior iliac spine below the iliopubic tract. Dissection, the use of electrocautery, and stapling in this area should be done cautiously to prevent injury to this nerve. Approximately 2% of early laparoscopic herniorrhaphies resulted in this injury because of lack of knowledge of the neuroanatomy. Fortunately, the majority of these injuries are transient, disappearing in 1 to 2 weeks. There have been many reported cases of pain in this area that was severe enough to compel the surgeon to remove the staples. Fortunately, this is the exception rather than the rule. If a patient complains of pain, paresthesia, or numbness immediately following surgery, the staple should be removed immediately from the lateral posterior portion of the mesh. If the patient was pain free until several days after the procedure, he or she may be observed; the symptoms will disappear in several months. This injury is usually due to edema, irritation from the mesh, or possibly electric current. Electric current is unnecessary and may even be contraindicated in laparoscopic herniorrhaphy. Certainly it should never be used below the iliopubic tract. Finally, if it is discovered several weeks following surgery that the patient had immediate postoperative pain that has not resolved, the area should be injected with cortisone. If the patient fails to respond, the clip will need to be localized with a computed tomography–guided needle and removed surgically through a transgroin approach.

Staples placed in the area of the iliac artery and vein below the iliopubic tract may injure the femoral nerve, resulting in both motor and sensory loss. Any motor loss should be explored immediately and the staple removed.

SCROTAL EMPHYSEMA

In the early plug and patch method, scrotal emphysema was not uncommon when the sac was reduced into the abdominal cavity. As more and more of the distal sacs are left in place, this complication is seen less frequently. It is a transient complication, and although the scrotum may become quite large, most of the emphysema can be reduced at the time of surgery with compression of the scrotal area. If most of this emphysema is reduced under anesthesia, by the time the patient is discharged the majority of the remaining portion will have dissipated. Scrotal emphysema also occurs to a large extent with the extraperitoneal repair, as does abdominal wall emphysema. CO_2 pressure should be below 8 mmHg when using the extraperitoneal approach to prevent abdominal wall and scrotal emphysema.

SUBCUTANEOUS EMPHYSEMA

Subcutaneous emphysema occurs most commonly with extraperitoneal dissection. A transient rise in CO_2 content may be observed; however, this has not been significant in the otherwise normal patient. Subcutaneous emphysema can be extensive, extending from the neck to the lower extremities, but it does not produce a significant complication. This complication is avoided by lowering the CO_2 pressure during extraperitoneal dissection to 8 mmHg or less.

Abdominal wall emphysema can extend from the neck down to the lower extremities but is more frightening than painful or disabling. No residual has been noted.

BOWEL OBSTRUCTION

There have been many reported cases of bowel obstruction resulting from incarceration of the small bowel between the peritoneum and the hernia repair. Meticulous closure of the peritoneum following transabdominal preperitoneal surgery is mandatory to prevent this complication. Staples should be placed approximately 1 cm apart and the peritoneum completely closed. The peritoneum may also be sutured with such devices as the Autostitch (USSC Norwalk, CT.).

The other common cause of bowel obstruction is a Richter's-type hernia through the 12-mm ports. All of these ports must be sutured.

If a patient presents with intestinal obstruction, examine the port sites. If the patient is too obese to allow these sites to be felt, a sonogram will reveal incarcerated bowel. If the port sites are clear, no other workup is necessary. The bowel is probably incarcerated between the peritoneum and the hernia repair. This bowel is in the extraperitoneal space and cannot be palpated. The patient should be examined laparoscopically. Usually the bowel can be reduced and the peritoneal defect repaired.

VASCULAR AND SPERMATIC CORD INJURIES

There have been at least two deaths from injuries of the iliac vessels during laparoscopic herniorrhaphy. It is imperative that the anatomy of the inguinal area be completely understood prior to attempting herniorrhaphy and that the triangle of doom be avoided during dissection in this area. On many occasions, the iliac vessels cannot be directly observed; therefore, sharp dissection or the use of energy sources in the posterior triangle of doom should be avoided. If the iliac artery or vein is injured during laparoscopic herniorrhaphy, the patient should be opened immediately to avoid mortality. Injury to the spermatic cord may also occur in dissection in the triangle of doom. Therefore, dissection in this area should proceed with caution. More commonly, spermatic cord injuries occur when the large scrotal sac is reduced into the abdominal cavity. For this reason, most surgeons choose to leave the distal sac in place.

EPIGASTRIC VESSELS INJURIES

Epigastric vessels which lie at the level of the umbilicus lateral to the rectus muscle may be injured during placement of the secondary trocars. These trocars must be placed under direct vision, identifying the epigastric vessels in the pelvis and noting their course across the abdominal wall. Any injury to a vessel during port placement should be repaired by suture at the end of the procedure or at its initiation if there is large blood loss.

The other common cause of epigastric injury is dissection of the pelvic floor. The epigastric vessels lie between the direct and indirect spaces and must be observed throughout the procedure. If the vessels are divided during herniorrhaphy, they must be ligated or stapled. It will not suffice to use electrical coagulation to control the bleeding. The epigastric vessels, after being dissected by the transperitoneal or extraperitoneal approach, will tend to form an hour-glass figure with the triangle of doom. This hourglass configuration will be helpful after the mesh has been placed during the stapling portion of the procedure.

The majority of surgeons leave the inferior epigastric vessels attached to the abdominal wall and avoid placing the mesh anterior to the vessels, which obviates unnecessary dissection of these structures.

On rare occasions, the epigastric vessels protrude into the abdominal cavity causing them to interfere with dissection and mesh placement. In such cases, the mesh will have to be placed behind these vessels. This is the exception rather than the rule.

COMPLICATIONS RELATED TO PROSTHETIC MATERIALS

Hernia repair depends on incorporation of fibrous tissue into the prosthetic material. It has, therefore, been recommended that a polypropylene mesh such as SurgiPro, Marlex, or Prolene be used during the transabdominal and extraperitoneal approaches. A new mesh by Gore-Tex (DualMesh) is now under consideration. This material has the ability to incorporate fibrous material on one side and to produce a "knotted hair" property on the other side. This mesh is being used mainly in the modifications of the onlay method.

There have been reports of bowel adhesions using a polypropylene mesh in the onlay technique. Therefore, most surgeons using this technique use a material which has been reported to avoid this complication. Inspection of patients undergoing a second operation for other reasons following laparoscopic herniorrhaphy has revealed minimal adhesions if any of these materials are placed in the extraperitoneal space. These materials appear to have no transperitoneal influence on adhesive properties.

There have been no cases of infection or rejection of any of these materials used in laparoscopic hernia approaches. A long-acting preoperative antibiotic is usually administered when anesthesia is induced, which may account for this excellent result. However, a long postoperative course of antibiotics is not indicated.

Acknowledgments

This chapter has been contributed to by the following surgeons (personal communications): M. Arregui, R. Bailey, C. Filipi, R. Fitzgibbons, Jr., M. Franklin, B. MacFadyen, Jr, J. McKernan, D. Olsen, E. Phillips, D. Rosenthal, L. Schultz, R. Sewell, R. Smoot, A. Spaw, F. Toy, K. Zucker, J. Payne, P. Go, and J. Gracia.

Over 4,000 cases of laparoscopic herniorrhaphy with as much as a 5-year follow-up have been reviewed to produce this chapter. The complication rates are approximate but substantially accurate and reliable.

REFERENCES

1. Lichtenstein IL, Shulman AG, Amid PK, et al: The tension-free hernioplasty. *Am J Surg* 157:188–192, 1989.
2. Nyhus LM, Pollak R, Bombeck TC, et al: The preperitoneal approach and prosthetic buttress repair for recurrent hernia. *Ann Surg* 208:733–737, 1988.
3. Stoppa RE, Warlaumont CR: The preperitoneal approach and prosthetic repair of groin hernia. In Nyhus LM, Condon RE (eds): *Hernia*. Philadelphia, Lippincott, 1989, pp 199–225.
4. Shultz L, Graber J, Pietrafitta J, et al: Laser laparoscopic herniorrhaphy: A clinical trial preliminary results. *J Laparoendosc Surg* 1:41, 1990.
5. Corbitt JD: Laparoscopic herniorrhaphy. *Surg Laparosc Endosc* 1:23–25, 1991.
6. Corbitt JD: Laparoscopic hernia repair. *Laparosc Focus* 1:1, 1992.
7. Corbitt JD: Laparoscopic preperitoneal tension-free herniorrhaphy. *Lasers Surg Med*, (Suppl 3):2, 1991.
8. Corbitt JD: Laparoscopic herniorrhaphy. *Lasers Med Surg* 4:27, 1992.
9. Corbitt JD: Laparoscopic herniorrhaphy. In Reddick E, Saye W, Corbitt JD (eds): *Atlas of Laparoscopic Surgery*. New York, Raven Press, 1992, pp 103–113.
10. Corbitt JD: Laparoscopic inguinal hernia repair. In Ballantyne GH, Leahy P, Modlin IM (eds): *Laparoscopic Surgery*. Philadelphia, Saunders, 1993, pp 625–639
11. Corbitt JD: Laparoscopic herniorrhaphy—a preperitoneal approach. In Welter R, Steichen F (eds): *Minimally Invasive Surgery and New Technology*. St Louis, Quality Medical, 1994, pp 334–337.

12. Corbitt JD: An update, laparoscopic herniorrhaphy. *Laparoscopy in Focus* 1:8,
13. Corbitt JD: Transabdominal preperitoneal herniorrhaphy. *Surg Laparosc Endosc* 3:328–332, 1993.
14. Ger R: The laparoscopic management of groin hernias. *Contemp Surg* 39:15–19, 1991.
15. Ger R: Personal communication.
16. Salerno GM, Fitzgibbons RJ Jr, Filipi CJ: Laparoscopic inguinal hernia repair. In Zucker KA (ed): *Surgical Laparoscopy*. St Louis, Quality Medical, 1991, pp 281–293.
17. Fitzgibbons RJ Jr, Annibali R, Litke B, et al: A multicentered clinical trial on laparoscopic inguinal hernia repair: Preliminary results. SAGES Scientific Session 1: abstract 118, 1993.
18. Toy FK, Smoot RT Jr: Toy-Smoot laparoscopic hernioplasty. *Surg Laparosc Endosc* 1:151–155, 1991.
19. Toy FK, Smoot RT Jr: Laparoscopic hernioplasty update. *J Laparoendosc Surg* 2:197–205, 1992.
20. Phillips EH, Caroll BJ: Laparoscopic inguinal hernia repair. *Gastrointest Endosc Clin North Am*
21. McKernan JB, Laws HL: Laparoscopic preperitoneal prosthetic repair of inguinal hernias. *Surg Rounds* 597–610, 1992.
22. McKernan JB, Laws HL: Laparoscopic repair of inguinal hernia using a totally extraperitoneal prosthetic approach. *Surg Endosc* 7:26–28, 1993.
23. Phillips EH, Carroll B, Fallas M, et al: Reasons for recurrence following laparoscopic hernioplasty. *Ann Surg* 1993.
24. Corbitt JD: Plug and patch repair: Lessons learned. In Arregui M, Rosin D (eds): *Inguinal Herniorrhaphy; A Modern Perspective*. Radcliffe Medical Press, 1995, pp
25. The 43rd Surgical Forum, University of Southern California Medical Center, March 18–21, 1993.

chapter fourteen
Extraperitoneal Herniorrhaphy

George S. Ferzli

INTRODUCTION

The open preperitoneal placement of prosthetic mesh for the repair of inguinal hernia has been popularized by Nyhus et al.,[1-3] Stoppa et al.,[4] and Wantz[5] and has an exceptionally low recurrence rate.[6] Recent advances in laparoscopic instrumentation and technology have made it possible to perform this time-honored repair endoscopically.

HISTORICAL REVIEW

Laparoscopic management of inguinal hernia was first suggested by Ger et al.[7] in 1983. Using a special stapling device called a *herniastat*, they reapproximated the internal ring. The closure of the ring did not address floor weakness, however, nor did it deal with concomitant hernia defects. It left the sac behind and was not a tension-free repair. Later that year, Popp[8] reported a case of endoscopic repair in a female patient using polypropylene mesh inserted into the defect after incising the overlying peritoneum. In the same year, Schultz et al.[9] presented early results of the use of an intraperitoneal approach to identify the defect, reconstructing it with two plugs and a patch of polypropylene mesh and reapproximating the edges of the peritoneum. The plug and patch graft combined with high ligation of the sac was also reported by Corbitt[10] in 1991. This technique, however, resulted in high failure and recurrence rates. The mesh plug in the inguinal canal resulted in a hard, uncomfortable mass in the groin. The plug migrated into the scrotum and in some cases eroded through the skin. In 1992, Gazayerli[11] attempted reconstruction of the floor through an intraperitoneal approach. This was technically difficult and time-consuming, and again was not a tension-free repair. During the same period, Toy and Smoot[12] described a technique using an expanded polytetrafluoroethylene (PTFE) patch. This was attached by an intraperitoneal onlay mesh technique (IPOM), a new approach that left the indirect sac behind, with an uncertain long-term fate as an intraperitoneal prosthetic material. Erosion into adjacent structures, formation of adhesions, and foreign body infection were of continuing concern.

A little later, the transabdominal preperitoneal repair (TAPP)[13] emerged, soon becoming the most popular procedure. In this repair, the peritoneum covering the entire myopectineal orifice on the side of the defect was stripped, and a large piece of mesh was inserted and fixed in place so that it covered the entire myopectineal orifice. The peritoneum was then closed over the mesh. Numerous complications were reported with the TAPP procedure.[14] Among them were neuralgias involving the femoral branch of the genital femoral nerve and the lateral femoral cutaneous nerve. Other complications included bowel and bladder injuries, adhesion formation, internal hernias, intestinal obstructions, and bleeding. A brief summary of the different methods employed for this purpose is presented in Table 14.1. In all of the previously described techniques, general anesthesia was used and the peritoneal cavity was entered, risking possible associated complications. Finally, in 1992, endoscopic extraperitoneal hernia repair (EEPH)[15] was first described. It is also known as the *laparoscopic extraperitoneal approach (LEP)* or the *total extraperitoneal approach (TEP)*.

Table 14.1. Laparoscopic Repair Methods

Technique	Disadvantages
Closure of neck using the herniastat (transperitoneal, 1990)	Floor weakness/leaves sac/ concomitant defects/not tension free
Plug and patch (transperitoneal, 1990–91)	Plug migrates to scrotum/painful lump in groin/high recurrence rate
Floor reconstruction (transperitoneal, 1991)	Difficult/cumbersome/not tension free
Intraperitoneal onlay mesh (IPOM) (transperitoneal, 1991)	Leaves indirect sac/longterm follow-up/adhesions/fistulas?
Transabdominal preperitoneal mesh placement (TAPP) (transperitoneal, 1991)	Bowel/bladder injury/intestinal obstruction/adhesions/intestinal hernias/bleeding/neuralgia

Note: All procedures are performed under general anesthesia.

TECHNICAL ASPECTS OF EEPH

The patient is placed in the supine position, and intravenous antibiotics are given. The skin of the abdomen, scrotum, and perineum is scrubbed, prepped and draped.

Anesthesia

General or epidural anesthesia is commonly used. Spinal, or more often epidural, anesthesia is especially useful in patients with respiratory problems.

Position

The video monitor, insufflation apparatus, and light source are positioned at the feet of the patient (Fig. 14.1). The surgeon stands on the side opposite the hernia. A slight Trendelenburg position is helpful.

Operation

A small incision is made in the inferior aspect of the umbilicus. Dissection is continued down to the rectus fascia. The fascia is secured on either side of the midline with 0-vicryl sutures, which are used later to anchor the blunt-tip cannula. The fascia is then incised in the midline. The linea alba is seen in the midline, along with the entrance to the preperitoneal space (Fig. 14.2). Dissection of this space can be done in three ways.

Operative scope dissection

Blunt finger dissection is initially performed extraperitoneally in the midline toward the pubic symphysis. This allows the placement of a 10-mm blunt-tip trocar, which is secured in place. The CO_2 insufflation tubing is attached to the cannula, and a pressure of 8 to 10 mmHg maintained. A 10-mm 0° operative scope with a 5-mm working channel is introduced in the trocar. A blunt probe or 5-mm cautery scissors are used to further develop the preperitoneal space in the midline down to the retropubic space of Retzius. It is important to stay in the midline in a plane parallel to the rectus muscles and as anterior as possible to avoid bleeding or peritoneal tearing (Fig. 14.3A).

The surgeon must stay posterior or through a thin, translucent, filmy fascial layer that represents the posterior lamina or the inner portion of the fascia transversalis, as described by Cooper.[16] Even though Nyhus[17] states that this layer has no practical value because it lacks sufficient strength (p. 63), it is impossible to overemphasize the importance of recognizing this layer, which is always present. Read[18] has stated, "it is only after this was disrupted, avoiding injury to the epigastric vasculature lying on it, that the finger could be passed freely outside the preperitoneal fat." To repeat, it is important to recognize the presence of this layer; if raw rectus muscle fibers are seen, the surgeon is in the wrong plane. The probe or scissors then continue laterally, dissecting the posterior portion of the rectus abdominis muscle on each side to develop the cavity further. This is continued medially into the

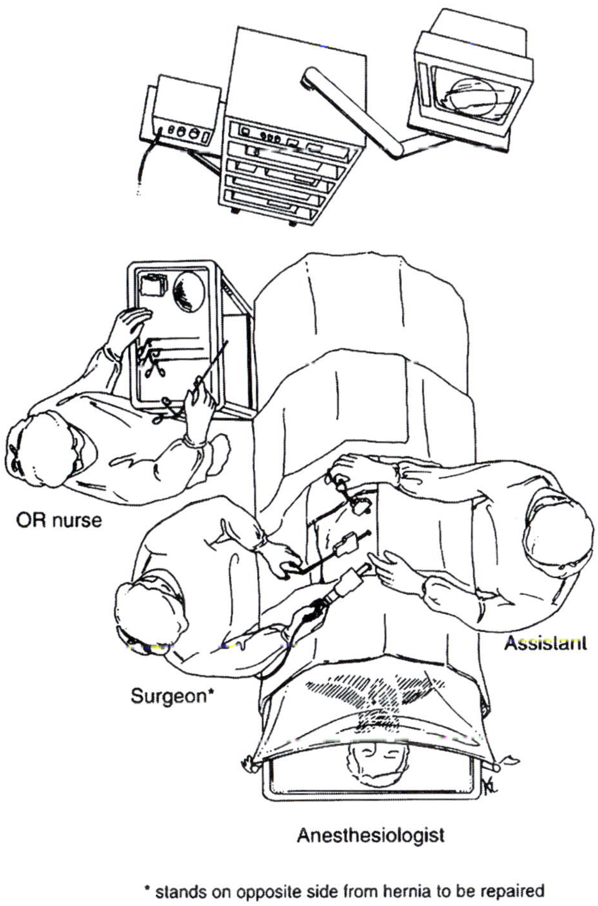

Figure 14.1. Position of the operating room staff and equipment for a right inguinal hernia.

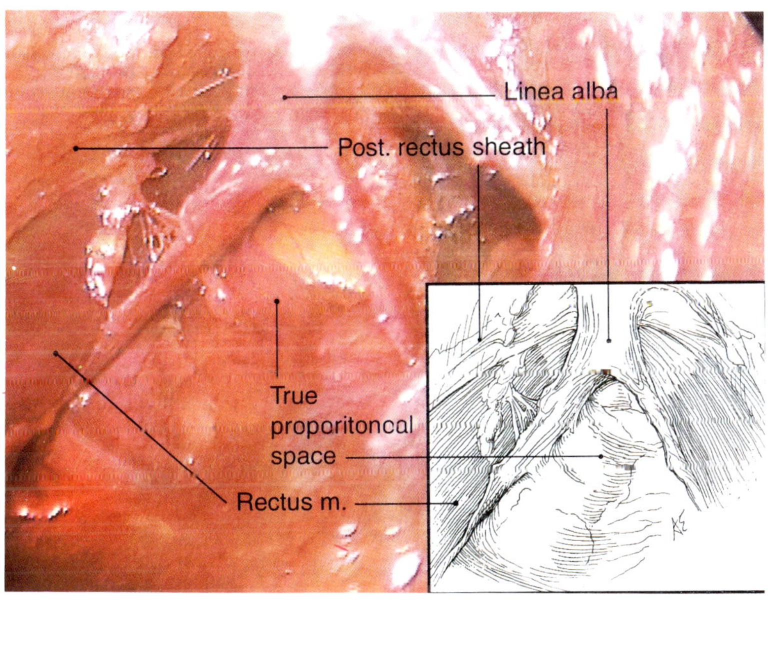

Figure 14.2. Entrance to the preperitoneal space.

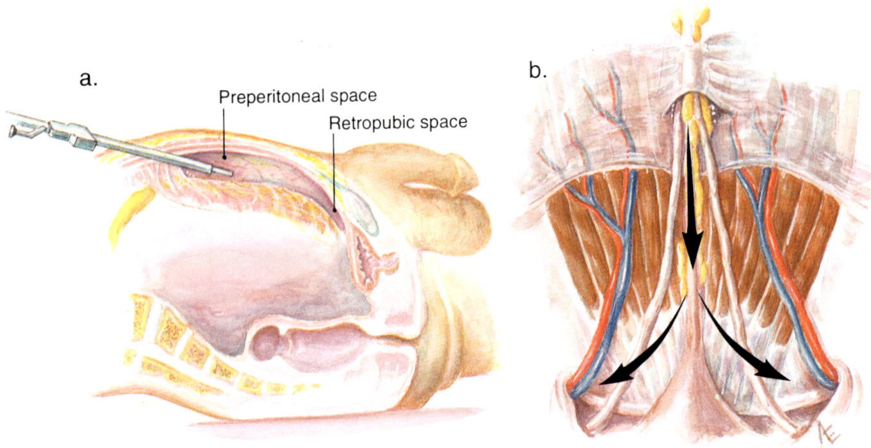

Figure 14.3. (a, b) Operative scope dissection of the preperitoneal space.

Retzius space and laterally into Bogros's space and the iliopsoas fascia (Fig. 14.3B).

Balloon dissection

Preperitoneal dissection can be done using a balloon dissector; two types are available. The first, the Origin Medsystems (Menlo Park, CA) balloon, is introduced on either side of the midline between the rectus muscle and the posterior rectus sheath. It is advanced to the pubis symphysis in the midline. A 10-mm endoscope, either 0° or 25°, is placed within the lumen of the balloon, which is then insufflated and used to dissect the preperitoneum, the space of Retzius, and the posterior aspect of the rectus abdominis muscle on either side, all under direct visualization. The second balloon available is marketed by USSC (Norwalk, CT) and is incorporated with a cannula that does not allow an endoscope to be placed within its lumen. It is introduced in a fashion similar to that of the previous balloon but is insufflated in a blind fashion to dissect the same preperitoneal space (Fig. 14.4).

Blunt finger dissection

The same results obtained with either the operative scope or the balloon can also be achieved using simple blunt finger dissection through the initial fascial incision in the midline. A gentle sweeping motion in the midline toward the pubis symphysis is initially employed, followed by lateral sweeping motions on each side, posterior to the rectus muscles. It is important to place the finger in the true preperitoneal midline space at the onset. If this is not possible, the surgeon should enter the space between the rectus muscle and the posterior rectus sheath on either side of the midline and then bluntly tear the insertion of the two posterior sheaths at the midline.

Placement of trocars

Once a preperitoneal space has been developed and kept open by CO_2 insufflation, two additional trocars are placed in the midline under direct visualization. A 10- or 12-mm trocar is placed infraumbilically, and a 5-mm trocar is placed in a suprapubic position. On rare

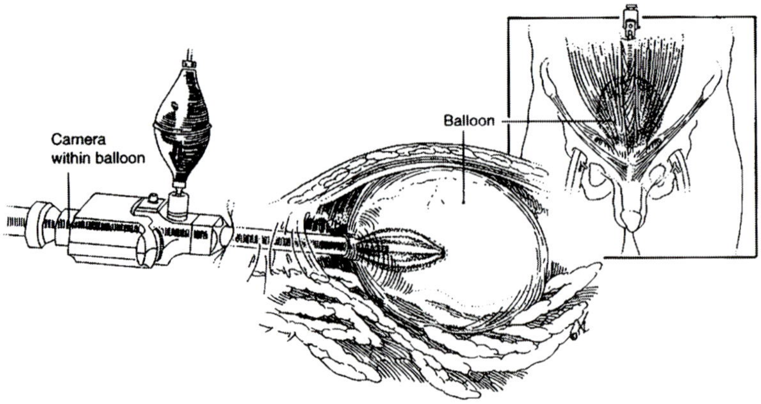

Figure 14.4. Balloon dissection of the preperitoneal space.

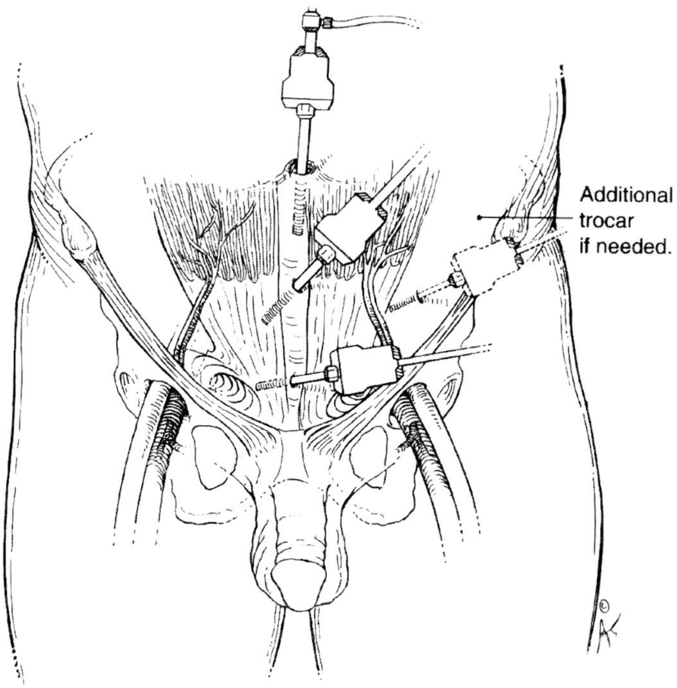

Figure 14.5. Placement of trocars.

occasions, such as the occurrence of a large sliding hernia or a giant scrotal one, an additional trocar may be needed. It is placed lateral to the rectus muscle below the linea semicircularis (Fig. 14.5).

Dissection

A 25° or 30° 10-mm lens is preferable to a 0° one. Two blunt-nose, nonlocking graspers are used, and laparoscopic scissors should be available. Suction/irrigation devices and electrocautery are not routinely set up, since they are rarely needed. Hemoclips are also rarely used.

The first and most important part of the dissection is to visualize the bone in the midline (step 1). This prevents any mishaps or potential injury to the bladder, bowel, or peritoneum. Once the bone is safely identified, the surgeon gently develops the retropubic space of Retzius, using blunt, gentle, short, sweeping moves. The surgeon stays along the bone on each side of the midline to identify Cooper's ligament (step 2). The pubic branch vein is frequently seen crossing over Cooper's ligament from the iliac vessels to the obturator fossa. At this point, attention is directed superiorly to the rectus abdominis muscle to identify the epigastric vessels (step 3). The direct space, or medial fossa, will be readily visible; it is bounded by the epigastric vessels superolaterally, the rectus muscle medially, and the iliopubic tract inferiorly.

An anteropubic branch of the iliopubic vein, originating from the epigastric vessels, is often seen as a blue line running along the iliopubic tract in a horizontal fashion, making this structure easily identifiable. Dissection continues posterior to the epigastric vessels (step 4), with one grasper retracting these vessels anteriorly while the other is gently sweeping in a horizontal right-to-left motion through the space lateral to the epigastric vessels (step 5). Dissection in this area should be particularly gentle to avoid tears in the peritoneum. It is continued superiorly to the anterosuperior iliac spine level (step 6). At this point, a small perforating vessel will be seen piercing the parietal peritoneum to the transverse muscle. Dissection should not be pursued above the linea semicircularis, where the peritoneum is adherent and might tear. In general, the surgeon can easily perform this dissection without causing hemorrhage. Any femoral defects can be seen medial to the femoral vessels, any direct ones medial to the epigastric vessels, and any indirect ones lateral to these vessels (Fig. 14.6).

DIRECT HERNIA

A direct hernia will be recognized immediately when the surgeon moves from the pubic symphysis in the

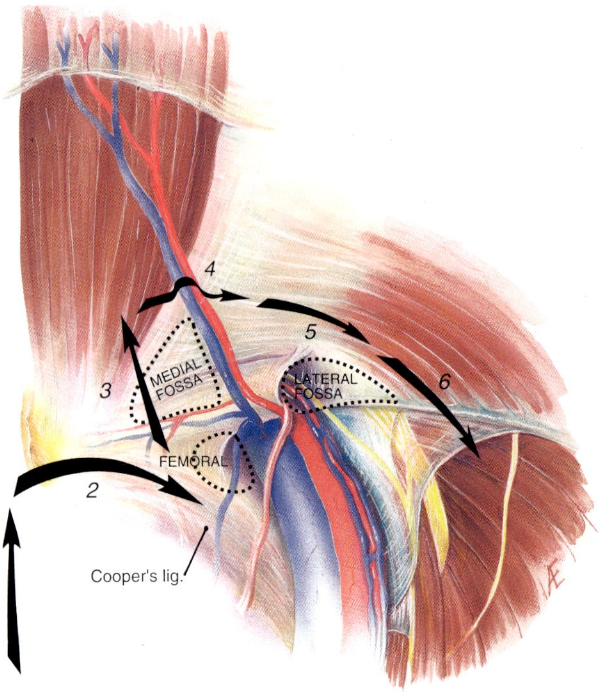

Figure 14.6. The six steps of the dissection.

midline along Cooper's ligament toward the femoral canal. Cooper's ligament and the femoral canal are usually obscured by the contents of the direct hernia defect. This material can almost always be freed with gentle traction and countertraction, rarely requiring sharp dissection. A rolled edge or fold nicely demarcates the separation between the redundant thickened transversalis and the peritoneal sac (Fig. 14.7A). Dissection continues along this fold, reducing the entire contents of the direct defect. Dissection utilizing gentle traction and countertraction is usually free of hemorrhage and avoids sharp dissection. The edges of the defect, the iliopubic tract, the epigastric vessels, and the iliac vessels in their sheath will all be readily visible. The margins of the direct hernia defect should be cleansed of preperitoneal areolar and fatty tissue.

Large hernia defects can be imbricated with suture material or staples to reduce the amount of dead space, thereby reducing the chance of a postoperative seroma. A direct hernia may occur as a small hole within the floor, as multiple defects, or solely as a widening of the floor.

Incarcerated Direct Hernia

When the hernia is incarcerated, or when the patient has had prior lower abdominal surgery such as a suprapubic cystostomy or a prostate procedure, extra care must be exercised during dissection to prevent damage to the bladder. It is also important to enlarge the opening of the defect to allow safe dissection of the contents. The releasing incision should be made at the anteromedial aspect of the defect to avoid injury to the epigastric or iliac vessels (Fig. 14.7B).

Femoral Hernia

The anterior margin is formed by the iliopubic tract and the posterior margin by Cooper's ligament. Dissection is mostly blunt, and is done along the supramedial and inframedial aspects of the femoral canal to avoid injury to the external iliac and femoral vessels. The sac is reduced by traction and countertraction. An aberrant obturator artery originating from the inferior epigastric vessels (corona mortis) or the external iliac vessels should be recognized and protected (Fig. 14.8). Cautery is not desirable.

Incarcerated Femoral Hernia

A releasing incision is often needed and is effected by carefully incising the insertion of the iliopubic tract into Cooper's ligament at the medial portion of the femoral ring. If needed, dissection can then be continued under visualization in the femoral canal to the level of the femoral canal orifice (Gimbernat's ligament).

INDIRECT HERNIA

For the inexperienced surgeon, the approach to the internal ring must start with identification of the epigastric vessels. The fascia transversalis sling of the internal abdominal ring will be seen immediately. Keeping in mind that the vas deferens is adjacent to the epigastric vessels and loops toward the space of Retzius, dissection should be started in the anterolateral aspect of the deep internal ring. (Fig. 14.9A) This has several advantages. It avoids injury to the cord structures and it allows identification of a preperitoneal cordal lipoma, which can be easily suppressed, allowing the surgeon to grasp the indirect sac, if present, without injuring its contents or the cord structures.

To avoid complications, it is mandatory to start dissection in the upper outer quadrant of the deep internal ring. Dissection of the sac off the cord structures is done in a direction perpendicular to the cord structures, sweeping them gently, medially and posteriorly,

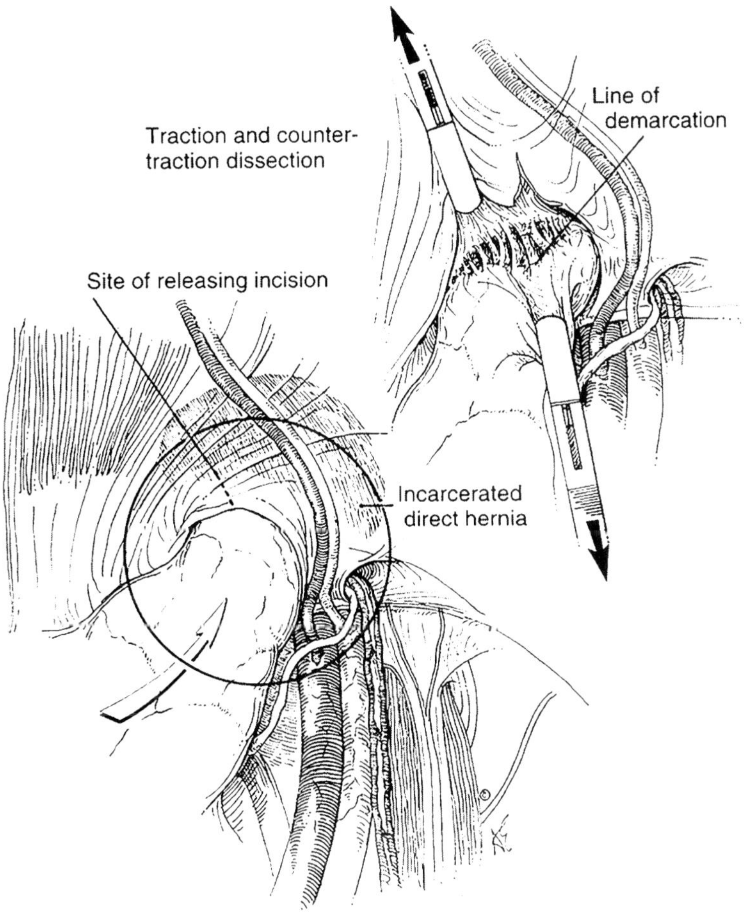

Figure 14.7. Direct hernia.

while holding the sac with the other grasper, laterally and superiorly (Fig. 14.9A). An alternative and certainly safer technique is to pivot the hernia sac medially and posteriorly and dissect the cord structures in a perpendicular fashion, sweeping in a lateral and posterior direction (Fig. 14.9B). An advantage of this approach is easy identification of a cord lipoma and the margins of the indirect sac, as well as avoidance of injury to the internal spermatic vessels. The surgeon can then alternate dissection between the medial and lateral approaches. A window is thus created between the cord structures and the sac. The latter is either totally invaginated and reduced or transected, leaving the distal blunt end in situ while suturing closed the proximal end after ensuring that the contents are not injured. Cord structures must be totally parietalized with the posterior wall so that no element crosses the preperitoneal prevesical space.

Incarcerated Indirect Hernia

In this situation, as with some large sliding hernias or giant scrotal ones, the large indirect sac encroaches on the posterior inguinal wall, causing the medial fossa to bulge inward. This bulge in the floor is always an indication of a large indirect hernia.

Certain steps must be taken to facilitate dissection; they are the same when dealing with large indirect, giant scrotal, incarcerated large indirect, or recurrent large indirect hernias.

1. The epigastric vessels may be divided to allow easier dissection of the sac.
2. An additional trocar placed laterally below the linea semicircularis (Fig. 14.5) will be needed for three reasons: The first is to facilitate dissection of the sac. The second is to keep the proximal part of the indirect sac occluded while it is being

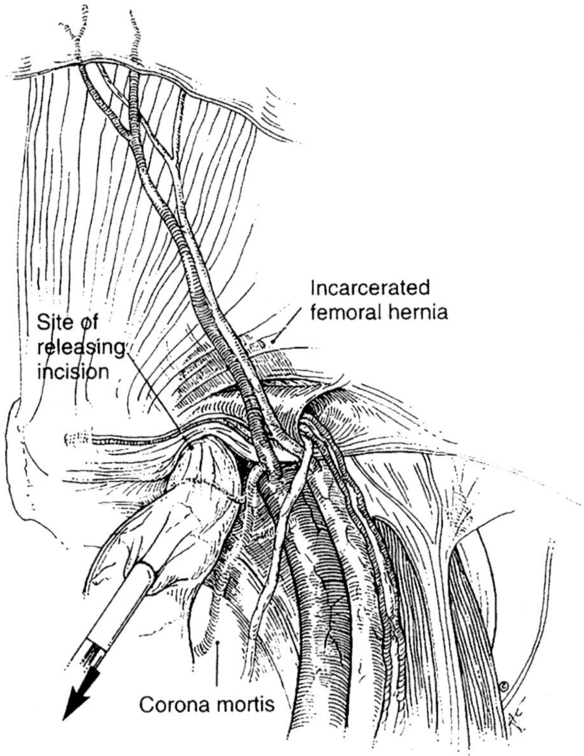

Figure 14.8. Femoral hernia.

divided distally. This minimizes the amount of CO_2 escaping into the peritoneal cavity. Occlusion of the sac is accomplished by gently pressing it between a blunt grasper anteriorly and the psoas muscle posteriorly. The third reason is to help in suturing closed the divided large indirect sac.

3. The six steps previously described in the dissection of EEPH are modified somewhat (Fig. 14.10). The surgeon identifies the midline pubic symphysis, Cooper's ligament, the medial aspect of the iliopubic tract, and the direct space. No further dissection is done from this point on. Instead, the surgeon moves proximally behind the rectus muscle, posterior to the epigastric vessels, laterally along the linea semicircularis to the level of the anterosuperior iliac spine. From there, the iliac fascia is dissected bluntly, in a horizontal fashion, identifying some of the lateral aspect of the iliopubic tract. The contents of the large indirect are now within two open spaces, Retzius and Bogros. It is important always to suppress the cord lipoma before approaching the sac. This will delineate the sac margins, giving more room to work on the anterolateral aspect of the indirect hernia sac. Cord lipoma dissection may also allow immediate identification of the internal spermatic vessels and occasionally the vas. Gentle, blunt and sharp dissection is carried out from

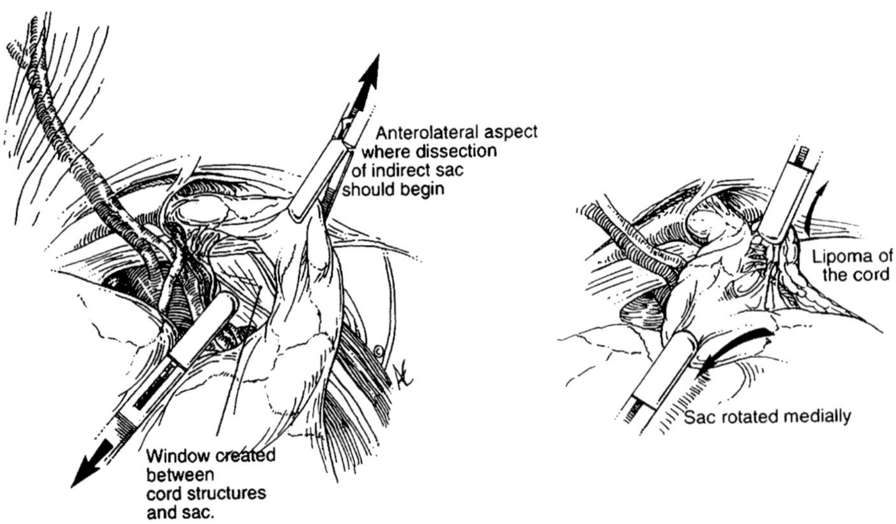

Figure 14.9. Indirect hernia.

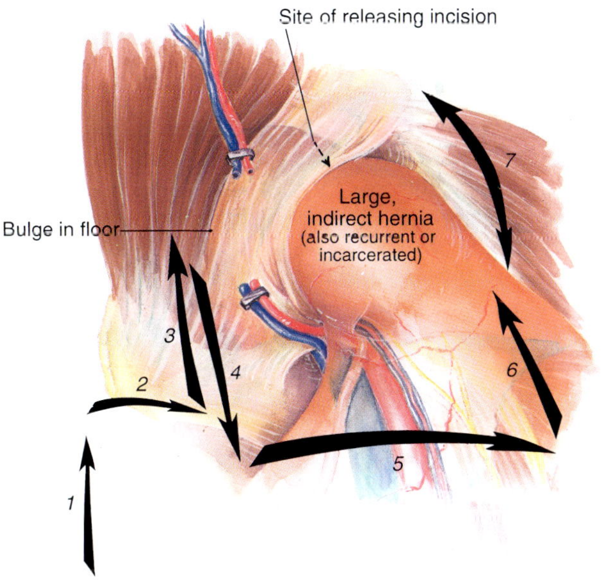

Figure 14.10. Steps of dissection in large indirect, incarcerated large indirect, giant scrotal, sliding, and recurrent large indirect hernias.

the lateral aspect toward the medial aspect; the surgeon trying first to identify the lateral aspect of the deep internal ring opening from the 12 o'clock to the 6 o'clock position in a clockwise direction (Fig. 14.10). The last part of the dissection should involve the medial aspect of the deep internal ring, where care should be taken not to injure the iliac vessels or the origin of the epigastric vessels.

In incarcerated hernias, as in giant scrotal ones, the deep internal ring is divided anteriorly at the 12 o'clock position toward the external ring, facilitating dissection of the indirect sac (Fig. 14.10). The site of the releasing incision is shown for these cases (Fig. 14.10).

RECURRENT HERNIA

Recurrent Direct Hernia

In general, these hernias are treated the same way as primary direct ones. Gentle traction and countertraction reduces the contents and delineates the margins of the defect. The contents can sometimes be very adherent, and scissors may be needed to complete the dissection. The same applies when the patient has lower abdominal incisions from appendectomy, bowel resection, suprapubic cystostomy, and so on. Suture material is often identified from previous anterior repairs. In the dissection of a recurrent hernia, a fundamental principle for avoiding bowel or bladder injury is to adhere to the posterior aspect of the rectus muscle anteriorly. From there, dissection is done in a horizontal fashion, from right to left or vice versa, to approach the direct defect.

Recurrent Indirect Hernia

The same considerations and procedures used with incarcerated indirect hernia apply to recurrent indirect hernias.

GENERAL CONSIDERATIONS

1. Multiple hernia sacs are sometimes encountered. They are dealt with individually, using the principles previously described. One great advantage of the preperitoneal approach is the impossibility of overlooking other hernias, regardless of their location. Many rare types are readily identifiable, including Velpeau's true prevascular, Serafini's retrovascular, Cloquet's posteromedial hernia emerging through the pectineus fascia, the obturator, Laugier's through the lacunar ligament, and Hesselbach's through the cribriform fascia.
2. The surgeon should not fear a tear in the peritoneum. With experience, exposure of the preperitoneal space need not be compromised, despite full pneumoperitoneum. When we encountered a rent in the peritoneum early in our clinical experience, we tried to close it with hemoclips, endoclips, or a piece of fat from the lipoma. Those methods were cumbersome and sometimes not successful, so we occasionally tried to vent the pneumoperitoneum through another port placed transperitoneally. But this again did not help much, and we now realize that this could be a very dangerous site for potential complications, since the venting process is not done under direct visualization.

We eventually became reconciled to performing dissection despite full pneumoperitoneum, merely lowering the CO_2 pressure to 8 or 9 mmHg and sometimes opting for a head-down position of about 15°. We found that dissection could continue because the weight of the preperitoneal fat kept the space open, especially in the midline and posterior to the pubic symphysis. Indeed, the pneumoperitoneum sometimes allowed better identification and delineation of an indirect hernia sac that, now being filled with CO_2, was much easier to dissect off the cord structures.

3. It is routine to verify the contralateral hernia orifice. This does not add much operative time and might preclude another complete procedure later on. The surgeon changes sides to do this dissection.
4. Associated extraperitoneal operations like varicocelectomy, vasectomy, pelvic lymph node dissection, and the like can be performed at the same time if no potentially septic maneuver will be required. There are reports of several varicocelectomies and pelvic lymph node dissections[19] having been done with no added morbidity. It is important, though, to dissect the hernia first and then proceed to the other surgery.

PROSTHESIS

A polypropylene mesh, previously cut in a diamond shape as described by Wantz,[20] and measured at the skin level, as described by Stoppa et al.,[21] Rives,[22] and Rignault,[23] is handled with a "no touch" technique. It is rolled like a cigarette, grasped at one end, and introduced via the umbilical trocar under the pubic symphysis in the midline. It is placed in a longitudinal fashion from head to toe in the space of Retzius (Fig. 14.11). It is then unrolled from the pubic symphysis laterally toward the anterosuperior iliac spine and posteriorly to the epigastric vessels. If a contralateral hernia also exists, the operator changes sides and proceeds as before. In this situation, two symmetrical pieces are placed, overlapping in the midline.

The mesh is secured in place with either sutures or staples. Whatever the size of the pieces, careful fixation is mandatory, especially on the medial and superior edges of the myopectineal orifice. The mesh is secured to Cooper's pectineal ligament, the pubic symphysis in

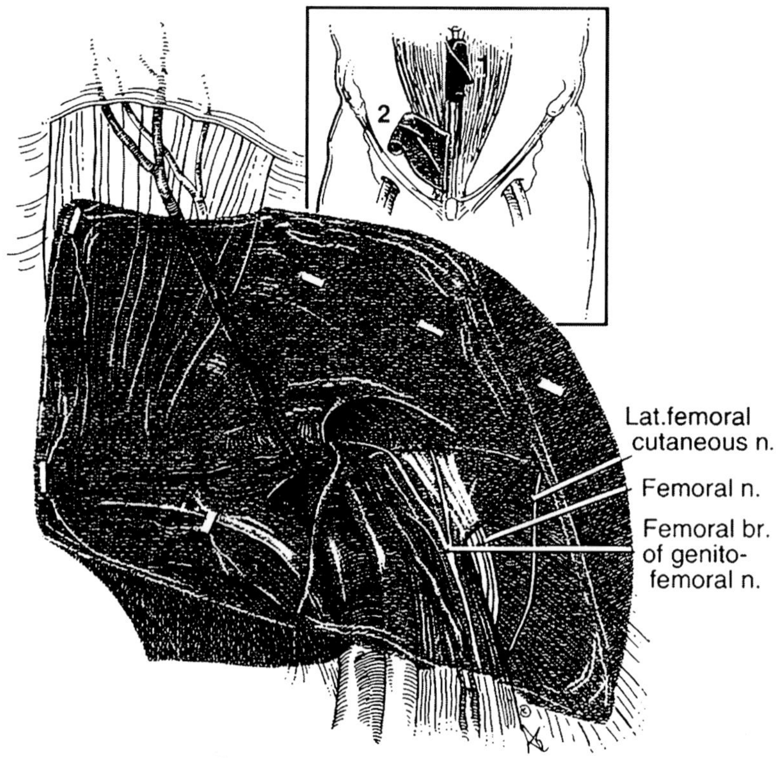

Figure 14.11. Placement and fixation of a prosthesis.

the midline, the rectus abdominis muscle medially, and laterally to the iliac fascia above and parallel to the iliopubic tract. This line is also parallel to the inguinal fold and 2 to 3 cm above it. It is identical in direction and latitude to the skin incisions made in standard open herniorrhaphy. It is vital to avoid stapling the femoral branch of the genital femoral nerve, lateral to the iliac vessel (Fig. 14.11), or the lateral femoral cutaneous nerve under the iliac fascia.[24] This area, lateral to the internal spermatic vessel, has been referred to as the *triangle of pain*[25]; by stapling as described, nerve injury can be avoided. Stapling should not be done in the iliopubic tract laterally, since the femoral branch of the genital femoral nerve is sometimes multiple, following the psoas muscle and piercing the iliopubic tract laterally and underneath to enter the leg. Stapling should also be avoided between the vas deferens medially and the internal spermatic vessels laterally, an area known as the *triangle of doom*.[26] The trapezoid area seen in Figure 14.12 outlines the triangles of doom and of pain.

Some surgeons prefer to slit the mesh either superiorly, parallel to the epigastric vessels,[27] or inferiorly around the cord structures. Others feel that with a large mesh and a total parietalization of the cord structures, a slit is not needed unless it is done to suppress folding of the mesh. In general, the type of mesh used is polypropylene. However, Mersilene (Dacron)[20,21] is a much softer material that will mold to the pelvic contours better than polypropylene, reducing the risk of folds, especially along the lateral edges, where there is a potential site for recurrence.

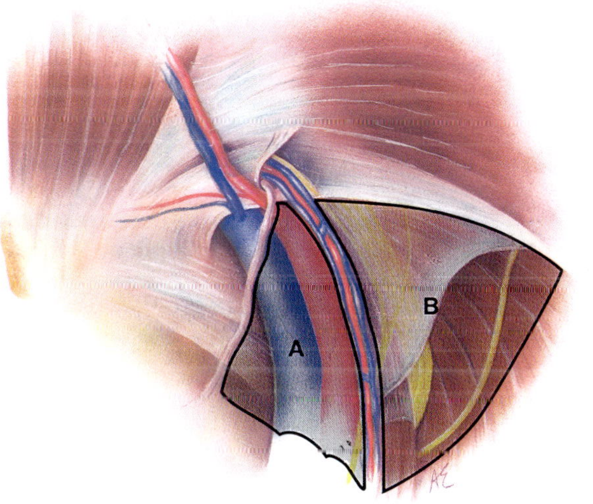

Figure 14.12. Right-sided inguinal anatomy as viewed during EEPH. The placement of staples in either the triangle of doom (A) or the triangle of pain (B) should be avoided.

In the extraperitoneal approach, a straight stapling device is all that is needed; the roticulator aspect that is useful for the transperitoneal approach is not necessary. It should be possible to see through the mesh so that staple placement can be done safely, especially when the surgeon is still inexperienced with the technique. The most important point is that the prosthesis, whether Prolene, Marlex, Gortex, Surgipro, or Mersilene, must extend broadly beyond the weak inguinal area, covering the entire myopectineal orifice in all directions, as described by Fruchaud.[28,29] Other alternatives are the use of a double buttress technique, as described by Felix and Michas,[30] and the placement of a Dudai Butterfly, as described by Dudai.[31]

Closure

Trocars are removed under direct visualization. The extraperitoneal space is emptied of CO_2 with gentle pressure applied to the lower abdomen. If pneumoperitoneum occurred, the surgeon should make sure that this is also evacuated. Fascial defects are repaired, and skin and subcutaneous fat are closed. A sterile dressing is applied. Drains are not considered necessary.

Postoperative Care

An ice pack and a scrotal support are recommended. Nonprescription pain medication is routinely given. Activities are not restricted unless there is postoperative discomfort. Hospital discharge occurs on the same day. The patient is told to expect some ecchymosis and swelling in the groin area and in the scrotum. A bulge or a cough impulsion in the immediate postoperative period is not worrisome; both will dissipate in 2 to 3 weeks.

SPECIAL CONSIDERATIONS

1. The patient is asked to void prior to surgery. A Foley catheter is not needed and is not routinely placed. However, in patients with giant scrotal or large indirect hernias, and in those with prior suprapubic cystostomy or prostatectomy, the Foley catheter is mandatory. In operating on

patients with prior bladder or prostate surgeries, great care must be taken to avoid bladder injury. This damage is easily recognizable, for the Foley drainage bag will be constantly filled with CO_2 under tension. It is then essential to identify the site of bladder perforation and to repair it.

2. If an umbilical hernia is present, it is dealt with as part of the same procedure but prior to the preperitoneal dissection. Similarly, if laparoscopy is desired, this is done first, the pneumoperitoneum evacuated, the peritoneal incision closed, and the preperitoneal dissection begun.
3. Large peritoneal tears must be closed to avoid exposure of the mesh to the bowel. If a sac is opened, the closure can be done either with pretied knots or with intracorporeal or extracorporeal suturing.
4. During initial dissection, fat surrounding the inferior epigastric vessels sometimes dangles and becomes cumbersome, interfering with visualization of the lateral components of the myopectineal orifice. This fat can be gently stripped without the need of cauterization or ligation. If a bleeder is encountered during fat dissection, the surgeon can place a grasper posterior to the epigastric vessels with the lower trocar and lift them anteriorly for a short time. This should stop bleeding from any of the epigastric vessels.

GASLESS ENDOSCOPIC REPAIR

In earlier years, when the peritoneum was torn while a patient was under regional anesthesia for EEPH, conversion to general anesthesia was mandated because of the resulting pneumoperitoneum. As a consequence of this problem, a gasless technique was developed by the author that avoided CO_2 insufflation.[32]

Technique

The patient is placed in the supine position. Once adequate epidural anesthesia has been administered, a Foley catheter is inserted to decompress the bladder.

An incision is made in the umbilicus, extended posteriorly to the level of the fascia, and incised without violating the peritoneum. Blunt finger dissection in the midline allows the insertion of a balloon trocar dissector just proximal to the level of the pubic symphysis. The balloon is inflated for further dissection of the preperitoneal space posterior to the symphysis pubis and lateral to the epigastric vessels. Two other incisions are made under direct visualization. The first is below the umbilicus, and the second is just superior to the pubic symphysis. Several methods can be used to retract the abdominal wall upward. One involves a Laparofan (Origin MedSystems, Menlo Park, CA) fan retractor, which is inserted through the umbilical incision and spread open under the rectus muscle. A Laparolift is then used to elevate the anterior wall via the fan retractor. Other methods include the use of suture material that elevates the abdominal wall or fine wire attached to a pulley system that lifts it. Through one of the other incisions, several devices may be used to push the peritoneum posteriorly. Among the options is an inflated 5-mm balloon trocar retractor, an insufflated Foley catheter, an insufflated Penrose drain, a sponge on a stick, or a fan retractor. The area of interest is observed from behind the lifting device, and the herniorrhaphy is performed under direct visualization using standard surgical tools (Fig. 14.13).

Results

The gasless herniorrhaphy technique has one major advantage over the traditional method. Large indirect hernia sacs are easier to dissect, since opening the sac does not risk leakage of CO_2 into the peritoneal cavity, with subsequent pneumoperitoneum. However, large direct defects require more experience to recognize because intracavity pressure does not increase, as it would if CO_2 were used for insufflation. The defect does not bulge outward, making it more difficult to identify. Even though standard surgical equipment can be used, eliminating the need for trocars and other laparoscopic equipment and thereby reducing the cost, the visibility and the exposure are, unfortunately, very compromised. Diffuse pinpoint peritoneal hemorrhage makes the field bloodier. In addition, excessive downward retraction of the parietal peritoneum is needed, which can lead to bowel, bladder, or peritoneal perforations. A number of surgeons, including the author, now feel that the advantages of the gasless technique are outweighed by its various disadvantages and no longer advocate its use.

BALLOON DISSECTION

As experience has been gained, shortcomings in the use of balloon dissection have also become more noticeable. The common purpose of the balloon dissector is to create asymmetric preperitoneal space. When the

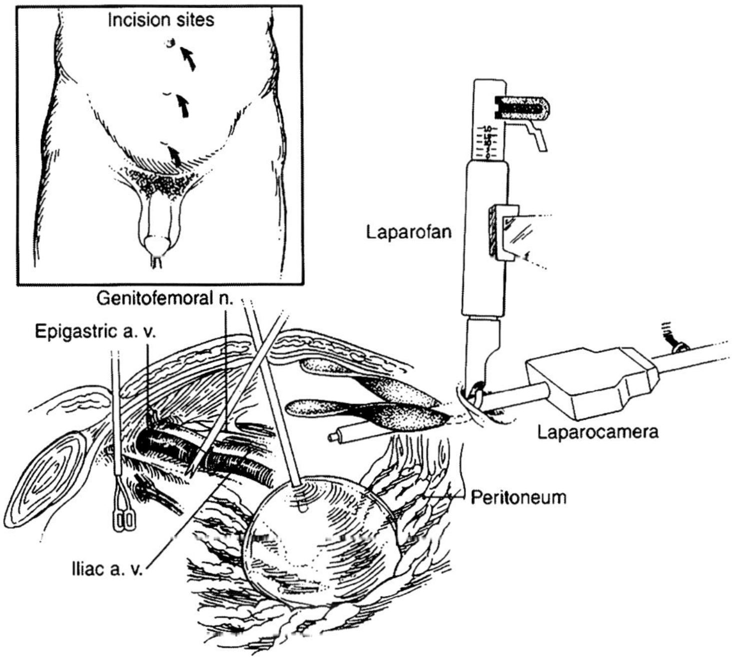

Figure 14.13. Gasless endoscopic repair.

balloon is introduced at the umbilical level on either side, between the rectus and the posterior rectus sheath, two things may happen: (1) trocar placement in the midline may be compromised (Fig. 14.14) and (2) one side of the linea alba is extended more than the other due to the persistent midline band below the linea semicircularis, which may cause a tear in the epigastric vessels, rents in the peritoneum, or bowel injuries (Fig. 14.14), especially when the patient has had prior lower abdominal incisions where the peritoneum is adherent.

If the balloon trocar dissector is used, its inflation in the extraperitoneal space must be done slowly. There are three reasons for this: (1) In patients with direct hernias, balloon inflation will push the hernia contents out of the canal. This must be done slowly to avoid

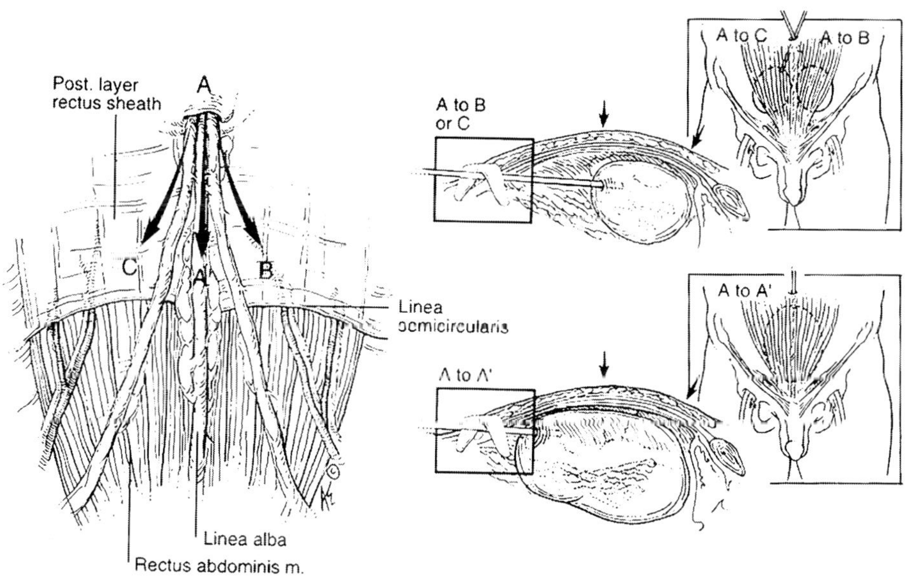

Figure 14.14. Balloon dissection. A to A′: proper placement. A to B and A to C: improper placement.

tearing the contents. (2) Patients with prior lower abdominal surgery probably have adhesions in the area of dissection that must be dealt with. (3) Slow inflation gives the surgeon time to identify landmarks essential to the repair (Cooper's ligament, symphysis pubis, etc.) and to ensure proper placement of the balloon trocar dissector.

However, many surgeons, including the author, now feel that once experience is gained, digital dissection offers much greater control and eliminates the need for the balloon and its extra cost.

CLINICAL EXPERIENCE

Between September 1991 and May 1994, 249 patients underwent EEPH in our clinic. All were male, ranging in age from 18 to 82 years (mean, 43.2 years). These patients had a total of 326 Nyhus type III and type IV hernia defects: 163 indirect, 148 direct, 11 pantaloon, and 4 femoral. Some 77 of these hernias were bilateral; 37 patients were operated on for recurrent hernia. Their earlier operations included 17 modified Bassini, 8 undetermined herniorrhaphy, 7 Lichtenstein, 4 Shouldice, and 1 laparoscopic plug and patch. Some 19 patients had incipient contralateral hernias diagnosed only at the time of endoscopy; 34 had previous abdominal surgery with a lower midline, paramedian, or Pfannenstiel incision. Conversion to another approach was required in seven patients (2.8%). Five of these conversions occurred in the first 100 patients who underwent the procedure and were due to rents in the peritoneum with subsequent pneumoperitoneum.[33] Of the subsequent 149 cases, only 2 required conversion.

Operating time ranged between 22 and 185 minutes (mean, 77 minutes). Some 26 patients underwent gasless repair. Polypropylene mesh was used with 243 patients and Mersilene mesh with six. Follow-up ranged from 9 to 42 months (mean, 22 months), and 15 patients were lost to follow-up. To date, there have been four recurrences, all dating from early in our experience, for a rate of 1.6%. The overall complication rate is calculated at 5.2%. This included five cases of urinary retention, four cases of fluid collection in the groin region requiring aspiration, one trocar site infection, one case of cardiac arrhythmia, one of laryngospasm, and one of lateral femoral cutaneous nerve neuralgia in a patient who was converted to a transabdominal preperitoneal repair with a concomitant left varicocelectomy on the side of the neuralgia. Herniorrhaphies performed concomitantly with other surgical procedures were included in our study. These included eight pelvic lymph node dissections, two varicocelectomies, one transurethral resection of the prostate, one cystoscopy, six umbilical herniorrhaphies, and one cervical node biopsy. The length of the hospital stay varied, 219 patients being discharged home in stable condition on the day of surgery (88%). Another 20 were discharged within 24 hr because they were operated on late in the day, while 10 required hospitalization for other simultaneous procedures, one TURP, one cystoscopy, and eight lymph node dissections.

Recurrence

Reported causes of recurrence reported in the literature include too small mesh, hernia never recognized and repaired, clips pulling through, and mesh never stapled in.[34]

In our clinic, the four recurrences occurred early in our experience, and all appeared within the first 3 months after repair. Three occurred in patients with large indirect hernias and one in a patient with large bilateral direct defects. In our opinion, these recurrences occurred for two reasons: (1) the mesh was too small, and (2) a split was made in the mesh inferiorly and passed below the cord structures. We have never questioned that recurrence after preperitoneal repair is always technical and depends on the operator.

OBSERVATIONS

As experience was gained, several modifications were made that lessened operating time and reduced operating room expenditure. In our earlier years, all patients were prepared as if undergoing peritoneal insufflation and cannulation, so Foley catheters and orogastric tubes were routinely placed. As the prospect of inadvertent peritoneal presentation lessened, these devices were no longer deemed necessary. Epidural regional anesthesia was more frequently used and better tolerated by the patient. Blunt digital dissection of the preperitoneal space eliminated the shortcomings in the use of the balloon dissector, as well as the need for the operative scope.

Special irrigation devices, electrocautery, endoscopic instruments, and hemoclip appliers were no longer needed, since the dissection of the preperitoneal space could again be done without significant bleeding. Also, as experience was gained, conversion to open herniorrhaphy was no longer necessary when tears in the peritoneum occurred. The surgeon could continue despite

Table 14.2. Operating Room Cost Comparison: Laparoscopic Herniorrhaphy

	Lap. A*	Lap. B†
OR cost (unilateral)	$1517 (~69 min)	$806 (~22 min)
OR cost (bilateral)	$1568 (~75 min)	$1091 (~40 min)

* A = early laparoscopic surgical experience.

† B = expanded experience (material no longer needed: irrigation setup, operative scope, balloon dissector, endoclip, Foley catheter, and long endoshears). Cost estimated as follows: first hour, $949; second hour, $338; third hour, $338.

a full pneumoperitoneum with a pressure of 8 to 9 mmHg and with enough room in the space of Retzius to introduce the mesh. In comparing the operating room cost of laparoscopic herniorrhaphy (Table 14.2), it can be seen that with expanded experience, the cost has substantially decreased compared with that of our earlier procedures.[35]

For inexperienced surgeons using this procedure, it is better to start with easy cases, including direct hernias (if a preoperative diagnosis can be made with certainty) and small indirect ones. After gaining experience, the surgeon can move to more difficult cases like large indirect, giant indirect scrotal, and incarcerated hernias, as well as those in patients with previous bladder surgery or prostatectomy. The last situation, however, is still a relative contraindication. There is an absolute technical contraindication to the extraperitoneal endoscopic approach in patients with prior radiation therapy to the pelvis for prostatic cancer. EEPH is very advantageous in patients having recurrent hernias and with those who have bilateral hernias; here there is a great advantage in being able to evaluate multiple regions without additional incision. If a previously unrecognized contralateral defect is noted, it can be repaired through the same incision in a very short period of time. To prevent complications, *good anatomic knowledge* remains the basic principle. As Sir Ashley Cooper put it in 1804, "No disease of the human body belonging to the province of the surgeons, requires in his treatment a greater combination of accurate anatomic knowledge, with surgical skill, than a hernia in all its varieties." This is as true today as it was almost 200 years ago. The location of the femoral branch of the genital femoral nerve must be known, as must the location of the lateral cutaneous femoral nerve and the rest of the myopectineal orifice, as described by Fruchaud.

Another important point to remember is the necessity of placing a *wide sheet of nonabsorbable mesh* between the muscle and the peritoneum, effectively reinforcing or replacing the fascia transversalis. Failure to adhere to this practice will lead to recurrence. *Staple placement over the mesh should be standardized* to avoid injury to vessels and nerves and to facilitate staple removal by other surgeons in the event of a future operation. It should also be noted that universal agreement on a hernia classification is needed to facilitate comparison of different methods and results; such a classification would include the height and weight of patients in all reports.

CONCLUSION

In conclusion, extraperitoneal herniorrhaphy clearly provides an alternative to other methods of hernia repair and their potential complications.[36,37] This approach avoids violation of the peritoneal cavity and is feasible under regional anesthesia. It maintains all the benefits of minimally invasive surgery, exactly reproducing the open preperitoneal Stoppa repair. It is a safe and cost-effective method for repairing both primary and recurrent defects, and with experience, operative time decreases, as does the rate of conversion.

REFERENCES

1. Nyhus L, Condon R, Harkins H: Clinical experiences with preperitoneal hernia repair for all types of hernia of the groin: With particular reference to the importance of transversalis fascia analogue. *Am J Surg*, 100:234–244, 1960.
2. Nyhus L, Pollak R, Bombeck CT, et al: The preperitoneal approach and prosthetic buttress repair for recurrent hernia: The evolution of a technique. *Ann Surg* 208(6): 733–737, 1988
3. Nyhus L: The preperitoneal approach and iliopubic tract repair of inguinal hernia. In Nyhus L, Condon R (eds): *Hernia*. Philadelphia, Lippincott, 1989, pp 154–176.
4. Stoppa R, Warlaumont CR: The preperitoneal approach and prosthetic repair of groin hernia. In Nyhus LM, Condon R (eds). *Hernia*. Philadelphia, Lippincott, 1989, pp 189–225.
5. Wantz G: Giant prosthetic reinforcement of the visceral sac. *Surg Gynecol Obstet* 169:408–417, 1989.
6. Greenburg AG: Revisiting the recurrent groin hernia. *Am J Surg* 154:35–40, 1987.

7. Ger R, Mishrick A, Hurwitz J, et al: Management of groin hernias by laparoscopy. *World J Surg* 17:46–50, 1983.
8. Popp L: Endoscopic patch repair of inguinal hernia in a female patient. *Surg Endosc* 4:10, 1990.
9. Schultz L, Graber J, Pietrafitta J, et al: Laser laparoscopic herniorrhaphy: A clinical trial—preliminary results. *J Laparoendosc Surg* 1(1):41–45, 1990.
10. Corbitt J: Laparoscopic herniorrhaphy. *J Laparoendosc Endosc* 1:23–25, 1991.
11. Gazayerli M: Anatomical laparoscopic hernia repair of direct or indirect inguinal hernias using the transversalis fascia and iliopubic tract. *Surg Laparosc Endosc* 2(1): 49–52, 1992.
12. Toy F, Smoot R Jr: Laparoscopic hernioplasty update. *J Laparoendosc Surg* 2(5):197–205, 1992.
13. Arregui M, Davis C, Yucel O, et al: Laparoscopic mesh repair of inguinal hernia using a preperitoneal approach: A preliminary report. *Surg Laparosc Endosc* 2(1):53–580, 1992.
14. MacFadyen B, Arregui M, Corbitt J, et al: Complications of laparoscopic hernia. *Surg Endosc* 7:155–158, 1993.
15. Ferzli GS, Massaad A, Albert P: Extraperitoneal endoscopic hernia repair. *J Laparoendosc Surg* 2:281–286, 1992.
16. Cooper AP: *The Anatomy and Surgical Treatment of Inguinal and Congenital Hernia*. London, Longman, 1804.
17. Nyhus LM: Editor's comments: The anatomy of the inguinal region and its relation to groin hernia. In Nyhus LM, Condon R (eds): *Hernia*, ed 4. Philadelphia, Lippincott, 1994, pp 16–72.
18. Read RD: The transversalis and preperitoneal fascia: a reevaluation. In Nyhus LM, Condon R (ed): *Hernia*, ed 4. Philadelphia, Lippincott, 1994, pp 57–63.
19. Ferzli GS, Raboy A, Albert P: Extraperitoneal endoscopic pelvic lymph node dissection (EEPLND). *Surg Endosc* 8:124–126, 1994.
20. Wantz G: Prosthesis and abdominal wall hernia. In Bendavid R (ed): Austin, TX, Lanoes, 1995, pp 399–405.
21. Stoppa RE, Rives JL, Warlaumont CR, et al: The use of Dacron in the repair of hernias of the groin. *Surg Clin North Am* 64(2):296–285, 1984.
22. Rives JL: Surgical treatment of the inguinal hernia with Dacron patch: Principles, indications, technique and results. *Int Surg* 47:360, 1967.
23. Rignault D: Preperitoneal prosthetic inguinal hernioplasty through a Pfannenstiel approach. *Surg Gynecol Obstet* 163:465–468, 1986.
24. Stashing JR: Genitofemoral neuralgia (special comments, complications of groin hernia). In Nyhus LM, Condon R (eds): *Hernia*, ed 4. Philadelphia, Lippincott, 1994, pp 278–282.
25. Annibali RG, Fitzgibbons R Jr, Fillipi C, et al: Laparoscopic hernia repair. In Green FL, Ponsky JL, Nealon WH (eds): *Endoscopic Surgery*, Philadelphia, Saunders, 1994, pp
26. Spaw AT, Ennis BW, Spaw LP: Laparoscopic hernia repair: The anatomic basis. *J Laparoendosc Surg* 1(5): 269–277, 1991.
27. McKernan JB, Laws HL: Laparoscopic repair of inguinal hernias using a totally extraperitoneal prosthetic approach. *Surg Endosc* 7:26–28, 1993.
28. Fruchaud H: *Anatomie chirurgicale de hernies de l'aine*. Paris, G Doin, 1956.
29. Fruchaud H: *Traitement chirurgicale de hernies de l'aine*. Paris, G Doin, 1957.
30. Felix E, Michas C: The double buttress laparoscopic herniorrhaphy. *J Laparosc Surg* 1:1–4, 1993.
31. Dudai ML: Laparoscopic hernia repair using the Dudai butterfly with or without mesh according to the Nyhus hernia type. In Nyhus LM, Condon R (eds): *Hernia*, ed 4. Philadelphia, Lippencott, 1994, pp 213–217.
32. Ferzli GS, Dysarz FA: Extraperitoneal endoscopic inguinal herniorrhaphy performed without carbon dioxide insufflation. *J Laparoendosc Surg* 4:301–304, 1994.
33. Ferzli GS, Massaad A, Dysarz FA, et al: A study of 101 patients treated with extraperitoneal endoscopic laparoscopic herniorrhaphy. *Am Surg* 59:707–708, 1993.
34. Philips E, Carrole BJ, Fallas MJ, et al: Reasons for recurrence following laparoscopic hernioplasty. In Arregui M, Nagan R (eds): *Inguinal Hernia Advances and Controversies*. New York, Radcliffe Medical, 1994, pp 297–301.
35. Ferzli GS, Massaad A, Albert P, et al: Endoscopic extraperitoneal herniorrhaphy vs conventional hernia repair. *Curr Surg* 50:291–294, 1993.
36. Wantz GL: Complications of inguinal hernia repair. *Surg Clin North Am* 64(2):287–297, 1984.
37. Wantz GE: Testicular atrophy as a risk of inguinal hernioplasty. *Surg Gynecol Obstet* 154:570–571, 1982.

chapter fifteen

Pelvic Lymphadenectomy and Surgery of the Genitourinary System

Peter G. Schulam
Louis R. Kavoussi

INTRODUCTION

Urologic laparoscopic surgery is truly in its infancy, having come to the urologic forefront only within the last 5 years. Scheussler et al. have been credited with heralding its arrival with their pioneering techniques of laparoscopic pelvic lymph node dissection.[1] The application of laparoscopy to urology has been a slow evolution punctuated by a sudden surge of interest within the last decade. Although the first laparoscopic procedure was performed by Kelling in 1901 using Nitze's cystoscope,[2] it was not until 1976, when Cortesi et al. used laparoscopy to identify an intra-abdominal testicle, that laparoscopy was employed in urology.[3] Wickham in 1979 described retroperitonescopy for the removal of ureteral calculi.[4] Then in 1985, Eshghi and his associates used a laparoscope for a percutaneous transperitoneal removal of a staghorn calculus from a pelvic kidney.[5] Since Scheussler et al.'s description in 1991 of their series of 12 consecutive patients who had undergone endosurgical lymphadenectomy, there have been many papers on laparoscopy in the urologic literature. In addition to pelvic lymph node dissection, laparoscopic approaches for the following have been described: bladder neck suspension,[6] bladder diverticulectomy,[7,8] cystectomy,[9] ureteral lithotomy,[10,11] ureteroureterostomy,[12,13] ureterolysis,[14] pyeloplasty,[12] nephropexy,[15] nephrectomy,[16] varicocelectomy,[17,18] partial nephrectomy,[19] ileal conduit formation,[20] retroperitoneal lymph node dissection,[21] Fowler-Stephens maneuver,[22] live-donor nephrectomy,[23] and dismembered pyeloplasty.[24]

The excitement over laparoscopic urology must be tempered by consideration of the cost, both financially and with respect to morbidity and mortality, that this new surgical approach carries. The general belief is that laparoscopy, when successful, offers the patient decreased morbidity and shortened convalescence. The majority of data on the incidence of complications related to laparoscopy have come from the gynecologic literature, with rates for major complications ranging from 0.3% to 2.8% and those for minor complications ranging from 1% to 4%.[25–29] These data cannot be easily transferred to urology because the patient population undergoing gynecologic laparoscopy is predominantly young and healthy. In addition, the procedures are primarily diagnostic, not therapeutic.[30] A better predictor of the risks of laparoscopy in the general population may come from data obtained from patients undergoing laparoscopic cholecystectomy. A review of over 1000 laparoscopic cholecystectomies by Cushieri et al. revealed no operative deaths and a total complication rate of 5.2%.[31] Regardless, it is imperative that if laparoscopy is to gain acceptance as the standard of care for a particular urologic disease process, we must understand the complications as they apply specifically to urologic laparoscopy.

The goal of this chapter is to define the complications of laparoscopic urologic surgery and their management. Unfortunately, because this is a relatively new technique being applied to several urologic processes, there is a paucity of literature on the overall incidence of complications. In addition, as one can imagine, the increasing number of surgeons performing laparoscopy, the increasing number of operations performed, and the dynamic field of laparoscopic instrumentation make assessment of the true incidence nearly impossible. Undoubtedly, it will be a while before the field of laparoscopy approaches a steady state comparable to that of open surgery. Nevertheless, within the past several years there have been many efforts to examine the complications and outcomes of laparoscopic urologic surgery. Much of the work has been done in relation to pelvic lymph node dissection simply because this is the area that most accurately reflects the limits of laparoscopic surgery when considering its steep learning curve. In addition, other areas in which data are just beginning to emerge, including retroperitoneal lymphadenectomy and nephrectomy, will be reviewed.

The most dangerous aspect of laparoscopic surgery is Veress needle and trocar insertion. Because Chapter 3 focuses on this problem, we will forgo its discussion here. Rather, we will focus on the specific complications of laparoscopy as they relate to urology.

PELVIC LYMPH NODE DISSECTION

Kavoussi et al.[32] reported on the complications in 372 patients from eight centers who had undergone laparoscopic pelvic lymph node dissection (LPLND) between 1989 and 1991. Among these 372 patients there were 55 complications, 14 noted intraoperatively and 41 postoperatively. The overall complication rate was 15%. In 13 patients the complication required open surgical intervention. Vascular injuries were the most common, with six injuries occurring during trocar placement and five during surgical dissection. The remaining complications, by category, included viscus-bowel, bladder (8); lymphocele (5); infection (5); gastrointestinal ileus obstruction (7); genitourinary retention, scrotal swelling (10); anesthetic (2); obturator nerve palsy (2); and deep venous thrombosis (5).

Parra and his associates reported on 98 cases of LPLND performed between 1990 and 1993.[33] Their overall complication rate was comparable at 16.6%.

Lang et al. reported the outcome of their first 100 consecutive LPLNDS, which were performed between 1990 and 1992.[34] Their overall complication rate was 9%. Interestingly, they also analyzed their complication rate by comparing the first 50 cases to the second 50 cases. As one might expect, there is a significant learning curve associated with laparoscopy. The complication rate during the second 50 cases was significantly lower than that of the first 50, 4% versus 14%.

Vascular Injury

The prevention of vascular injuries depends on the laparoscopic surgeon's knowledge of anatomy and understanding of the laparoscopic perspective.

To prevent intraoperative and/or postoperative bleeding, small vessels should be cauterized or clipped before transection. In addition, attention to hemostasis is imperative because significant bleeding distorts surgical planes and hemoglobin absorbs the incident laparoscopic light, so that visualization is impaired. When a vessel is ligated or clipped, it should always be transected sharply because electrocoagulation of a clipped or ligated vessel can lead to local tissue necrosis and delayed bleeding.[35] This occurs because the thermal effect along the path of the vessel is related to local current density (LCD). LCD is related to the cross-sectional area of the vessel. Therefore, ligating or clipping a vessel decreases the cross-sectional area while increasing LCD and the thermal effect (the relationship is such that if the cross-sectional area is decreased by half, the thermal effect is increased by a factor of 4).

In performing LPLND, the obliterated umbilical artery may need to be transected. One must remember that the umbilical artery is one of the first branches of the hypogastric artery and gives rise to the superior vesical artery. Distal to the take-off of the superior vesical artery, the umbilical artery is an obliterated fibrous cord, but in the area where it branches, it is patent.[36] Therefore, the umbilical artery should be clipped prior to transection to avoid bleeding.

Injuries to thin-walled great veins are difficult to manage. We have used the Endostitch (Autosuture, Norwalk, CT) to repair vascular injuries laparoscopically in five patients. In all cases, we were successful in repairing the vessel, and only one patient required a transfusion.[37] If a more significant venous injury occurs and attempts at primary repair are unsuccessful, then the inferior vena cava below the renal vein can be ligated.[38]

Finally, at the end of a laparoscopic procedure, the field should be carefully inspected for injured vessels. Because the pneumoperitoneum can tamponade an injured vessel, the insufflation pressure should be decreased to 6 to 8 mmHg prior to inspecting the field for bleeding.

Lymphocele

In a review, Parra and his associates noted that among 96 laparoscopic lymphadenectomies, the most common complication was lymphocele formation.[33] The lymphoceles in four patients were symptomatic. Three of the four were managed by laparoscopic marsupialization. The other patient underwent percutaneous drainage.

Parra et al. analyzed the lymphocele data and found that when all lymphoceles (symptomatic and incidental) were considered, the incidence of formation was significantly increased in those patients in whom the peritoneum was approximated. In addition, the incidence was increased in patients receiving total pelvic radiation versus spot radiation.[33,35] The current recommendation is to leave the peritoneum open to allow lymphatic fluid to drain into the peritoneal cavity.[32,33]

Gastrointestinal Injuries

Gastrointestinal injuries related to laparoscopic surgery include perforation and mechanical obstruction due to herniation. Bowel perforation can occur during trocar insertion and while dissecting, either as an enterotomy with sharp dissection or as a thermal injury.

Bowel perforation secondary to sharp dissection, if noted during the procedure, can be repaired either laparoscopically or in an open manner. Thermal injury to the bowel is the most serious complication of laparoscopic surgery and can be associated with significant morbidity and mortality. A limitation of laparoscopic surgery is that the surgeon's field of view is limited by the camera. As a result, instruments outside the field of the camera can cause unrecognizable damage. This is particularly true for electrocautery. It is imperative that any uninsulated portion of the electrocautery be in full view during the entire laparoscopic procedure.

The incidence of thermal bowel injuries is rare, with a reported incidence of 2.2 per 1000 cases.[39] Wheeless reported on 33 patients who had intraoperative thermal injuries.[40] The first six patients who had sustained thermal bowel injuries underwent immediate laparotomy. Of these, only two had an actual bowel perforation. The next 27 patients were managed conservatively, and none required laparotomy. These data indicate that conservative management is a viable treatment plan.

In a review by Gomella et al., a treatment plan was outlined based on the visual appearance of the burn at the time of laparoscopy.[41] If the serosa is whitened but intact, then laparotomy is not usually required. Laparotomy is indicated if the serosa is separated and muscularis, mucosa, or lumen is evident.

Unfortunately, the injury may not be noticed at the time of surgery. In such a patient, the immediate postoperative period may be unremarkable. However, 2 to 7 days postoperatively, the patient may present with abdominal pain, nausea, low-grade fever, and a moderate leukocytosis. The delay is due to the time it takes for the burned bowel to undergo necrosis and subsequent perforation. If such a patient does not respond to intravenous antibiotics and/or if peritonitis develops, laparotomy is indicated. Resection of a bowel burn is rather extensive. Tissue damage secondary to electrocautery can be detected as far as 5 cm from the area burned.[42] Wheeless et al. suggest that a 6-cm margin on either side of the injury should be resected.[42]

An additional complication of laparoscopy involving the bowel is herniation of omentum or small intestine into a trocar site. The time of presentation varies from 3 to 7 days postoperatively.[30] The patient may present with signs and symptoms of either complete or incomplete bowel obstruction. Making the diagnosis of an incarcerated loop of small bowel into a trocar site may not be obvious by physical examination alone.[43] Burney and his associates believe that computed tomography of the abdomen for patients with abdominal pain following laparoscopy will greatly improve diagnostic accuracy.[44] Once the diagnosis has been made, conventional teaching is that immediate laparotomy is indicated. Kreutzer et al. have recently described two cases in which herniation of small bowel into a trocar site was managed with a laparoscopic technique.[43] It is universally agreed that to avoid this complication, all trocar sites 10 mm or more should be closed under direct laparoscopic control; in children, the recommendation is that all trocar sites be closed.

Recently, instrument companies have made several advances in the development of instrumentation to facilitate fascial closure. One such device is the spring-loaded needle. This instrument allows straight needles to be placed on either side of the trocar incision. Then, under laparoscopic guidance, the needles can be accurately positioned and suture placed, allowing adequate closure of the trocar site.[45]

Genitourinary Injuries

Damage to the urinary tract during laparoscopy is relatively uncommon. In a large series in the gynecology literature, the reported incidence of urinary tract injuries was 0.2 per 1000 cases.[26] Injuries to the urinary tract include both bladder perforation and ureteral injury. A majority of injuries to the bladder occur during Veress needle and trocar placement. By decompressing the bladder during laparoscopy with a Foley catheter, one can greatly reduce the likelihood of bladder injury. In addition, with a Foley catheter in place, one can watch for signs of bladder injury during surgery. Indications of bladder injury include hematuria, passage of significant amounts of clear fluid into the operative field, and pneumaturia. If a bladder injury is suspected, instillation of indigo carmine or methylene blue through the catheter into the bladder may help locate the injury. Once a bladder injury is identified, it is reasonable to attempt a laparoscopic repair.[46,47]

Ureteral injury is a rare event during laparoscopic urologic surgery. Kavoussi et al.[32] reported two cases of ureteral injury out of a total of 372 patients who had undergone LPLND. In one case, the injury was noted at the time of surgery and repaired immediately. In the second case, the patient developed a fever 3 days postoperatively; computed tomography revealed a urinoma. During exploration, the transected ureter was repaired. Ureteral injuries are serious complications of laparoscopy and, as demonstrated in the second case, their diagnosis is often made in the postoperative period.

Ureteral injuries usually are manifested 1 to 5 days after surgery.[30] Common presenting symptoms are abdominal pain with peritonitis, leukocytosis, and fever; less common are flank tenderness and hematuria.[41] Diagnosis is usually made by intravenous urography or retrograde ureterography.

The management of ureteral injuries depends on the extent and location of the injury and the time of diagnosis. For injuries identified intraoperatively, immediate repair should be performed. If the injury consists of a small laceration or burn, then ureteral stenting may be adequate. However, if the injury is significant, then reanastamosis or reimplantation may be necessary.

Prevention of ureteral injury depends on a thorough knowledge of the anatomy of the ureter. During LPLND, the ureter should be identified as it crosses over the common iliac artery. The ureters usually run medial to the medial umbilical ligament; therefore, the dissection should be kept lateral to the obliterated umbilical artery. In addition, during dissection of the medial border of the nodal packet, sharp dissection should be avoided to prevent incidental ureteral injury.

Obturator Nerve Injuries

Injury to the obturator nerve during either laparoscopic or open pelvic lymph node dissection is a rare event. In a review of the literature, Fishman et al.[48] reported 11 obturator nerve injuries during 1681 open lymphadenectomies, with an incidence of 0.7%. In contrast, a total of 434 laparoscopic cases resulted in 2 obturator nerve injuries (0.5%). The nerve injuries which occurred during laparoscopic lymphadenectomy were due to inadvertent fulguration leading to transient weakness of the adduction muscles of the thigh. Both patients, however, recovered completely within 3 weeks.[32] During open lymphadenectomies the obturator nerve injuries ranged from inadvertent clipping and fulguration to complete transection. Partial nerve injuries were conservatively managed, and complete transections were primarily anastomosed. Of these patients, two had no significant functional deficits.[49]

The obturator nerve is an important landmark during pelvic lymphadenectomy. However, due to lack of depth perception, injury may occur. Transection is unlikely, but damage to the nerve secondary to thermal injury is of great concern. Monopolar electrocautery can lead to thermal injury distant from the area targeted because the heat is dissipated through adjacent tissue. Interestingly, in the report by Fishman et al.,[48] one patient did not report a motor deficit until the night of discharge. This delay in presentation may be explained by delayed necrosis and injury secondary to thermal injury. The recommendation would be to employ the electrocautery judiciously when dissecting close to the nerve. In the absence of transection, obturator nerve injuries can be followed conservatively and will usually resolve completely.

Deep Venous Thrombosis

Deep venous thrombosis, a serious complication of surgery, does not appear to be increased in incidence during laparoscopic surgery. The reported incidence in one series was 0.2 per 1000 cases.[26] To minimize the risks of this complication, we routinely employ pneumatic compression boots and/or subcutaneous heparin until the patient is fully ambulatory.

RETROPERITONEAL LYMPHADENECTOMY

Laparoscopic retroperitoneal lymph node dissection was first described by Rukstalis et al. for stage I testicular cancer in 1992.[50] Gerber et al. reported on the experience at five institutions where modified unilateral retroperitoneal lymph node dissections were performed laparoscopically.[51] The procedure was attempted in 20 patients and completed in 18. Complications occurred in 6 of the 20 patients, including gonadal vessel injury (two), myonecrosis of flank musculature (one), injury to the inferior mesenteric artery secondary to retraction (one), retroperitoneal lymphocele (one), and bleeding at a trocar site (one). One of the two patients who suffered an injury to the gonadal vessel required an open procedure.

The overall complication rate in this study was 30%. Published series on open lymphadenectomy report incidences of major complications ranging from 6% to 19%.[52–54] This indicates that we are not yet as far along on the learning curve for laparoscopic retroperitoneal lymphadenectomy as we are for other laparoscopic procedures.

It is important to note that most patients were hospitalized for 3 days or less and returned to normal activity by 2–3 weeks. In addition, all 20 patients maintained antegrade ejaculation. Laparoscopic retroperitoneal lymphadenectomy may well become a viable staging procedure and treatment modality as experience is gained.

NEPHRECTOMY

The first laparoscopic total nephrectomy was performed in 1991 by Clayman and his associates.[55] Since then, laparoscopic approaches to both total and partial nephrectomies have evolved.

Kerbl et al. published a report comparing laparoscopic to open nephrectomy for benign disease.[56] They compared 20 patients undergoing laparoscopy for benign disease to 23 patients who underwent open surgical nephrectomy and 29 patients who underwent donor nephrectomy. The complications associated with the laparoscopic technique included retroperitoneal hematoma (one), mild congestive heart failure (two), and pulmonary embolism (one). Their overall complication rate for laparoscopy was 15%. Based on published reports, the complication rate for open surgical nephrectomy ranges from 6% to 25%.[57,58] The complications associated with an open procedure include wound-related problems such as fasciitis, infection, and hematoma. Other complications associated with an open nephrectomy are related to organ retraction, such as pneumonia, pleurotomy, and incidental splenectomy. One should note that many of these complications rarely occur in laparoscopy.

Kavoussi et al. reported on eight patients who underwent radical laparoscopic nephrectomy for renal tumors.[59] They reported complications in three patients (38%) postoperatively. The complications were congestive heart failure, congestive heart failure associated with atrial fibrillation and ileus, and urinary retention. Interestingly, there were no late complications 7 to 35 months postoperatively. In addition, during their follow-up, there was no clinical or radiographic evidence of tumor recurrence. These findings were compared to those in 58 patients who underwent conventional radical nephrectomy during the same period. Complications occurred in 34% of these patients, an incidence similar to that in the laparoscopic group. In contrast, 11 of the patients undergoing standard nephrectomy had long-term complications, including incisional hernia and parasthesia. These complications were not observed in the laparoscopic group.

Compared to total nephrectomy, partial nephrectomy is more difficult. A recent report from Winfield's group presented the feasibility of laparoscopic partial nephrectomy.[60] They attempted laparoscopic partial nephrectomies in six patients and were successful in four of those cases. They employed the argon beam coagulator and found it successful in controlling hemorrhage from the kidney. They did report, however, that prior to incision of the kidney, they attempted to stabilize the kidney and tamponade bleeding with a modified Remel tourniquet, but they were unsuccessful. This particular step will require further development before this procedure can routinely be performed. An additional step of the procedure which is impossible laparoscopically is palpation of the kidney. Winfield et al. claimed that this caused their two failures, which consisted of a residual stone in one case and failure to isolate the tumor in the other. They attempted to overcome this deficit by employing a 7.5 MHz ultrasonic sector scanning system, but this did not provide an optimal image. Further development of laparoscopic ultrasonic and Doppler equipment is crucial to the success of this procedure.

CONCLUSION

It is difficult to predict the future of laparoscopic urologic surgery. If we consider laparoscopic cholecystectomy as a model and heed the data which underscore the apparent learning curve of laparoscopy, no one can deny that further investigation and time should be granted to this exciting field of surgery. One must also be cognizant of the significance of technological advances which will affect both laparoscopic instrumentation and imaging.

The learning curve of laparoscopic urologic surgery is a dynamic field which is slowly reaching its steady state. Gomella et al.[61] recently reported on an ongoing prospective study which reveals the outcome assessment of laparoscopic procedures performed at various times during a laparoscopic surgeon's experience. The predominant procedure was the laparoscopic pelvic lymph node dissection. They presented the data in three phases: prior to 1991, 1991–92, and 1993–94. All three phases had more than 100 cases enrolled. The following were their results for each phase, respectively: operative time—162, 125, and 91.4 min; major complications—11.3%, 6.0%, and 0.8%; minor complications—11.3%, 10.1%, and 1.6%; cases requiring laparotomy—2.9%, 1.5%, and 2.0%. These data undoubtedly demonstrate the learning curve associated with laparoscopy.

One of the greatest arguments used against laparoscopy is the long operative time. If, however, we assume that is there is a steep learning curve, then eventually the disparity in operative times will become negligible. Parra et al.[62] compared standard flank versus laparoscopic nephrectomy for benign disease in a comparable group of patients. The operative time ranged from 105 to 360 min (mean, 145 min) for the laparoscopic group and 60 to 240 min (mean, 156.6 min) for the open group. There were two complications in the laparoscopic group. The first was a vascular injury that required laparotomy. The other was a small enterotomy which was repaired laparoscopically. Needless to say, the laparoscopic group had minimal surgical scars and shorter hospitalizations, required less analgesia, and had a significant shorter convalescence.

REFERENCES

1. Schuessler WW, Vancaillie TG, Reich H, et al: Transperitoneal endosurgical lymphadenectomy in patients with localized prostate cancer. *J Urol* 145:988–991, 1991.
2. Kelling G: Zur Colioskopic. *Arch Klin Chir* 126:226–229, 1923.
3. Cortesi N, Ferrari P, Zambarda E, et al: Diagnosis of bilateral abdominal cryptorchidism by laparoscopy. *Endoscopy* 8:33–34, 1976.
4. Wickham JEA: The surgical treatment of renal lithiasis. In *Urinary Calculus Disease*. New York, Churchill Livingstone, 1979, pp 145–198.
5. Eshghi AM, Roth JS, Smith AD: Percutaneous transperitoneal approach to a pelvic kidney for endourological removal of staghorn calculus. *J Urol* 134:525–527, 1985.
6. Albala DM, Schuessler WW, Vancaillie TG: Laparoscopic bladder neck suspension. *J Endourol* 6:137–141, 1992.
7. Das S: Laparoscopic removal of bladder diverticulum. *J Urol* 148:1837–1839, 1992.
8. Parra RO, Jones JP, Andrus CH, et al: Laparoscopic diverticulectomy: Preliminary report of a new approach of the treatment of bladder diverticulum. *J Urol* 148: 869–871, 1992.
9. Parra RO, Andrus CH, Jones J, et al: Laparoscopic cystectomy: Initial report on a new treatment for the retained bladder. *J Urol* 148:1140–1144, 1992.
10. Garden R, Shemtor M, and Stone N: Laparoscopic ureterolithotomy (abstr. v-67). *J Urol* 147:204A, 1992.
11. Lipsky H, Wuernschimmel E: Laparoscopic lithotomy for ureteral stones. *Min Invasive Ther* 2:19–22, 1993.
12. Schuessler WW, Vancaillie TG, Preminger GM: Laparoscopic dismembered pyeloplasty. *Min Invasive Ther* (Suppl) 1(Suppl):68, 1992.
13. Nezhat C, Nezhat F, Green B, et al: Laparoscopic ureteroureterostomy. *J Endourol* 6:143–145, 1992.
14. Kavoussi LR, Clayman RV, Brunt LM, et al: Laparoscopic ureterolysis. *J Urol* 147:426–429, 1992.
15. Urban DA, Clayman RV, Korbl K, et al: Laparoscopic nephropexy for symptomatic nephroptosis: Initial case report. *J Endourol* 7:27–30, 1993.
16. Clayman RV, Kavoussi LR, Soper NJ, et al: Laparoscopic nephrectomy (letter). *N Engl J Med* 324:1370–1371, 1991.
17. Donovan JF, Winfield HN: Laparoscopic varix ligation. *J Urol* 147:77–81, 1992.
18. Mehan DJ, Hagood PG, Worischeck JH, et al: Laparoscopic varicocelectmy: Preliminary report of a new technique (abstract 117). *J Urol* 145:242A, 1991.
19. Winfield HN, Donovan JF, Godet AS, et al: Human laparoscopic partial nephrectomy, case report. *Min Invasive Ther* 1(Suppl):66, 1992.
20. Kozminski M, Partamian KO: Case report of laparoscopic ileal loop conduit. *J Endourol* 6:147–150, 1992.
21. Hulbert JC, Fraley EE: Laparoscopic retroperitoneal lymphadenectomy: A new approach to pathologic staging of clinical stage I germ cell tumors of the testis. *J Endourol* 6:123–125, 1992.
22. Bloom DA: Two-step orchiopexy with pelviscopic clip ligation of the spermatic vessels. *J Urol* 145:1030–1033, 1991.
23. Ratner L, Cisek L, Moore RG, et al: Laparoscopic live donor nephrectomy. *Transplantation* 60:1047–1049, 1955.
24. Schuessler WW, Grune MT, Tecuanhuey LV, et al: Laparoscopic dismembered pyeloplasty. *J Urol* 150: 1795–1799, 1993.
25. Peterson HB, Hulka JF, Phillips JM: American Association of Gynecologic Laparoscopists' 1988 membership survey on operative laparoscopy: *J Reprod Med* 35:587–589, 1990.
26. Chamberlain GVP, Carron-Brown J: *Gynaecological Laparoscopy*. London, Royal College of Obstetricians and Gynecologists, 1978.
27. Riedel HH, Lehman-Willenbrock E, Conrad P, et al: Ger-

man pelviscopic statistics for the years 1978–1982. *Endoscopy* 18.219–222, 1986.

28. Cuschieri A: Laparoscopy in general surgery and gastroenterology. *Br J Hosp Med* 24:255–258, 1980.
29. Hulka JF, Soderstrom RM, Corson SL, et al: Complications Committee of the American Association of Gynecologic Laparoscopists, First Annual Report. *J Reprod Med* 10:301–306, 1973.
30. Capelouto CC, Kavoussi LR: Complications of laparoscopic surgery. *Urology* 42(1):2–12, 1993.
31. Cushieri A, Dubois F, Moviel J, et al: The European experience with laparoscopic cholecystectomy. *Am J Surg* 161:385–387, 1991.
32. Kavoussi LB, Sosa E, Chandhoke P, et al: Complications of laparoscopic pelvic lymph node dissection. *J Urol* 149:322–325, 1993.
33. Parra RO, Hagood PG, Boullies JA, et al: Complications of laparoscopic urological surgery: Experience at St. Louis University. *J Urol* 151:681–684, 1994.
34. Lang GS, Ruckle HC, Hadley HR, et al: One hundred consecutive laparoscopic pelvic lymph node dissections: Comparing complications of the first 50 cases to the second 50 cases. *Urology* 44:221–225, 1994.
35. Hunter JG: Laser use in laparoscopic surgeries. *Surg Clin North Am* 72:655–664, 1992.
36. Stanley KE: Management of laparoscopic vascular injuries in urology. *Atlas Urol Clin North Am* 1:103–116, 1993.
37. Kavoussi LR: Personal communication, 1995.
38. Malinak LR, Wheeler JM, Simolka G: Vascular injuries at laparoscopy. In Nichols DH (ed): *Clinical Problems, Injuries, and Complications of Gynecologic Surgery*. Baltimore, Williams & Wilkens, 1988, pp 58–61.
39. Lofler FD, Pent D: Statistics In Phillips JM (ed): *Laparoscopy*. Baltimore, Williams & Wilkins, 1977, pp 242–246.
40. Wheeless CR: Thermal gastrointestinal injuries. In Phillips JM (ed): *Laparoscopy*. Baltimore, Williams & Wilkins, 1977, pp 231–235.
41. Gomella CG, Lotfi MA, Ruckle HC: Management of laparoscopic complications. In Gomella CG, Kozminski M, Winfield HN (eds): *Laparoscopic Urologic Surgery*. New York, Raven Press, 1994, pp 257–266.
42. Wheeless CR Jr, et al: Gastrointestinal injuries associated with laparoscopy. In Phillips JM (ed): *Endoscopy in Gynecology*. American Association of Gynecologic Laparoscopists, Baltimore, MD, 1978, pp 317–324.
43. Kreutzer ER, Lerner JE, Kahan NZ, et al: Laparoscopic treatment of small-bowel obstruction following laparoscopic lymphadenectomy. *Urology* 44:768–770, 1994.
44. Burney TL, Jacobs SC, Naslund MJ: Small bowel obstruction following laparoscopic lymphadenectomy. *J Urol* 150:1515–1517, 1993.
45. Grice DO, Garzotto MG, Newman RC, et al: Closure of laparoscopic trocar sites using a spring loaded needle (abstract 939). *J Urol* 151.462A, 1994.
46. Font GE, Brill AL, Stuhldreher PV, et al: Endoscopic management of incidental cystotomy during operative laparoscopy. *J Urol* 149:1130–1131, 1993.
47. Reich H, McGlynn F: Laparoscopic repair of bladder injury. *Obstet Gynecol* 76:909–910, 1990.
48. Fishman JR, Moran ME, Carey RW: Obturator neuropathy after laparoscopic pelvic lymphadenectomy. *Urology* 42:198–200, 1993.
49. Fowler JE, Barzell W, Hilaris BS, et al: Complications of ^{125}I implantment and pelvic lymphadenectomy in the treatment of prostate cancer. *J Urol* 121:447–451, 1979.
50. Rukstalis DB, Chodak GW: Laparoscopic retroperitoneal lymph node dissection in a patient with stage I testicular carcinoma. *J Urol* 148:1907–1909, 1992.
51. Gerber GS, Bissada NK, Hulbert JC, et al: Laparoscopic retroperitoneal lymphadenectomy: Multi-institutional analysis. *J Urol* 152:1188–1191, 1994.
52. Skinner DG, Melamud A, Lieskovsky G: Complications of thoracoabdominal retroperitoneal lymph node dissection. *J Urol* 127:1107–1110, 1982.
53. Donohue JP, Rowland RG: Complications of retroperitoneal lymph node dissection. *J Urol* 125:338–340, 1981.
54. Sago AL, Ball TP, Novicki DE: Complications of retroperitoneal lymphadenectomy. *Urology* 13:241–243, 1979.
55. Clayman RV, Kavoussi LR, Soper NJ, et al: Laparoscopic nephrectomy: Initial case report. *J Urol* 146:278–282, 1991.
56. Kerbl K, Clayman RV, McDougall EM, et al: Transperitoneal nephrectomy for benign disease of the kidney: A comparison of laparoscopic and open surgical techniques. *Urology* 43:607–613, 1994.
57. Schiff MS, Glazier WB: Nephrectomy: Indications and complications in 347 patients. *J Urol* 118:930–931, 1977.
58. Scott RF, Selzman HM: Complications of nephrectomy: Review of 450 patients and a description of a modification of the transperitoneal approach. *J Urol* 95:307–312, 1966.
59. Kavoussi LR, Kerbl K, Capelouto CC, et al: Laparoscopic nephrectomy for renal neoplasms. *Urology* 42:603–609, 1993.
60. Winfield HN, Donovan JF, Lund GO, et al: Laparoscopic partial nephrectomy: Initial experience and comparison to the open surgical approach. *J Urol* 153:1409–1414, 1995.
61. Gomella LG, Abdel-Meguid T, Hirsch II, et al: Laparoscopic urologic surgery: Continued improvement in outcome. *Proc Am Urol Assoc* 153:518A, 1995.
62. Parra RO, Perez MG, Boullier JA, et al: Comparison between standard flank versus laparoscopic nephrectomy for benign renal disease. *J Urol* 153:1171–1174, 1995.

section four

Laparoscopy in Gynecology

chapter sixteen

Complications and Their Management During Laparoscopic Pelvic Surgery

Camran Nezhat
Farr Nezhat
Ceana H. Nezhat
Daniel S. Seidman

INTRODUCTION

The progress in operative laparoscopy has, to a large extent, been made by gynecologic surgeons.[1–4] The routine use of diagnostic laparoscopy to assess infertility patients led to the development of techniques to treat these patients. One of the most challenging disease processes found in infertility patients is endometriosis. It causes severe adhesions, complete obliteration of the cul-de-sac, and deep infiltration of the pelvic and abdominal walls. By adapting and creating techniques to treat endometriosis, any abdominal surgical procedure can be performed laparoscopically, including bowel resection[5,6] and extensive urinary tract operations.[7,8]

As gynecologists have the most experience with laparoscopy, they are particularly aware of complications and their avoidance.[9,10] Increases in the number of advanced endoscopic procedures performed are associated with a significant complication rate.[11,12] The risk of complications is strongly related to the operator's experience, that is, the learning curve. As the results show, in the hands of highly experienced surgeons, operative laparoscopy is generally at least as safe as laparotomy.[13]

The known rate of intraoperative and postoperative complications is less than 1% (Table 16.1), but this probably does not reflect the risk of complications for the average gynecologic surgeon. Most reports are from large practices with experienced gynecologists,[13] surveys of members of the American Association of Gynecologic Laparoscopists (AAGL),[14,15] and reports from tertiary referral clinics.[16]

From July 1982 to December 1993 at the Center for Special Pelvic Surgery (CSPS) in Atlanta and at Stanford University in Palo Alto,[13] 6949 advanced operative laparoscopies were performed, with a complication rate of 3.08%, significantly lower than that expected from laparotomy (Table 16.2). The most common complication was abdominal wall vascular injury (inferior epigastric vessels); none of these complications required laparotomy. Intestinal and urinary tract injuries were the second most common complication. Severe adhesions and endometriosis were the main factors contributing to these injuries. Laparotomy used to manage complications was only 0.23%; most cases occurred early in the experience with operative laparoscopy. For example, in the last 5000 operations performed, only one laparotomy was necessary to control bleeding. To date, no fatalities have occurred.

Complication rates associated with operative laparoscopy appear to be low when procedures are performed by an experienced laparoscopist. The incidence of complications is related directly to the severity of pelvic and abdominal pathology. Adhesions and endometriosis are contributing factors to urinary tract and intestinal injury. Certain complications are unavoidable, and surgeons must be prepared to manage them by laparotomy or laparoscopy. The incidence of conversion to laparotomy to manage complications or to complete a procedure tends to be higher early in one's experience.[17]

Table 16.1 Major Complications per 1000 Operative Laparoscopies

By instrument	
Veress needle	2.7
Large trocar	2.4–2.7
Accessory trocar	2.5–6
Electrocautery	0.5–2.8
Laser	1.2
Pneumoperitoneum	7.4
By site of injury	
Vessels/bleeding	2.6–11.0
Bowel	0.6–2.0
Genitourinary	0.6–1.6
Nerve	6.1
Uterine perforation	3.7
Other indicators	
Death	0.054–0.3
Hospitalization >72 hr	4.2–27.0
Hospital readmission	3.1–5.0
Persistent βHCG titers	63.2–144.0
Infection	1.4–6.5
Febrile	2.0

Sources: Refs. 15 and 16; Goodman

In a study encompassing 17,521 diagnostic and operative procedures performed at seven centers, an overall complication rate of 3.2/1000 was found (Table 16.3).[18] The rate for diagnostic and minor procedures was 1.1/1000, and for major and advanced operations it was 5.2/1000. Laparotomies were performed for hemorrhage (17) or visceral complications (40), and injury was most common following extensive adhesiolysis and advanced laparoscopic surgery; 1 fatality was reported.

In this chapter, the focus will be the prevention, diagnosis, and management of injuries involving the pelvic organs, including the uterus, ureters, urinary bladder, and bowel.

INTRAOPERATIVE COMPLICATIONS

Uterus

Complications involving the uterus include cervical lacerations or uterine perforation from sounding the uterus or from the use of the uterine dilator or uterine manipulator. Cervical lacerations are managed with pressure from a sponge stick or suture. Bleeding from uterine perforations is controlled with bipolar electrocoagulation. Occasionally, the uterus is repaired using laparoscopic suturing. A CO_2 laser beam can lacerate the uterine serosa, and the uterus should not be used as a backstop.

Table 16.2 Complications in a Series of 6949 Laparoscopic Operations

Injuries and Complications	Vascular		Gastrointestinal		Genitourinary		
	Abd. Wall	Intra-Abd.	Small Bowel	Large Bowel	Bladder	Ureter	Other*
Intraoperative	117	6	22	9	8	3	3
Laparoscopy	116	2	15	8	5	2	0
Minilaparotomy	1	0	3	1	0	0	0
Laparotomy	0	4	4	0	2	0	0
Medical	0	0	0	0	1	1	3
Postoperative	12	5	6	5†	3	1	17‡
Laparoscopy	6	2	1	1	1	1	3
Laparotomy	1	2	1	3	0	0	3
Medical	5	1	4	1	2	0	12

* Includes pelvic infection, subcutaneous emphysema, pulmonary edema, incisional hernia, deep vein thrombosis, pleural effusion, vaginal cuff dehiscence, and severe dehydration.

† Some patients had a combination of laparoscopy and laparotomy or laparoscopy and medical treatment.

‡ Three women had more than one complication.

Table 16.3 Complications of Gynecologic Laparoscopic Surgery

Laparoscopic Procedures	No. of Procedures	Laparotomies for Complications	Rate/1000
Diagnostic	4130	7	1.7
Minor	4213	2	0.5
Major extensive adhesiolysis	1910	16	8.4
Other	6370	24	3.8
Advanced	898	8	8.9

Bladder Injuries

Prevention

Bladder injury is rare and usually occurs in patients who have had laparotomies[15] or whose bladder is not empty.[19] Under these conditions, sharp instruments such as trocars and uterine anteverters can perforate or lacerate the bladder, electricity and lasers can cause thermal injury, and blunt instruments can lacerate the bladder. Certain laparoscopic procedures increase the risk of bladder injury. The Veress needle can perforate a distended bladder. A misplaced Rubin's cannula can perforate the vagina and bladder with upward pressure.[20] Accessory trocar insertion can injure a full bladder; one with anatomy distorted by previous pelvic surgery, endometriosis, or adhesions; or if insertion is less than 4 cm above the pubic symphysis. Coagulation or laser ablation of endometriosis implants or adhesiolysis in the anterior cul-de-sac can predispose the patient to bladder injury unless hydrodissection or a backstop is used with the CO_2 laser. During a laparoscopic hysterectomy (LH) or a laparoscopy-assisted vaginal hysterectomy (LAVH), the bladder may be lacerated or torn if blunt dissection is used to free the bladder from the pubocervical fascia, particularly in women with prior cesarean section, severe endometriosis, or lower segment myomas. If sutures are placed in the bladder during LH or LAVH, a vesicovaginal fistula may develop. Also, bladder injury can occur while entering and dissecting the space of Retzius before laparoscopic bladder neck suspension.

To prevent injuries, a Foley catheter is placed to drain the bladder. The position of the bladder should be assessed during the initial examination with the laparoscope. If the boundaries of the bladder are not clear, particularly when pelvic anatomy is distorted, the bladder should be filled with 350 mL of normal saline to delineate its position. Care should be used when performing LH or LAVH, and the assistant should push the uterus up during bladder dissection.

Recognition

Intraoperative recognition of a bladder injury is important to prevent long-term sequelae. Signs of intraoperative bladder injury include (1) air in the urinary catheter and bag during insufflation; (2) a bladder that appears to be pushed by the accessory trocar as the latter is advanced through the abdominal wall; (3) blood in the urine; (4) urine drainage from the accessory trocar incision; (5) postoperative urinary retention, particularly if the amount of urine obtained during catheterization is less than anticipated; (6) postoperative signs of peritonitis; and (7) leakage of indigo carmine from the injured site. Because trocar injury often involves entry and exit punctures, locating both is important.

Some bladder complications become apparent postoperatively, particularly those caused by electrocoagulation. Signs and symptoms include decreased urine output, hematuria, suprapubic bruising, a mass in the abdominal wall or pelvis, abdominal swelling, azotemia, and peritonitis. If a bladder injury is suspected, a retrograde cystogram may demonstrate a bladder leak.

Management

Small holes generally heal without sequelae. However, trocar injuries to the bladder dome require closure followed by urinary drainage for 5 to 7 days. Drainage promotes healing, encourages spontaneous closure, and minimizes further complications.

Lacerations may require a laparotomy, although some surgeons can repair them laparoscopically. After identifying the injury and removing any endometriosis, adhesions, or necrotic tissue, the laceration is repaired in one layer, using 0 polyglactin (Vicryl; Ethicon, Somerville, NJ) or chromic suture.[7] The suture is placed through the serosa, muscularis, and mucosa. Small injuries (less than 0.5 cm) may be repaired by placing one Endoloop around the injury. Cystoscopy is performed to be sure that there is no damage to the ureteral orifices and the repair is watertight. In a series of eight intraoperative bladder injuries, five were repaired laparoscopically using one layer suturing (Table 16.2).

Nezhat and associates reported successful laparoscopic partial resection and repair of the bladder wall for severe vesical endometriosis without complications.[7] Recently, while removing an excised ovary through a 10-mm trocar, blood and CO_2 gas were noted in the urine bag. The trocar was removed and cystoscopy was performed immediately. A perforation was found on the anterior and posterior walls of the bladder dome. The ureteral orifices were not injured, and there was no bleeding. A Foley catheter was inserted and remained in place for 7 days. Prophylactic antibiotics were given. After 7 days, a cystogram showed complete healing.

Ureter Injuries

The development of the ureter is associated embryologically with the development of the female genital tract. This close association persists postnatally, predisposing women to ureteral injury.

Prevention

Knowledge of the ureter's path through the pelvis and the vulnerable points are key to preventing injuries. The intrapelvic segment of the ureter is near the broad ligament, ovaries, and uterosacral ligaments, and injuries occur often in these areas.[21] The surgeon should note the ureter's course through the peritoneum. Endometriosis and severe pelvic adhesions can thicken the peritoneum, obscuring the location of the ureter, especially near the uterosacral ligaments.

If the ureter cannot be identified clearly through the peritoneum, it must be located by retroperitoneal dissection. Using hydrodissection, a horizontal incision is made in the peritoneum midway between the ovary and the uterosacral ligaments. The lower edge of the peritoneum is grasped and pulled medially. Blunt dissection with the suction-irrigator probe helps locate the ureter lateral to the peritoneum. If the peritoneum is involved with endometriosis and there is retroperitoneal fibrosis, the ureter can be attached to the peritoneum. The horizontal incision in the peritoneum is extended as necessary.

Until recently, most reported cases of ureteral injury during laparoscopy involved electrocoagulation because this is the technique most commonly used to arrest bleeding. As the use of stapling devices increases, additional injuries to the ureters are being reported.[22–24]

Ureteral injury can occur during sharp dissection of an ovary adherent to the pelvic sidewall; in uterosacral transection; with ligation, transection, or coagulation of the uterine arteries; when removing endometriosis implants or fibrosis from the ureter;[25–27] and while trying to control bleeding vessels. Nezhat et al. reported six ureteral injuries involving endometriosis and fibrosis (five) or adhesion (one).[28] Four of the six injuries were intentional and were performed to treat partial or complete obstruction. Unrecognized anomalies in ureteral location may predispose the patient to injury.[29] To avoid such injuries, the tissue being destroyed or removed and the location of the ureter must be identified before irreversible action is taken. Meticulous and continuous attention to the location of the ureter will reduce complications.

Methods to protect the ureter include using hydrodissection and resecting the affected peritoneum.[30] A small opening is made in the peritoneum, and 50 to 100 mL of lactated Ringer's solution is injected along the course of the ureter. This displaces the ureter laterally, providing a plane for safe ablation of endometriotic implants, lysis of adhesions, and resection of the involved peritoneum. The fluid absorbs the CO_2 laser energy, decreasing the risk of thermal damage to underlying tissue.[31] This procedure is applicable only when the peritoneum is not densely adherent to the underlying ureter. During uterosacral transection, a backstop can be placed between the lateral aspect of the uterosacral ligament and the ureter. Before using the bipolar forceps during adnexectomy, the infundibulopelvic ligament is put under traction to identify the ureter and avoid thermal damage.

The routine use of preoperative intravenous pyelography (IVP) is not recommended, and no prospective study substantiates that this prevents ureteral injury. However, for selected patients, it may help diagnose ureteral obstruction and allow appropriate surgical planning. The routine use of ureteral catheters is not warranted, but we find it useful in cases of severe endometriosis and adhesions.

Recognition

It is reported that a favorite quote of Dr. Thomas Green of Boston was, "The venial sin is injury to the ureter; the mortal sin is failure of recognition."[32] Early recognition is critical to successful management. Intraoperative ureter damage is suspected when urine leakage or blood-tinged urine is noted and indigocarmine dye is spilled intraperitoneally following intravenous administration. When surgical procedures involve the ureter, postoperative ureteral integrity can be ascertained by cystoscopy, ureteral catheterization, or intravenous retrograde pyelography (IVP). Stenting of the ureter or repair by laparotomy generally is indicated, but laparoscopic repair of partial and full-thickness injuries is an option for some laparoscopists.[26,29]

Unfortunately, a diagnosis of ureteral injury usually is made postoperatively by IVP.[21] Fever, flank pain, peritonitis, and abdominal distention within 48 to 72 hours postoperatively should alert the clinician to possible ureteral injury. Leukocytosis and hematuria may be present. Because the patient's symptoms may be indistinguishable from those of ileus or bowel injury, an IVP is indispensable for differential diagnosis.

Management

Whether the discovery of ureteral complications is immediate or delayed, a urologist should be consulted. If the IVP indicates ureteral injury, initial therapy should involve attempts at either retrograde or antegrade stenting. Therapeutic options by laparotomy include ureteroureterostomy and ureteroneocystostomy. Both require stenting and drainage with a ureteral catheter. There have been several recent reports of conservative management of ureteral injuries as well as laparoscopic management. Winslow and associates[33] reported the conservative management of a patient who sustained an electrical burn to the left ureter secondary to laparoscopy performed for an infertility evaluation. Postoperative retrograde ureteral stenting was performed for 18 days. Following removal of the catheter, an IVP demonstrated grade III left hydronephrosis secondary to ureteral stricture, which developed at the pelvic brim. The patient eventually underwent cystoscopy and left retrograde catheterization with placement of a J-stent. Her renal function improved markedly.

Gomel and James[29] reported ureteral injury that occurred during needle electrosurgical ablation of the left uterosacral ligament. When the pelvic structures were examined at the end of the procedure, a transverse laceration was found over the anterior aspect of the ureter extending over one-half of its circumference. Notably, the ureter was medial to the uterosacral ligament, a significant variation from its normal lateral position. The edges of the laceration appeared healthy, with no blanching or irregularity. Interestingly, no leakage of blue-stained urine was observed after the intravenous injection of methylene blue. A whistle-tip ureteral catheter was introduced through a cystoscope. The edges of the laceration were approximated with a single 4-0 plain catgut suture. Pelvic drainage was not used, and the patient was given prophylactic antibiotics. Two weeks following the procedure, the stent was removed. An IVP performed 10 weeks postoperatively did not indicate ureteral dilations or stenosis.

Nezhat and Nezhat managed a case of long-term ureteral obstruction caused by endometriosis and incidental partial resection of the ureter laparoscopically.[26] The ureter's course was distorted by a 2-cm fibrotic nodule on the ureter, approximately 4 cm above the bladder, corresponding to the level of obstruction. Hydrodissection aided in entering the retroperitoneal space at the pelvic brim. The ureter was dissected with the CO_2 laser. Under cystoscopic guidance, a No. 7 French ureteral catheter was passed through the ureterovesical junction. The catheter was advanced through the proximal portion of the ureter to the left renal pelvis. The edges of the ureter were reapproximated using four interrupted 4-0 polydioxanone sutures. The postoperative course was uncomplicated, and 6 weeks postoperatively the stent was removed. An IVP confirmed ureteral patency. Five years after surgery, this patient is doing well

In one case, during the treatment of severe pelvic wall endometriosis, a 1.5-cm segment of the ureter was unintentionally completely resected midway between the pelvic brim and the ureterosacral ligament. After the location of the injury was identified by injecting indigo carmine intravenously, 2 to 3 cm of the proximal and distal ureteral ends were freed from the periureteral attachments. After the ends were approximated with a 4-0 polydioxanone suture, a stay ureteral stent was introduced cystoscopically and passed through the proximal end of the injury into the renal pelvis. The stent was secured outside, and the patient was placed on continuous drainage. The ureter was repaired by placing four 4-0 polydioxanone sutures at 12, 6, 9, and 3 o'clock. The lacerated edges were approximated. A Jackson-Pratt drain was inserted, and an indwelling Foley catheter was introduced into the bladder. The duration of the entire procedure was 187 min, and the repair took 35 min. Cefoxitin (1 g) was given preoperatively and continued postoperatively (1 g every 6 hr) until the patient was discharged from the hospital.

On the first postoperative day, there was no drainage from the Jackson-Pratt drain and it was removed. No postoperative complications were noted. The patient remained afebrile, with normal renal function tests and sterile urine. Although the ureteral stent stayed in place, the Foley catheter was removed. The patient was discharged on the second postoperative day and prescribed prophylactic antibiotics (Septra DS: Burroughs Welcome, Research Triangle Park, NC). Six weeks postoperatively, the ureteral catheter was removed and no evidence of ureteral dilation or stenosis was found. An IVP revealed no leakage or stricture.

We have treated 12 additional cases of severe ureteric endometriosis causing partial or complete obstruction. All patients had histories of endometriosis with failed surgical and medical treatments.

In four women, the ureteral endometriosis was completely removed without entering the ureteral lumen. Three women required a complete segmental resection. One right and one left ureteroureterostomy and one reanastomosis of the left ureter to the bladder (ureteroneocystostomy) were performed using four through-and-through interrupted 4-0 polydioxanone sutures to reapproximate the edges over the uretal catheter.

In five women, the ureter was partially involved. The severe retroperitoneal and ureteral endometriosis was excised or vaporized, using a CO_2 laser, until ureterotomy occurred. In three of these patients, the ureterotomy was small and was detected by intravenous injection of indigo carmine. A uretal stent was left in place, and no suture was required. In two patients, the ureterotomy was repaired using 4-0 polydioxanone sutures to overlap the resected portion. Pathology revealed fibrosis, endometriosis, or both in all women. A rare case of endometriosis with focal severe, atypical hyperplasia was found in a 46-year-old women. She had total abdominal hysterectomy and bilateral salpingo-oophorectomy followed by hormonal replacement therapy at another institution. All patients had uneventful intra- and postoperative courses and reported symptomatic relief. Imaging techniques demonstrated patent ureters with functioning kidneys in all patients except one. She was 24 years old and several months earlier had been diagnosed with pelvic endometriosis, which was partially treated at initial laparoscopy followed by gonadotropin-releasing hormone agonist analogue. During a second laparoscopy, severe left ureterosacral and left pelvic sidewall endometriosis causing complete obstruction of the ureter was found. Segmental resection and ureteroureterostomy were performed (Fig. 16.1A–E). Intraoperative intravenous injection of indigo carmine did not reveal leakage from the ureter and raised the question of a nonfunctioning kidney. Postoperative follow-up and imaging revealed a 5–10% functioning kidney and a patent ureter.

Three patients had severe right pelvic sidewall-endometriosis with ureteral involvement resulting in some degree of stenosis and hydroureter. The endometriosis and fibrosis were excised and removed but required ureteral resection. In two cases, the ureter was repaired with two sutures. In one, the perforation was small and was managed by inserting the ureteral stent, which remained for approximately 2 weeks. In a 2- to 4-year follow-up period, no long-term complications were reported. A surgeon familiar with delicate laparoscopic suturing can repair ureteral injuries laparoscopically with good results.

Small Bowel

In general, small bowel injuries occur if the bowel is immobilized by adhesions. The bowel can be injured during Veress needle or trocar insertion, bowel manipulation, or enterolysis. Electrosurgery and stray laser beams can result in unrecognized thermal injuries to the bowel. Injury to the gastrointestinal tract is a serious complication. Whether discovered intraoperatively or several days following surgery, small bowel injuries result in unplanned laparotomy, serious morbidity, and even death.[15]

Prevention

Direct mechanical injury to the gastrointestinal tract is less common than electrical injury. Intestinal lacerations can occur when using scissors, the laser, or electricity. The risk of injury is higher when adhesions are dense and tissue planes poorly defined. In addition, traction on the bowel with serrated graspers may cause abrasions and lacerations. A case of inadvertent small bowel biopsy, unfortunately diagnosed by the pathologist, has been reported.[34] Bowel inspection following sharp dissection or in the presence of bleeding or hematoma should alert the operator to bowel trauma. Manipulation of the bowel such as displacement of the bowel from the pelvis with a blunt metal probe, should be done with care and blunt dissection of the bowel

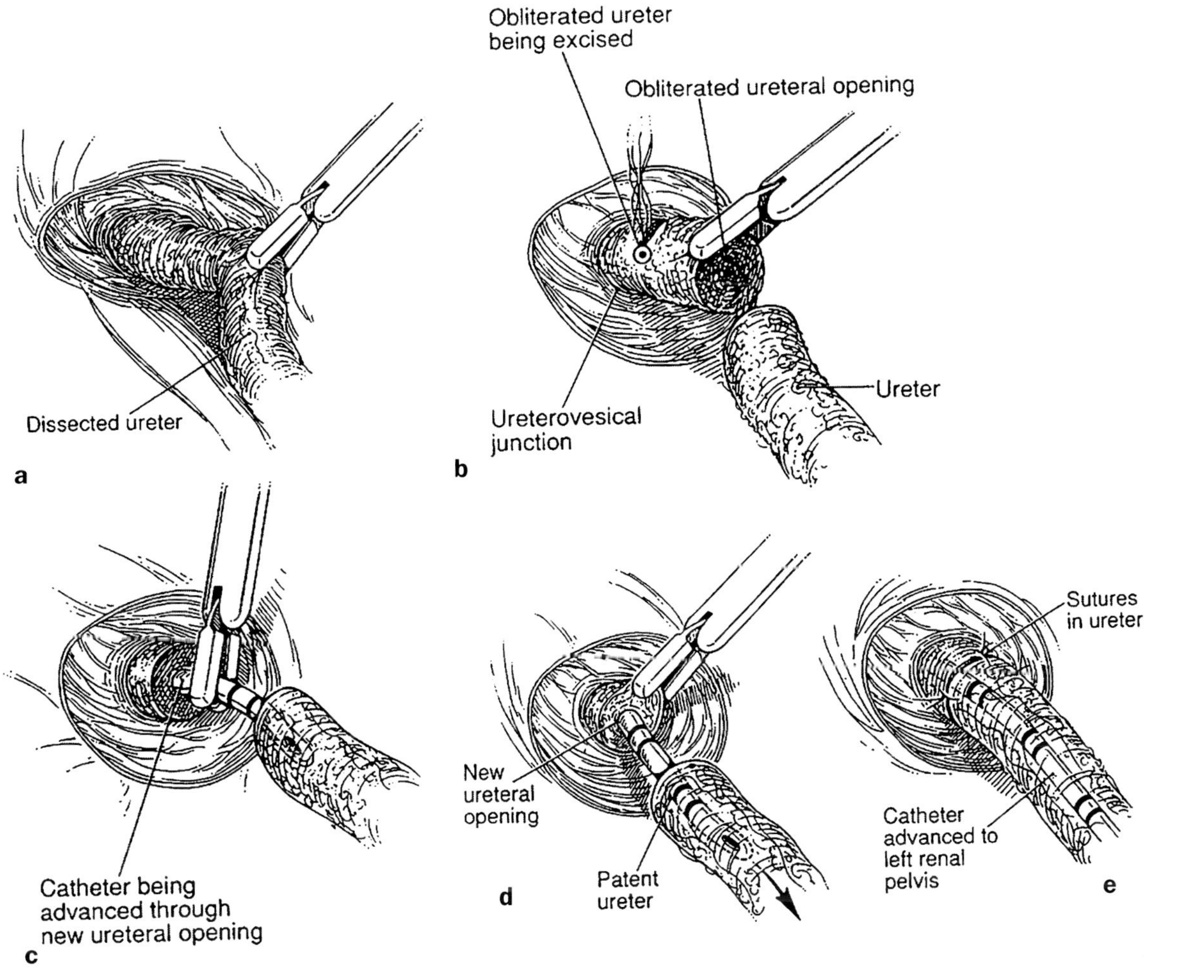

Figure 16.1. (a) The portion of the ureter to be resected is dissected. (b) The obliterated portion of the ureter is excised with the CO_2 laser. (c) A No. 7 French ureteral catheter is passed through the ureterovesical junction. (d) The catheter is advanced through the proximal portion of the ureter to the renal pelvis. (e) The edges of the ureter are approximated at the 12, 3, 6, and 9 o'clock positions using four interrupted 4-0 polydioxanone sutures.

avoided. The bowel can be trapped in an incision as trocars are withdrawn, placing the patient at risk for a small bowel obstruction.[35] For this reason, some advocate opening the valve of the umbilical trocar as it is withdrawn to prevent creation of a vacuum that may draw the bowel into the incision. Using a Z-track insertion may eliminate this complication.[36]

Adhesions between the small bowel and the anterior abdominal wall are associated with a risk of trocar injury, especially in patients who have had a bowel resection or exploratory laparotomy for trauma. (Figs. 16.2A,B). Women who undergo a second-look laparoscopy following treatment of ovarian carcinoma by laparotomy may have adhesions from previous abdominal surgery with omentectomy and debulking.[37]

Despite the use of open laparoscopy, bowel lacerations can occur on entering the peritoneum.[38] It is difficult to decide which patients should have an open laparoscopy. In a series of 22 patients who had small bowel injuries, all had previous laparotomies and small

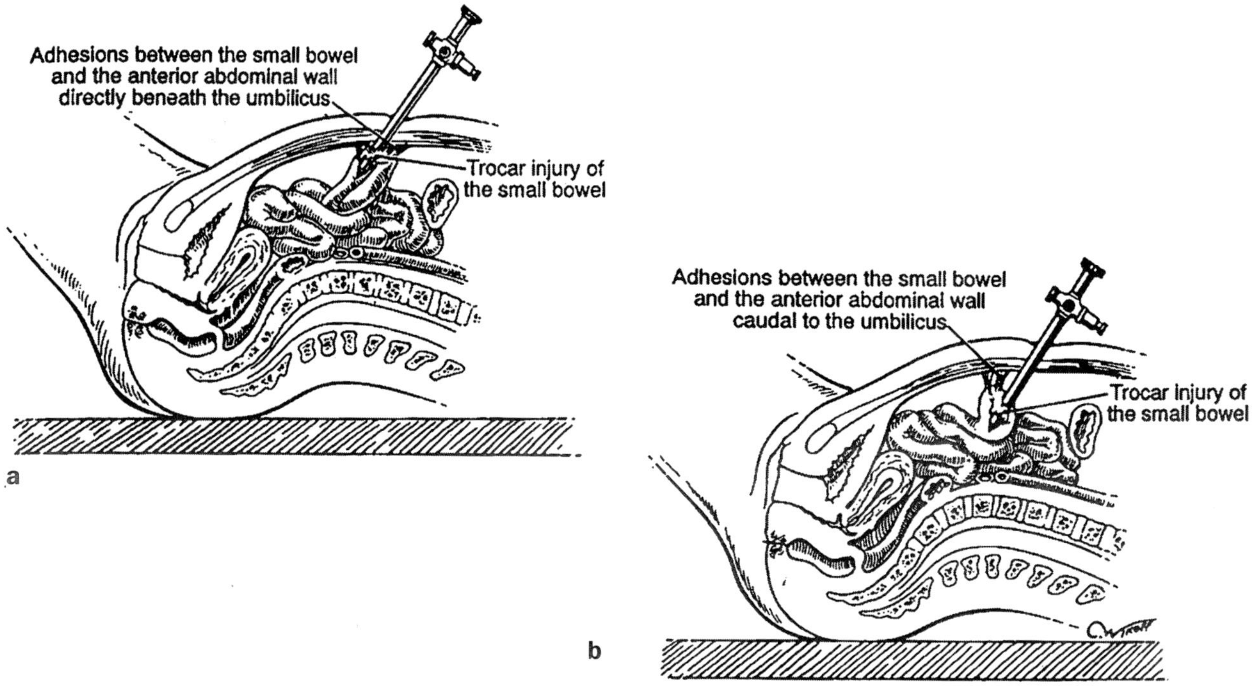

Figure 16.2. The bowel is attached to the anterior abdominal wall (a) directly under the umbilicus and (b) below and distal to the umbilicus.

bowel adhesions.[13] Seven were trocar injuries, 13 occurred during adhesiolysis, and 2 developed during open laparoscopy (Table 16.2).

In a study of 360 patients with prior single or multiple laparotomies, adhesions to the omentum and bowel were found in 128.[39] Laparoscopy was performed with a standard closed technique after establishing a pneumoperitoneum with a Veress needle in 328 (91%) women; in the remaining 32 (9%) patients, trocar insertion was by an open technique. Twenty-one (6%) sustained injury to the small bowel or omentum related to the presence of adhesions to an old scar. Two of these women underwent trocar insertion by the open technique.

Patients at risk for bowel adhesions should undergo preoperative mechanical and antibiotic bowel preparation to eliminate bowel contents, decompress the bowel, and prevent infection.

Recognition

Electrical injuries to the bowel are not always apparent intraoperatively or their appearance may lead the surgeon to choose conservative management. Most intestinal burns less than 5 mm in diameter can be managed expectantly. If the area of blanching on the intestinal serosa exceeds 5 mm, the extent of thermal damage will probably exceed the apparent damage and therapy should be instituted immediately. The injured area can extend up to 5 cm from the evident injury.[30]

If the small bowel has been lacerated by a trocar, the surgeon initially may view a mucosal surface or notice a foul smell when the laparoscope is inserted. Small bowel contents may be observed leaking from a laceration or a hematoma may be present on the small bowel serosa.

If the injury is not recognized intraoperatively, the patient generally presents on the third or fourth postoperative day with lower abdominal pain, mild fever, slight nausea, and anorexia. By the fifth or sixth postoperative day, symptoms include fever, severe abdominal pain, nausea, vomiting, constipation, increased white blood cell count, and peritonitis.[30] Radiographs reveal multiple air-fluid levels or air under the diaphragm.

Management

Complications from small bowel injury are related to the extent of damage and the time elapsed before the injury is discovered. Sharp trocar injuries to the bowel can be limited to the serosa or involve the entire wall. Small punctures or superficial lacerations seal readily and require no further treatment, assuming that careful inspection of the affected bowel reveals no leakage of bowel contents or bleeding. Small (less than 5 mm), superficial lacerations need to be inspected to ensure that only the serosa is involved. In these cases, the patient may be treated conservatively and discharged the day of surgery, with instructions to report any untoward reaction.

Patients with obvious peritoneal soiling require intervention and perhaps laparotomy. The bowel should be inspected on both sides to detect through-and-through injuries, especially if produced by a trocar. If only one entry is found and repaired, peritonitis may develop postoperatively. If the laparoscope has been inserted through the bowel laceration and laparotomy is performed, the defect is identified and closed by a purse-string suture as the laparoscope is withdrawn to minimize peritoneal contamination.[40]

Small bowel injuries should be repaired in one or two layers by placing an initial row of interrupted sutures of 3–0 chromic catgut to approximate the mucosa and muscularis. A reinforcing layer of 3–0 silk Lembert sutures is used to approximate the muscularis and serosal edges.[41] All lacerations should be closed transversely to minimize stenosis of the bowel lumen. This closure is appropriate only if the laceration is less than one-half the diameter of the bowel. If the laceration exceeds one-half the diameter of the lumen, segmental resection and anastomosis should be performed. If the mesenteric blood supply is interrupted by the puncture, a resection must be performed, regardless of the size or length of the laceration to maintain the blood supply to that particular segment of bowel.[40] Intraoperative consultation with a general surgeon is appropriate whenever significant bowel trauma occurs. Small bowel injuries caused by trocars or the CO_2 laser can be repaired in one layer using 3-0 silk or 4-0 polydioxanone without complications or laparotomy.[42] Injuries smaller than 2 cm (small or large bowel) may be repaired transversely or longitudinally. However, injuries larger than 2 cm should be repaired transversely.

Following is a simple technique used to repair bowel injuries caused by sharp instruments of the CO_2 laser if the perforation is less than 1 cm. After the edge of the perforation is cleaned of debris, a grasping forceps is used to bring the perforation inside a 0 polydioxanone or polyglactin Endoloop suture and tie the loop around the perforation (Fig. 16.3A,B). To evaluate the repair, the abdomen and posterior cul-de-sac are filled with lactated Ringer's solution. A sigmoidoscope is used to insufflate the bowel, which is pushed under the fluid. The presence of air bubbles indicates inadequate repair (Fig. 16.3C). We have used this technique to repair 12 cases of small and large bowel injuries without complication.

Following repair of a bowel laceration, the entire abdomen is irrigated. A nasogastric tube may be placed and removed when drainage has decreased, indicating that bowel function has resumed. The patient is not given anything by mouth until she passes flatus.

When possible bowel laceration becomes apparent after discharge, conservative management is successful in patients who have not developed peritonitis.[43] In-hospital management consists of hydration, nothing by mouth, and close observation, with monitoring of the white blood cell count and a physical examination every 6 hr. Wheeless[40] reported that over one-half of patients treated conservatively required no surical intervention. Those whose condition deteriorated during observation underwent laparotomy and had no complication attributable to delayed surgery.

Immediate surgical intervention and possible laparotomy may be indicated in patients who present with fever, severe abdominal pain, nausea, vomiting, obstipation, or peritonitis or in those whose clinical condition worsens. Surgical considerations for managing bowel injuries discovered postoperatively differ somewhat from considerations regarding injuries discovered and managed intraoperatively. The damaged bowel must be repaired or resected. In addition, resection of all necrotic tissue in the pelvis is mandatory even if this requires a hysterectomy and bilateral salpingo-oophorectomy. If burned or necrotic tissue which has been bathed in intestinal contents, blood, or serum is not excised, a pelvic abscess will develop.[43]

In a recent AAGL membership poll, the two deaths reported from 36,928 procedures were attributed to bowel injuries. In one instance, the patient had extensive adhesions from the abdominal wall to the bowel. Although the bowel injury was recognized and repaired, the patient developed persistent postoperative ileus and died of peritonitis. The second death was attributable to sepsis after an unrecognized small bowel perforation.[15]

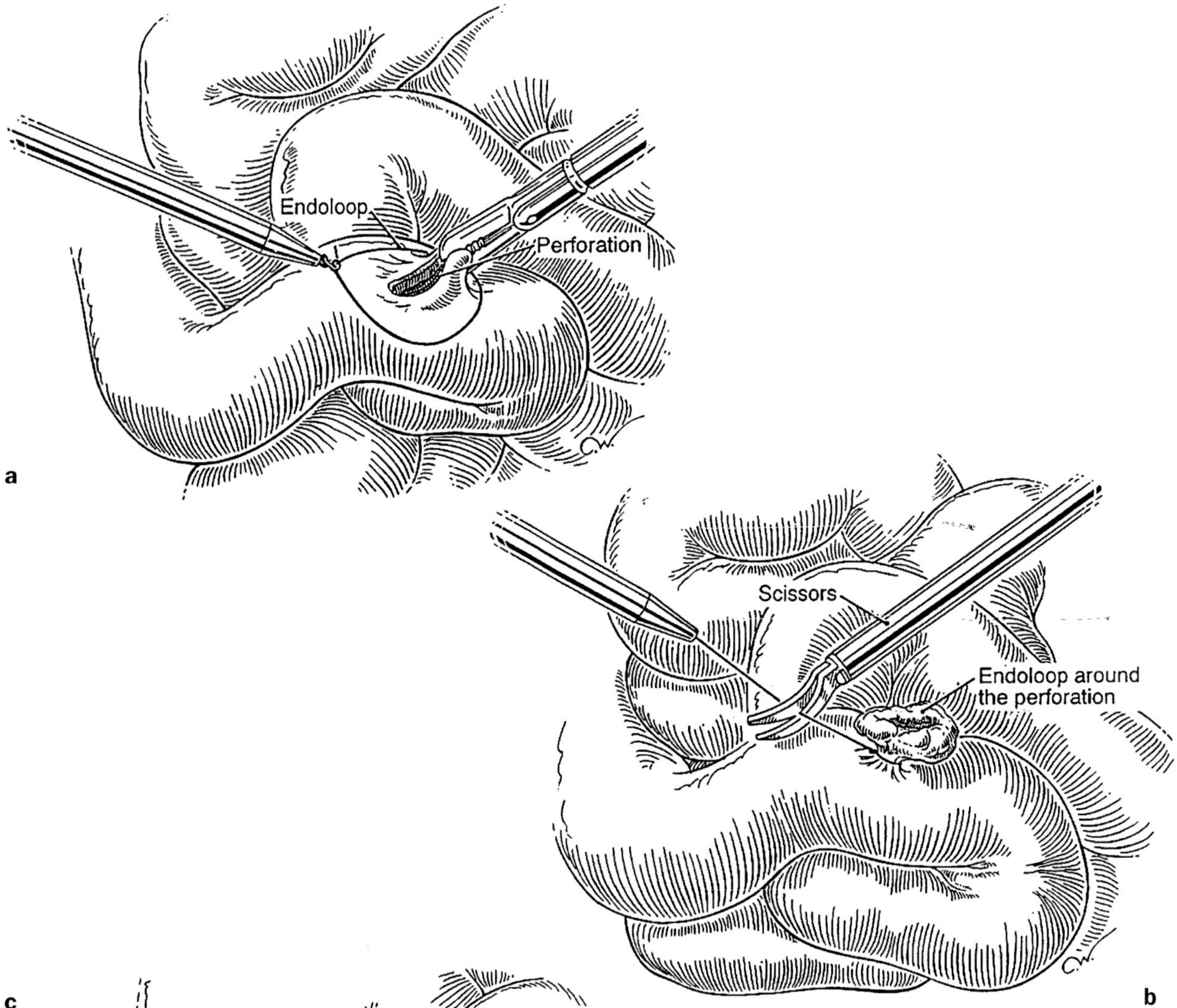

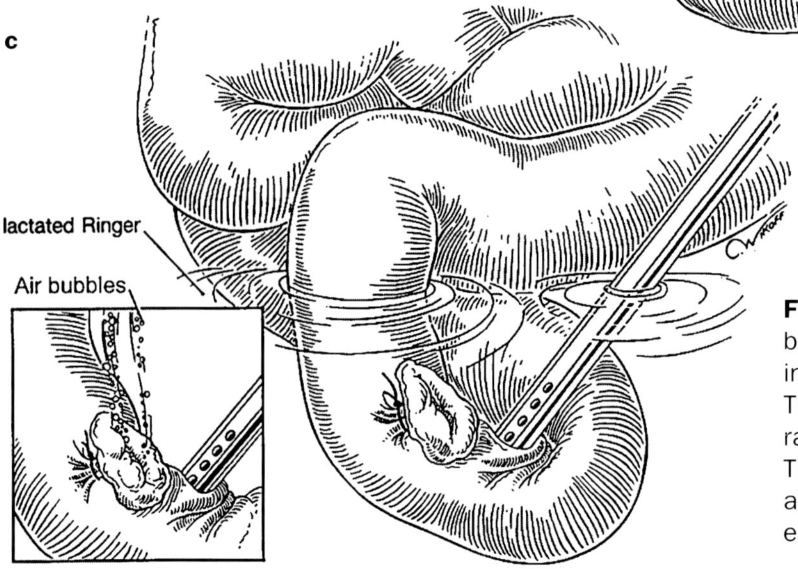

Figure 16.3. (a) Forceps are used to bring a small (<1 cm) bowel perforation inside a 4-0 PDS or 0 Vicryl Endoloop (b) The Endoloop is tied around the perforation, leaving an adequate stump (c) The repair is examined under fluid for air bubbles (inset), which indicate inadequate repair.

Large Bowel

Colon entry is a major complication, particularly if the bowel is unprepared or if the injury is not recognized. Even small perforations, such as those from the Veress needle, require attention because the high bacterial concentration of minor leaks can cause infection and abscess formation.

Prevention

Factors that contribute to an increased risk of large bowel injuries include (1) failure to establish an adequate pneumoperitoneum; (2) the use of dull trocars that require excessive force; (3) uncontrolled, sudden entry of sharp instruments; and (4) gastric distention. Poorly controlled or sudden trocar entry can result in rectosigmoid laceration. Gastric distention can displace the transverse colon toward the pelvis, where it can be punctured by the Veress needle or lacerated with the trocar. This complication can be eliminated by using a nasogastric tube intraoperatively.

The rectosigmoid colon can be injured if the depth of penetration by endometriosis is underestimated or the cul-de-sac is obliterated. When the rectum is adherent to the posterior aspect of the cervix or uterosacral ligaments, blunt dissection may lacerate the rectum. Sharp dissection with scissors or the CO_2 laser is recommended. The combination of a high-power superpulse or ultrapulse CO_2 laser and hydrodissection is relatively safe for working around the bowel.

When the cul-de-sac is dissected, identification of the vagina and rectum is facilitated by placing a probe or an assistant's finger in both the vagina and rectum. Dissection should begin lateral to the uterosacral ligaments, where anatomy is less distorted, and proceed toward the obliterated cul-de-sac.[44,45] Similarly, when posterior culdotomy is performed for tissue removal or during laparoscopic hysterectomy, correct identification of the vagina and rectum is important.[22,46]

When a difficult pelvic operation is contemplated, such as cul-de-sac nodularity in a patient with endometriosis or a history suggesting significant pelvic adhesions, preoperative bowel preparation is indicated.

Recognition

Perforation of the large bowel with the Veress needle can sometimes be recognized by the saline aspiration test the recovery of brownish fluid is pathognomonic. A fecal odor may be detected. If large bowel entry is suspected based on these two tests, the needle should be promptly withdrawn and another sterile Veress needle reinserted. Once the laparoscope is inserted, the entry site should be sought and examined. Because of the high bacterial concentration, minor leaks of fecal material into the peritoneal cavity can be the source of serious infection. Underwater examination is recommended following the treatment of severe endometriosis and adhesions of the rectum and rectosigmoid colon.

Large bowel injuries can be serious because they may not be recognized at surgery. Under these circumstances, the patient generally presents on the third or fourth postoperative day with lower abdominal pain, mild fever, slight nausea, and anorexia. By the fifth or sixth postoperative day, these symptoms progress to include fever, severe abdominal pain, nausea, vomiting, obstipation, an increased leukocyte count, and peritonitis.[43] An upright x-ray may show changes consistent with an ileus.[47] The patient appears ill with no clear explanation.

Management

For small enterotomies associated with minimal contamination, laparotomy with primary suture closure has been the accepted therapy. In addition, copious lavage of the peritoneal cavity, broad-spectrum antibiotics, and drainage minimize the risk of infection. Under the proper circumstances, certain enterotomies may be closed through the laparoscope (Fig. 16.4A–G). This procedure was performed in 25 to 26 large bowel injuries without complication.[48]

Electrical injury to the right colon is managed by resecting the injured segment and primary anastomosis. Diverting ileostomy facilitates healing and reduces morbidity and mortality. Injury to the descending colon, sigmoid, or rectum in unprepared bowel may not be amenable to primary closure or resection with primary anastomosis. Diverting colostomy with resection of the injured portion is recommended. Colonic lacerations in prepared bowel can be repaired laparoscopically after excising endometriosis nodules and identifying the extent of the laceration. A single-layered repair using 2–0 silk, 0 polydioxanone, or 0 polyglactin sutures is performed.

In a series of 100 consecutive rectosigmoid planned and unplanned enterotomies, repair was completed with single-layer suture and an Endoloop.[48] Complications included one fistula and one pelvic infection with abscess. The fistula was managed by drainage under computed tomography (CT) scan guidance and antibiotic therapy. The pelvic abscess was managed by drainage under CT scan guidance and laparoscopy after failed treatment with antibiotic therapy. Neither pa-

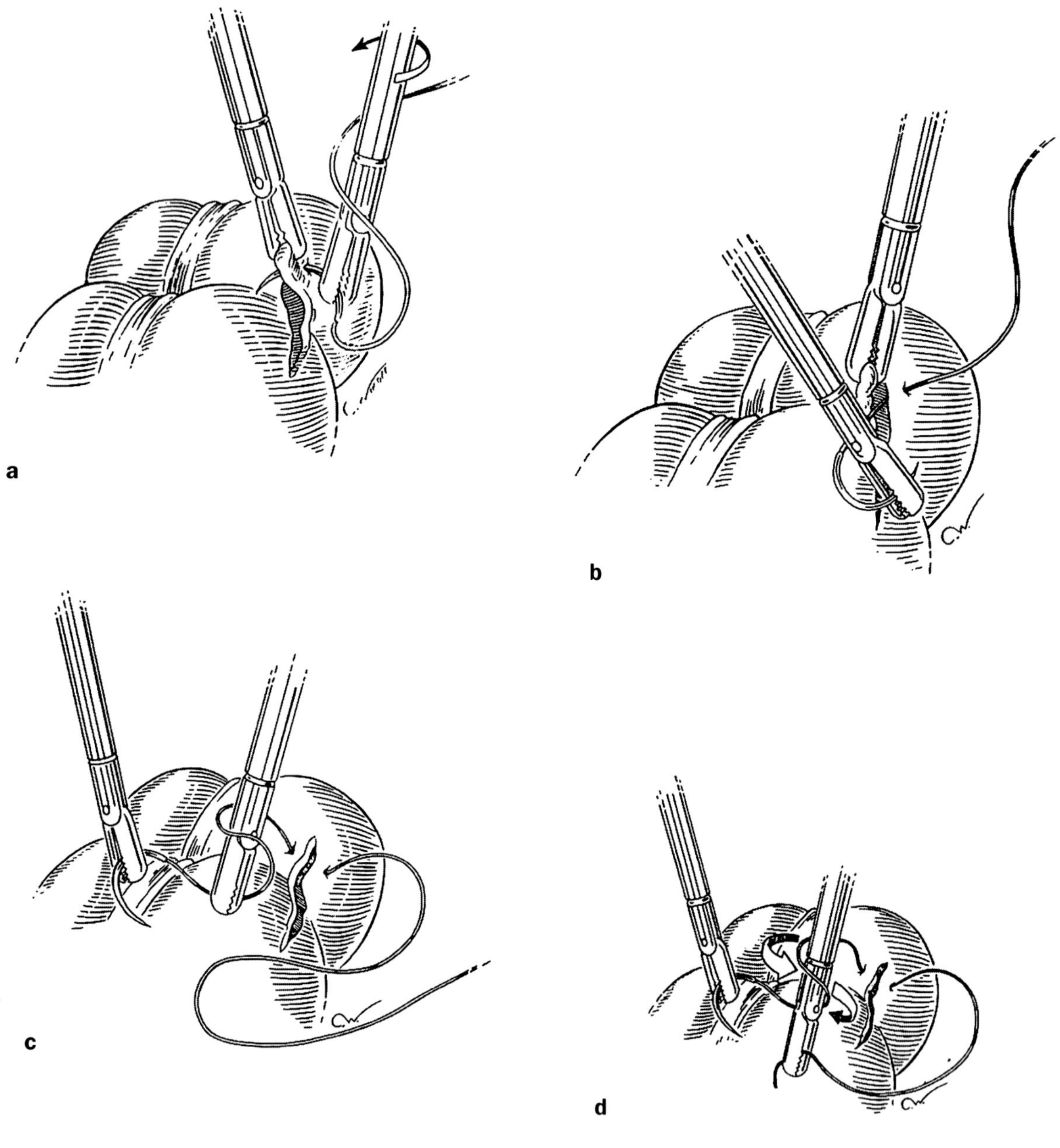

Figure 16.4. (a–d) A small perforation is repaired laparoscopically using intracorporeal knot tying.

tient required laparotomy. Both patients underwent anterior bowel disk excision for full-thickness endometriosis.

The knowledge that the bowel can be repaired successfully using laparoscopic techniques in the properly prepared patient should increase the confidence of the surgeon operating in the deep pelvis.

POSTOPERATIVE COMPLICATIONS

The unique postoperative care of patients undergoing extensive laparoscopic surgery is often neglected in physician training. The rapid convalescence of these patients, combined with their early discharge, often misleads those who are used to caring for patients after laparotomy. In fact, patients who have undergone extensive laparoscopic surgery involving multiple organ systems always require meticulous postoperative care. Unfortunately, physicians are not always aware of this. For instance, increasing abdominal pain after laparoscopic procedures demands an evaluation, even if it requires a repeat laparoscopy with negative findings.[49] There is a very limited place for in-hospital observation of patients who have had laparoscopy and fail to improve postoperatively.[49] Hesitating to rescope a patient suspected of having a postoperative complication, such as blood vessel injury or bowel perforation, may have serious consequences.

Bleeding

Hemostasis that appears adequate before closure because of the Trendelenburg position, high intra-abdominal pressures, and relative hypotension may change once the patient resumes an upright position. If the patient does not respond to intravenous hydration, a repeat hematocrit may suggest hemorrhage and physical examination may reveal abdominal distention.

Nezhat and colleagues[13,40] reported 17 complications involving postoperative bleeding. Only three patients required laparotomy. Location of the bleeding included nine from the anterior abdominal wall (seven from the suprapubic incision and two from the umbilical incision), three from the vaginal cuff after LH and LAVH, and five cases of intra-abdominal bleeding (Table 16.2). Vaginal cuff bleeding was managed by vaginal repair and packing without reexploration or transfusion.

Of five cases of intra-abdominal bleeding,[13] one was caused by persistent ectopic pregnancy, three resulted from blood disorders, and no source of bleeding was found for the fifth. One patient with persistent ectopic pregnancy presented at another center with signs of intra-abdominal bleeding and underwent laparotomy. She had a leaking, persistent ectopic pregnancy, which was removed. Another patient with storage pool disease presented with intra-abdominal bleeding 24 hr postoperatively. At laparoscopy, we were unable to locate the source of bleeding, so laparotomy was performed. However, laparotomy also failed to reveal the site. It was generalized oozing from the pelvic cavity. Postoperatively, the patient was treated with blood products and coagulation factors.

Small Bowel

In our series, we had six postoperative admissions due to small bowel complications (Table 16.2). Only one patient required laparotomy. This patient developed peritonitis 1 day after laparoscopic treatment of endometriosis and adhesions. Exploratory laparotomy showed severe bowel strangulation due to a congenital malrotation of the mesentery but no bowel perforation. The patient required extensive bowel resection and postoperative dietary adjustment.

Three patients with small bowel ileus were managed by conservative therapy, and one underwent laparoscopy to rule out pelvic infection. One patient was admitted for hydration and antibiotic therapy for severe gastroenteritis.

Large Bowel

Postoperative large bowel complications occur after unrecognized intraoperative bowel injuries, delayed necrosis caused by excessive thermal damage, and ischemia after enterotomy and bowel resection. Postoperative abdominal pain, fever, constipation, and peritoneal signs should alert the physician. Patients who have had excessive posterior cul-de-sac dissection, treatment of endometriosis, and lysis of severe large bowel adhesions should be given specific instructions regarding the avoidance of constipation and not using an enema, which can contribute to bowel perforation.

In our series, we encountered five postoperative complications involving the large bowel (Table 16.2). All patients had a history of rectal and rectosigmoid colon endometriosis and underwent different forms of bowel resection. Two women developed leaks and pelvic infections. One required laparoscopic temporary colostomy, with subsequent takedown and repair by laparotomy. One was managed by prolonged drainage under CT scan guidance and antibiotic therapy. One woman had bowel stricture after complete segmental resection, requiring resection and reanastomosis by laparotomy. One patient developed a pelvic abscess and subsequently underwent right salpingo-oophorectomy. The abscess was drained laparoscopically and under CT scan guidance. One patient with a history of endometriosis and constipation, as well as anterior wedge resection of rectal endometriosis, had an immediate postoperative rectal prolapse, which was reduced without surgical management. Her bowel symptoms persisted, and she subsequently had a colectomy at another center.

Bladder and Ureter

Patients who have postoperative genitourinary complications can present with peritoneal signs such as small bowel ileus, peritonitis, abdominal and flank pain, or fistula formation. Thorough postoperative evaluation including IVP and cystogram, pelvic ultrasound, or a CT scan should be implemented if injury is suspected.

In our series of 6949 operative laparoscopies,[13] we had three significant genitourinary complications, including one ureteral injury. One patient with a history of recent previous cervical conization underwent total LH and bilateral salpingo-oophorectomy. Three days postoperatively, she presented with right hydroureter and hydronephrosis with a ureterovaginal fistula. After placement of ureteral stents failed, she underwent laparoscopic evaluation. The distal portion of the right ureter was found to be obstructed by conization hemostatic suture. The suture apparently became loose and a fistula formed. Laparoscopic adhesiolysis and ureterolysis were performed, and the injury site was identified close to the bladder. After a ureteral stent was inserted cystoscopically, ureteroureterostomy was performed using 4-0 polydioxanone suture. An abdominal drain was inserted, and the patient was treated with antibiotic therapy. There were no postoperative complications. Follow-up studies showed a mild stricture of the distal portion of the ureter, which responded to conservative ureteral dilation.

Two patients developed vesicovaginal fistulas. One underwent extensive pelvic adhesiolysis and removal of an ovarian remnant from the rectum, right ureter, and bladder. Partial cystectomy was performed to remove the entire lesion. The bladder was repaired and drained with an indwelling Foley catheter. Unfortunately, the patient stopped using the Foley catheter less than a week postoperatively and developed a vesicovaginal fistula 1 week later. She did not respond to prolonged bladder drainage, but laparoscopic vesicovaginal fistula repair was successful. Since then, she has done well. The other woman developed a vesicovaginal fistula 2 weeks after total LH. She was managed with 2 weeks of bladder drainage and antibiotic therapy without sequelae.

Nerve Injury

Common postoperative neurologic syndromes include sciatic nerve injury, brachial palsy (shoulder-hand syndrome), and perineal nerve palsy. Allowing the buttocks to protrude too far off the end of the operating table may cause back injury.

Shoulder Pain

The CO_2 commonly used for insufflation is a peritoneal irritant. Intraoperatively, this irritation can manifest itself as a vasovagal reaction. Postoperatively, residual gas accumulates under the diaphragm when an upright position is maintained, thus irritating the diaphragm. The pain is referred to the shoulder by the phrenic nerve.

Complete removal of intra-abdominal CO_2 is difficult but may be improved by leaving the patient in the Trendelenburg position. Pressure exerted on the abdomen toward the symphysis allows the gas trapped in the lower abdomen to be expressed through the umbilical or suprapubic trocars. If pain develops, the patient can assume a supine position and use a pillow to elevate the lower abdomen, allowing gas to accumulate in the pelvis.

Infection

Postoperative infection is unusual following laparoscopic procedures, although the risk appears to be higher following prolonged, intricate surgery. Most infections are limited to skin or stitch abscesses and require incision and drainage. Occasionally, a pelvic infection occurs following tubal surgery, but it is not clear whether this is caused by a preexisting condition or contamination, or if it is secondary to tissue destruction and necrosis. Urinary tract infections can be caused by instrumentation or asymptomatic bacteria.

Nezhat and colleagues reported six pelvic infections.[13] Only two required laparotomy for management. All infections except one occurred in patients who had bowel surgery for the treatment of severe endometriosis, bowel adhesions, appendectomy, or bowel resection. This patient had a history of pelvic infections, and in spite of prophylactic antibiotic therapy, she still developed a postoperative pelvic infection.

Incisional Hernia

Herniation of the omentum or small bowel at the umbilical incision site has been reported with 7-mm or larger trocars. Patients at increased risk are those who are very thin (especially those who are elderly), have a chronic cough, or have a history of hernias. Possible preventive measures, although not proven, include Z-track insertion, avoiding trocar insertion directly through the umbilicus, and careful withdrawal of the umbilical trocar.

A subclinical hernia with adhesions between the peritoneal incision site and the bowel may place a patient at significant risk of bowel perforation if she requires another laparoscopy. Some surgeons advocate removing the umbilical trocar under laparoscopic observation to avoid entrapment of the bowel, or removing the trocar with the valve open to avoid negative pressure, which could draw omentum or small bowel into the defect. Nezhat and colleagues reported two incisional hernias in their series.[13] One involved the omentum and the other involved the small bowel. Neither required bowel resection.

SUMMARY

Laparoscopic surgery has been criticized as having a high risk of complications.[11] It has recently been noted that risk managers were informing hospital administrators that they were witnessing a rapidly increasing number of claims alleging the improper performance of endoscopic procedures by surgeons.[50] However, it has been well established that the degree of surgical risk is strongly related to the learning curve, that is, the operator's skill and experience.[51] Avoiding surgical complications requires careful use of instrumentation to prevent direct trauma to the abdominal organs by trocars, lasers, electricity, and stapling devices.[24,52] Recognition of these complications is of the utmost importance, demanding a high level of suspicion and careful examination of the patient once the surgical procedure has been completed. These diagnostic steps include cystoscopy to evaluate the integrity of the urinary bladder, observation for stitches in the bladder wall, and verification of the function of the ureters following the administration of intravenous indigo carmine. The surgeon should be able to apply ureteral stents in cases of suspected damage to the ureter. Sigmoidoscopy should be performed routinely following any procedure necessitating dissection of the rectosigmoid colon to identify disease involvement or damage to the bowel wall. Insufflation of the bowel via the sigmoidoscope allows the early recognition of bowel perforation by observing the fluid-filled rectum for air bubbles with the laparoscope. The ability to perform colonoscopy may also be helpful when lesions higher in the colon are suspected.

The need for surgical expertise is especially apparent when complications occur during laparoscopy, including damage to the bowel, ureter, or bladder. It has been shown that many of these complications can be safely repaired laparoscopically.[26,29,53] In our series of almost 7000 cases of operative laparoscopy, laparotomy was necessary in fewer than 20.[13] Only an expert laparoscopic surgeon should attempt to manage complications at laparoscopy. However, this allows the patient to enjoy the benefits of laparoscopy and may avoid the litigation commonly associated with unplanned laparotomy.

REFERENCES

1. Semm K: New methods of pelviscopy (gynecologic laparoscopy) for myomectomy, ovariectomy, tubectomy and adnexectomy. *Endoscopy* 11:85–93, 1979.
2. Bruhat MA, Mahnes H, Mage G, et al: Treatment of ectopic pregnancy by means of laparoscopy. *Fertil Steril* 33:411–414, 1980.
3. Gomel V: Laparoscopic tubal surgery in infertility. *Obstet Gynecol* 46:47–48, 1975.
4. Nezhat C, Crowgey SR, Garrison DP: Surgical treatment of endometriosis via laser laparoscopy. *Fertil Steril* 45:778–783, 1986.
5. Nezhat C, Pennington E, Nezhat F, et al: Laparoscopically assisted anterior rectal wall resection and reanastomosis for deeply infiltrating endometriosis. *Surg Laparosc Endosc* 1:2:106–108, 1991.
6. Nezhat F, Nezhat C, Pennington E: Laparoscopic proctectomy for infiltrating endometriosis of the rectum. *Fertil Steril* 57:1129–1132, 1992.
7. Nezhat F, Nezhat C: Laparoscopic segmental bladder resection for endometriosis: A report of two cases. *Obstet Gynecol* 81:882–884, 1993.

8. Nezhat C, Nezhat F, Green B: Laparoscopic treatment of obstructed ureter due to endometriosis by resection and ureteroureterostomy. A case report. *J Urol* 148:865–868, 1992.
9. Palmer R: Technique et instrumentation de la coelioscopie gynecologique. *Gynecol Obstet (Paris)* 46:420, 1947.
10. Frangenheim H: Die *Laparoskopie und die Culdoskopie in der Gynaecologie*. Stuttgart, Georg Thieme, 1959.
11. Smith DC, Donohue LR, Waszak SJ: A hospital review of advanced gynecologic endoscopic procedures. *Am J Obstet Gynecol* 170:1635–1640, 1994.
12. Assimos DG, Patterson LC, Taylor CL: Changing incidence and etiology of iatrogenic ureteral injuries. *J Urol* 152:2240–2246, 1994.
13. Nezhat F, Nezhat C, Nezhat CH: Complications of gynecologic operative laparoscopy in 6949 patients. Presented at the Society of Laparoendoscopic Surgeons Meeting, Seattle, June 10–11, 1994.
14. Phillips JM, Hulka JF, Hulka B, et al: 1979 AAGL membership survey. *J Reprod Med* 26:529–533, 1981.
15. Peterson HB, Hulka JF, Phillips JM: American Association of Gynecologic Laparoscopists' 1988 membership survey on operative laparoscopy. *J Reprod Med* 35: 587–589, 1990.
16. Lehmann-Willenbrock E, Riedel HH, Mecke H, et al: Pelviscopy/laparoscopy and its complications in Germany 1949–1988. *J Reprod Med* 37:671–677, 1992.
17. Levinson CJ, Hulka JF, Richardson DC: Laparoscopy. In Schaefer G, Graber EA, (eds): *Complication in Obstetric and Gynecologic Surgery*. Philadelphia, Harper & Row, 1981, p 281.
18. Querleu D, Chapron C, Chevallier L, et al: Complications of gynecologic laparoscopic surgery—a French multicenter collaborative study (letter). *N Engl J Med* 328:1355, 1993.
19. Georgy FM, Fetterman HH, Chefetz MD: Complication of laparoscopy: Two cases of perforated urinary bladder. *Am J Obstet Gynecol* 120:1121–1122, 1974.
20. Sherer DM: Inadvertent transvaginal cystotomy during laparoscopy. *Int J Gynecol Obstet* 32:77–79, 1990.
21. Granger DA, Soderstrom RM, Schiff SF, et al: Ureteral injuries at laparoscopy: Insights into diagnosis, management and prevention. *Obstet Gynecol* 75:839–843, 1990.
22. Nezhat C, Nezhat F, Gordon S, et al: Laparoscopic versus abdominal hysterectomy. *J Reprod Med* 37:247–250, 1992.
23. Woodland MB: Ureter injury during laparoscopy-assisted vaginal hysterectomy with the endoscopic linear stapler. *Am J Obstet Gynecol* 176:756–757, 1992.
24. Nezhat C, Nezhat F, Bess O, et al: Injuries associated with the use of a linear stapler during operative laparoscopy: Review of diagnosis, management, and prevention. *J Gynecol Surg* 9:145–150, 1993.
25. Cheng YS: Ureteral injury resulting from laparoscopic fulguration of endometriotic implant. *Am J Obstet Gynecol* 126:1045–1046, 1976.
26. Nezhat C, Nezhat F: Laparoscopic repair of resected ureter during operative laparoscopy to treat endometriosis. A case report. *Obstet Gynecol* 80:543–544, 1992.
27. Chaffkin L, Luciano LA: Ureteral injuries. In Corfman RS, Diamond WP, DeCherney AH (eds): *Complications of Laparoscopy and Hysteroscopy*. Cambridge, MA, Blackwell Scientific, 1993, p 134–140.
28. Nezhat C, Nezhat F, Nezhat C: Operative laparoscopy (minimally invasive surgery): State of the art. *J Gynecol Surg* 8:111–141, 1992.
29. Gomel V, James C: Intraoperative management of ureteral injury during operative laparoscopy. *Fertil Steril* 55:416–419, 1991.
30. Nezhat C, Nezhat F: Safe laser excision or vaporization of peritoneal endometriosis. *Fertil Steril* 52:1:149–151, 1989.
31. Cook AS, Rock JA: The role of laparoscopy in the treatment of endometriosis. *Fertil Steril* 55:663–680, 1991.
32. Nichols DH: *Clinical Proglems, Injuries and Complications of Gynecologic Surgery*, ed 2. Baltimore, Williams & Wilkins, 1988, p 181–182.
33. Winslow PH, Kreger R, Effesson B, et al: Conservative management of electrical burn injury of ureter secondary to laparoscopy. *Urology* 27:60–62, 1986.
34. Gentile GP, Siegler AM: Inadvertent intentional biopsy during laparoscopy and hysteroscopy: A report of two cases. *Fertil Steril* 36:402–404, 1981.
35. Sauer M, Jarrett JC: Small bowel obstruction following diagnostic laparoscopy. *Fertil Steril* 42:653–654, 1984.
36. Corson SL, Bolognese RJ: Laparoscopy overview and results of a large series. *J Reprod Med* 9:148–157, 1972.
37. Loffer FD, Pent D: Indications, contraindications and complications of laparoscopy. *Obstet Gynecol Surv* 30: 407–427, 1975.
38. Penfield AJ: However to prevent complications of open laparoscopy. *J Reprod Med* 30:660–663, 1985.
39. Brill AI, Nezhat F, Nezhat CH, et al: The incidence of adhesions after prior laparotomy: A laparoscopic appraisal. *Obstet Gynecol* 85:269–272, 1995.
40. Wheeless CR: Gastrointestinal injuries associated with laparoscopy. In Phillips JM (ed): *Endoscopy in Gynecology*. 1978, p 317–324.
41. DeCherney AH: Laparoscopy with unexpected viscus penetration. In Nichols DH (ed): *Clinical Problems, Injuries and Complications of Gynecologic Surgery*. Baltimore, Williams & Wilkins, 1988, pp 62–63.
42. Borton M: In *Laparoscopic Complication: Prevention and Management*. Philadelphia, BC Decker, 1986, pp 317–329.
43. Nezhat C, Nezhat F, Ambroze W, et al: Laparoscopic repair of small bowel, colon, and rectal endometriosis: A report of twenty-six cases. *Surg Endosc* 7:88–89, 1993.

44. Nezhat C, Nezhat F, Pennington E: Laparoscopic treatment of lower colorectal and infiltrative rectovaginal septum endometriosis by the technique of videolaseroscopy. *Br J Obstet Gynaecol* 99:664–667, 1992.
45. Redwine D: Laparoscopic en bloc resection for treatment of the obliterated cul-de-sac in endometriosis. *J Reprod Med* 37:696–698, 1992.
46. Nezhat F, Brill AI, Nezhat CH, et al: Adhesion formation after endoscopic posterior colpotomy. *J Reprod Med* 38:534–536, 1993.
47. Thompson BH, Wheeless CR Jr: Gastrointestinal complications of laparoscopic sterilization. *Obstet Gynecol* 41:669–676, 1973.
48. Nezhat C, Nezhat F, Luciano AA, et al: Complications. In *Operative Gynecologic Laparoscopy: Principles and Techniques*. New York, McGraw-Hill, 1995, pp 287–310.
49. Soderstrom RM: Bowel injury litigation after laparoscopy. *J Am Assoc Gynecol Laparosc* 1:74–77, 1993.
50. Keye WR Jr: Hitting a moving target: Credentialing the endoscopic surgeon. *Fertil Steril* 62:115–117, 1994.
51. Hatlie MJ: Climbing "the learning curve." New technologies, emerging obligations. *JAMA* 270: 1364–1365, 1993.
52. Khare VK, Martin DC, Kaigh J: Buttonhole ulceration and perforation of the rectum. *J Am Assoc Gynecol Laparosc* 1:12–15, 1993.
53. Nezhat F, Brill A, Nezhat C, et al: Traumatic hypogastric artery bleeding controlled with bipolar desiccation during operative laparoscopy. *J Am Assoc Gynecol Laparosc* 1:171–173, 1994.

chapter seventeen

Complications of Laparoscopic Hysterectomy: Avoidance, Recognition, and Management

C.Y. Liu

INTRODUCTION

The use of operative laparoscopy for the treatment of nonmalignant intra-abdominal and pelvic diseases began in the late 1970s and early 1980s in France, Germany, and the United States as gynecologists lysed adhesions, removed ectopic pregnancies, and treated ovarian cysts and endometriosis. This laparoscopic use exploded in the late 1980s when first laparoscopic hysterectomy and then cholecystectomy were accomplished using laparoscopic techniques. Published reports regarding the complications of these procedures are still limited. The reported surgeries were performed by experienced laparoscopic surgeons but nonetheless were associated with some serious complications. Operative laparoscopy is not an innocuous procedure; for example, laparoscopic hysterectomy carries the combined risks of laparoscopy and hysterectomy. In our (Liu and Reich personal communication) series of 518 cases of laparoscopic hysterectomy and total laparoscopic hysterectomy, the complication rate was 5.7%. These complications included febrile morbidity (2.1%), injury to the urinary tract system (1.3%), injury to the bowel (1.1%), delayed postoperative vaginal cuff bleeding (0.5%), unanticipated blood transfusion (0.3%), and pulmonary embolism (0.2%) (Table 17.1). As a rule, the more complex the pathology and the more technically difficult the procedure, the more likely that serious complications will occur. This chapter will systematically address the possible sites of complications, precautionary measures for avoiding intraoperative complications, and, should they occur, the management of the complications.

VESSEL INJURY

Perforation of Abdominal Wall Vessels

The likelihood exists that every gynecologist will perforate one or more of the major abdominal wall vessels if he or she performs enough laparoscopic surgery. Of primary concern are the deep and superficial epigastric vessels of the abdominal wall when secondary trocars are placed in the lower abdomen. The deep inferior epigastric artery arises from the external iliac artery just before the latter enters the femoral canal. Then, shortly after coming out of the external iliac artery, the deep inferior èpigastric artery branches out into the rectus abdominus muscle, where it usually has a tributary running along the lateral border of the rectus muscle. The superficial epigastric artery arises from the femoral artery near the inguinal ring and courses medially over the rectus muscle toward the midline. Since the deep inferior epigastric vessels traverse beneath the rectus muscle and immediately above the parietal peritoneum, they usually can be readily seen through the laparoscope. The superficial epigastric vessels usually can also be seen through the transillumination of the abdominal wall when the tip of the laparoscope is placed near or against the abdominal wall. However, in obese patients and in those with surgical scars in the

Table 17.1. Complications of 518 laparoscopic hysterectomies and concomitant surgeries

Complication	No. of patients	Rate (%)	Rate Per 100 Women*
Febrile morbidity	11		2.12
Pneumonia†	1	0.19	
Pelvic hematomas	4	0.77	
Dehydration	1	0.19	
Transient febrile episodes	5	0.96	
Urinary tract system	7		1.35
Bladder injury	5	0.96	
Vesicovaginal fistula	1	0.19	
Ureterovaginal fistula	1	0.19	
Intestinal complications	6		1.15
Small bowel enterotomy	2	0.38	
Thermal injury of sigmoid colon	1	0.19	
Partial bowel obstruction	1	0.19	
Ritcher's hernia‡	2	0.38	
Vaginal cuff bleeding	3		0.57
Unanticipated blood transfusion	2		0.38
Pulmonary embolism	1		0.19
Total	30		5.7

* Rate per 100 women who underwent hysterectomy and concomitant surgery.
† This patient later developed adult respiratory distress syndrome and died.
‡ Ritcher's hernia occurred at the 12-mm trocar puncture site.

lower abdomen, especially a Pfannenstiel incisional scar, these vessels may be obscured. When these vessels are not visible, the risk of vessel injury will be increased; however, injury may be minimized by placing the trocars *medial* to the obliterated umbilical artery or *lateral* to the site where the round ligament inserts into the inguinal canal. The obliterated umbilical artery and the round ligament can always be identified even in very obese patients. When the secondary trocar is placed near the level of the umbilicus, the inferior epigastric vessels are much more difficult to identify. However, because the rectus muscle is more obvious, the trocar should be placed lateral to that muscle to avoid puncturing the tributaries of the inferior epigastric vessels. All the secondary trocars should always be inserted under direct visualization, never placed blindly; they should be placed perpendicular to the fascia to avoid lacerating the vessels close to the trocar insertion sites.

If vessel injury is noted at the time of trocar insertion, it is important to remember that the trocar sleeve should be left in place. *Do not remove the sleeve.* Because the sleeve is the only marker for the location of that injured vessel, removal would make it difficult to find the bleeding vessel within a large hematoma. Furthermore, the sleeve acts as a drain, allowing the blood to escape into the peritoneal cavity, thus preventing large hematoma formation. The deep inferior epigastric vessels lie just above the perietal peritoneum. Unless the artery is completely severed and retracted, bipolar forceps inserted from the other side of the abdomen are used to compress and desiccate the vessel and the tissues adjacent to the sleeve. This is usually able to control the bleeding. It is important to remember that the deep inferior epigastric vessels have significant anastomosis with internal mammary vessels and deep circumflex iliac vessels. Both ends of the injured vessel must be desiccated to achieve adequate hemostasis. When bipolar coagulation around the trocar sleeve fails to control the bleeding and the hematoma is rapidly increasing in size, the blood vessel is most likely completely severed and retracted. In that case, the skin incision around the trocar sleeve should be enlarged longitudinally and the dissection carried down, following the tract of the sleeve. The bleeding vessel should be secured and ligated on both ends. The popular method of using an inflated Foley catheter tip to compress the bleeding site may not work if the artery is completely severed and retracted. Large trocars (>10 mm) are more likely than small trocars (5 mm or less) to sever the vessel completely. Therefore, whenever possible, a smaller trocar (5 mm or less) with a conical tip, instead of a pyramidal tip with three sharpened edges, should be used to avoid lacerating or completely severing the vessel. Instruments designed to close the fascial layer of the large trocar puncture site are available. These instruments can also be used to control bleeding from a lacerated epigastric vessel.

Intraoperative Hemorrhage

Massive, troublesome intraoperative hemorrhage can occur with a slipped ligature tie or hemoclips, large ovarian or uterine artery injury, or premature division before the vessels are completely desiccated. The principles which follow in regard to dealing with massive bleeding laparoscopically are the same as those used during open surgery. These basic principles are *compression, suction and irrigation of the bleeding site, and clear identification of the bleeder.* After the bleeder is clearly identified, it can be controlled by suture ligation, electrodesiccation, or hemoclip application. The majority of bleeding can be controlled by bipolar desiccation alone. However, the surrounding anatomy needs to be checked prior to the initiation of electrodesiccation in order to avoid thermal injury to vital structures such as the ureter, bladder, or bowel. Such ligation or application of hemoclips is more appropriate when the bleeder is close to vital structures. The key to preventing premature division before the large vessels are completely desiccated is to have the assistant or circulating nurse carefully observe the ammeter on the generator of the electrosurgery unit to make sure that the flow of the electric current between the prongs of the bipolar forceps has completely ceased. If the vessels are not completely desiccated and occluded, the electric current will continue to flow between the tips of the forceps, and the needle of the ammeter will not return to the 0 position. If a large vessel still cannot be desiccated after 8–10 sec of application of the bipolar forceps, the two prongs of the forceps have not grasped it completely, in which case the forceps must be reapplied. Injury to external iliac vessels, aorta, or vena cava requires immediate laparotomy an intraoperative consultation with a vascular surgeon.

URINARY TRACT SYSTEM INJURY

Bladder Injury

Bladder injury occurs in approximately 0.5–1% of all major pelvic surgeries. Laparoscopic hysterectomy should carry about the same incidence of injury as other major pelvic surgeries. However, in our series of 518 laparoscopic hysterectomies, 6 (1.5%) bladder injuries occurred, which is slightly higher than those figures reported for abdominal hysterectomy.

Basically two types of bladder injury may occur during laparoscopic hysterectomy—intraperitoneal and extraperitoneal. Intraperitoneal bladder injury involves perforation of the bladder and its covering peritoneum, which results in urine leakage into the peritoneal cavity. In extraperitoneal bladder injury, the peritoneum remains intact, and the urine leaks into the space of Retzius. Bladder injury during laparoscopic hysterectomy is always caused either mechanically by instruments, such as an improperly placed trocar or scissors, or thermally from electrosurgery and/or laser use.

Recognition

Intraoperative recognition Intraperitoneal bladder injury can be easily recognized by the observation of leakage of instilled indigocarmine dye. However, on rare occasions with a small trocar injury, there may be no leakage of dye. A high degree of suspicion is needed to make the proper diagnosis. If the trocar tip appears to be pushing through the muscular organ, bladder injury should be ruled out by performing a cystoscopic examination. Cystoscopic examination is also necessary when excessive electrosurgery has been performed around the bladder.

Postoperative recognition Unexplained hematuria found in postoperative catheterization, decreased urine output, anuria, suprapubic swelling and pain, and abdominal distention with an elevated blood urea nitrogen level may be indicative of bladder injury. A cystogram and a cystoscopic examination should be performed to make the proper diagnosis. Thermal injury to the bladder wall usually does not manifest itself immediately after surgery. Sudden hematuria or a vesicovaginal fistula 7–14 days postoperatively may be the first sign of thermal injury to the bladder. Cystoscopic examination should be performed to confirm the diagnosis.

Prevention

We find the following steps very helpful to prevent injury to the bladder during laparoscopic hysterectomy.

Step 1. The bladder should be emptied prior to surgery. We routinely instill 15–20 mL of concentrated indigocarmine dye into the bladder after it is emptied. This facilitates early recognition of bladder injury during surgery. It is not necessary to leave the Foley catheter in the bladder during prolonged, complicated laparoscopic procedures, which usually require extensive uterine or vaginal manipulation by the assistant from below. The catheter may inadvertently be pulled and tucked by the assistant while manipulating the uterus or vagina, thereby bruising the trigone area of the bladder by the balloon tip of the catheter. If the bladder becomes distended during surgery, it can be emptied with a straight catheter.

Step 2. Insert all secondary trocars under direct visualization. This is especially important when the anatomy is distorted due to infection, extensive endometriosis, or previous surgery.

Step 3. Separate the bladder from the low uterine segment by using sharp dissection. *Never dissect the bladder bluntly.* This is especially important when the patient has had a previous cesarean section, infection, or endometriosis.

Step 4. If an automatic multifire stapling device is to be used during the hysterectomy, make sure that the bladder is not inside the jaws of the device before firing it.

Step 5. Avoid using electrosurgery extensively around the bladder, especially monopolar electrosurgery in a coagulation mode. Brisk bleeding from around the bladder usually indicates injury to the muscular layer of the bladder wall. Hemostatic suturing, rather than electrocoagulation, will reduce the possibility of bladder injury.

Management

Any bladder injury must be evaluated cystoscopically. The integrity of both ureters needs to be confirmed. For a small extraperitoneal bladder injury, catheterization with a Foley catheter for 10–14 days should be adequate. However, for a larger injury, a mini-laparotomy with standard two-layer repair using absorbable sutures should be done, followed by 10–14 days of catheterization. For intraperitoneal bladder lacerations of less than 1 cm, a two-layer pursestring suture with 2-0 absorbable sutures can be used. The first pursestring suture includes the muscular and mucosal portions, and the second includes the serosa and the muscular layer. If the laceration of the bladder is more than 1 cm, the bladder is mobilized to ensure that the suture site is free from tension. Then a standard two-layer closure should be done. We recommend using a 3-0 delayed absorbable suture with an SH needle for the first layer closure, which includes the muscular and mucosal portions of the bladder, with continuous nonlocking running stitches. From 250 to 300 mL of indigocarmine dye or sterile infant formula should be instilled into the bladder after the first layer is closed to ensure that the repair is watertight. If any leakage from the suture line is observed, the bladder is deflated and a figure-of-eight suture is placed at the leakage site. The bladder is reinflated with 250–300 mL of dye or infant's formula and checked for leakage. If there is no leak from the suture line, the bladder is deflated and a second layer of stitches, including the serosa and the muscular portion of the bladder, is placed with 2-0 delayed, absorbable sutures, using either interrupted or continuous stitches. The bladder is then drained with a Foley catheter for 10–14 days. Finally, a cystoscopic examination is performed at the end of any bladder repair to ensure that the complete bladder injury is repaired and the integrity of the ureters is not compromised. The intraperitoneal bladder injury can always be performed laparoscopically without any difficulty. If the injury is caused by a through-and-through thermal burn, the devitalized tissue of the thermal injury of the bladder wall must be excised and the defect repaired with the two-layer technique, as described above.

Ureteral Injury

The incidence of ureteral injury in laparoscopic hysterectomy is unknown at present. In the (Liu and Reich personal communication) series of 518 laparoscopic hysterectomies, there was only one ureteral injury. However, our private correspondence with gynecologic laparoscopists throughout the world leads us to believe that the incidence of ureteral injury in laparoscopy-assisted hysterectomy is higher than in traditional abdominal or vaginal hysterectomy, which is reported to vary from 0.4% to 1.5%. Most ureteral injuries during laparoscopic hysterectomy occur in the area between the ureteric canal and the bladder base. Patients at risk for ureteral injury should be recognized prior to surgery. Those with a history of extensive pelvic inflammatory disease or endometriosis, preoperative findings of a large pelvic mass, intraligamentary leiomyomas, obliterated cul-de-sac, and induration in the paracervical area should arouse the suspicion of ureteral involvement. Preoperative evaluation with intravenous pyelograpy (IVP) is helpful in patients with these conditions.

Prevention of ureteral injury

The best way to prevent ureteral injury during laparoscopic hysterectomy is to be certain of the location of the ureter at all times during the procedure. With laparoscopic surgery, one loses the ability to palpate the pelvic organs but gains greatly improved visibility of the pelvic structures. This is precisely the reason we are not in favor of using preoperative ureteral catheterization in high-risk patients. One may argue that transillumination of the ureter through the recently developed lighted ureteral catheter makes the course of the ureter obvious during laparoscopy. However, the presently available lighted ureteral catheters are all rather rigid and have a large caliber. Thus, the mucosa of the ureter can be easily damaged by the heat emitted from the lighted catheter and from intraoperative manipulation of the catheter against the ureter. Ureteral injury can be especially severe in cases of preexisting periureteral fibrosis and scarring, which may be secondary to previous infection or endometriosis. We recommend routine identification and dissection of the pelvic ureters at the beginning of the hysterectomy; this procedure clarifies the ureteral locations throughout the entire surgical procedure. Using ureteral identification and dissection as the first step of any laparoscopic hysterectomy, we have avoided ureteral injury.

Recognition of ureteral injury

Intraoperative recognition Ureteral injuries have the best prognosis when they are recognized and repaired intraoperatively. A delay in diagnosis can lead to the development of progressively decreased renal function. As many as 25% of unrecognized ureteral injuries result in eventual loss of the affected kidney. Any complicated laparoscopic pelvic surgery should prompt the surgeon to look for possible ureteral injury, even though no obvious damage has been recognized.

Postoperative recognition Patients with undetected ureteral injuries will present with various signs and symptoms, such as flank pain, tenderness, unexplained fever and chills, abdominal distention, and ileus. A high suspicion of ureteral injury and prompt investigation with IVP is crucial for diagnosis of the postoperative ureteral injury. Cystoscopy and retrograde pyelography are often needed to determine the exact location of the lesion or obstruction.

Treatment

As soon as intraoperative ureteral injury is detected, immediate laparotomy with ureteral repair is recommended. Although a few gynecologists can effectively repair ureteral injury laparoscopically, one must consider one's own experience and skills and maintain caution about one's own limits, especially when laparoscopic repair of ureteral injury is intended. Consultation with colleagues experienced in ureteral repair is highly recommended. The timing of the repair of postoperatively recognized ureteral injuries is more complicated. The patient's general condition, the degree of edema, and the associated local inflammation should be carefully evaluated, since the surgery for this type of ureteral reconstruction is usually more difficult and lengthy. Some authors suggest that early intervention, as soon as ureteral injury is diagnosed, does not increase the postoperative complications or sequelae. However, in the presence of edema, local inflammation, and poor general condition of the patient, we believe that surgery for ureteral reconstruction should be postponed for 4 to 6 weeks unless a percutaneous nephrostomy cannot be done or there is evidence of progressively deteriorating renal function in spite of intensive conservative treatments.

Surgical considerations Regardless of whether the injury is detected intraoperatively or postoperatively, surgery for ureteral reconstruction should adhere to the following principles:

1. Have adequate debridement, and use only healthy ureter for reanastomosis.
2. Avoid using too many sutures.
3. Avoid any tension on the site of anastomosis.
4. Obtain complete hemostasis if possible.
5. Insert an indwelling ureteral catheter and place a retroperitoneal drain.

There are essentially three options for ureteral repair:

1. *End-to-end reanastomosis:* If the site of ureteral injury is above the midpelvis and the injury is not extensive, end-to-end anastomosis of the ureter

can be performed easily, first debriding the injured portion and then mobilizing the ureter to avoid undue tension on the anastomosis site. A double-J ureteral catheter is inserted and some type of extraperitoneal suction drain, such as a Jackson-Pratt drain, is placed close to the anastomosis site. The bladder is drained with a urethral or suprapubic catheter.

2. *Ureteroneocystostomy:* Most ureteral injuries in laparoscopic hysterectomy occur around the area of the ureteric canal or along the site of the cardinal ligament between the ureteric canal and the base of the bladder. This area is located deep in the pelvis. After resection of the damaged segment of the ureter, the continuity of the urinary tract can best be restored by performing a ureteroneocystostomy rather than an end-to-end ureteroureterostomy. To avoid any tension on the anastomosis site, the bladder must be mobilized from the back of the pubis. An anterior cystostomy is performed and the ureter is brought through the wall of the bladder by means of a submucosal tunnel. An end-to-side mucosa-to-mucosa anastomosis between the end of the ureter and the side wall of the bladder is then performed. A double-J ureteral catheter is inserted and a Jackson-Pratt drain is inserted retroperitoneally, close to the anastomosis site but not touching it. If adequate mobilization of the bladder is difficult, a bladder hitch can be done by simply displacing the bladder upward and attaching it to the fascia of the iliopsoas muscle. Similarly, the upper segment of the ureter can be further mobilized to reduce the tension on the anastomosis site.
3. *Transureteroureterostomy:* If a large segment of the ureter has been damaged and a ureteroneocystostomy is not possible, a transureteroureterostomy by an experienced urologist is advised.

Bowel Injury

Bowel injury during laparoscopic hysterectomy is uncommon. When it occurs it is usually associated with trocar insertion, extensive intraperitoneal adhesions, or endometriosis. In our series of 518 cases of laparoscopic hysterectomy, two small bowel injuries occurred during enterolysis due to extensive adhesions. One superficial thermal injury of the anterior wall of the sigmoid colon occurred. Two intentional anterior rectal wall resections for full-thickness endometriosis were performed. Two patients developed Richter's hernia at the 12-mm trocar sites postoperatively. Early recognition of the bowel injury is crucial, preferably during surgery, so that immediate implementation of appropriate treatment can reduce morbidity.

Small Bowel Injury

Most small bowel injuries during laparoscopic hysterectomy are caused by trocar insertion and enterolysis secondary to extensive adhesions. Patients with a history of multiple laparotomies, prior ruptured appendix, inflammatory bowel disease, previous pelvic inflammatory disease, and extensive endometriosis are particularly at risk for bowel adhesions. Trocar injury of the small bowel usually occurs when there are bowel adhesions to the anterior abdominal wall, especially around the umbilical area.

Recognition There are basically three different causes of small bowel injuries during laparoscopic hysterectomy

1. *Trocar injury:* If the umbilical trocar has made a large laceration in the small bowel, the surgeon may be able to view the mucosal surface of the small bowel laparoscopically. Also, small bowel contents may be seen leaking from the laceration or a hematoma may be present on the surface of the small bowel. If adhesions are detected around the umbilical area, even if there is no evidence of bowel injury, inspection of the umbilical trocar in its entirety, with a 5-mm laparoscope through a secondary trocar sleeve, must be performed to ensure that there is no occult or through-and-through small bowel laceration. If a trocar or laparoscope is detected inside the lumen of the small bowel, *do not remove it* before laparotomy or laparoscopic repair of the injury, for it will seal the puncture and identify the site of laceration.
2. *Injury secondary to enterolysis or electrosurgery:* When dense adhesions exist and require extensive enterolysis and electrosurgery for hemostasis, small bowel injury is usually obvious. Monopolar electrosurgery should not be used around the small bowel unless the surgeon possesses the highest level of expertise. Another drawback in the wide use of electrosurgery is that through the discharge of static electric, energy from the trocar sleeve or instruments can produce bowel injury. In such cases, electrical burns can be difficult to detect and evaluate because the

injury is usually outside the laparoscopic viewing field. Furthermore, monopolar electrical injury of the small bowel often appears smaller than it actually is.

3. *Richter's hernia:* Due to manipulation of the trocar sleeve during laparoscopy, fascia and peritoneal defects can easily become enlarged, often allowing a loop of small intestine to herniate into this defect and become incarcerated. Therefore, any fascia defect of the puncture site for any trocar greater than 10 mm should be closed to prevent formation of Richter's hernia. Various instruments are available for this purpose. Richter's hernia usually presents as signs and symptoms of small bowel obstruction within 48 hr of surgery.

Avoiding small bowel injury Most small bowel injuries occur during insertion of the Veress needle for pneumoperitoneum or the initial trocar insertion. Unintentional preperitoneal insufflation can complicate the initial trocar insertion; this is more common with the obese patient. *Do not attempt to reinsert the trocar in the face of preperitoneal insufflation.* The risk of injuring the intra-abdominal organs is much higher, since the ballooned-out peritoneum is now much closer to the abdominal organs, and small bowel injury with the tip of the trocar can easily occur. Preperitoneal gas should be emptied through the trocar sleeve, after which pneumoperitoneum can be reestablished.

Factors that may cause the surgeon to perform an uncontrolled, sudden trocar entry into the abdominal cavity include an inadequate umbilical incision, scar tissue from a prior laparoscopy or laparotomy, and a dull trocar. These problems can occur in the absence of intra-abdominal adhesions or other predisposing pelvic pathology.

Trocar insertion in patients at risk for small bowel adhesions to the anterior abdominal wall should follow the techniques described in Chapter 7.

Treatment Small bowel injury caused by the Veress needle usually is innocuous as long as no leakage of bowel contents is observed and the laceration does not involve the mesenteric vessels. Superficial bowel injury caused by the trocar seals readily and requires no further treatment. When the lacerations involve the muscularis or mucosa, repair with sutures is needed. When the lacerations are small, they can be repaired through either laparoscopy or laparotomy. However, if the laceration exceeds one-half the diameter of the lumen, or if the mesenteric blood supply is interrupted or damaged, a segmental resection and anastomosis should be performed through laparotomy. For small lacerations that do not compromise the mesenteric blood supply, we recommend the use of a two-layer closure. The first layer is with 3-0 absorbable sutures, including the muscularis and mucosa, either with interrupted or continuous running, nonlocking stitches. A second layer of reinforcing sutures of 3-0 silk Lembert stitches is used to approximate the muscularis and the serosal edges. However, some surgeons repair small bowel injuries with a single-layer closure using absorbable suture material. All lacerations should be closed transversely to prevent the possibility of narrowing the bowel lumen. Thorough lavage of the entire abdomen and pelvis with copious amounts of Ringer's lactate solution after the bowel repair is completed is essential to reduce the possibility of peritonitis. A nasogastric tube should be placed and removed postoperatively when the patient starts to pass flatus. Our experience shows that the postoperative recovery for patients with laparoscopic small bowel repair is short. Bowel function is resumed quickly; however, the nasogastric tube should stay in place until the patient passes flatus or has a bowel movement. Patients with small bowel injuries should not be fed orally too soon. Food could stimulate peristalsis of the small bowel, raising its intraluminal pressure. This could jeopardize the healing process.

When the patient presents with signs and symptoms of possible small bowel obstruction or peritonitis after discharge from the hospital, *immediate* second-look laparoscopy or laparotomy should be done as soon as the patient is stabilized. This is done to rule out an unrecognized intestinal perforation or Richter's hernia. The prognosis is usually favorable if intervention occurs before the incarcerated bowel is damaged or before extensive peritonitis has developed in the case of undetected bowel perforation. For a Richter's hernia, the trapped loop of small bowel can usually be pulled out of the previous trocar puncture site. Active peristalsis of the bowel usually can be observed immediately after the bowel is pulled out. The abdominal wall defect can usually be sutured laparoscopically with various newly developed instruments.

Wheeless has presented a seven-point plan for the management of patients with peritonitis secondary to unrecognized bowel perforation:

1. Preoperative stabilization with fluids, electrolytes, and nasogastric suction.
2. Exploratory laparotomy with repair or resection of the injured bowel.
3. Resection of all necrotic tissue.
4. Copious, repeated lavage of the abdomen with saline.
5. Pelvic drainage through the vagina using a closed drainage system.
6. Aggressive antibiotic therapy.
7. Starting mini-dose heparin (5000 units every 8 hr) for embolus prophylaxis.

Large Intestine Injury

Injury to the colon during laparoscopic surgery is uncommon. The actual incidence is unknown at present. In the Liu and Reich series of 518 cases of laparoscopic hysterectomy, we have had one case of superficial thermal injury of the sigmoid colon and two cases of intentional resection of the anterior rectal wall due to full-thickness bowel wall infiltration of the endometriosis. We do not consider the latter two cases as complications, but rather as part of the therapeutic process.

Recognition and prevention

Colon injury due to trocar insertion Most injuries to the large intestine occur during trocar insertion. The incidence is estimated to be about 0.1%. The transverse and sigmoid colons are most commonly traumatized by trocar insertion, usually during blind insertion of the umbilical trocar. This fact can be explained by consideration of the anatomy of the large intestines. Because the ascending and descending colons are on the lateral sides of the abdominal cavity and are retroperitoneally located, there is no medial displacement by intraperitoneal adhesions. In contrast, the transverse colon is the most mobile portion of the colon, and the entire length is attached to the greater curvature of the stomach by the gastrocolonic ligament. The upper end of the omentum apron is attached to the anterior aspect of the transverse colon. Therefore, the transverse colon can be easily displaced inferiorly to the middle of the abdominal cavity when there is omental adhesion to the anterior abdominal wall or gastric distention secondary to mask ventilation prior to a difficult intubation during the initial stage of anesthesia. The sigmoid colon is also at risk because of its midline location in the path of the uncontrolled advancing trocar.

The diagnosis of colon injury is obvious if fecal material is noted on the tip of the trocar or in the abdomen during the procedure. However, if the injury to the bowel is not a full-thickness perforation or if the colon is empty, the only sign may be a rent and bleeding from the site of injury. Therefore, it is important to conduct a systematic and thorough inspection of the abdominal organs during the initial viewing through the laparoscope in order to rule out any injury that might have been sustained during trocar insertion. A distended stomach and anterior omental adhesions should draw special attention to the possibility of colon injury.

To prevent trocar injury to the large intestine during laparoscopic hysterectomy, careful review of the patient's history is necessary. This will usually reveal those patients at risk. The risk of bowel injury is increased in patients with previous abdominal surgery, including bowel resection, colostomy, appendectomy for ruptured appendix, or a history of intestinal obstruction or inflammatory bowel disease. A nasogastric tube should always be used in patients known to have difficulty with endotracheal intubation in the initial stage of anesthesia. Ideally, a nasogastric tube should be used in all cases to prevent gastric distention and subsequent inferior displacement of the transverse colon. The importance of having an adequate umbilical incision and a sharp trocar to prevent injury to the bowel was emphasized in the section on avoiding small bowel injury.

Colon injury secondary to electrosurgery and laser Laparoscopic hysterectomy requires the extensive use of electrosurgical or laser devices for hemostasis and tissue division, which can produce thermal injury to the bowel. The rectosigmoid colon is especially vulnerable because of its close proximity to the uterus and ovaries. The inherent risk of burn injury to the bowel, ureter, and skin necessitates the use of bipolar rather than unipolar electrosurgical devices. Burn injury to the rectosigmoid colon from bipolar forceps is almost always caused by poor exposure. That is, the surgeon did not see the prong tips of the forceps touch the rectosigmoid colon when he or she stepped on the pedal. Therefore, the surgeon must first make sure that both prongs are clearly in view and away from the bowel before stepping on the pedal. Viewing the magnified operative field on the video monitor is not only less fatiguing for the surgeon but is also valuable in reducing the incidence of bowel injury. Colon injury caused by bipolar electrocoagulation can be readily identified by viewing the area of blanching on the surface of the bowel.

Colon injury caused by unipolar electrosurgery can be difficult to detect and evaluate. This injury is usually due to a direct burn or discharge of static electricity built up in the trocar sleeve. According to Thompson and Wheeless, the signs and symptoms of electric bowel burns appear 3 to 7 days postoperatively. Wheeless also reported that only 2 out of 33 known bowel burn patients developed perforation. With the exception of the cecum, the wall of the colon is much thicker than the wall of the small bowel. This accounts for the fact that the large intestine is more resistant to thermal injury than the small bowel.

Although there is a theroretical risk of colon injury by laser energy, in reality the risk is extremely low, especially in the hands of a well-trained laser surgeon. The only laser which may potentially inflict significant trauma to the colon is the Nd-YAG laser delivered through the bare fiber tip as a result of deep penetration of the energy, which may be unrecognized at surgery. The use of sapphire tips practically eliminates the risk of colon injury by the laser if used judiciously.

Colon injury related to the obliterated cul-de-sac

Cul-de-sac obliteration, caused either by endometriosis or by previous pelvic inflammatory disease, is a difficult challenge for the gynecologic surgeon. The sigmoid colon and rectum are at risk with an obliterated cul-de-sac. Accidental entry into the rectum or sigmoid colon during their separation from the posterior wall of the uterus and cervix, or during excision of infiltrating endometriosis on the rectal wall, can cause a major complication if the bowel is unrepaired or improperly repaired. Intentional bowel entry for adequate excision of full-thickness infiltrating endometriosis of the bowel wall seldom results in any complication. This probably reflects the expertise of the surgeon who has experience and skill in performing this difficult surgery.

After extensive dissection of the cul-de-sac, a careful inspection for complete hemostasis and evidence of possible bowel injury should be done. It is also prudent to perform a thorough rectovaginal examination to ensure that all of the infiltrating endometriosis has been excised and to be certain that no rectal injury has occurred during the dissection.

Management

Early recognition of large bowel injury, preferably before the patient leaves the operating room, is crucial to avoid catastrophic consequences. Patients at risk for large bowel injury are those who have had previous bowel surgery, such as resections and colostomies. Also at risk are patients who have the following conditions: a history of bowel obstruction and extensive intra-abdominal adhesions, a history of bowel inflammatory disease, or a history of or evidence (by clinical examination) of an obliterated cul-de-sac with rectal nodules. These patients should be recognized preoperatively, and standard bowel preparation should be implemented prior to surgery. Our standard bowel preparation includes the following:

1. Neomycin 1 g every 4 hr, and erythromycin, 500 mg every 6 hr by mouth starting 48 hr before surgery.
2. Clear liquid diet starting 36 hr before surgery.
3. GoLytely, 4 L by mouth, beginning the afternoon before surgery.

This bowel preparation regimen has worked well for us both in open laparotomy and in laparoscopic surgery.

BIBLIOGRAPHY

Ball TL, Platt MA: Urological complications of endometriosis. *Am J Obstet Gynecol* 84:1516–1518, 1962.

Barnhill D, Doering D, Remmenga S, et al: Intestinal surgery performed on gynecologic cancer patients. *Gynecol Oncol* 40:38–41, 1991.

Bradford JA, Ireland EW, Warwick BG: Ureteric endometriosis: Three case reports and a review of the literature. *Aust NZ J Gynecol* 29:421–424, 1989.

Case AS: Diagnostic studies in bladder rupture. *Urol Clin North Am* 16:267–273, 1989.

Corriere JN Jr, Sandler CM: Management of the extraperitoneal bladder rupture. *Urol Clin North Am* 16:275–277, 1989.

Corson SL: Major vessel injury during laparoscopy. *Am J Obstet Gynecol* 138:589, 1980.

Fry DE, Milholen L, Harbrecht PJ: Iatrogenic ureteral injury. Options in management. *Arch Surg* 118: 454–457, 1983.

Gambee LP, Garnjobst W, Hardwick CE: Ten years' experience with a single layer anastomosis in colon surgery. *Am J Surg* 92:222–227, 1956.

Gomel V, James C: Intraoperative management of ureteral injury during operative laparoscopy. *Fertil Steril* 55:416 419, 1991.

Grainger DA, Soderstrom RM, Schiff SF, et al: Ureteral injury at laparoscopy: Insights into diagnosis, management, and prevention. *Obstet Gynecol* 75:839– 843, 1990.

Harrow BR: A neglected maneuver for ureterovesical implantation following injury at gynecological operations. *J Urol* 100:280–287, 1968.

Hoch WH, Kursh ED, Persky L: Early aggressive management of intraoperative ureteral injuries. *J Urol* 114:530–532, 1975.

Hulka JF: Major vessel injury during laparoscopy. *Am J Obstet Gynecol* 138:590, 1980.

Hurd WW, Pear ML, DeLancey JOL: Laparoscopic injury of abdominal wall blood vessels: A report of three cases. *Obstet Gynecol* 82:673–676, 1993.

Mann WJ, Arato M, Pastiner B, et al: Ureteral injuries in an obstetric and gynecology training program: Etiology and management. *Obstet Gynecol* 72:82–85, 1988.

Montz FJ, Holschneider CH, Munro MG: Incisional hernia following laparoscopy: A Survey of the American Association of Gynecologic Laparoscopists. *Obstet Gynecol* 84: 881–884, 1994.

Neto WA, Lopes RN, Cury M, et al: Vesical endometriosis. *Urology* 24:271–274, 1984.

Penfield AJ: Trocar and needle injury. In Phillips JM (ed): *Laparoscopy*. Baltimore, Williams & Wilkins, 1977, pp 236–241.

Peters PC: Intraperitoneal rupture of the bladder. *Urol Clin North Am* 16:279–282, 1989.

Phillips JM, Julka JF, Peterson HB: American Association of Gynecologic Laparoscopists' 1982 membership survey. *J Reprod Med* 29:592–594, 1984.

Reich H, McGlynn F: Laparoscopic repair of bladder injury. *Obstet Gynecol* 76:909–910, 1990.

Shah PM, Kim K, Ramirez-Schon G, et al: Elevated blood urea nitrogen: An aid to the diagnosis of intraperitoneal rupture of the bladder. *J Urol* 122: 741–743, 1979.

Shin CS: Vascular injury secondary to laparoscopy. *New York State J Med* 82:935–936, 1982.

Symmonds RE: Ureteral injuries associated with gynecologic surgery: Prevention and management. *Clin Obstet Gynecol* 19:623:644, 1976.

Tarkington MA, Dejter SW Jr, Bresette JF: Early surgical management of extensive gynecologic ureteral injuries. *Surgery* 173:17–21, 1991.

Thompson BH, Wheeless CR Jr: Gastrointestinal complications of laparoscopic sterilization. *Obstet Gynecol* 41:669–676, 1973.

Wheeless CR Jr: Gastrointestinal injuries associated with laparoscopy. In Phillips JM (ed): *Endoscopy in Gynecology*. Downey, CA: American Association of Gynecologic Laparoscopists, 1978, pp 317–324.

Yuzpe AA: Pneumoperitoneum needle and trocar injuries in laparoscopy. A survey on possible contributing factors and prevention. *J Reprod Med* 35: 485–490, 1990.

Zinman LM, Libertino JA, Roth RA: Management of operative ureteral injury. *Urology* 12:290–303, 1978.

chapter eighteen

Management of Adnexal Masses and Myomas

Fred Marion Howard

INTRODUCTION

As surgical skills with operative laparoscopy have improved, it has become apparent that laparoscopy represents another incisional approach for most surgical procedures. Thus, the gynecologic surgeon must be familiar with four surgical approaches to pelvic surgery—vaginal, abdominal, hysteroscopic, and laparoscopic. Although much of the gynecologic literature debates the merits of each approach in a global or universal manner, the choice of surgical approach is best individualized. It should take into account many factors, including:

- Specific patient wishes and characteristics, such as cosmetic concerns, fertility, obesity, medical conditions, and previous surgery.
- The expertise of the surgeon with each surgical approach.
- The surgical condition(s) necessitating surgery and the need for any additional procedures.
- The potential for complications and their management with each approach.

The potential complications of laparoscopic treatment of gynecologic pelvic masses are the subject of this chapter. Currently, the laparoscopic approach to both adnexal masses and leiomyomas is controversial. Concerns about complications are a major part of the ongoing controversy.

This controversy is unfortunate, as it appears that endoscopic surgery may represent a major improvement in the surgical care of many women with pelvic masses. However, the widespread application of laparoscopic surgery for an increasingly broad range of procedures has been pushed vigorously much faster than peer-reviewed, scientific studies can be published to allow solid, evidence-based practice.[1] For pelvic masses, current evidence seems ample to allow us to state that laparoscopic management is usually less expensive, allows shorter hospital stays (usually ambulatory surgery), and results in a more rapid recovery than laparotomy. However, there are concerns when this comparison is made from the perspective of outcomes and complications.

Operative feasibility is a legitimate concern in some cases. For example, in expert endosurgical hands, difficult cases such as ovarian retention syndrome, ovarian remnant syndrome, or advanced endometriomas have been handled. However, in the hands of a less skilled endoscopic surgeon, an incomplete and inadequate operation may be done. Another worry is the potential length of the operations. In particular, early on, a surgeon's operative time may be quite long. The rates of intraoperative and postoperative complications are also a worry. Currently, there is inadequate prospective study of the occurrence of complications when advanced operative laparoscopic procedures are performed by the practicing general obstetrician-gynecologist rather than restricted to a few experts. Some have suggested that the rate of complications may be unacceptable when these operations are more generally performed.[2] Another concern is the potential for treatment of insignificant pathology through the unnecessary utilization of operative laparoscopy. This fear arises because most gynecologists are accustomed to the liberal use of laparoscopy for diagnosis and, with newly acquired operative skills, may be tempted at the time of diagnostic laparoscopy to treat normal, functional ovarian cysts or asymptomatic, small leiomyomas. Finally, and possibly most important, are concerns regarding patients with ovarian cancer. First is the worry of inadequate endosurgical procedures that may worsen the prognosis of patients with malignant ovarian neoplasms falsely diagnosed as benign.[3,4] Second is the possibility of worsening the prognosis due to spill with unexpected ovarian carcinoma during laparoscopic ovarian cystectomy.[5,6]

Additionally with leiomyomas, excessive blood loss, inadequate uterine repair, uterine dehiscence, and severe adhesive disease are concerns. If hysteroscopic myomectomy is done, added to these worries is the risk of hyponatremia and water intoxication.

Clearly, some of these concerns represent prejudice against new ideas and approaches. Unfortunately, there are many examples to support such prejudice supplied by a very few surgeons unwilling to obtain adequate surgical knowledge and skills before attempting to use an endoscopic approach. There is no technologic substitute for sound clinical judgment. In competent and knowledgeable hands, the incisional approach, whether endoscopic, vaginal, or abdominal, should rarely be an impediment to proper surgery.[7] It is worth while to point out that poor judgment may result in incomplete intraoperative management regardless of the operative approach. For example, one published study reports that 65% of patients initially operated on by laparotomy for ovarian carcinoma require a second laparotomy for appropriate staging and that 95% of those with an early stage carcinoma have incomplete staging at the initial laparotomy.[8] Whether approaching the patient with a pelvic mass through a laparoscopy or a laparotomy incision, it is imperative that the surgeon know and perform the appropriate procedure or have an appropriate consultant readily available to help in the event that the mass turns out to be more than the primary surgeon is capable of managing.

GENERAL COMMENTS ABOUT COMPLICATIONS

The ideal way to manage surgical complications, an ideal that is not always attainable, is to avoid them completely. A basic tenet of avoiding complications is to avoid operating when surgery is not indicated. For that reason, in the subsequent sections on complications of laparoscopic surgery for adnexal masses and leiomyomas, discussions of the indications for surgery are included. Also helpful is extensive knowledge of the observed and potential complications of any surgical procedure. This includes knowledge of the pertinent anatomy and physiology, the usual ways that specific complications occur, and alternative approaches when the routine or usual approach is impossible.

Table 18.1. General Categories of Complications at the Time of Laparoscopic Surgery

Laparoscopy-specific complications
Procedure-specific complications
Laparoscopic procedure-specific complications

For advanced operative laparoscopic procedures, categorizing complications into three broad categories may be helpful (Table 18.1). First are *laparoscopy-specific* complications. These are complications that may occur due to the laparoscopic approach, regardless of the actual operation being performed. Examples are trocar injuries to the great vessels of the abdomen or to bowel. Second are *procedure-specific* complications. These are complications that may arise with a given surgical procedure, regardless of the incisional approach. An example is ureteral injury near the uterine vessels, a complication that occurs with abdominal, vaginal, and laparoscopic hysterectomies. Third are *laparoscopic procedure-specific* complications. Some of these are complications that arise only with the laparoscopic approach to a particular operation. Others are complications that may arise with other approaches, but occur either in a specific way with laparoscopic technology or occur with a markedly different frequency due to the laparoscopic approach. Examples of the former are the loss of a portion of an ovarian mass within the abdominal wall during an attempt to extract it through a trocar incision site or the loss of a myoma in the abdominal cavity during morcellation. Examples of the latter are ureteral transection with an endoscopic stapler-cutter or intra-abdominal spill of ovarian cyst contents.

LAPAROSCOPY-SPECIFIC COMPLICATIONS

Although not the primary focus of this chapter, a few comments about laparoscopy-specific complications in gynecologic surgery are pertinent, as this category continues to constitute a significant proportion of reported complications with laparoscopic surgery for pelvic masses. The most serious complications in this category are injuries of the great vessels of the abdomen or pelvis, the vessels of the abdominal wall, or the bowel due to introduction of trocars at the umbilicus or lower abdomen.

Introduction of the trocar and cannula for the laparoscope may be done with either closed or open techniques. The usual closed methods are direct trocar insertion without first establishing a pneumoperitoneum or insertion of a Verres needle to establish a pneumoperitoneum followed by insertion of a trocar. Traditionally, gynecologists have performed diagnostic laparoscopy with the latter technique, usually inserting the Verres needle and trocar at the umbilicus. Classical thinking is that initially establishing a pneumoperitoneum with a Verres needle allows protection of the great vessels of the abdomen and avoids inadvertent bowel injury. Such thinking has been questioned, as evidence suggests that this approach does not always provide these benefits. In fact, the majority of reported injuries to the aorta, vena cava, and iliac vessels have been from the Veress needle. Although great vessel injuries are rare, better knowledge of anatomy may decrease the risk of this complication. Hurd and coworkers[9] have illustrated the importance of recognizing the variations in location and distance to the great vessels as a function of the patient's body habitus (Fig. 18.1). Based on findings of computed tomography (CT) and magnetic resonance imaging, they recommend angles of insertion based specifically on the patient's body mass (Table 18.2).

Bowel injuries also occur from trocar insertions, even with Veress needle techniques of irrigation, aspiration, and hanging drop that supposedly detect bowel at the site of abdominal entry. If bowel is adherent at the umbilicus, the Veress needle often is passed through the bowel, a pneumoperitoneum is successfully established, and there is no suspicion of bowel adherence and injury until bowel mucosa is seen on insertion of the trocar and laparoscope or, even worse, the bowel injury is unrecognized until the patient develops postoperative symptoms (Fig. 18.2).

As injuries occur in spite of (or even because of) Veress needle use, some gynecologists recommend direct trocar insertion without establishing a pneumoperitoneum. Proponents of direct trocar insertion point out that it replaces two blind insertions into the abdominal cavity with only one, albeit with a larger-diameter device. Current data suggest that the potential for serious consequences from puncture of the aorta, vena cava, or iliac vessels is as great with a Veress needle as with a shielded, disposable trocar. Also, there is the concern that inserting both instruments may double the chance of a major vascular injury. Another argument for direct trocar insertion is that abdominal entry is immediately confirmed and the occasional complication of preperitoneal insufflation is avoided.

Open laparoscopy is proposed as a method that prevents both major vascular and bowel injuries. Even without specific supportive data, it seems apparent that if properly done, an open laparoscopy obviates any risk of great vessel injury. This represents one of the best arguments for its use. However, data regarding open laparoscopy and bowel injury suggest that open laparoscopy does not prevent bowel injury, although it probably ensures prompt recognition. For example, the rate of bowel injuries with open laparoscopy was 1.2%, compared to 0.15% with closed laparoscopy, in the 1991 survey of members of the American Association of Gynecologic Laparoscopists. Overall, 71% of all bowel injuries involved closed laparoscopy and 10% involved open laparoscopy (19% were not specified).[10] Combining the above data on rates of bowel injuries shows that gynecologists perform closed laparoscopy about 60 times more often than open laparoscopy. Thus, it could be that gynecologists' inexperience with open laparoscopy accounts for the eightfold higher rate of bowel injury, but this seems unlikely, as most gynecologists use the same incisional approach for postpartum tubal sterilizations, with a very low incidence of bowel injury. It seems more likely that open laparoscopy is more commonly used in difficult cases with prior abdominopelvic surgery and is not completely effective in avoiding bowel injury when bowel is adherent to the anterior abdominal wall.

In patients with histories of prior abdominopelvic surgery, it may not be wise to use the umbilicus for the introduction of the laparoscopic trocar, whether using an open or closed technique. Utilization of an upper abdominal entry site may be the best way to avoid bowel injury in cases with significant risk of periumbilical adhesions. Additionally, in patients with large cystic masses or uterine myomas approaching the level of the umbilicus, this site minimizes the chance of inadvertently rupturing the cyst or impaling the uterus during entry.[4] Figures 18.3 and 18.4 illustrate the left upper quadrant site for trocar insertion. Most experience has been with left upper quadrant entry, but either the left or right upper abdomen may be used, with the side determined by the anticipated pathology and diagnosis. Entry is at the midclavicular line,

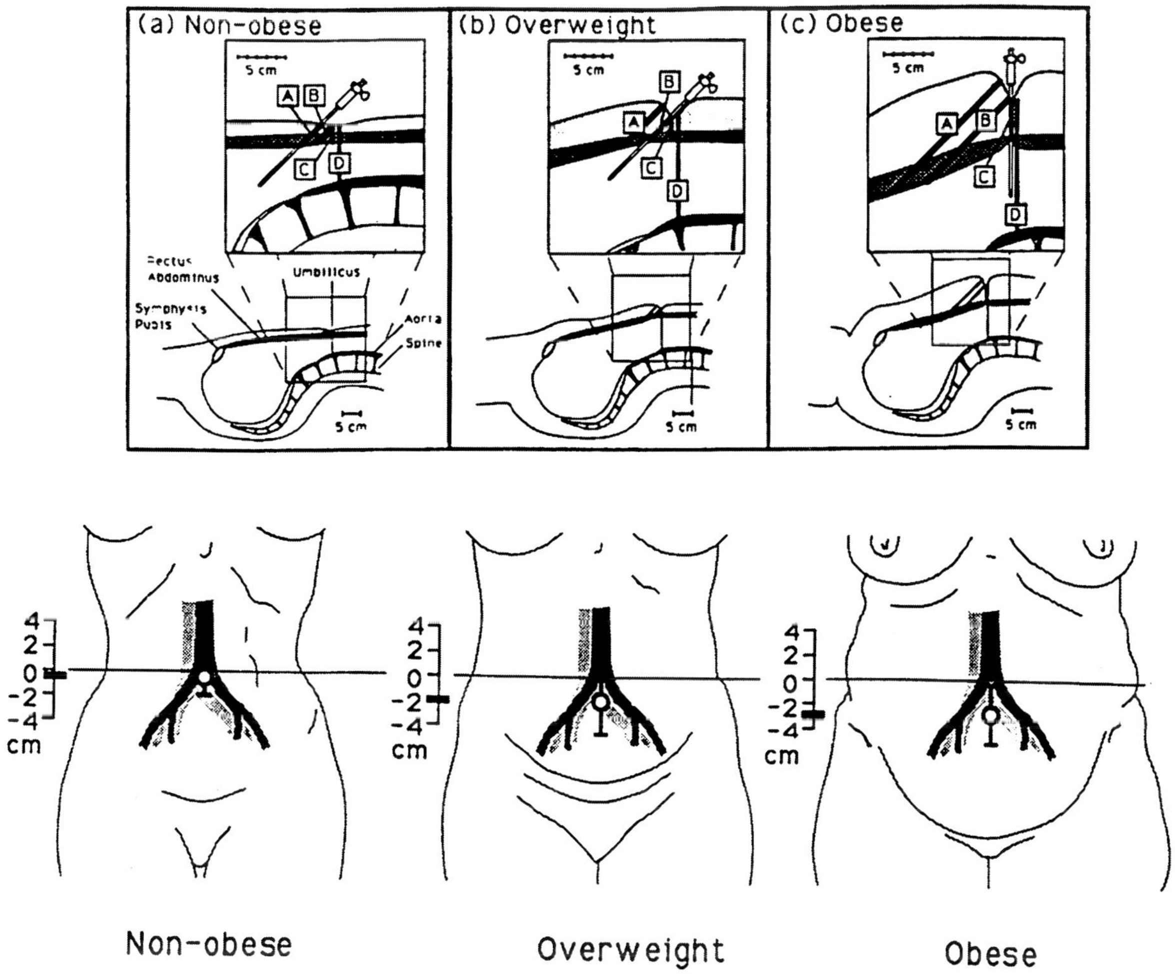

Figure 18.1. Average location of the umbilicus and peritoneum in relation to the major vessels in non-obese, overweight, and obese patients. In nonobese patients the umbilicus is 0.4 cm caudal to the bifurcation and 6 cm anterior to the great vessels. In overweight patients the umbilicus is 2.4 cm caudal to the bifurcation and 10 cm anterior to the great vessels. In obese patients the umbilicus is 2.9 cm caudal to the bifurcation and 13 cm anterior to the great vessels. Of course, there are inherent variations among individuals. (Adapted from Ref. 9.)

Table 18.2. Anatomic Measurements and Suggested Angles of Instrument Insertion at the Umbilicus for Laparoscopy Based on the Patient's Body Habitus (see also Fig. 18.1)

Group	Distance from Umbilicus to Peritoneum at 45° (cm)	Distance from Umbilicus to Vessels at 90° (cm)	Suggested Angle of Instrument Insertion
Nonobese (160 lb)	2 ± 2	6 ± 3	45°
Overweight (160–200 lb)	2 ± 1	10 ± 2	45°–90°
Obese (>200 lb)	12 (median)	13 ± 4	Near 90°

Source: Adapted from Ref. 9.

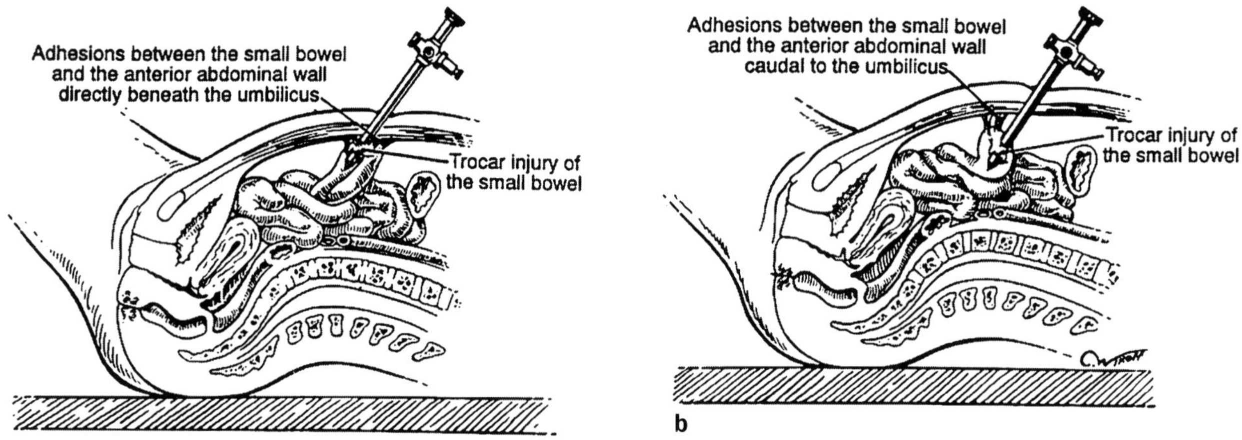

Figure 18.2. Attachment of the bowel to the anterior abdominal wall as a cause of trocar injury. (a) The bowel is attached directly under the umbilicus. (b) The attachment is below and distal to the umbilicus. (Modified from Ref. 51.)

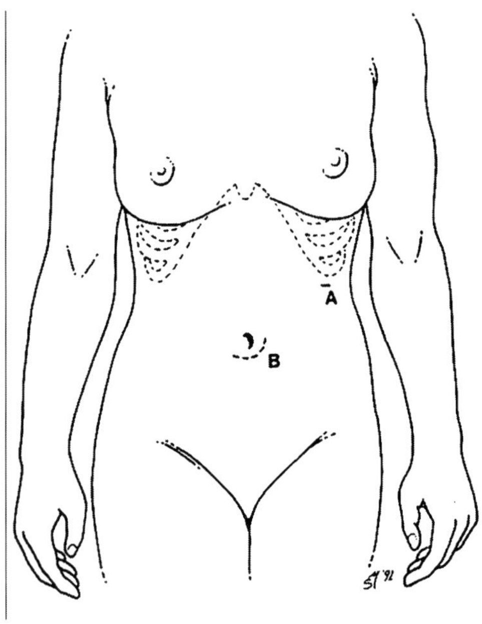

Figure 18.3. Use of the left upper quadrant (a) for Veress needle and/or trocar insertion may be preferable to the umbilicus (b) in patients with a risk of periumbilical bowel adhesions. (Adapted from Ref. 52.)

2–3 cm below the costal margin. Of course, a Veress needle may be inserted at either of these sites to establish a pneumoperitoneum prior to trocar entry or direct trocar insertion may be done. Several special precautions need to be mentioned regarding these entry sites.

- The stomach should be empty. It advisable to pass a nasogastric tube to empty the stomach, regardless of the anesthesiologist's opinion about the introduction of air into the stomach during induction of anesthesia.
- There must be no hepatomegaly or splenomegaly.
- Entry should be at the midclavicular line, lateral to the rectus sheath, to minimize the risk of abdominal wall vascular injury (superior epigastric artery and branches) or trauma to the rectus muscle.
- Ideally, the uterine fundus or adnexal mass should be more than 4 cm below the entry site.
- The patient should not have a history of upper abdominal surgery.

Unfortunately, there are no large series that allow objective substantiation of the theoretical advantages of this method.

Lower abdominal ports are needed for operative laparoscopic treatment of adnexal masses and leiomyomas, and these are also significant sources of compli-

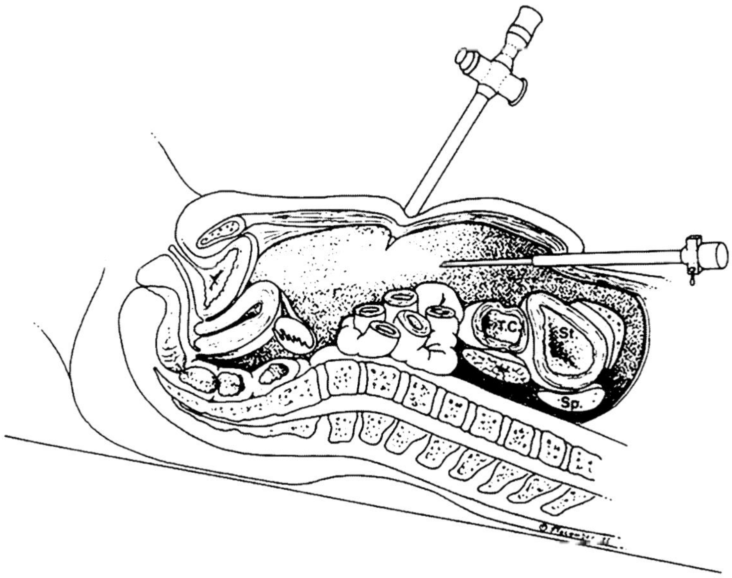

Figure 18.4. Upper abdominal introduction of the laparoscope. This allows inspection of the umbilical area and umbilical insertion of the trocar under direct visualization. Alternatively, surgery may be done with the laparoscope left at the upper abdomen (see also Figure 18.3). (Adapted from Ref. 51.)

cations. In particular, lacerations of the bladder, a persistent urachal cyst, the rectus muscles, or the inferior epigastric vessels may occur. As larger, sharper trocars are used for newer, larger instruments, these complications seem to be occurring more frequently. Bladder perforations usually occur with midline suprapubic trocar insertions, especially in patients with prior surgeries or significant adhesive disease. This can be avoided in two ways. One method is needle tracking. In this technique, a spinal needle is inserted into the abdominal cavity at the planned insertion site. Direct visualization confirms intra-abdominal entry. The needle is then slowly withdrawn while aspirating and observing for urine in the syringe. Of course, there must be some urine in the bladder for this technique to work. The trocar is then inserted through the exact path of the needle. The other technique is direct visualization. The bladder can almost always be directly visualized at laparoscopy. Pressing with the surgeon's finger, the back of the knife handle, or a hemostat on the midline suprapubic abdominal wall at the planned site of entry identifies the eventual site of penetration. The resulting indentation can be clearly seen laparoscopically and can be noted to be above the bladder. If not, then the same procedure is repeated in a slightly more cephalad location until a position is reached that is clearly above the bladder.

To avoid the rectus muscles and epigastric vessels, a very similar technique is useful. Knowledge of the normal anatomy of the anterior abdominal wall as seen laparoscopically is very useful (Figs. 18.5 and 18.6). If the midline is located first, then movement of the laparoscopic visual field laterally in either direction demonstrates the medial umbilical ligaments. The novice laparoscopist not uncommonly identifies these as the epigastric vessels and inserts the trocar just lateral to them, a disastrous error. The epigastric vessels are always lateral to the medial umbilical ligaments, although their exact location varies greatly. Usually these vessels can be easily visualized laparoscopically. In obese patients they may be difficult to see directly. In these cases, the above described technique of indenting the anterior abdominal wall with a pointed instrument (the back of the knife handle works well) will often reveal a V formed just lateral to the medial umbilical ligament that, with experience, can be identified as the vessels (Figs. 18.7 and 18.8). Confirmation can often be obtained by observing arterial pulsations of this V. When using this technique, it is important to be sure that the trocar is inserted directly and straight below the site selected for introduction. Often there is a tendency to aim the trocar in a medial direction. In an obese patient with a thick abdominal wall, this may carry the trocar sufficiently medial to the skin site to end up in the inferior epigastric vessels by the time the peritoneum is reached. With trocars 10 mm or larger, this occurs more easily than one may think. It is crucial to insert all ancillary trocars under full control and

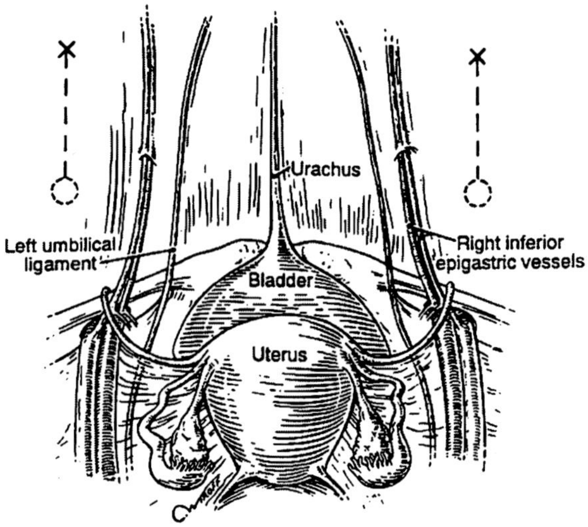

Figure 18.5. Diagram of the anatomy of the anterior abdominal wall below the umbilicus. (Adapted from Ref. 52.)

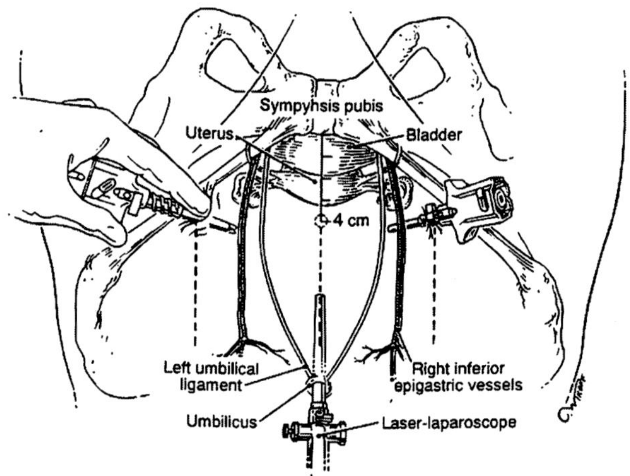

Figure 18.6. Diagram of possible insertion sites for accessory trocars lateral to the inferior epigastric vessels and rectus muscles. (Adapted from Ref. 51.)

direct visualization, lest bowel or the common iliac vessels be perforated.

Transillumination is sometimes advised and may occasionally be useful, but more often than not, the vessels seen by transillumination are the superficial, not the inferior, epigastric vessels. Although these two sets of vessels may lie directly over one another, this is not always the case, and reliance on the findings at transillumination may still lead to laceration of the inferior epigastric vessels. Transillumination is not possible in obese patients.

Hernias may also be considered a laparoscopy-specific complication, as they usually result not from breakdown of the fascial closure, but rather from nonclosure of the fascia. Traditionally, gynecologists have not closed the fascia at the time of diagnostic laparoscopy or laparoscopic tubal sterilization, as herniation at the 5-mm lower trocar or 10-mm umbilical trocar sites is infrequent (but both have been reported). However, with the use of larger trocars in the lower abdomen and at the umbilicus, herniation is a significant problem. Currently, the best advice is to ensure fascial closure on any laparoscopic incision greater than 5 mm. Several commercially available devices are available to assist with this. A simple, inexpensive method is illustrated in Figure 18.9.

ADNEXAL MASSES

Indications for Surgery

Women with adnexal masses may require surgical evaluation and treatment for any of the following indications:

- Acute or persistent abdominopelvic pain.
- Torsion, hemorrhage, or rupture.
- Infertility and a persistent cystic mass.
- Prophylaxis for complications such as torsion, hemorrhage, or rupture.
- Concern about possible malignancy.

Although there are minor differences of opinion, most gynecologists agree that in premenopausal women with the last two indications, asymptomatic masses should be examined surgically and pathologically for any of the following reasons:

- Occurrence in nonovulating women.
- A solid or mixed ultrasonographic appearance.
- Diameter of 8 cm or more (some use 6 cm or more).
- Failure to resolve after a full menstrual cycle (4 to 6 weeks) or during oral contraceptive treatment.
- Persistent pain that is resistant to other therapy for 6 months.[11,12]

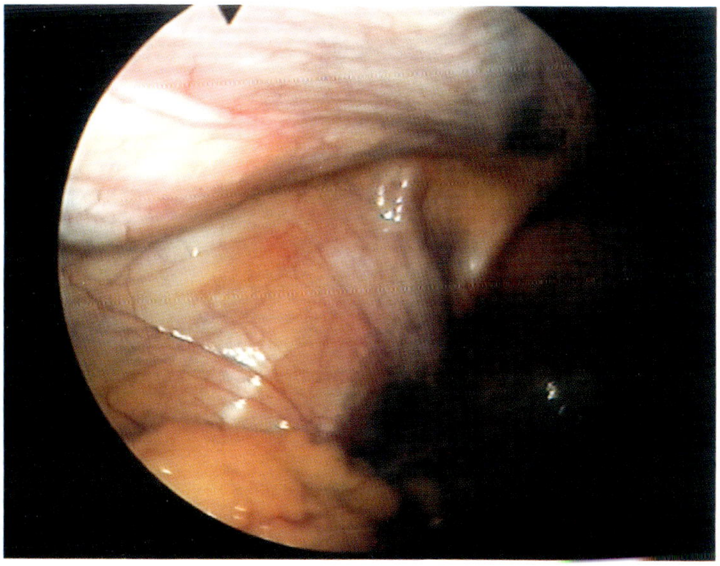

Figure 18.7. Laparoscopic view of the left anterior abdominal wall. Indentation of the anterior abdominal wall made by the surgeon with a knife handle, demonstrating the location selected for insertion of an accessory trocar. The inferior epigastric vessels. The round ligament. The medial umbilical ligament.

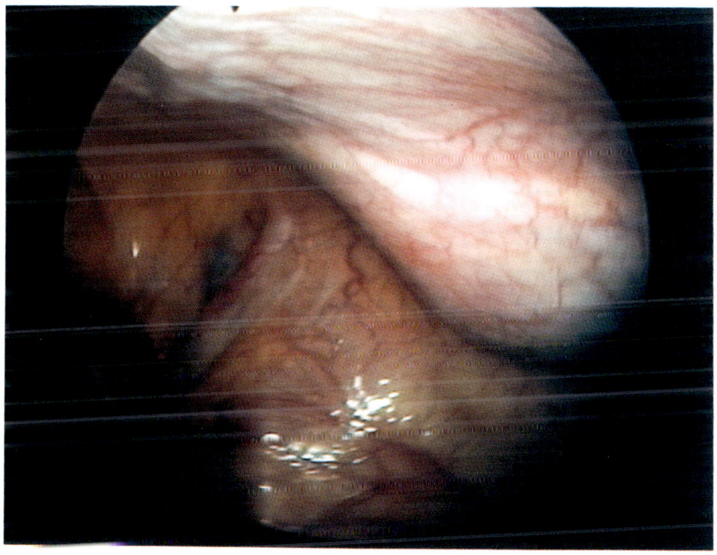

Figure 18.8. Laparoscopic view of the right anterior abdominal wall. Indentention of the anterior abdominal wall made by the surgeon with a knife handle, demonstrating the location selected for insertion of an accessory trocar. The inferior epigastric vessels. The round ligament. The medial umbilical ligament.

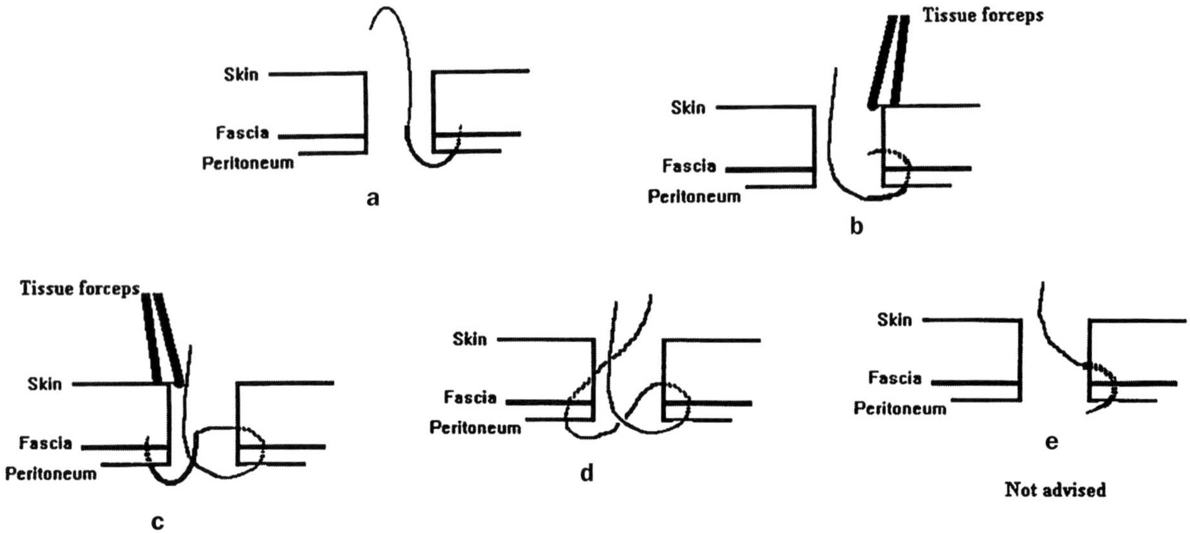

Figure 18.9. (a) A urology needle (UR-6) with more than a 180 degree curve is used. The needle is placed completely into the incision as shown, then lifted and driven through the peritoneum and fascia. Carbon dioxide is lost during this maneuver, but with practice steps, (a) and (b) can be done without complete loss of the pneumoperitoneum. (b) While retracting the skin edge with tissue forceps, the needle is driven in the direction of its curve so that it is exposed in the subcutaneous fat. It can then be released from the needle driver, and the needle driver can be used to grasp the pointed end and retrieve it from the incision. (c) Between steps (b) and (c), a finger is placed over the incision to reestablish the pneumoperitoneum if necessary. Step (c) is then a duplication of step (a) on the opposite side of the incision. (d) The suture is tied after pulling the needle through the second side of the incision. Although this technique pulls one peritoneal edge toward the opposite subcutaneous tissue, this is of no consequence with these small incisions that require a single suture for closure; the fascial edges are well approximated. (e) Many surgeons attempt to use a normal closure, as shown here. This is not advised on either fascial surface. The incision is too small to allow visualization and retrieval of the needle tip in the peritoneal cavity. This method increases the possibility of incorporating the bowel or omentum into the closure.

In postmenopausal women, any cystic mass more than 3 cm in diameter by ultrasound and pelvic examination should be evaluated surgically and pathologically via oophorectomy. As functional cysts occasionally develop postmenopausally, it is not unreasonable to observe a postmenopausal woman with a small cyst (3 cm or less) for spontaneous resolution for 4 weeks prior to surgical evaluation. More recently, it has been suggested that cysts up to 5 cm may be observed for resolution for several weeks before surgical exploration is necessary. Despite progress with tumor markers and ultrasound, none have sufficient accuracy to preclude surgical and pathologic examination to distinguish benign and malignant adnexal neoplasms.[4] It seems prudent to do bilateral oophorectomies when surgery is indicated in postmenopausal women even if the findings are benign.[13]

Generally, ovarian cystectomy is the preferred procedure in premenopausal women. However, oophorectomy may be indicated for evaluation and treatment of ovarian masses in premenopausal women for the following conditions:

- Chronic abdominopelvic pain, especially with ovarian retention syndrome (residual ovary syndrome), tubo-ovarian abscess, pelvic congestion syndrome, or a large endometrioma with ovarian destruction.

- Torsion, hemorrhage, or rupture if the ovary is not reparable or salvageable.
- Serious concern that the ovary is malignant, so that avoidance of rupture may be important.

The decision to perform an oophorectomy in a young woman (less than 40–45 years old) should never be made casually. If technically possible, it is best to preserve the ovary unless the clinical situation contraindicates conservation.[12]

Surgical Techniques

Ovarian Cystectomy

Figure 18.10 summarizes the cogent steps in managing a patient by ovarian cystectomy. This scheme refers to premenopausal women with cystic adnexal masses, as cystectomy should rarely if ever be done for adnexal masses in postmenopausal women. It is important to avoid mismanagement of the rare case of ovarian cancer, as such mismanagement is one of the most significant complications of laparoscopic ovarian cystectomy. Unfortunately, examples of this complication have been documented in a disturbing report by Maiman et al.[3] In a survey of 156 gynecologic oncologists, they identified 42 cases of laparoscopic management of ovarian cysts subsequently found to be malignant. In only 12 (29%) of the cases was a complete excision of the cyst done. In 14 (33%) cases a partial excision was done, and in 16 (38%) cases the procedure was aborted without a histologic diagnosis. An immediate laparotomy was done in only 7 (17%) cases, and only 17 (40%) had a frozen section at the time of surgery. In 30 cases laparotomy for definitive staging and debulking was delayed for a mean period of 4.8 weeks after laparoscopy. Laparotomy was never performed in five cases. Characteristics of the cysts preoperatively were not helpful. Sixty-seven percent were less than 8 cm in size, 48% were unilocular, 81% were unilateral, and 31% were less than 8 cm, unilateral, and unilocular. Clearly benign sonographic characteristics preoperatively are not a guarantee of benign disease. Therefore, any cystic adnexal mass should be approached via a laparoscopic incision in the same manner that it is approached via laparotomy.

Accordingly, simple aspiration of an ovarian cyst is almost never an appropriate laparoscopic procedure. First, cytology of aspirated ovarian cystic fluid is not reliable as a diagnostic test for malignancy. Although the results vary somewhat, the sensitivity of cyst fluid cytology for cancer is about 25% (i.e., it diagnoses cancer in 25 of 100 cancer cases) and the negative predictive value is about 75% (i.e., it is wrong 25 out of 100 times when it indicates that there is no malignancy).[14]

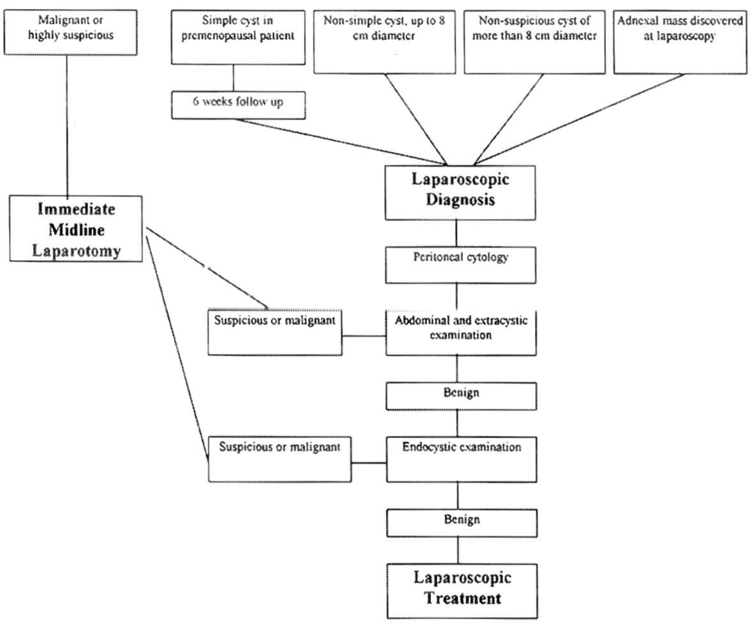

Figure 18.10. A schema for laparoscopic management of adnexal cystic masses.

Second, the recurrence rate of benign ovarian cysts after aspiration is 30–60%.[15] This is too high a failure rate for an invasive surgical procedure when there is an alternative with similar morbidity but much higher cure rates (i.e., ovarian cystectomy).

A possible exception to this prohibition against simple aspiration of adnexal cysts may be torsion during pregnancy. Of 16 reported cases of adnexal torsion during pregnancy treated laparoscopically, in only 1 was the cyst or mass causing the torsion biopsied or excised.[16–21] Two concerns about this approach are those already discussed. First, the experience with simple aspiration is that there is a significant chance of recurrence of the cyst, with the potential of retorsion due to recurrence. However, in the 15 cases managed with simple aspiration and untwisting, no instances of retorsion occurred during the pregnancy. A second concern is the worry about inappropriate management of ovarian carcinoma. Cytology of aspirated cyst fluid, as already noted, is not always diagnostic and may be misleading. Additionally, a benign appearance of the external capsule of an ovarian cyst is not always diagnostic. However, with the relatively low risk of ovarian cancer during pregnancy (less than 5% of adnexal masses), with careful preoperative ultrasound evaluation, and with meticulous intraoperative evaluation of the abdomen and pelvis, the risk is low that an ovarian cancer would be misdiagnosed during laparoscopic treatment of torsion during pregnancy. This simple approach may have particular advantages during pregnancy, as it minimizes abdominal and uterine manipulation and shortens operative time. Thus, although further study is needed, it currently seems reasonable to recommend simple aspiration and untwisting at the time of laparoscopy during pregnancy for adnexal torsion. However, in cases with any degree of uncertainty, the usual protocol for management of an ovarian cyst is advisable (see Table 18.8).

Sonography should be done preoperatively in any premenopausal woman with an adnexal mass that may require surgical treatment, but CA-125 testing is not particularly useful in this age group. If ultrasound or CT scans show apparent signs of cancer, such as ascites, matted bowel, an omental mass, an upper abdominal mass, liver metastases, or lymphadenopathy, then laparoscopy is not indicated. Although laparoscopic staging and treatment of ovarian cancer have been attempted and may in the future be useful, they cannot be recommended at this time. Laparoscopy has no current role in primary surgical evaluation and treatment of ovarian cancer.

If there are no overt signs of cancer, then most women may be approached laparoscopically, regardless of the sonographic appearance of the mass. In other words, the presence of complex or bilateral masses per se is not a contraindication to laparoscopy. Peritoneal fluid or washings of the peritoneal cavity should be obtained on initial entry into the abdominal cavity in all cases. This fluid may not need to be sent for cytologic examination if the adnexal disease is subsequently determined to be benign. Next, inspection of the ovary, pelvic peritoneum, contralateral ovary, colic gutters, diaphragm, omentum, liver, and bowel for any tumor masses, ascites, excrescences, or other suspicious findings is done.[4] If any findings suggest a malignancy, then a midline laparotomy should be done immediately. Puncture and aspiration of the cyst should not be done in such cases. Even though there is controversy about the influence on survival of surgical rupture of a malignant ovarian cyst, the prognosis cannot be improved by puncture of a malignant ovarian tumor.

If there is no evidence of cancer, then either of two approaches may be chosen. If the size and nature of the cyst allow an intact ovarian cystectomy, then this may be attempted (Fig. 18.11). Realistically, this is usually difficult to accomplish without inadvertent rupture of the cyst. The other option is to aspirate the cyst contents prior to starting the cystectomy. Several techniques are possible. One is the use of laser energy, electrical energy, or scissors to open the cyst, followed by immediate introduction of a suction irrigator into the cyst cavity. With practice this can be done with minimal spill. Stabilizing the cyst with two grasping instruments may facilitate this maneuver (Fig. 18.12). After the cyst is completely evacuated, the cavity should be irrigated and aspirated many times, taking care not to spill the irrigant. Washing with large amounts of irrigant minimizes any subsequent spill of contents during cystectomy. Simple needle aspiration of the cyst contents is another technique. This is not always feasible with benign cystic teratomas or mucinous cystadenomas because of the tenacity and thickness of the cyst fluid. However, it works well for simple cysts and cystomas. Another technique is the introduction of a large endoscopic bag into the abdomen to catch the cyst contents as the cyst is opened.

Whichever method is used to open benign-appearing lesions, it is important to minimize spillage and to lavage the pelvic cavity with copious amounts of irrigant if any spill does occur.[4] With benign cystic teratomas this is particularly important, as postoperative

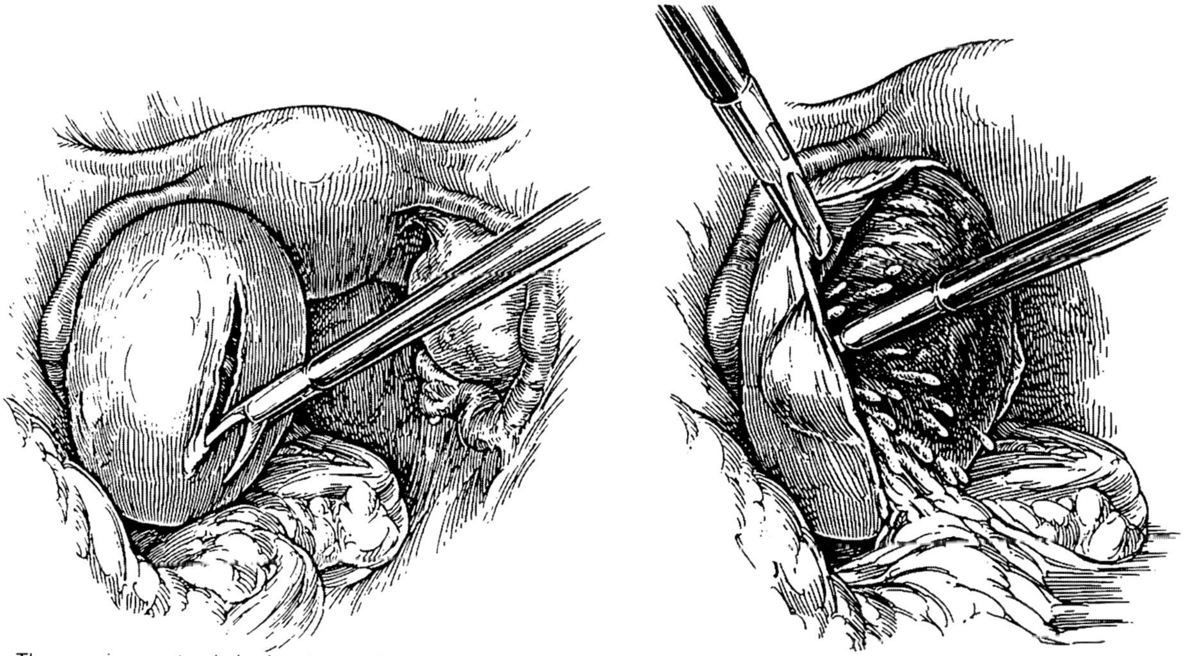

The ovarian cortex is incised revealing the underlying cyst wall.

The irrigating instrument is used at high pressure to separate the cyst wall from the ovary (aquadissection).

Figure 18.11. The initial steps in laparoscopic ovarian cystectomy without rupture of the cyst. (From Ref. 53.)

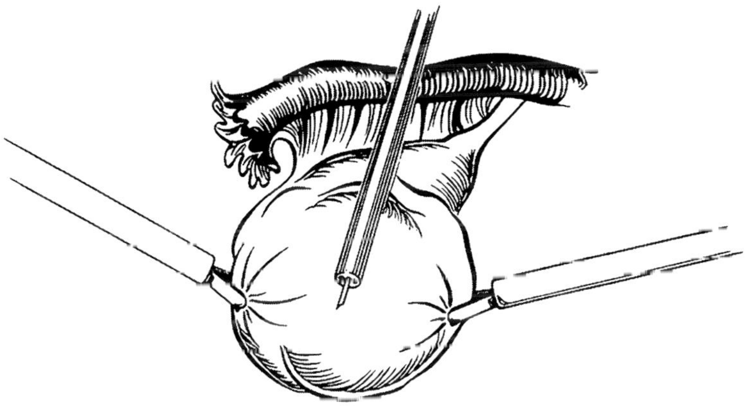

Figure 18.12. A cannula with irrigation and suction channels and a retractable diathermy needle is inserted into the cyst to allow immediate suction and irrigation, minimizing intraperitoneal spill. (From Erian MM, Goh TW: A new laparoscopic aspiration technique for ovarian dermoid cysts. *J Am Assoc Gynecol Laparosc* 2:71–73, 1994.)

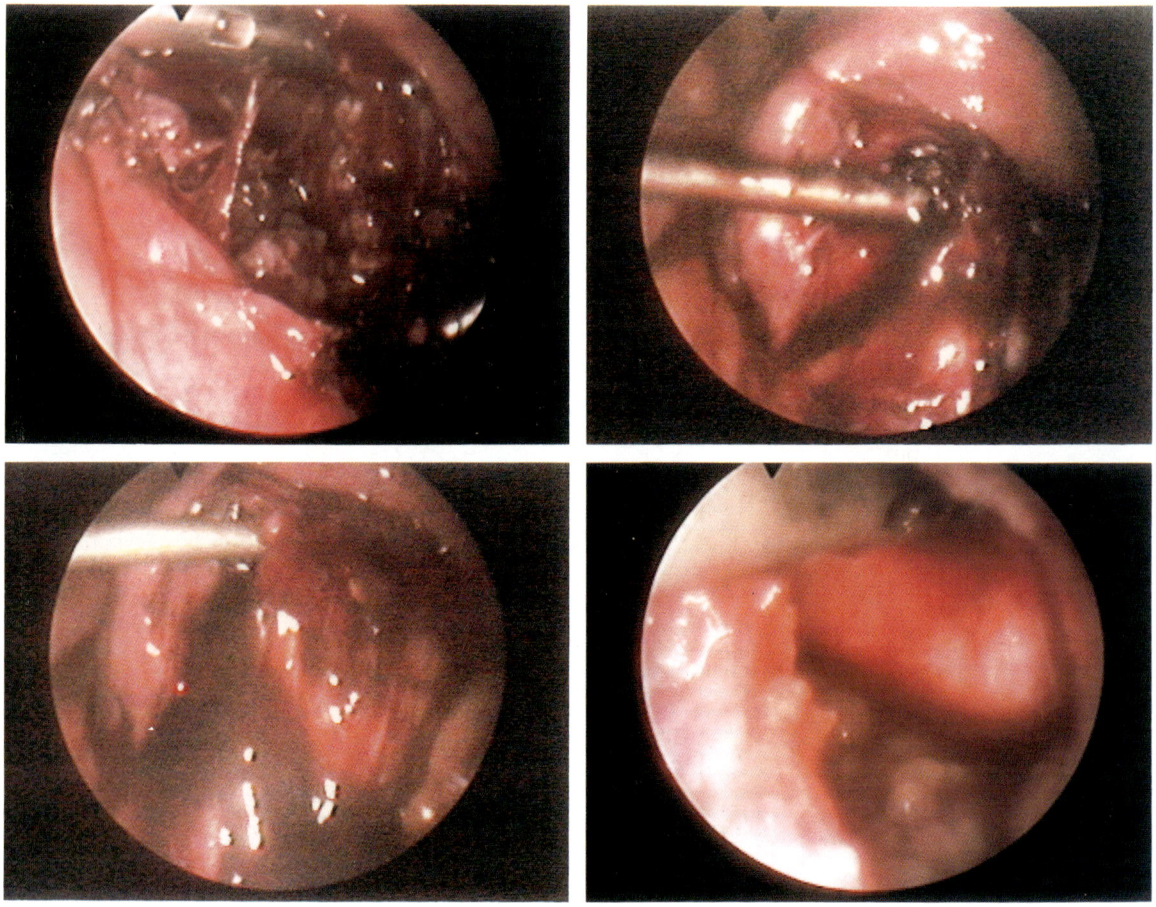

Figure 18.13. Excrescences in the cyst cavity of an apparent endometrioma. Immediate laparotomy was done, and well-differentiated endometrioid adenocarcinoma was diagnosed.

complications have been reported when less than 10 L of irrigant was used or when irrigation was not continued until the spilled sebaceous material was totally removed.[4,22]

The next step is to evaluate the entire cyst lining endoscopically, looking for any papillary excrescences (Fig. 18.13). If the lining clearly appears consistent with cancer, laparotomy should be done. Currently, there is some debate as to the proper approach if minimal excrescences are found that are not clearly suggestive of malignancy. Some recommend biopsies and frozen sections in uncertain cases, particularly as most such cysts are benign in young women and these tests may avoid unnecessary laparotomies. Others believe that biopsies of excrescences should not be done at laparoscopy. A concern is that the effects of positive intra-abdominal pressure, the carbon dioxide environment, and the inability to protect the upper abdomen at the time of laparoscopic biopsies of malignant lesions have not been addressed and could, at least theoretically, worsen the prognosis.[4] Another concern is the uncertain accuracy of frozen section diagnoses with small biopsy specimens obtained laparoscopically. Information from studies of intraoperative consultation when the entire ovarian tumor is evaluated suggests that there may be significant errors in frozen section diagnosis of ovarian tumors. For example, one study from the University of Massachusetts covering 10 years of intraoperative consultations shows a sensitivity of frozen section diagnosis of malignant ovarian tumors of 92.5%, a sensitivity of diagnosis of borderline ovarian tumors of 45%, and a sensitivity of diagnosis of benign ovarian tumors of 99%.[23] To illustrate the predicament that the gynecologic surgeon may encounter, of all cases diagnosed as benign at the time of pathologic intraoperative consultation and frozen section, about 6% will be low malignant potential tumors and 2% will be malignant tumors at the time of permanent section diagnosis. Errors are particularly common in frozen section diagnoses of large ovarian tumors with a small focus of malignant tumor.

In cases with a smooth cyst lining or findings consistent with endometriosis or benign cystic teratoma, as much of the cyst wall as possible should be removed and sent for histologic evaluation. Although uncommon, the possibility of a focus of cancer in an apparently benign cyst makes this policy prudent. For example, apparently benign cystic teratomas may contain malignant elements in 1–3% of cases.[24] Of course, complete removal of the entire cyst lining and its contents is also essential to prevent recurrence or other sequelae. Occasionally, but particularly in cases of endometriomas, complete removal is quite difficult. In these cases, very generous specimens still should be obtained and the remainder of the lining destroyed with laser or electrical energy. If this is not possible via laparoscopy, then a laparotomy should be done. Partial removal of an ovarian mass that would be unacceptable at laparotomy is also unacceptable at laparoscopy.

The most common technique used for removal of an ovarian cyst is stripping. This method requires at least two accessory cannulas so that the cyst lining can be stripped from the ovary with one grasper while countertraction is applied by holding the ovarian tissue with another grasper (Fig. 18.14). It is advisable to place the cyst in an endoscopic bag for removal via one of the cannulas, a minilaparotomy incision, or a culpotomy. Ordinarily, using one of the larger cannula incisions seems preferable to doing a culpotomy or enlarging the laparoscopic incisions. With this method, the purse string of the endoscopic bag is brought to the skin as the cannula is withdraw from the incision (Fig. 18.15). The top of the bag that is extending through the incision is cut and spread open with hemostats or similar clamps. This allows introduction of a Kocher or Allis clamp into the bag to grasp the specimen. The specimen can be pulled and morcellated within the bag, allowing its extraction without enlarging the incision. The intra-abdominal portion of the bag is observed with the laparoscope to avoid puncture. Attempts to remove an ovarian cyst directly through the abdominal or vaginal wall without placing it in a bag may lead to

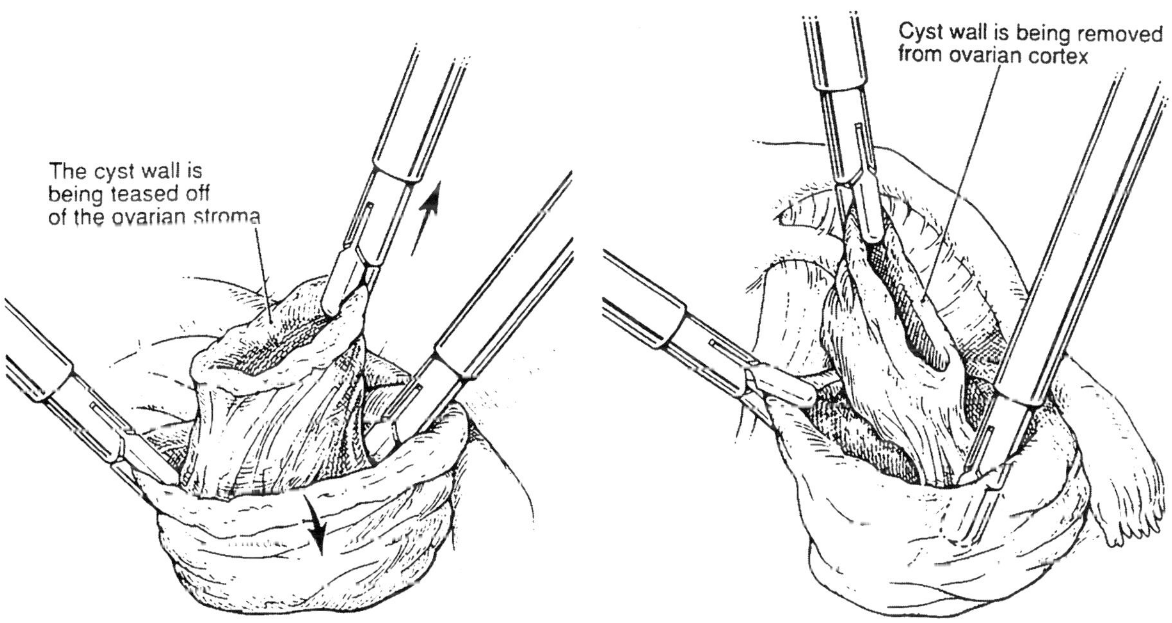

Figure 18.14. A technique for stripping the entire capsule of an ovarian cyst from the ovarian stroma using two or three grasping forceps for traction and countertraction. The capsule should be submitted for histologic evaluation. (From Ref. 51.)

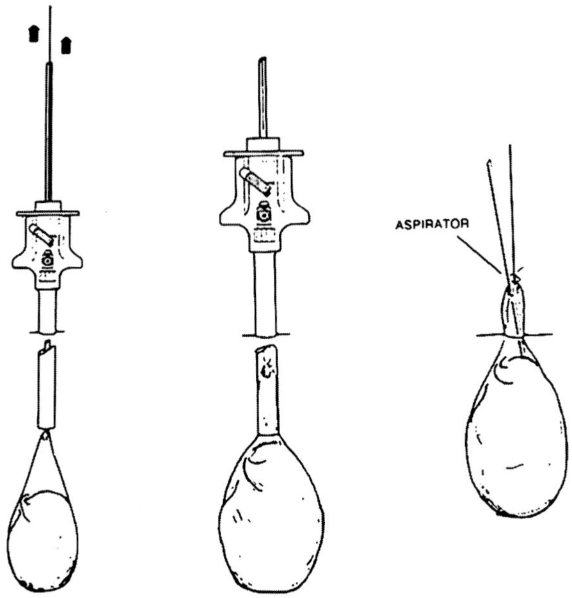

Figure 18.15. A technique to remove an ovarian cyst via a laparoscopic port using an endoscopic bag. The bag is pulled to the base of the trocar sleeve until resistance is felt. Then the whole trocar and bag are pulled through the incision, bringing the bag to the abdominal wall. At this point, the cyst may be aspirated and morcellated in the bag to allow removal. (Modified from Ref. 51.)

loss of part or all of the specimen in the abdominal wall or result in implantation of endometriosis, teratomas, or malignancy in the abdominal or vaginal wall.

Two large series have been reported using laparoscopy to treat patients with cystic adnexal masses, both using approaches similar to that suggested in Figure 18.8. One is by Bruhat's group in France, reporting the results from 757 patients with 819 masses[4] (Table 18.3). Nineteen (2.5%) of the 757 women had ovarian cancers, 12 with low malignant potential tumors and 7 with invasive cancers. The incidence of malignant ovarian lesions was 7.6% among women 50 years of age or older (7 of 92) and 1.8% among women less than 50 years old (12 of 665). Tumor size was not predictive of malignancy. Of cysts less than 5 cm in size, 2.7% were malignant; of those 5 to 10 cm, 1.9% were malignant; and of those 10 cm or greater, 2.9% were malignant.

Table 18.3. Results of Laparoscopic Management of 819 Cystic Adnexal Masses in 757 Patients: Occurrence of Malignancy

	Mean (cm)	Range	Number
Cyst size	6.0 + 2.7	1–20	819
Cancers	6.6 + 4.6	1–20	19
LMP*	—	—	12
Invasive	—	—	7

LMP = low malignant potential tumors (Ref. 4).

Using this approach, Bruhat and coworkers had a sensitivity of 100% for ovarian cancer, performing immediate midline laparotomies on 19 of 19 patients with malignancies (true positives). They also did 27 laparotomies for suspected cancers that were subsequently found to be benign (false positives) (Table 18.4). Ten of the 19 patients with malignant tumors underwent laparoscopic puncture of their tumors, 2 with invasive cancers and 8 with low malignant potential tumors. In this series, laparoscopy's positive predictive value was 41.3% (19 of 46) and its negative predictive value was 100% for cancer. Intraoperative management was based on visual findings, and frozen sections were not done in this study.

The other large series is from Nezhat and coworkers in the United States[7] (Table 18.5). They reported their findings based on 1011 patients with 1209 adnexal masses managed laparoscopically. Although they did ultrasound scans and determined CA-125 levels preoperatively, no patients were excluded based on preoperative findings. The other major difference in their protocol compared to that of Bruhat's group was that they performed laparoscopic biopsies and frozen sections on suspicious lesions. They found only four ovarian malignancies. However, none of these four patients had immediate laparotomy. Definitive surgery via laparotomy was done 3 days to 2 months after the laparoscopy (the 2 months' delay was due to the patient's delay). Four patients had immediate laparotomys for suspicious but benign lesions (one teratoma, one mesothelioma, one serous cystadenoma, and one degenerating leiomyoma), giving a positive predictive value of 50% (quite similar to the 41.3% of Bruhat's group, even though the absolute numbers are quite different). In this study, cysts ranged from 2 to 25 cm and included cystic, complex, and solid masses. Nezhat and coworkers concluded that only frozen and permanent

Table 18.4. Characteristics of 46 Patients with Cystic Adnexal Masses Who Underwent Laparotomy Based on Laparoscopic Findings

	Cancer	LMP Tumors	Falsely Suspicious Masses
Total	7	12	27
Punctured	2	8	10
Not punctured	5	4	17
Suspicious ultrasonography findings*	1	1	4
Extraovarian signs of malignancy	4	3	13
Peritoneal metastases	2	3	0
External ovarian vegetations	4	3	12
Turbid fluid	0	3	0
Abnormal vessels	0	1	1
Intracystic vegetations	2	6	10

*There were no extraovarian signs of malignancy, but once an ovarian origin of the mass was established, a laparotomy was done based on preoperative ultrasound findings thought to be consistent with cancer.

Source: Ref. 4.

Table 18.5. Diagnoses in 1011 Women with Operative Laparoscopies for Treatment of Adnexal Masses

Diagnosis	Number	Percent	Age Range (yr)	Size Range (cm)	No. Bilateral
Ovarian cancer	4	0.4	33–44	2–13	1
Endometrioma	457	45.2	16–54	2–25	162
Functional cyst	358	35.5	11–47	2–12	27
Benign cystic teratoma	35	3.4	17–44	2–14	6
Mucinous cystadenoma	12	1.1	31–35	2–13	0
Serous cystadenoma	17	1.6	33–40	3–15	0
Hydrosalpinx	26	2.5	26–45	5–8	2
Leiomyoma	16	1.5	33–50	5–8	0
Paratubal-paraovarian cyst	39	3.8	22–45	2–8	0
Ovarian remnant	10	0.9	25–40	2–5	0
Miscellaneous	37	3.6	22–45	2–17	0

Source: Ref. 7.

pathology distinguish cancer patients from those with benign ovarian cysts. Age, cyst size, CA-125 levels, ultrasound findings, and peritoneal cytology did not distinguish patients with cancer from those with benign disease.

Table 18.6 summarizes the results from these two large series. The average incidence of ovarian cancer was 1.3%, and the average incidence of laparotomy for benign disease was 1.8%. Overall, 23 (43%) of 51 laparotomies were performed for cancer, and unnecessary laparotomies were avoided in 97% of women with cystic adnexal masses.

Table 18.6. Summary of Two Large Series of Laparoscopically Managed Patients with Cystic Adnexal Masses: Ovarian Cancers and Laparotomies for Suspicious But Benign Disease

Series	Total No. of Patients	No. of Cancers	% of Cancers	No. of Noncancer Laparotomies	% of Noncancer Laparotomies
Canis et al.[4]	757	19	2.5	27	3.6
Nezhat et al.[7]	1011	4	0.4	4	0.4
Total	1768	23	1.3	31	1.8

Complications

Reported complications are uncommon with laparoscopic ovarian cystectomy. For example, in the large series from Bruhat's group, there were eight complications in 757 cases (1.1%).[4] The complications were:

- Gastric laceration by umbilical trocar (one case).
- Unexplained acute abdominal pain requiring a second laparoscopy (one case).
- Peritonitis from undiagnosed sigmoid laceration (one case).
- Ovarian abscess after aspiration (two cases).
- Abdominal wall endometrioma at 18 months (one case).
- Peritonitis subsequent to teratoma (two cases).

Of these eight complications, the first is a laparoscopy-specific complication, that is, it may occur with any laparoscopy, even a diagnostic one. The second complication, acute abdominal pain, cannot be classified, as the cause was undetermined. The third, fourth, and fifth groups of complications represent procedure-specific complications. Bowel injury with adhesiolysis and infection after ovarian aspiration are both complications that could occur with ovarian cystectomy or cystotomy, regardless of how they are done. Abdominal wall endometrioma also represents a complication that can occur with ovarian cystectomy for endometriosis by laparotomy or laparoscopy. Whether it is more common with the laparoscopic approach is not known, as it has been infrequently reported with either laparoscopy or laparotomy. The final complication, peritonitis after cystectomy for teratoma, represents laparoscopic procedure-specific complications. Both of the cases of peritonitis are attributed to spillage of cyst contents, and although spillage may occur at laparotomy, it is much more easily avoided than at laparoscopy. In the first case, reexploration was done five days postoperatively, and no explanation for peritonitis was found. In the second case, reexploration was done 12 months postoperatively, and adhesions and granulomatous peritonitis were found. In this case, the authors state that there was a breakdown of the aspiration lavage system during the laparoscopic cystectomy that probably accounted for the development of granulomatous peritonitis.

A brief pause to discuss the laparoscopic management of benign cystic teratomas is appropriate. It is possible to remove benign cystic teratomas laparoscopically, but as previously stated, it is quite difficult to remove ovarian cysts without some spillage of cyst contents. Traditionally, great care has been taken to avoid intra-abdominal spillage of cystic teratomas, as development of granulomatous peritonitis is a serious sequela. For that reason, many have considered benign cystic teratoma a contraindication to laparoscopy. However, in the large series from Bruhat's group there were only two cases of peritonitis (2.1% of all cases with benign cystic teratomas), only one of which was confirmed as due to spillage. In that case the complication appears to have been due to incomplete lavage of the peritoneal cavity. Keil and Juilian have also reported a serious complication, a case of serious granulomatous peritonitis with subsequent fistulae.[22] In this case, intraperitoneal lavage was with only 3000 mL of fluid for an 8-cm teratoma, and it is not stated whether visual confirmation of complete removal of all sebaceous material and hair was documented. Reich et al.,[25] Nezhat et al.,[26] Howard,[27] and Albini et al.[28] all report successful management of benign cystic teratomas via laparoscopy with intraperitoneal spillage without sequelae. These reports suggest that techniques to minimize spillage (as discussed previously) and copious irrigation to remove any spilled material are adequate to prevent postoperative peritonitis. It is not uncommon to need to lavage with more than 10 L of irrigant to ensure complete removal of all spilled material.[7] However, in view of the two reported cases of serious complications, further study needs to be done to ensure that there are no long-term sequelae.

Surgical Techniques

Oophorectomy

Oophorectomies and salpingo-oophorectomies are two of the most commonly performed gynecologic operative laparoscopic procedures. They accounted for 10.5% of the operative laparoscopies performed by members of the American Association of Gynecologic Laparoscopists surveyed in 1993, a significant increase from the 5.9% performed in 1991.[10] Endoscopic pretied loop ligatures, bipolar electrocoagulation, and stapler-cutter instruments are the usual techniques used for laparoscopic oophorectomy or salpingo-oophorectomy. Extensive comparisons of these modalities have not been done, but evidence from Daniell et al. suggest that all three are equally efficacious, although stapler-cutters make the procedure more expensive.[29] Nezhat et al.[30] suggest that the loop ligature technique may increase the possibility of ovarian remnant syndrome. They base this concern on a history of oophorectomy via loop ligatures in 2 of 13 patients with this syndrome.

Regardless of the technique used, it is important that the anatomy of the pelvic brim be carefully identified, including the bifurcation of the common iliac vessels, the internal and external iliac vessels, the ureters, and the infundibulopelvic ligaments. On the left side, this is sometimes difficult due to the overlying rectosigmoid colon. At times it is necessary to mobilize the rectosigmoid colon to allow adequate exposure of the infundibulopelvic ligament. Figure 18.16 shows ligation of the infundibulopelvic ligament with its ovarian vessels with an endoscopic stapler-cutter, and Figure 18.17 shows coagulation with bipolar cautery. Semm's triple loop technique that ligates en masse the infundibulopelvic ligament, fallopian tube, and mesovarium is common when endoscopic loop ligatures are used (Fig. 18.18). Another technique is creation of a window in the infundibulopelvic ligament below the ovarian vessels that allows suture to be passed to ligate the vessels.

After detaching the adnexae from their vessels and

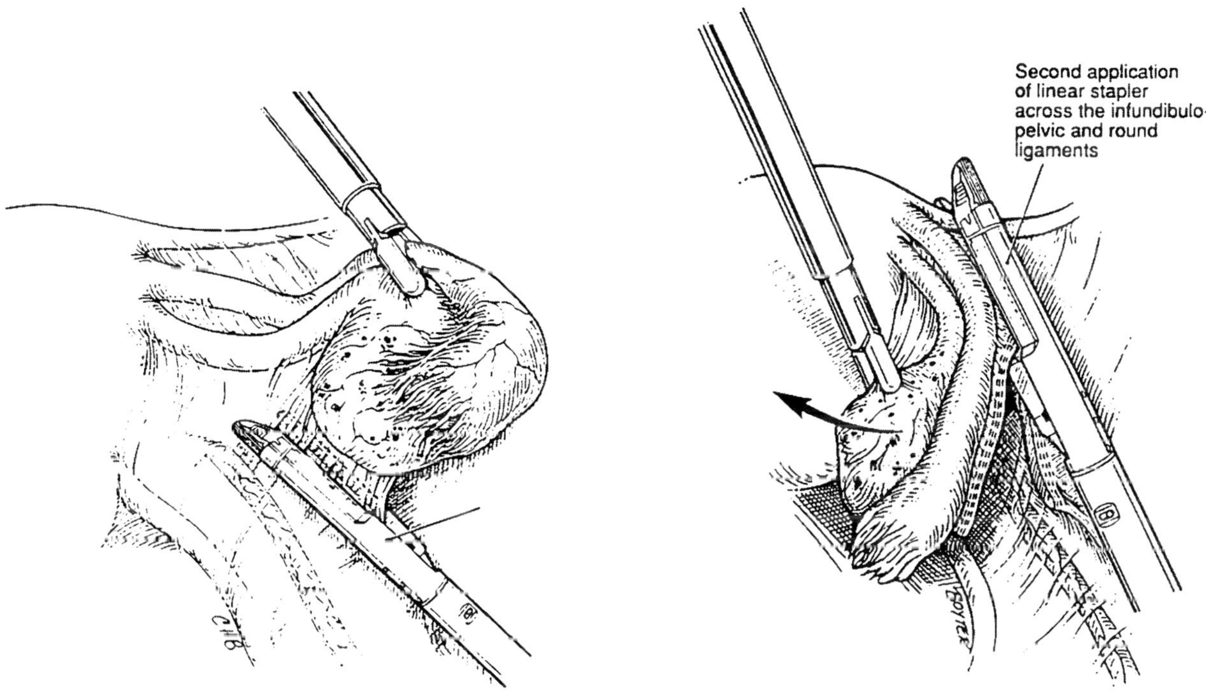

Figure 18.16. Salpingo-oophorectomy with an endoscopic stapler-cutter. Defining the anatomic location of the ureter is crucial. The salpingo-oophorectomy is completed (not shown) by firing the stapler-cutter across the uterovarian ligament and fallopian tube. (Modified from Ref. 51.)

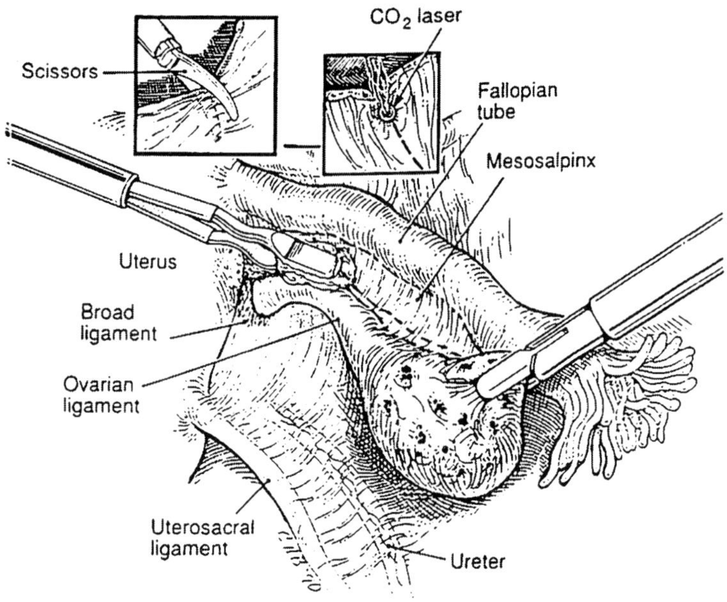

Figure 18.17. Oophorectomy using bipolar cautery. (Modified from Ref. 51.)

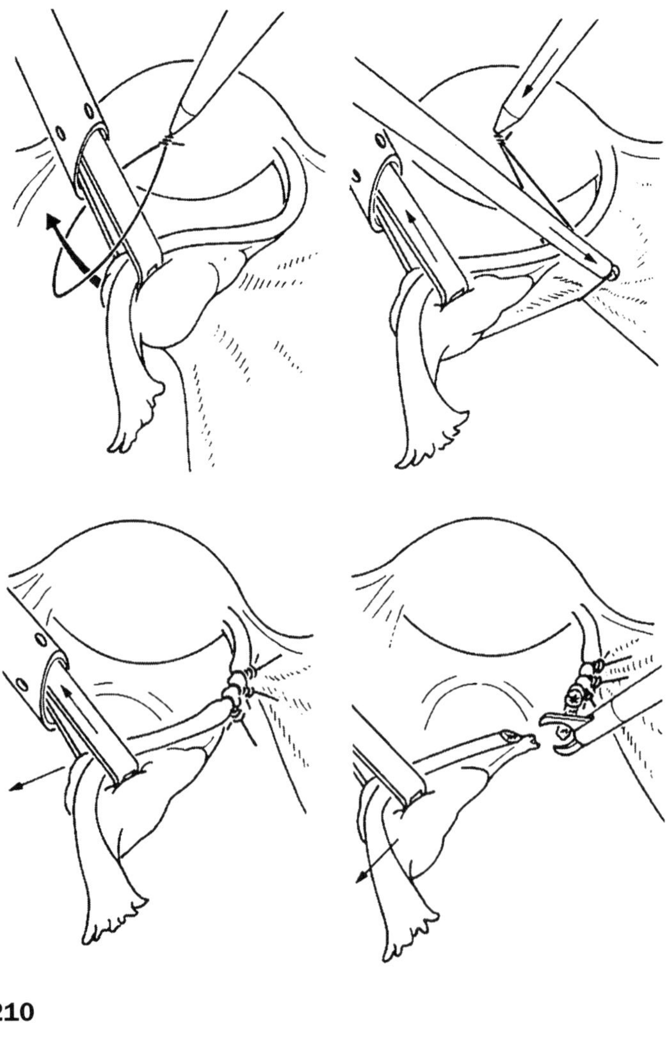

Figure 18.18. Triple-loop technique of salpingo-oophorectomy using endoscopic loop ligatures.

ligaments, it is best to remove the specimen by placing it in an endoscopic bag (Fig. 18.19). This prevents spillage from inadvertent rupture of any ovarian cysts or seeding of the incision by unsuspected cancer or endometriosis. It also minimizes the chance of losing the specimen in the peritoneal cavity. Intact removal can be done via a colpotomy or minilaparotomy incision. Removal may also be accomplished through a trocar incision site by morcellating the ovary within the bag, as described for ovarian cystectomy.

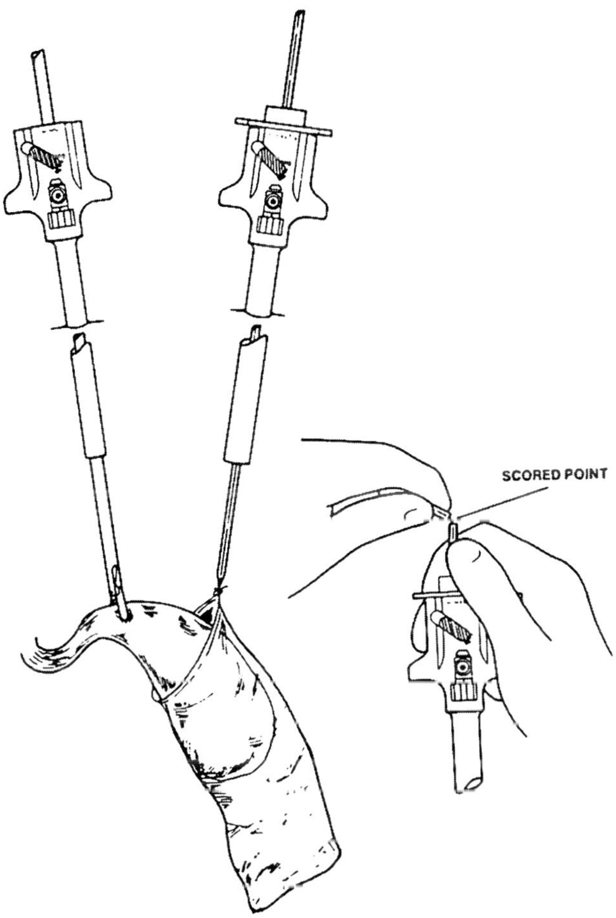

Figure 18.19. Placing a specimen into an endoscopic bag for removal from the abdomen (see also Figure 18.15). (Modified from Ref. 51.)

Complications

Patients with indications for oophorectomy, salpingo-oophorectomy, or ovarian cystectomy often have significant pelvic disease, especially adhesions or endometriosis, that must also be treated at the time of surgery.[29] It is crucial that the ovary and fallopian tube be freed from any adhesions and that normal anatomy be restored. The requisite adhesiolysis is often itself a source of complications. Not surprisingly, bowel injury or inability to free the adnexae may result. In one series of 420 patients with surgery for ovarian cystic masses, 61 required a laparotomy and in about 42 of these the laparotomy was necessary due to dense adhesions.[11] In a smaller series reported by Perry and Upchurch, 6 of 23 patients who underwent pelviscopic adnexectomy required a laparotomy to complete the surgery due to inability to free the adnexa or to visualize the ureter.[31] If bowel injuries occur, they may be repaired laparoscopically in some cases (see Chapters 20, 21, and 22), but often they require a laparotomy.

Ureteral injury also represents a significant risk during adnexectomy; in fact, adnexectomy is one of the most common causes of operative injury to the ureter. A published review of 5 years of experience with gynecology-related ureteral injuries particularly illustrates this point.[32] Ureteral injuries occurred in 1.5% of gynecologic operations over the period 1980–85 at two teaching hospitals (16 injuries in 1093 cases). One injury occurred at laparoscopy and 15 at laparotomy. Seventy-five percent (12 of 16) of the ureteral injuries occurred at the pelvic brim with adnexectomy (Fig. 18.20). These injuries were related to dense adhesions in 10 of the 12 cases. The adhesions were due to ovarian retention syndrome after previous hysterectomies in eight cases, endometriosis in one case, and endometrial cancer in one case. Although most of these cases occurred during laparotomy, it is probable that as more experience is obtained with similarly complicated adnexectomies done laparoscopically, the complication rates will be comparable.

Particular risk factors for ureteral injury during adnexal surgery are:

- Previous operation in the pelvis.
- Distorted anatomy at the pelvic sidewall and pelvic brim.
- Removal of the adnexa remaining after a prior hysterectomy.
- Removal of an ovarian neoplasm.
- Intraoperative hemorrhage at the pelvic brim.

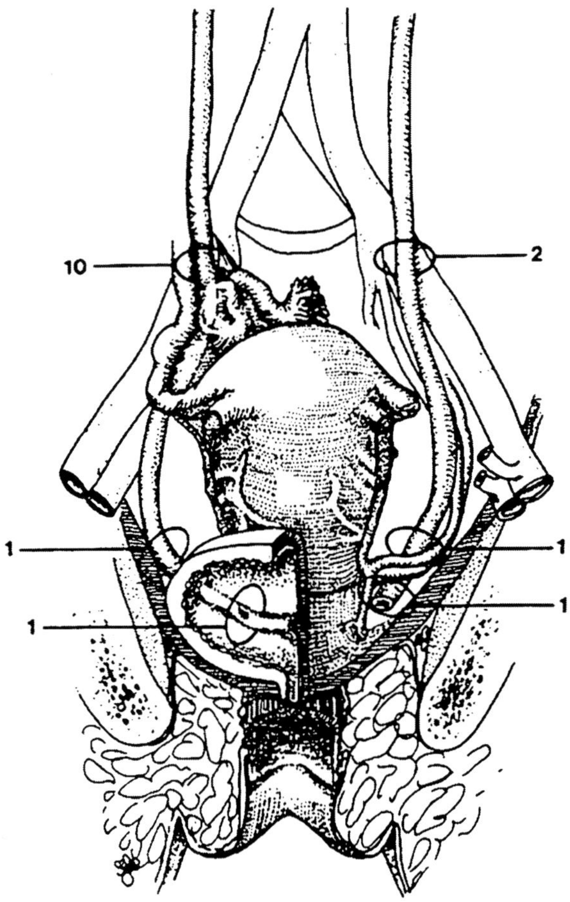

Figure 18.20. Sites of 16 ureteral injuries during gynecologic surgery. The numbers represent the actual number of injuries at each site. (Adapted from Ref. 32.)

In all cases the ureter should be clearly identified as free of the surgical field, but especially so with any of these risk factors. Sometimes this can be accomplished by transperitoneal visualization. However, if because of fibrosis, scarring, or obesity this is not possible, then the lateral pelvic peritoneum should be opened and the ureter surgically identified. This advice is particularly crucial in cases of bleeding at the pelvic brim. Positive identification of the ureter and the bleeding point must be obtained before cautery, clips, or sutures are placed.

Published series of laparoscopic adnexectomies with details about complications are few. Daniell et al. reported their experience with 65 difficult cases but had only two complications, both inferior epigastric artery lacerations that were treated with pressure using insertion of a Foley balloon to tamponade the vessels.[29] Perry and Upchurch reported 10 complications (43%) in 23 patients who underwent laparoscopy for adnexal pathology.[31] Six of the complications were simply conversions to laparotomies due to inability to free the adnexa or to visualize the ureter. The other complications, one each, were pain of 2 weeks' duration postoperatively, hemorrhage postoperatively requiring transfusion (reported as two complications), and urinary retention. Smith et al. report the experience of 42 surgeons performing 11 ovarian cystectomies, 8 oophorectomies, and 11 salpingo-oophorectomies.[2] There were five complications (17%) in this series: two borderline tumors that required laparotomy, one abdominal wall hematoma; one case in which they could not retrieve the ovary; one case of technical difficulty with an endoscopic stapler; and one unplanned hospitalization for fever and ileus postoperatively. From the experience reported so far, most of the complications with laparoscopic adnexectomies are laparoscopy specific, not procedure specific or laparoscopic procedure specific. In spite of that, with the known experience with difficult adnexectomies via laparotomy, all patients should be counseled about the potential for either bowel or ureteral injury, or significant bleeding complications, with laparoscopic oophorolysis and oophorectomy.

Another complication reported with laparoscopic surgery for malignant adnexal masses is tumor implantation at the trocar insertion site.[33–35] Currently, Childers et al. have reported data that allow the best estimate of the potential for this complication.[36] Retrospectively, they reviewed 105 laparoscopic procedures (96 patients) for intraperitoneal or retroperitoneal cancer at the University of Arizona from November 1990 to February 1994. These 105 procedures used 437 different trocar or Veress needle punctures. One patient developed abdominal wall tumor implantation. This occurred after a second-look laparoscopy for stage IIa, grade 3 serous papillary adenocarcinoma of the ovary with grossly negative findings but positive peritoneal washings and positive peritoneal biopsies. From these data, the estimated risk of abdominal wall tumor implantation is 0.2% per puncture site and 1.0% per procedure. Based on these data and other case reports, Childers et al. draw the following conclusions regarding abdominal wall tumor implantation:

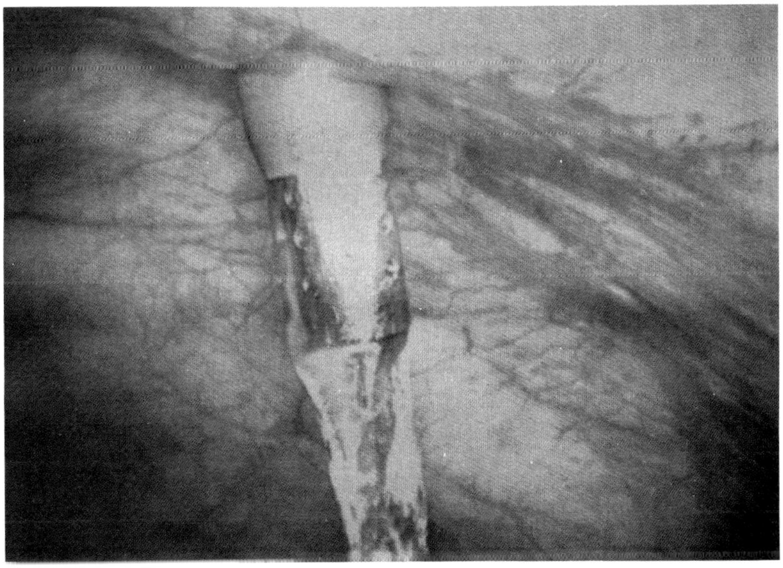

Figure 18.21. Laparoscopic port sites can be irrigated using the 5-mm irrigator-aspirator to decrease the risk of tumor metastases at the site. First, the instrument is placed into the laparoscopic sleeve and irrigation is started. (From Ref. 36.)

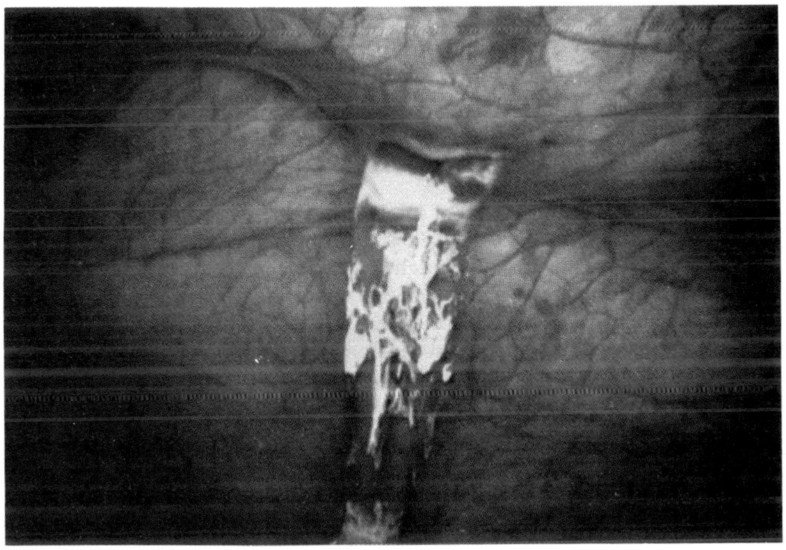

Figure 18.22. (Continued from Figure 18.21) As the port sleeve is withdrawn from the abdomen, irrigation is continued, forcing irrigation fluid into the abdominal cavity.

- Implantation can occur at any abdominal puncture site.
- Implantation has occurred only with adenocarcinoma but may involve any grade thereof.
- Ascites is not necessary for implantation.
- Abdominal wall implantation generally appears to grow rapidly and is recognized promptly.
- Implantation can occur with nonovarian malignancies (e.g., gastric, gallbladder, pancreatic).

Childers et al. make the following recommendations to decrease the likelihood of abdominal wall implantation of tumor:

- Irrigate all abdominal wall puncture sites (Figs. 18.21 and 18.22).
- Reexamine all patients within 2–3 weeks postoperatively.
- Excise any implantation sites promptly, as they appear to grow rapidly.

MYOMECTOMY

Indications for Surgery

Surgery for leiomyomas may be indicated for:

- Pelvic pain.
- Abnormal bleeding.
- Rapidly increasing tumor size.
- Infertility.[37]

Obviously, in younger women desiring preservation of fertility, myomectomy is preferred to hysterectomy. When fertility is not an issue, it is not clear whether morbidity with myomectomy is less than with hysterectomy or whether myomectomy has any advantages over hysterectomy (laparoscopic hysterectomy is discussed in Chapter 17). However, if a woman prefers to avoid hysterectomy, for whatever reason, myomectomy is usually a medically acceptable alternative. If hysteroscopic myomectomy for submucosal leiomyomas is compared to abdominal hysterectomy, the morbidity of the endoscopic procedure appears to be much less. Clearly, when medically indicated, hysteroscopic myomectomy is preferable to hysterectomy.

Because of the technical difficulties sometimes associated with laparoscopic myometocomy, Parker and Rodi have tried to determine if preoperative evaluations can predict successful treatment.[37] They suggest the following contraindications to attempted laparoscopic myomectomy:

- Myomas adjacent to the uterine vessels.
- Myomas with submucous extension.
- Total uterine size larger than 14 weeks' gestation.
- Individual myoma larger than 7 cm.
- Myoma in proximity to the tubal cornua if fertility is desired.
- Less than 50% of the myoma is subserosal.

These contraindications can be ascertained by clinical examination, ultrasound, magnetic resonance imaging, and laparoscopic visualization. Using these criteria, Parker and Rodi prospectively selected 19 of 41 patients who were considered appropriate for laparoscopic myomectomy, and all 19 had successful laparoscopic myomectomies. The contraindications in their patients were as follows: more than 50% intramural extension, eight; submucous myomas and had hysteroscopic resection, two; individual myomas greater than 8 cm or uterine size greater than 14 weeks' gestation even after gonadotropin-releasing hormone agonist (GnRHa), six; elected hysterectomy during GnRHa therapy, two; laparoscopy showed myoma over uterine vessels, one; laparoscopy showed myoma beneath the tubal cornua, one; and more than 50% intramural component of myoma, two.

It is not clear whether myomectomy for infertility should be done laparoscopically. Evidence is not currently available to show that pregnancy rates after laparoscopic myomectomy are similar to those after open myomectomy. Concerns have been voiced even by ardent supporters of laparoscopic surgery that the repair of the uterus after laparoscopic myomectomy is inferior, leading to significant adhesive disease and incomplete uterine healing.[38] Obviously, these problems could decrease successful establishment of fertility and could lead to uterine rupture with any subsequent pregnancy.

Surgical Techniques

Preoperative treatment for 3 months with GnRHa may be helpful with endoscopic myomectomy. If the patient has bleeding and anemia, several months of GnRHa treatment generally stops the bleeding and allows reestablishment of a normal hemoglobin level (Fig. 18.23).[39] If the uterus is more than 16 weeks' gestation in size, its volume may decrease by 30–50% (Fig. 18.24). This may allow a faster, easier myomectomy and decrease intraoperative blood loss.[40]

Intraoperatively, many techniques have been utilized. For pedunculated myomas, the simplest technique is bipolar coagulation of the stalk, followed by transection at the uterine junction with scissors, electrocautery, or laser. Small bleeders can be controlled with cautery or laser, and repair is usually not necessary.

Subserosal and intramural leiomyomas are more difficult. Five to 10 cc of dilute vasopressin can be injected at the base of each myoma to decrease deep myometrial bleeding, but this is not without risk. Another 3 to 5 cc of dilute vasopressin can also be injected at the capsule where the incision into the uterus and myoma is planned. One 1-cc ampule of vasopressin (20 units) in 100 cc of lactated Ringer's or another electrolyte solution appears to give adequate potency to decrease bleeding. Many surgeons choose not to use vasopressin. Other options are use of an endocoagulator, unipolar current, or bipolar current to decrease bleeding at the incision site. A longitudinal or vertical incision is made using either electrical or laser

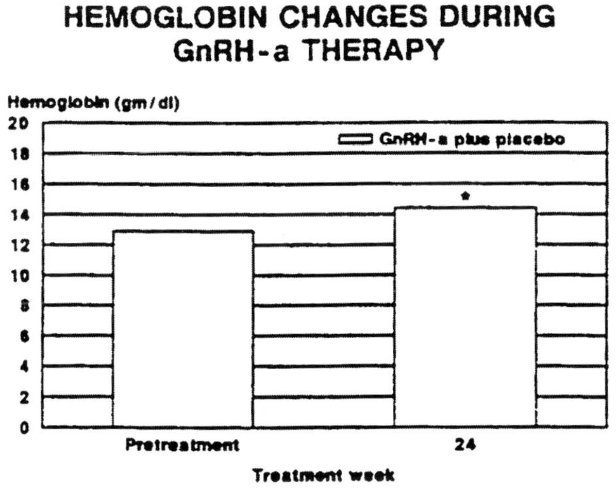

Figure 18.23. Significant hemoglobin elevations can be achieved with GnRHa therapy for 3 to 6 months. This may improve the patient's preoperative status. (From Ref. 50.)

energy. A laparoscopic knife may be used instead, but this is uncommon in the United States. The actual instrument to deliver cutting electrical current is a matter of personal preference and is usually a needle electrode, spatula, or scissors tip. The laser preference also varies, but carbon dioxide, KTP, and argon are the most commonly used. Enucleation of the myoma is not dissimilar to the methods used at laparotomy, but manipulation of the myoma may be difficult and is greatly aided by the use of a laparoscopic myoma screw. Bleeding is best prevented, if possible, with endocoagulation or cautery. Significant bleeding deep in the bed of a leiomyoma can be very difficult to control laparoscopically. Both closure and nonclosure of the defects created by myomectomy have been evaluated. When no closure is done, notable indentations and persistent patency of the defects have been observed, suggesting poor healing. Uterine dehiscence with subsequent pregnancy has been reported. When closure is done, it is generally difficult and less meticulous than that accomplished microsurgically at laparotomy. Severe adhesions have been observed at second-look procedures after laparoscopic suturing.

Intraligamentous leiomyomas are removed much as described for intramural myomas, with the caveat that the ureters, bladder, and major pelvic vessels must be identified and protected from injury. Submusocal leiomyomas are best removed hysteroscopically, not laparoscopically.

Several methods can be used to remove myomas from the abdominal cavity after their excision from the uterus. Often a culdotomy or colpotomy is done. This allows removal of fairly large leiomyomas without the need for morcellation, but very large tumors may still require vaginal morcellation to permit extraction. Additionally, the culdotomy or colpotomy can lengthen the surgical time and increase potential morbidity due to infection or rectal injury. Smaller leiomyomas can be removed without morcellation through a minilaparotomy incision, but this detracts from the minimally invasive advantages of laparoscopy. Intra-

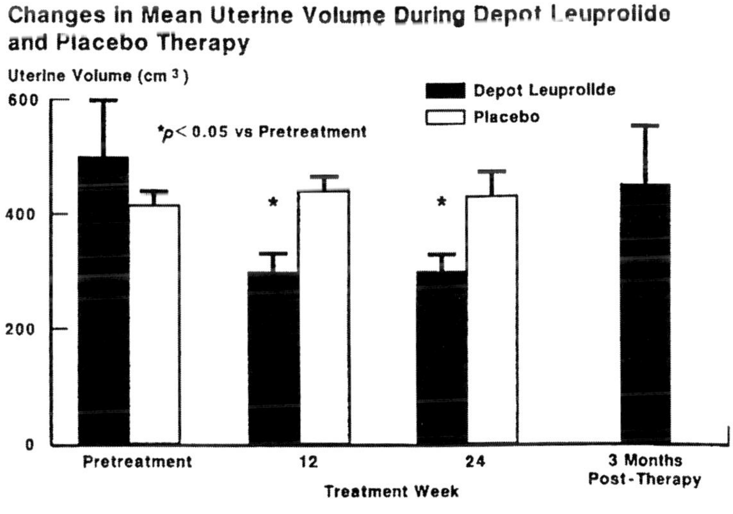

Figure 18.24. GnRHa treatment significantly reduces uterine size in women with leiomyomas. However, return to pretreatment size occurs after discontinuation of treatment. (From Ref. 39.)

abdominal morcellation can be done to allow extraction via a 12- to 15-mm port. The serrated edge macromorcellator (SEMM) is a particularly useful instrument for this procedure and allows fairly rapid morcellation of even large myomas. Clearly, as can be noted by the operative times given in Table 18.7, laparoscopic myomectomy can be challenging and time-consuming.

A new laparoscopic technique for the treatment of leiomyomas is myoma coagulation or myolysis, performed with the Nd:YAG laser or with bipolar needle electrical energy. With this operation too, pretreatment with GnRHa may facilitate the procedure. At surgery the myoma is drilled with either the Nd:YAG fiber or the bipolar needle and coagulated (Fig. 18.25). The coagulation usually extends to a diameter of about 5 mm round the needle or fiber. A 5-cm myoma may require 50 to 75 punctures. Preoperative evaluation with sonography, hysteroscopy, and endometrial biopsy is important. If the patient has significant uterine bleeding abnormalities, an endometrial ablation may also be needed. Intraoperatively, care must be taken to protect the rectum, bladder, and uterine vessels. Initial results with this method seem promising. Tumor regression by 50% or more is usually obtained. Regrowth has not yet been observed. A major limitation is that this technique is not recommended for women who wish to preserve fertility, as uterine cavity shrinking and adhesions may occur.[41] In fact, based on second-look laparoscopy, it appears that most women develop severe bowel or omental adhesions to the myolysis site postoperatively.[42] An advantage of myolysis over myomectomy may be the shorter surgery time. For example, in one reported series of 48 cases, myolysis required only 20 to 45 minutes, which is noticeably shorter than the usual operative times for laparoscopic myomectomy (Table 18.7).

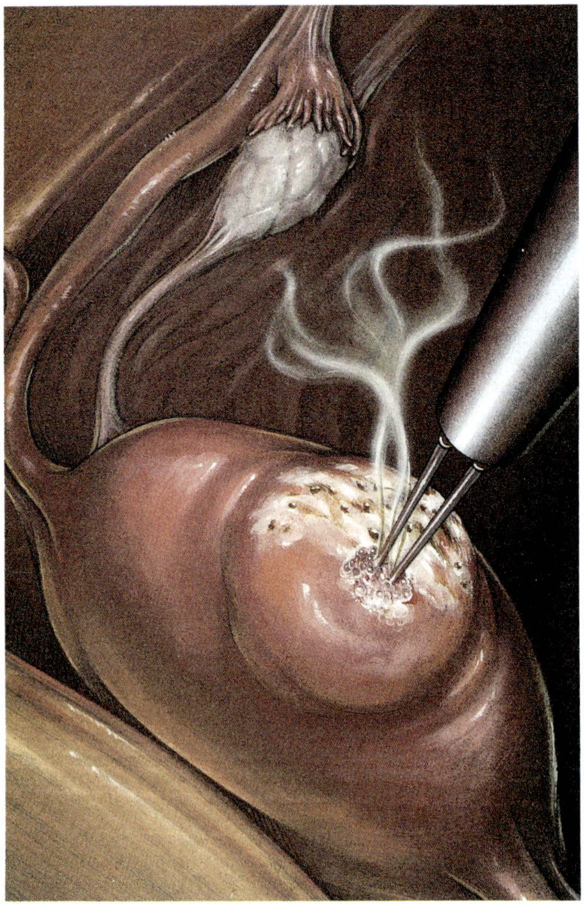

Figure 18.25. Myolysis with the bipolar needle for laparoscopic treatment of leiomyomata uteri. (From Ref. 41.)

Recurrences have not been reported with either laparoscopic myomectomy or myolysis after up to 4 years of follow-up. There is no reason to expect the recurrence rate to be any different from the 10-year 20–30% rate with myomectomy via laparotomy.[43]

Complications

Excessive blood loss and transfusions have been the major complications reported with laparoscopic myomectomy. This is a procedure-specific complication related to myomectomy, probably occurring with similar frequency at the time of abdominal myomectomy.[44] It does not appear that the laparoscopic approach increases the occurrence of this complication. In Parker and Rodi's series, 2 of 19 women with laparoscopic myomectomies required transfusion of autologous blood due to intraoperative blood loss. In Nezhat's et al.'s series, 2 of 154 women required transfusions. Other series of laparoscopic myomectomies have not reported the need for transfusions. (Table 18.7).

The technical difficulty of retrieving myomas after laparoscopic myomectomy, although not a complication per se, does complicate the performance of the procedure. This may have been the cause of the five cases of abdominal wall ecchymosis and one case of postoperatively recognized inferior epigastric artery laceration that occurred in the 154 cases reported by Nezhat et al. It also appears to be the major reason

Table 18.7. Data on Laparoscopic Myomectomy and Myolysis

	Nezhat[38]	Daniell[46]	Dubuisson[47]	Hasson[45]	Parker[37]	Nisolle[42]
Procedure	Myomectomy	Myomectomy	Myomectomy	Myomectomy	Myomectomy	Myolysis
Size of myomas (cm)	2–15	3–7	1–11	3–16	5–7 cm	3–8
Operative time (min)	50–190	30–180	25–240	45–443	60–270 min	20–45
Blood loss	10–600	5–200	—	10–400	50–750 ml	<50
Hospital stay	7–48	<24	24–96	<24–96	3–96 hrs	≤24
Return to normal activity	—	—	—	—	3–14 days	—
Complications	4	0	0	4	2	0
Number of patients	154	17	43	56	19	48

for the long operative times needed for laparoscopic myomectomies. In addition to the previously mentioned SEMM instrument, the "orange-peel" technique used by Hasson et al. may help to speed morcellation and retrieval of large myomas without the need to do culdotomy, colpotomy, or minilaparotomy[45] (Fig. 18.26).

Another complication of laparoscopic myomectomy is the severity of adhesions formed postoperatively. Adhesions to the myomectomy site are observed in more than one-half of the patients and appear to be worse if suture repair of the uterine defect is done. In Nezhat's et al.'s series, 17 of 19 cases with suturing of the defect had severe adhesions at the time of second-look laparoscopy or laparotomy.[38] They suggested that placing Interceed over the myomectomy site may decrease adhesions, but no data were presented. In Daniell and Gurley's series, the one patient in whom Interceed was used had severe adhesions at second-look laparoscopy.[46] Although the long-term sequelae of adhesions are difficult to predict, this approach seems contraindicated in cases with infertility as the primary indication for surgery. With improved techniques and adhesion barriers this situation may improve, but evidence supporting such improvement has not yet been published. The pregnancy rate in the series from Hasson et al., with 12 of 17 women with infertility conceiving during the 2–36 months of follow-up after laparoscopic myomectomy, is higher than that of other series.[45] The authors did second-look procedures in 21 of their 56 myomectomy cases; it is difficult to discern whether this improved their pregnancy rate. Eleven of the 21 women were found to have severe adhesions at the time of second-look surgery. Nezhat et al. had only 6 of 38 infertile patients with myomectomies become pregnant during 3 months to 3 years of follow-up.[38] Dubuisson et al. had only 3 pregnancies in 21 infertile patients after laparoscopic myomectomy (the duration of follow-up was not specified).[47] Further concerns about performing laparoscopic myomectomies in infertility patients are raised by a report of uterine dehiscence after this procedure.[48]

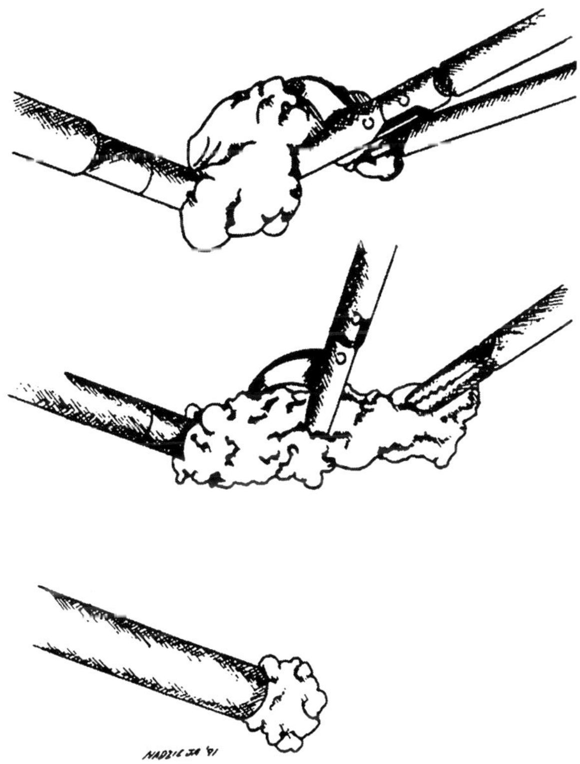

Figure 18.26. Converting a myoma into a narrow strip with the orange-peel technique to allow removal from the abdomen via laparoscopic ports. (From Ref. 45.)

This patient, who conceived 3 months after a laparoscopic myomectomy, had a 3-cm uterine dehiscence that presented with severe hemorrhage at 34 weeks' gestation. There was no premature rupture of membranes, and the infant did well except for respiratory distress syndrome. The laparoscopic myomectomy may have extended into the endometrial cavity, but this was unclear. At the time of the laparoscopic myomectomy, the uterus was repaired with 4–0 polyglycolic suture.

Although vasopressin is commonly used and has been shown to decrease intraoperative blood loss with myomectomies,[49] it is not without risk. For example, Nezhat et al. report a case of severe hypotension and bradycardia secondary to left ventricular hypokinesis with decreased cardiac output and a reduced cardiac index after a uterine injection of vasopressin. After complete recovery, laparoscopic myomectomy was again attempted without vasopressin and without complication.[50] Vasopressin is not FDA approved for local injection as it is used at laparoscopy. Approved indications are prevention and treatment of postoperative abdominal distention, in abdominal roengenography to dispel interfering gas shadows, and in diabetes insipidus. If vasopressin is to be used for endoscopic surgery, it should be used in dilute solution (e.g., 20 units in 60–100 mL of normal saline) and sparingly (e.g., 3–5 mL per injection). Additionally, care should be taken to avoid intravascular injection.

Other complications that have been reported after laparoscopic myomectomy have not been serious. Some examples are subcutaneous emphysema, febrile morbidity, intraperitoneal loss of a small myoma, abdominal wall ecchymoses, and superficial wound infections.

CONCLUSION

It must be recognized that as more complicated surgical procedures are done via laparoscopic incisions, the complication rates of laparoscopy will increase. This trend is demonstrated by the 1988–93 data from the American Association of Gynecologic Laparoscopists (Table 18.8). Although at first review these data appear disquieting, they do not represent a worsening of clinical practice as more surgeons utilize operative laparoscopy, nor are they an indictment of laparoscopy itself. Had there been a similar historical progression for laparotomy, without doubt the same complication trends would have been noted as laparotomy progressed from a diagnostic procedure to a sterilization procedure to an operative procedure. Again alluding to the previously proposed classification of complications, to the inherent risk of *laparotomy-specific complications* would have been added the risks of *procedure-specific complications* and *laparotomy procedure-specific complications*. This, of course, never happened with laparotomy. However, with gynecologic laparoscopy in the United States, this has been well documented as laparoscopy has gone from a diagnostic to a sterilization to an operative procedure. It has been shown that operative laparoscopy adds to the baseline rate of laparoscopy-specific complications, the rate of procedure-specific complications, and the rate of laparoscopic procedure-specific complications.

The challenge with current laparoscopic procedures, and as new procedures develop in the future, is to evaluate them critically, especially with regard to complications, to ensure that the risk to patients is not

Table 18.8. Complications Associated with Operative Laparoscopy by AAGL Members in 1988–93

Complication	1993 Rate/1000	1991 Rate/1000	1988 Rate/1000
Hospital readmission	5.2	4.2	3.2
Unintended laparotomy	13.6	8.9	5.9
Hemorrhage	12.8	6.8	2.6
Transfusion for hemorrhage	5.1	2.7	NA
Bowel or urinary tract injury	8.9	2.8	1.6
Nerve injury	0.5	0.5	0.5
Death	0	1.8/100,000	NA

Source: Refs. 10 and 54.

increased. It appears that the rate of laparoscopy-specific complications is generally less than the rate of laparotomy-specific complications. Procedure-specific complications are by definition not different for different incisional approaches. The crux of the challenge, then, is to elucidate laparoscopic procedure-specific complication rates compared to laparotomy procedure-specific or vaginotomy procedure-specific complication rates. This can only be done by treating new surgical procedures and approaches as what they are—research. If this is done, it means adhering to the ethical principle of telling the patient of the inherent uncertainty of the outcome of the new procedure. It also means that sufficient record keeping and reporting are done to allow objective evaluation. In some cases, this will mean a specific research protocol that allows epidemiologically valid means of analysis. As can be seen from the scarcity of scientifically valid publications referenced in this chapter, this has not yet been done for many laparoscopic procedures. For example, it is not known if the laparoscopy-specific technique of using a stapler-cutter on the infundibulopelvic ligament at salpingo-oophorectomy has fewer or more complications than using suture, as is traditionally done at laparotomy. Nor is it known if rupturing a malignant cyst at the time of laparoscopic ovarian cystectomy worsens the prognosis compared to intact cystectomy or inadvertent rupture at laparotomy. Although the history of medicine is one of trial and error, this is no longer acceptable on a widespread basis. The ability exists to evaluate new treatments and technologies before they are universally applied. It is each practitioner's responsibility, as much as possible, to be sure that such evaluations are done before he or she incorporates a new treatment into daily practices so that epidemics of iatrogenic complications are avoided.

REFERENCES

1. Grimes DA: Frontiers of operative laparoscopy: A review and critique of the evidence. *Am J Obstet Gynecol* 166:1062–1071, 1992.
2. Smith DC, Donohue LR, Waszak SJ: A hospital review of advanced gynecologic endoscopic procedures. *Am J Obstet Gynecol* 170:1635–1642, 1994.
3. Maiman M, Seltzer V, Boyce J: Laparoscopic excision of ovarian neoplasms subsequently found to be malignant. *Obstet Gynecol* 77:563–565, 1991.
4. Canis M, Mage G, Pouly JL, et al: Laparoscopic diagnosis of adnexal cystic masses: A 12-year experience with long-term follow-up. *Obstet Gynecol* 83:707–712, 1994.
5. Dembo AJ, Davy M, Stenwig AE, et al: Prognostic factors in patients with stage I epithelial ovarian cancer. *Obstet Gynecol* 75:263–273, 1990.
6. de la Cuesta RS, Goff BA, Fuller AF, et al: Prognostic importance of intraoperative rupture of malignant ovarian epithelial neoplasma. *Obstet Gynecol* 84:1–7, 1994.
7. Nezhat F, Nezhat C, Welander CE, et al: Four ovarian cancers diagnosed during laparoscopic management of 1011 women with adnexal masses. *Am J Obstet Gynecol* 167:790–796, 1992.
8. Trimbos J, Schueler J, van Lent M, et al: Reasons for incomplete staging in early ovarian carcinoma. *Gynecol Oncol* 37:374–377, 1990.
9. Hurd WH, Bude R, DeLancey JOL, et al: Abdominal wall characterization with magnetic resonance imaging and computed tomography. The effect of obesity on the laparoscopic approach. *J Reprod Med* 36:473–476, 1991.
10. Levy BS, Hulka JF, Peterson HB, et al: Operative laparoscopy: American Association of Gynecologic Laparoscopists, 1993 membership survey. *J Am Assoc Gynecol Laparosc* 1:301–305, 1994.
11. Mage G, Canis M, Manhes H, et al: Laparoscopic management of adnexal cystic masses. *J Gynecol Surg* 6:71–79, 1990.
12. Deckardt R, Saks M, Graeff H: Comparison of minimally invasive surgery and laparotomy in the treatment of adnexal masses. *J Am Assoc Gynecol Laparosc* 1:333–338, 1994.
13. Parker WH, Levine RL, Howard FM, et al: A multicenter study of laparoscopic management of selected cystic adnexal masses in postmenopausal women. *J Am Coll Surg* 179:733–737, 1994.
14. Moran O, Menczer J, Ben-Baruch G, et al: Cytologic examination of ovarian cyst fluid for the distinction between benign and malignant tumors. *Obstet Gynecol* 82:444–446, 1993.
15. Lipitz S, Seidman DS, Menczer J, et al: Recurrence rate after fluid aspiration from sonographically benign-appearing ovarian cysts. *J Reprod Med* 37:845–848, 1992.
16. Shalev E, Peleg D: Laparoscopic treatment of adnexal torsion. *Surg Gynecol Obstet* 176:448–450, 1993.
17. Garzarelli S, Mazzuca N: One laparoscopic puncture for treatment of ovarian cysts with adnexal torsion in early pregnancy. A report of two cases. *J Reprod Med* 39:985–986, 1994.
18. Shalev E, Rahav D, Romano S: Laparoscopic relief of adnexal torsion in early pregnancy. Case reports. *Br J Obstet Gynaecol* 97:853–854, 1990.
19. Bider D, Ben-Rafael Z, Goldenberg M, et al: Outcome of pregnancy after unwinding of ischemic hemorrhagic adnexum. *Br J Obstet Gynaecol* 96:428–431, 1989.
20. Wittich AC, Lockrow EG: Laparoscopic management of adnexal torsion in early pregnancy: A case report. *Milit Med* 159:254–255, 1994.

21. Howard FM, Vill M: Laparoscopic adnexal surgery during pregnancy. *J Am Assoc Gynecol Laparosc* 2:91–93, 1994.
22. Keil KH, Julian TM: Trichuria, pneumaturia, urosepsis, and bowel fistulization after pelviscopic cystectomy of a mature ovarian teratoma. *J Gynecol Surg* 9:235–239, 1993.
23. Rose PG, Rubin RB, Nelson BE, et al: Accuracy of frozen-section (intraoperative consultation) diagnosis of ovarian tumors. *Am J Obstet Gynecol* 171:823–826, 1994.
24. Herbst AL: Neoplastic diseases of the ovary. In Herbst AL, Mishell DR, Stenchever MA, et al (eds): *Comprehensive Gynecology*. St Louis, Mosby Year Book, 1992, pp 937–988.
25. Reich H, McGlynn F, Sekel L, et al: Laparoscopic management of ovarian dermoid cysts. *J Reprod Med* 37:640–644, 1992.
26. Nezhat C, Winer WK, Nezhat F: Laparoscopic removal of dermoid cysts. *Obstet Gynecol* 73:278–291, 1989.
27. Howard FM: Surgical management of patients with benign cystic teratoma: Laparoscopy versus laparotomy. *J Reprod Med* 40:495–499, 1995.
28. Albini SM, Benadiva CA, Haverly K, et al: Management of benign ovarian cystic teratomas: Laparoscopy compared with laparotomy. *J Am Assoc Gynecol Laparosc* 3:219–222, 1994.
29. Daniell JF, Kurtz BR, Lee JY: Laparoscopic oophorectomy: Comparative study of ligatures, bipolar coagulation, and automatic stapling devices. *Obstet Gynecol* 80: 325–328, 1972.
30. Nezhat F, Nezhat C: Operative laparoscopy for the treatment of ovarian remnant syndrome. *Fertil Steril* 57:1003–1007, 1992.
31. Perry CP, Upchurch JC: Pelviscopic adnexectomy. *Am J Obstet Gynecol* 162:79–81, 1990.
32. Daly JW, Higgins KA: Injury to the ureter during gynecologic surgical procedures. *Surg Gynecol Obstet* 167:19–22, 1988.
33. Hsiu JG, Given FT Jr, Kemp GM: Tumor implantation after diagnostic laparoscopic biopsy of serous ovarian tumors of low malignant potential. *Obstet Gynecol* 68: 90S–93S, 1986.
34. Miralles RM, Petit J, Gine L, et al: Metastatic cancer spread at the laparoscopic puncture site. Report of a case in a patient with carcinoma of the ovary. Case report. *Eur J Gynaecol Oncol* 10:442–444, 1989.
35. Stockdale AD, Pocock TJ: Abdominal wall metastasis following laparoscopy: A case report. *Euro J Surg Oncol* 11: 373–375, 1985.
36. Childers JE, Aqua KA, Surwit EA, et al: Abdominal-wall tumor implantation after laparoscopy for malignant conditions. *Obstet Gynecol* 84:765–769, 1994.
37. Parker WH, Rodi IA: Patient selection for laparoscopic myomectomy. *J Am Assoc Gynecol Laparosc* 2:23–26, 1994.
38. Nezhat C, Nezhat F, Silfen SL, et al: Laparoscopic myomectomy. *Int J Fertil* 36:275–280, 1991.
39. Friedman AJ, Fine C, Barbieri RL, et al: A randomized, double-blind trial of a gonadotropin releasing-hormone agonist (leuprolide) with or without medroxyprogesterone acetate in the treatment of leiomyomata uteri. *Fertil Steril* 49:404–409, 1988.
40. Friedman AJ, Garfield JM, Rein MS, et al: A randomized, placebo-controlled, double-blind study evaluating leuprolide acetate depot treatment before myomectomy. *Fertil Steril* 52:728–733, 1989.
41. Goldfarb HA: Removing uterine fibroids laparoscopically. *Contemp Ob/Gyn* 50–72, 1994.
42. Nisolle M, Smets M, Malvaux V, et al: Laparoscopic myolysis with the Nd:YAG laser. *J Gynecol Surg* 9:95–99, 1993.
43. Candiani GB, Fedele L, Parazzini F, et al: Risk of recurrence after myomectomy. *Br J Obstet Gynaecol* 98: 385–389, 1991.
44. LaMorte A, Lalwani S, Diamond MP: Morbidity associated with abdominal myomectomy. *Obstet Gynecol* 82: 897–900, 1993.
45. Hasson HM, Rotman C, Rana N, et al: Laparoscopic myomectomy. *Obstet Gynecol* 80:884–888, 1992.
46. Daniell JF, Gurley LD: Laparoscopic treatment of clinically significant symptomatic uterine fibroids. *J Gynecol Surg* 7:37–40, 1991.
47. Dubuisson JB, Mandelbrot L, Lecuru F, et al: Myomectomy by laparoscopy: A preliminary report of 43 cases. *Fertil Steril* 56:827–830, 1991.
48. Harris WJ: Uterine dehiscence following laparoscopic myomectomy. *Obstet Gynecol* 80:545–546, 1992.
49. Frederick J, Fletcher H, Simeon D, et al: Intramyometrial vasopressin as a haemostatic agent during myomectomy. *Br J Obstet Gynaecol* 101:435–437, 1994.
50. Nezhat F, Admon D, Nezhat C, et al: Life-threatening hypotension after vasopressin injection during operative laparoscopy, followed by uneventful repeat laparoscopy. *J Am Assoc Gynecol Laparosc* 2:83–85, 1994.
51. Cohen MR, Scoccia B: Double laparoscopy: An alternative two-stage procedure to minimize bowel and blood vessel injury. *J Gynecol Surg* 7:203–206, 1991.
52. Nezhat CR, Nezhat FR, Luciano AA, et al: *Operative Gynecologic Laparoscopy. Principles and Techniques*. New York, McGraw-Hill, 1995.
53. Parker WH: Laparoscopic management of ovarian cysts. *Contemp Ob/Gyn* 47–58, 1991.
54. Hulka JF, Peterson HB, Phillips JM, et al: Operative laparoscopy. American Association of Gynecologic Laparoscopists 1991 membership survey. *J Reprod Med* 38:569–573, 1993.

section five

Surgery of the Gastrointestinal Tract

chapter nineteen

Laparoscopic Appendectomy: Avoiding Complications

Eddie Joe Reddick
Michael O'Reilly
William B. Saye

Appendectomy was first performed just over a century ago,[1] and except for a few minor variations, it is still performed much the same way as it was then. In 1983, Kurt Semm[2] offered an alternative method to appendiceal removal by utilizing a laparoscope for visualization and minimally invasive techniques for the mobilization and removal of the organ. The early appendiceal removals were for nonacute disease, usually associated with gynecologic procedures. In 1987 Schrieber[3] reported the first removal for acute appendicitis utilizing laparoscopic techniques. A few scattered reports of laparoscopic appendectomies followed,[4,5] but it was not until the introduction of laparoscopic cholecystectomy[6,7] that general surgeons became adept enough with the equipment to begin performing these operations with more regularity.[8,9]

Laparoscopic access has very definite advantages in cholecystectomy[10] since it changes a large upper abdominal incision which transects major muscle groups and causes considerable postoperative pain into an operation with three to five incisions measuring 1-cm or less which are muscle splitting and create minimal pain. Patients with less pain recover more quickly, leading to shorter hospital stays and a faster return to activities. Fortunately, most cholecystectomies are performed electively for nonacute disease.

Appendectomy, on the other hand, is usually performed for acute disease as an emergency operation. When it is performed using an open technique, a small muscle-splitting incision in the lower abdomen is utilized, minimal pain is encountered, the hospital stay is usually short, and patients are not usually debilitated for long periods. The obvious advantages of the laparoscopic approach, as demonstrated by laparoscopic cholecystectomy, are less evident with laparoscopic appendectomy. The average hospital stay after an open operation for acute appendicitis is 2.8 days compared to 2.0 days after a laparoscopic appendectomy.[8] This difference is even less pronounced with a ruptured appendix or appendiceal abscess since most patients require parenteral antibiotics after operations for these diseases, regardless of the operative approach.

Laparoscopic evaluation of right lower quadrant pain does have some definite diagnostic advantages, however. The diagnosis of appendicitis is in doubt 20% of the time. This has led to the use of many nonspecific tests for diagnosis prior to surgery,[11] including barium enema,[12] computed tomography,[13] ultrasound,[14,15] Meckel's scan, and repeated white blood cell counts and chemistries.[16] This, in turn, has led to expensive extra hospital inpatient days, delays in diagnosis, and escalated laboratory expenses. Laparoscopy can be used in lieu of these expensive and delaying tests to confirm or refute the diagnosis.[17] As an added benefit, laparoscopy can be used to treat most pathologies causing right lower abdominal pain. Ovarian cysts, tubo-ovarian abscesses, endometriosis, Meckel's diverticulum, perforated peptic ulcer, obturator and inguinal hernias, torsed ovaries, and tubal pregnancies have been successfully treated with laparoscopy. Laparoscopy can facilitate the diagnosis of diverticular disease, Crohn's disease, mesenteric adenitis, and retroperitoneal diseases of the pelvis. Laparoscopic exploration eliminates the need for extensions of right lower quadrant incisions when the diagnosis of appendicitis is in error.

Laparoscopic appendectomy has been associated with a lower wound infection rate in several series when compared to the open technique, with some series reporting no wound infection.[18,19] In a properly performed operation, the appendix never touches the skin, subcutaneous tissue, or the muscle and fascial layers.[20] It is either pulled into a trocar or, more recently, placed in a plastic bag prior to removal,[21] eliminating any contamination as it is pulled through the abdominal wall.

Theoretically, the surgeon should be able to visualize the abdominal cavity better with laparoscopy and laparoscopy should allow for better irrigation and suctioning of remaining debris in the peritoneal cavity. However, there is no convincing evidence that laparoscopic appendectomy has a lower incidence of postoperative intraabdominal infection than does open appendectomy, each ranging from 0-20% in selected series.[21–23]

Appendectomy performed laparoscopically can be much more cosmetically pleasing then open appendectomy when the trocars are properly placed. Although various trocar locations have been utilized, the most aesthetic method utilizes a trocar in the umbilicus for the camera, a 10- or 12-mm trocar in the midline, 2 cm suprapubic but still below the hairline, and a 5-mm trocar in the hairline just lateral to the inferior epigastric vessels. Utilizing this trocar placement, all incisions are hidden either by the umbilicus or by the pubic hairline, giving essentially a scarless appendectomy. Other techniques which place the trocars outside the hairline have less cosmetic benefit.[20]

INDICATIONS

The indications for appendectomy have not changed with the introduction of laparoscopy. A patient with the classic symptoms should be resuscitated and taken immediately to the operating room. There is no accepted medical therapy for appendicitis.

Classic symptoms include localized right lower quadrant pain or epigastric or periumbilical pain rapidly migrating and localizing to the right lower quadrant over McBurney's point (a point 5 cm medial on a line drawn from the right anterior superior iliac spine to the umbilicus). Mild fever, an elevated white blood cell count with a left shift, nausea, and vomiting usually accompany the physical symptoms. High fever and a markedly elevated white blood cell count (above 16,000) usually point to another diagnosis. Over 90% of patients have a white blood cell count above 10,000, a left shift, or both. In 95% of cases, anorexia occurs. Examination reveals localized tenderness, rebound, and guarding over McBurney's point. Rectal exam may elicit tenderness on the right side. A psoas sign is evoked by having the patient lift the extended right leg against resistance by the surgeon. The obturator sign can be elicited by passive rotation of the right leg, with the patient lying supine and the knee and hip flexed. Both cause pain when an inflammatory process lies near the tested muscle. The single most valuable sign is localized tenderness.

Patients who present with classic symptoms should be fluid resuscitated and taken to the operating room for appendectomy shortly after admission. Although data suggest that most perforated appendices rupture prior to hospital admission, in-hospital delay may cause rupture and nothing is gained by delaying the operative intervention once the diagnosis is made.[24–26]

Patients who do not have classic symptoms pose more of a problem. Retrocecal appendicitis and pelvic appendicitis can alter the presentation of abdominal pain simply by their altered position. The retrocecal appendix is shielded from the abdominal wall by the cecum, thereby causing less tenderness to palpation and less pain overall. Rebound may be diminished due to its protected position. The pelvic appendix may cause left-sided pain and may be associated with the urge to urinate or defecate. The pelvic appendix may also cause pain on pelvic exam, mimicking gynecologic disease. Pain patterns may vary with a high cecum, a malrotated cecum, or an exceptionally long appendix, causing tenderness in an abdominal quadrant.

The pregnant patient has a baseline leukocytosis, and the enlarged uterus may displace the cecum and appendix, causing an abnormal pain presentation. Due to the reluctance to operate on a pregnant patient for fear of harming the fetus or causing premature labor, the pain of appendicitis may be mistakenly attributed to stretching of the uterine ligaments. Failure to make the diagnosis and give appropriate surgical therapy will almost certainly result in premature labor, possible miscarriage, and endangering of the mother's life.

Appendicitis in very young and very old patients may be difficult to diagnose. Elderly patients have minimal pain and minimal or no elevation of temperature. Children probably have classic symptoms, but these may be hard to elicit. Patients who are immunosuppressed or have the acquired immunodeficiency syndrome usually present with abdominal pain without leukocytosis.

The differential diagnosis includes many gynecologic diseases, gastrointestinal diseases, urinary tract disorders, and systemic diseases. Salpingitis usually does not produce the shift of pain seen in appendicitis; in addition vomiting is rare, the pain is bilateral, and the temperature is markedly elevated. The cervix may be tender on pelvic exam, and gram-negative intracellular diplococci may be seen on the vaginal smear. A ruptured ectopic pregnancy, a twisted ovarian cyst, and a rupture of an ovarian follicle (*Mitelschmerz*) may all cause sudden pain and may be difficult to differentiate from acute appendicitis. With a ruptured ectopic pregnancy, the patient may show signs of hypovolemic shock. Gastrointestinal symptoms are usually not prominent in any of these processes.

Mesenteric lymphadenitis may closely mimic appendicitis; however, there is usually no left shift. Diarrhea usually occurs with associated adenitis and pharyngitis. Headache, malaise, and myalgias may be present. Meckel's diverticulum cannot routinely be differentiated from appendicitis preoperatively, and diverticulitis, Crohn's disease, intestinal obstruction, perforated peptic ulcer, and cholecystitis closely mimic appendicitis.

Ureteral stones cause pain which radiates into the groin and causes little or no direct abdominal tenderness. Although red blood cells may frequently be found in the urine with appendicitis, they are copious with ureteral colic. Pyelonephritis demonstrates pyuria, urinary bacteria, and white blood cell casts. Pain is usually localized more in the flank and costovertebral angles.

TECHNIQUE

General endotracheal anesthesia is considered the anesthetic of choice for laparoscopic appendectomies. A nasogastric or orogastric tube is placed for gastric decompression, and a catheter is placed in the urinary bladder. A single dose of preoperative antibiotics covering colonic bacteria should be administered to decrease the chances of wound infection. If perforation or abscess is discovered, antibiotics should be continued for a full course after surgery and adjusted based on sensitivity.

Females should be placed in the low lithotomy position to facilitate examination and treatment if the diagnosis is in error and gynecologic pathology is discovered. Males may be placed supine. After standard preparation and draping, laparoscopic access is attained using either the open (Hasson technique)[22,23,27] or the closed technique with an insufflation needle. Since peritonitis may decrease intestinal mobility and make the bowel more friable, the open technique is preferred to decrease the chance of inadvertent intestinal puncture with either the Veress needle or the initial trocar. The use of the open technique also decreases the chances of a retroperitoneal vascular injury.

Once the abdomen has been entered by either technique, it should be insufflated with CO_2 to a pressure of 15 mmHg. A 10-mm trocar should be placed in the umbilicus after insufflation with a needle or a 10- or 12-mm Hasson trocar should be used. Removal of the inflamed appendix is facilitated by the use of a 12-mm trocar.

If the surgeon is using a stapling instrument to transect the appendix and mesentery, a 12-mm trocar should be placed in the midline 2 cm cephalad to the symphysis pubis below the hairline. If ties are being used to ligate the appendix, a 10-mm trocar is adequate in this position. A third trocar (5 mm) is placed in the right lower quadrant, just lateral to the inferior epigastric vessels below the hairline. This trocar set gives the most cosmetically pleasing result. Alternative sites for the right lower quadrant trocar, or for additional sites, include a 5-mm trocar midway between the umbilicus and the suprapubic trocars or in the right upper quadrant 4–6 cm below the costal margin in the midclavicular line. When using the intestinal stapler, some surgeons will place a 12-mm trocar in the right upper quadrant. This is as cosmetically unpleasing as the incision used for open surgery and should be avoided whenever possible.

The surgeon and the camera operator stand on the patient's left. The surgeon's right hand controls the dissecting and clipping instruments through the suprapubic port. The left hand controls the tip of the appendix through the 5-mm trocar in the right lower quadrant. The patient may be placed in a head-down position and rotated slightly to the left to facilitate exposure. An assistant other than the camera holder is usually not needed.

After initial evaluation of the trocar puncture sites, attention should be directed to the right lower quadrant to verify that the appendix is the offending organ. The appendix is located at the confluence of the tenaie coli and the ligament of Trieves (the sail-like, fatty projection from the distal ileum pointing to the base of the appendix). If the appendix is not the diseased organ, further search of the abdominal cavity can be completed laparoscopically. The uterus, ovaries, sigmoid colon, and retroperitoneal pelvic area can be examined by placing the patient in the steep Trendelenburg position, allowing the intestine to fall cephalad. In the female, pushing up on the uterus with an intravaginal sponge stick will allow posterior evaluation of the cul-de-sac and the sigmoid colon. The small intestine can be evaluated by identifying the ileocecal valve and tracing the intestine cephalad for 90 cm. This will identify a Meckel's diverticulum, which routinely occurs on the antimesenteric border 40–90 cm from the distal ileum. The examination may be continued to the ligament of Trietz if indicated. The bowel should be grasped gently when using regular graspers, prohibiting injury from their crushing jaws. Intestinal clamps, either Babcock or Allis clamps, may be utilized. To prevent crossing instruments during the small bowel examination, the bowel should be picked up with two instruments and examined. Then the distal clamp should be released and replaced where the proximal clamp is holding. The proximal clamp can then be moved more proximally.

The liver may be lifted with a fan retractor. Lifting with a 5-mm instrument may cause inadvertent puncture of the capsule, with resultant bleeding. If bleeding is encountered, it may be controlled with topical agents and/or pressure. To rule out perforated peptic ulcer, the anterior stomach wall can be visualized by retracting caudad on the greater curvature with a Babcock clamp.

The right colon can be mobilized to search for a retrocecal appendix. One of the teniae is grasped with the left hand through the right lower port and pushed cephalad, exposing the lateral peritoneal reflection. The reflection can be incised with scissors. There is minimal bleeding when only the peritoneum is incised, and all important structures (ureter, vessels) should be medial to this dissection.

If the appendix is the offending organ, it may be removed by clipping and tying or with a multifire stapling device. There is general concern about the cost of the stapler,[8,24,28] but when the base of the appendix is necrotic, the stapler can facilitate the procedure by allowing the surgeon to staple across the cecum above the necrotic base, eliminating the need for inversion of the stump. The stapler is also advantageous when the mesoappendix is markedly thickened and the vessels cannot be readily identified. The vascular stapler can be utilized to ligate and transect the mesoappendix.

With either technique, the appendix is grasped at its tip, with the surgeon's left hand through the right lower port. This places the mesoappendix on tension and allows easy dissection with the surgeon's right hand through the suprapubic port. When using the stapler, only enough dissection need be done to identify the mesoappendix, distal small bowel, and cecum. Individual vessels need not be dissected. The stapler is placed in the abdomen through the suprapubic port and placed across the mesoappendix (Fig. 19.1). It may require two applications of vascular (2.5-mm) staples to transect the entire mesoappendix. Larger staples should not be used since bleeding from small mesoappendiceal vessels may occur through them. If bleeding from the staple line does occur, a clip or stitch should be placed for control. Electrocautery should not be utilized since it may heat up the entire staple line and cause its necrosis.

Once the mesoappendix is controlled and divided, the appendix can be transected with the linear stapler utilizing 3.5-mm staples (Fig. 19.2). Smaller staples may tear the appendiceal base and cause leakage. The stump should not be cauterized with electrical current because the current will heat the staples and cause necrosis of the stump, leading to delayed perforation and its attendant problems of peritonitis, abscess, or fecal fistula. There is also no need to invert the stump in uncomplicated cases. If an inversion is desired, a purse string or Z-stitch can be placed manually or with the Endo-Stitch (U.S. Surgical Corp., Norwalk, CT) to hold the buried stump in place.

Prior to dividing the appendix, a bag should be introduced into the abdomen through one of the ports and placed under the appendix to control any potential contamination. Once transected, the appendix should be dropped into the bag and the bag removed through one of the 10- or 12-mm ports (Fig. 19.3). Utilizing the bag decreases the chance of infection by isolating the appendix from the abdominal contents and the skin and subcutaneous tissues through which it is extracted. In the authors series of 291 cases,[19] there have been no wound infections.

The appendix may also be removed by using a clip and tie technique. The appendix is grasped by the tip with the left hand through the right lower quadrant port. If the appendix is difficult to grasp due to inflammation, a pretied suture loop may be placed through the right lower port and tied around the tip of the appendix. Care must be taken to apply only gentle tension to this tie to avoid avulsing the end of an inflamed

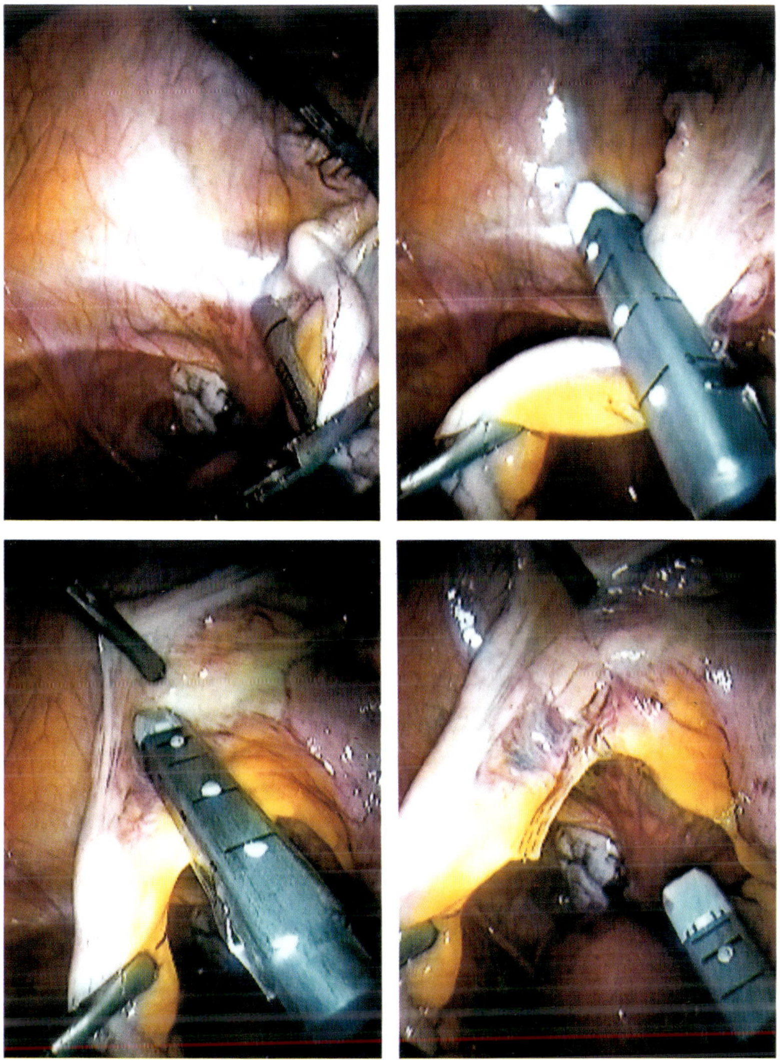

Figure 19.1. The mesoappendix is divided with a linear stapling device placed through the suprapubic port while the appendix is stablized with a grasper through the right lower quadrant port.

appendix. The appendix may also be grasped on the mesoappendix near its tip for control.

The vessels of the mesoappendix, and specifically the marginal artery, should be identified by dissecting windows in the mesoappendix with a dissector or the blunt tips of scissors. The vessels are double clipped with 9-mm clips. Double clipping will decrease the chance of having a vessel in the fatty inflamed mesentery slip through a clip. Clips need not be placed on the appendiceal side of the vessel. There will be some back bleeding when the clipped vessels are cut with the scissors, but this will be minimal. Once the mesoappendix is divided, three pretied sutures of 2-0 chromic or 2-0 Vicryl should be placed through the suprapubic port and tied around the appendiceal base. Two ties should be at the base, with the third about 1 cm distal to the initial two. After a bag is placed in the abdomen, the appendix can be transected between the second and third ties with scissors. No cauterization is needed. Cauterization of the tip with monopolar electrical current may heat the suture until it melts, allowing a leak from the stump. The stump does not need inversion.

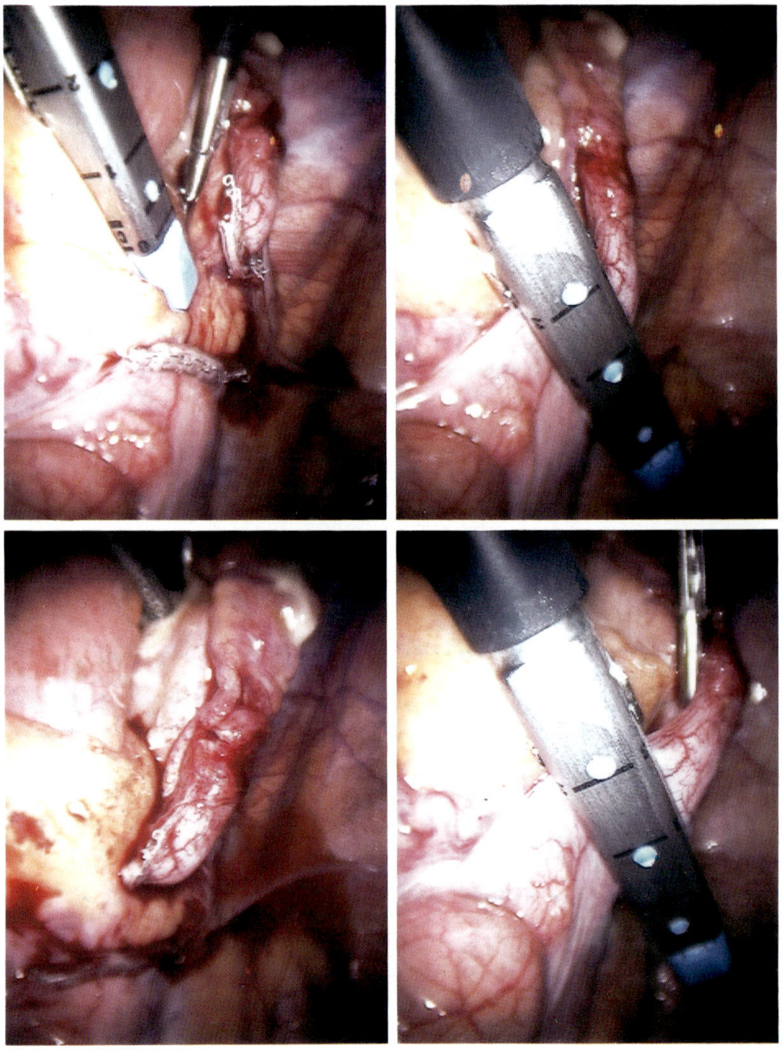

Figure 19.2. The appendix is divided with the linear stapler using 3.5-mm staples. The anatomy is well delineated so that the entire appendix can be removed.

The appendix is removed within a bag, as described above.

If there has been gross spillage or if there is pus in the peritoneal cavity, irrigation with saline or an antibiotic solution followed by vigorous suctioning may be performed. In the absence of spillage or contamination, minimal irrigation of the local area is indicated, with suctioning of the pelvis and gutters. The abdominal pressure should be reduced to 9 mmHg and the surgical site is checked for hemostasis (Fig. 19.4). High intra-abdominal pressures can mask venous bleeding. If there is bleeding along the clip line, vessels should be tied individually with pretied loops.

Occasionally an appendix may be so small that it can be pulled into a trocar sleeve and extracted without contaminating the surrounding tissues (Fig. 19.5). Although this technique is not as controlled as using a bag, it is acceptable in selected instances.

All trocar puncture sites larger than 5 mm should have a fascial closure with a figure of eight 2-0 absorbable suture. Although hernias occur at 5-mm trocar sites, they are much more rare than hernias through larger port openings, and closing 5-mm port incisions can be difficult in heavy patients. Most hernias through 5-mm trocar sites occur from rapid removal of the trocar sleeve, creating suction and

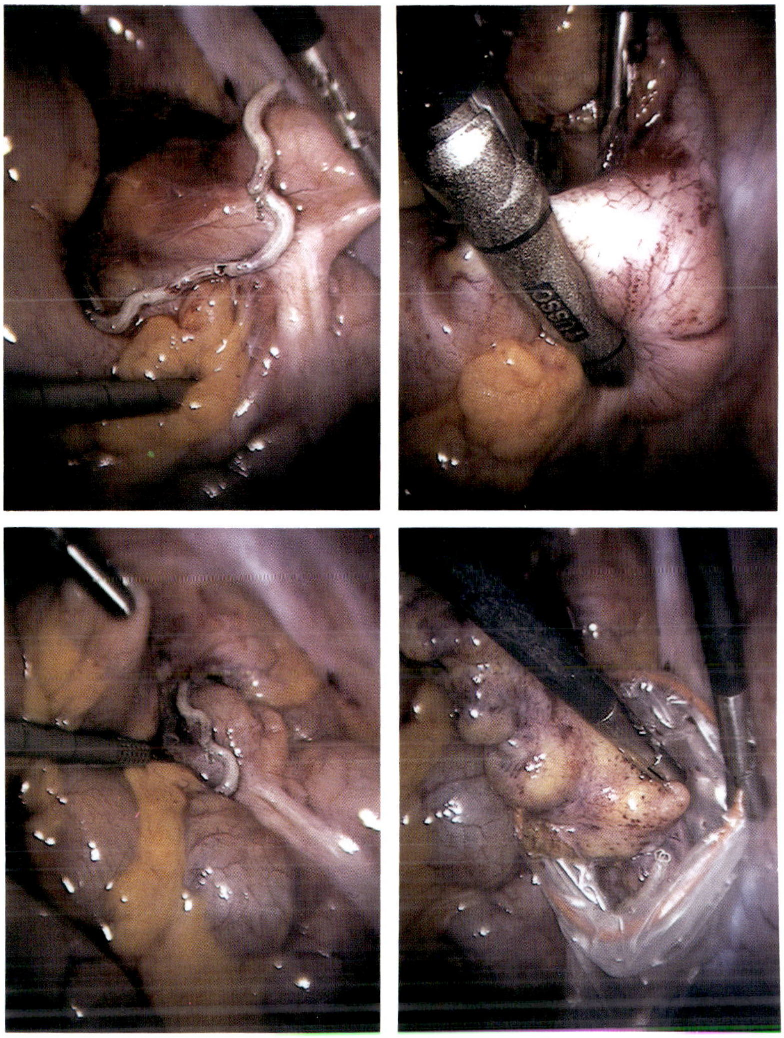

Figure 19.3. The appendix is placed in the Endobag (Dexide, Ft. Worth, TX) prior to removal from the abdomen to decrease the chances of contamination of the subcutaneous tissues.

pulling the intestine into the defect. A Richter's hernia is more common in this scenario. The skin can be closed with the surgeon's choice of methods.

Perforated appendicitis and appendiceal abscess can make identification of the appendiceal stump difficult in both open and laparoscopic cases. If the surgeon encounters difficulty identifying the anatomy, conversion to an open technique is indicated. Most cases (90–99%) can be performed laparoscopically.[8,9,18,22] The technique is predicated on finding normal anatomy and progressing from known tissue planes to areas of inflammation. Blunt dissection utilizing two opposing graspers can mimic the action of blunt finger dissection used in the open technique. Liberal use of the suction irrigator will help visualization since considerable oozing may occur during the dissection. It may be easier to identify the base of the appendix than the tip. In that circumstance, a window can be dissected in the mesentery at the base of the appendix, and a stapling device can be used to divide the base of the appendix so that the appendix can be removed antegrade. There is greater potential for contamination utilizing this technique, but it may be necessary in some cases.

Postoperative management does not differ from that of open appendectomy. For cases of perforation and

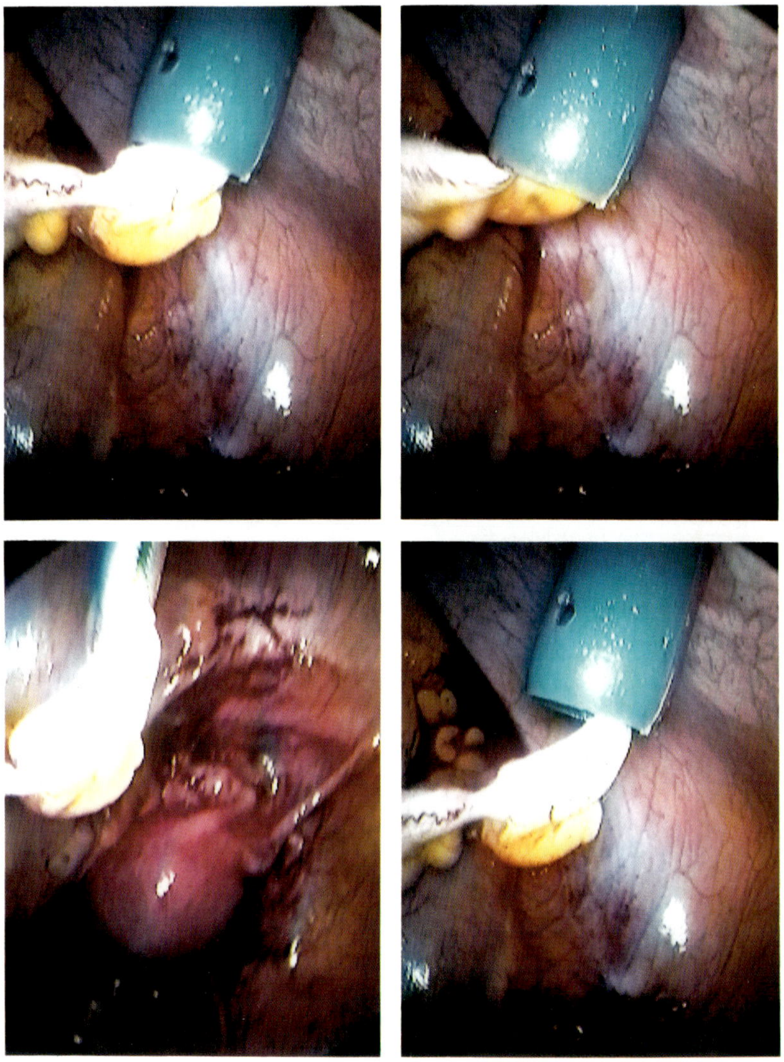

Figure 19.4. The appendix is removed from the abdomen through a trocar sleeve. When the appendix is small, it may be pulled into the sleeve and the entire sleeve removed instead of utilizing a bag.

abscess, 7–10 days of IV antibiotics covering *Bacteriodes fragilis, Escherichia coli, Klebsiella,* and *Enterobacter* should be utilized. The patient may eat whenever nausea subsides, usually in 6–8 hr. Nasogastric tubes and urethral catheters should be removed in the recovery room. Ambulation should begin in the first 12 hr. Narcotics may be needed for pain during the first 24 hr, but milder analgesics should be used as soon as possible to decrease the chance of ileus. Patients may be discharged when they become afebrile and can receive oral antibiotics. There are no postoperative activity restrictions on patients undergoing laparoscopic appendectomy.

COMPLICATIONS

The reported morbidity following open appendectomy ranges from 5% to 20%, and mortality is less than 1%.[25] It appears to be somewhat less after laparoscopic appendectomy. Postoperative complications are usu-

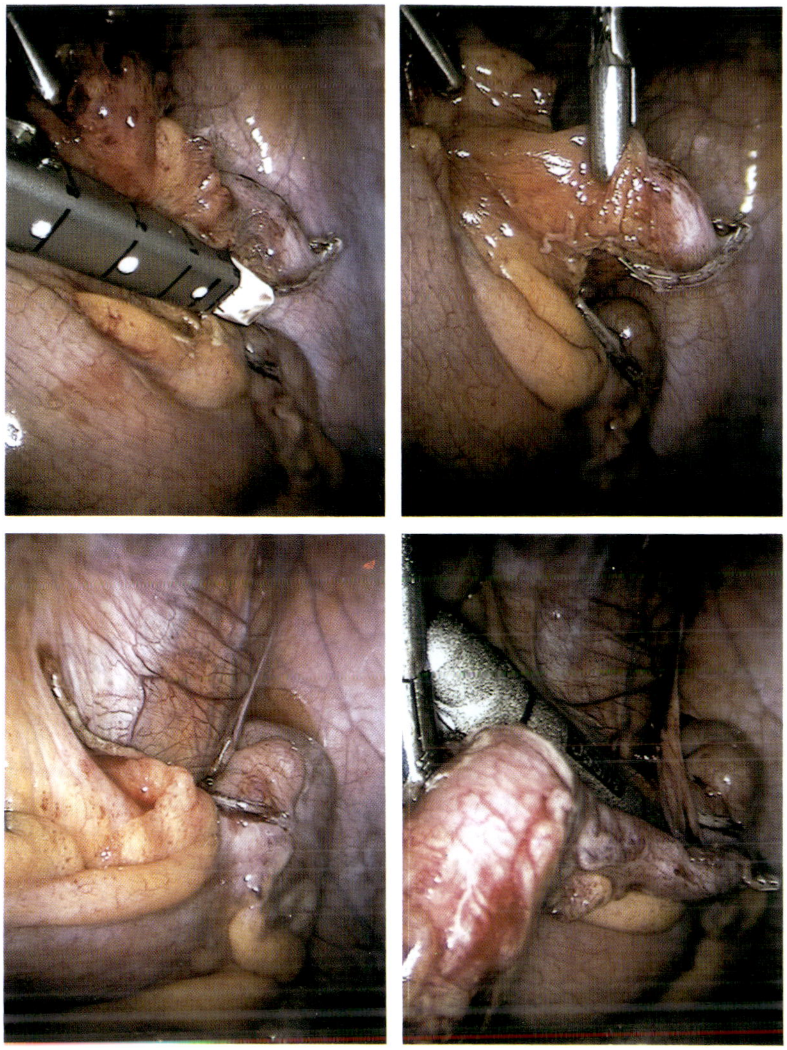

Figure 19.5. Inspection of the staple line at the termination of the procedure ensures hemostasis.

ally infectious. They occur in 5% of patients if the appendix is not ruptured and in over 30% of those with a ruptured or gangrenous appendix. Since the incidence of perforation is less than 20% in the first 24 hr of complaints and rises to over 70% after 48 hr, it is imperative to make a timely diagnosis and treat appropriately. Laparoscopy offers the surgeon a timely, effective, and minimally invasive method of evaluating the patient with a difficult diagnosis. Nonspecific tests such as barium enema and ultrasound have little indication today.

Subcutaneous wound infection is the most common complication following appendectomy. This can be markedly reduced utilizing the bag removal method described above.[19,21] The infected wound presents with mild swelling edema, and pain. Pus may not be present, with infection manifest by serosanguinous fluid. The skin and subcutaneous tissue should be opened and allowed to heal by secondary intention. Packing the wound may aid in debridement.

Intra-abdominal abscesses (pelvic, subphrenic, or abdominal) occurs in 20% of patients with perforation.

An abscess may form from preoperative leakage, or spillage during surgery, or it may stem from a retained fecalith. Its incidence can be reduced by performing surgery before the appendix ruptures, careful attention to technique intraoperatively (including the use of a bag), and meticulous irrigation suctioning of contamination. An abscess usually presents as malaise, abdominal pain, fever, and anorexia beginning 1 week after surgery. Low abdominal and pelvic abscesses cause diarrhea, while subphrenic collections cause pleural effusions. The site of the abscess is confirmed by computed tomography or ultrasound.[29] Although surgical drainage is still an accepted method of managing these complications, percutaneous drainage has become the mainstay of treatment.[30] Some presumed abscesses may be phlegmons and may respond to antibiotics. If a mass is present without clear-cut evidence of fluid and air, a course of antibiotics is indicated.

Pylephlebitis presents with jaundice, fever, and chills and is due to infection of the portal venous system. This infection, caused by *E. coli,* may result in multiple liver abscesses. Utilization of preoperative antibiotics and postoperative antibiotics in cases of rupture or gangrene has made this complication rare.

Postoperative bowel obstruction from adhesions is believed to be lessened with laparoscopy since laparoscopy forms fewer adhesions. However, this hypothesis has not been proven.

Hemorrhage is an unusual complication, and unless the patient has coagulation dysfunctions, it is nearly always attributable to poor operative technique. The mesoappendix should be doubly clipped and checked at the end of surgery to ensure that no clips have been dislodged. Clips placed on the fatty mesoappendix may easily be loosened by vigorous suctioning. The pressure should be dropped to 9 mmHg to allow the surgeon to observe venous bleeding which might be masked from the elevated intraperitoneal pressure. Bleeding sites should be managed by reclipping or placing a suture, but they should never be cauterized with electricity. Cauterization will heat the clips, necrosing the tissue underneath and possibly leading to postoperative hemorrhage.

With the use of laparoscopy, major vessel injury from trocar insertion should always be suspected when the patient presents with postoperative or intraoperative hypotension, tachycardia, and a falling hematocrit. The abdominal wall should be examined to ensure that there is no enlarging intramuscular hematoma from a trocar insertion injury. The retroperitoneal area under each insertion site should be examined with either repeat laparoscopy or laparotomy to ensure that a retroperitoneal vessel was not injured during insertion. The use of safety shield trocars has led to a more cavalier attitude toward trocar insertion. If the abdominal wall is pushed posteriorly during the insertion, the trocar may not activate quickly enough to prevent retroperitoneal injury. Intestinal mesentery may also be injured during insertion. This should be sought with thorough intestinal visualization. Retroperitoneal and intestinal vessels may also be injured by a scalpel cutting too deeply when making the skin incision. This occurs most commonly in very thin patients.

Reexploration should be done immediately when the diagnosis of postoperative hemorrhage is made, either by laparoscopy or laparotomy. Usually there is too much bleeding to evaluate with the laparoscope, and laparotomy is required. However, if only a mesenteric bleeder needs control, laparoscopy may avoid a major surgical procedure. If a retroperitoneal vessel has been injured, both the anterior and posterior walls should be examined. It is highly likely that a trocar injury will be discovered on both walls of the vessel. Failure to diagnose a posterior wall injury could lead to further bleeding, arteriovenous fistula formation, or pseudoaneurysm.

Trocar injuries can easily be avoided by utilizing the open technique for initial insertion and visually observing all secondary trocars as they enter the abdomen.

Stump disruption may cause intra-abdominal abscess or fecal fistula. It can be prevented by utilizing the correct staple size in the linear stapler and avoiding the use of electrical current on the stump. A staple that is too short will tear through the serosa and muscularis, causing a leak. A 3.5-mm staple is usually adequate for all appendix and cecal transections. The smaller vascular staples (2.5 mm) should not be used when transecting the appendix. Cautery should never be used on the stump since it will necrose the staple line or melt the ties.

Incisional hernias may present with partial or total bowel obstruction or absence of bowel obstruction. A tender lump in the incision shortly after surgery is the most common complaint, but it may occur several weeks or months postoperatively. It is repaired by operatively reducing the mass and closing the defect. The incidence of hernia can be reduced by careful fascial closure in all ports larger than 5 mm.

Recurrent appendicitis has been seen after laparoscopic appendectomy.[26] This usually occurs during the surgeon's learning curve when the anatomy is not precisely delineated and only a partial appendectomy is performed. It requires repeat appendectomy and can be avoided by careful attention to anatomic landmarks, ensuring that the entire appendix is removed.

Urologic injury is a rare complication. It presents with fever, flank pain, and hematuria. Abdominal pain and ileus may occur with bladder injury. Intravenous pyelography confirms the diagnosis. Cystoscopy will confirm bladder injury. Exploration should be performed for ureteral injury. Either primary repair (if no tissue is missing) or the creation of a bladder flap may be needed. Bladder injuries may be treated with catheter drainage (posterior injuries) or by direct repair (anterior injuries).

CO_2 embolization may occur when high intraperitoneal pressures (greater than 20mmHg) are used, when major venous injury occurs, or by direct injection into the venous system. The patient presents intraoperatively with rapid onset of hypotension. A murmur may be heard over the precordium or with an esophageal stethoscope, and bubbles may be visualized in large vessels. Treatment consists of immediate release of the pneumoperitoneum, positioning the patient left side down in the Trendelenberg position to force the bubble to the base of the right ventricle, administration of 100% O_2, and placement of a central venous line to aspirate the bubble from the right side of the heart.

Embolization can be prevented by aspirating the insufflation needle before insufflation to ensure that it is extravascular, maintaining a pressure of 15 mmHg or less, and avoiding major venous injury with careful dissection technique and immediate cessation of pneumoperitoneum when a venous injury is suspected.

Laparoscopic appendectomy is quickly becoming accepted as a treatment for acute appendicitis, especially in the female. It is associated with many of the same complications seen with open appendectomy, but is also has some morbidity associated only with this approach. As with open surgery, complications can be minimized by attention to detail, using excellent operative technique and correctly identifying anatomy. With the large array of laparoscopic instruments currently available, it is imperative the surgeon choose the least dangerous instrument in any given situation to minimize the opportunity for injury.

REFERENCES

1. Berry JJ, Malt RA: Appendicitis near its centenary. *Ann Surg* 200:567, 1984.
2. Semm K: Endoscopic appendectomy. *Endoscopy* 15:59–64, 1983.
3. Schreiber JH: Early experience with laparoscopic appendectomy in women. *Surg Endosc* 1:211–216, 1987.
4. Leahy PF: Technique of laparoscopic appendectomy. *Br J Surg* 76:616–617, 1989.
5. Brown DS: Laparoscopic guided appendectomy. *Aust NZ J Obstet Gynecol* 30:231–233, 1990.
6. Reddick EJ, Olsen DO, Saye WB, et al: Laparoscopic laser cholecystectomy. *Laser Med Surg News Adv* 7:38–40, 1989.
7. Reddick EJ: Laparoscopic laser cholecystectomy. *Curr Laser Monthly* 1988.
8. Frazee RC, Roberts JW, Symmonds RE, et al: A prospective randomized trial comparing open versus laparoscopic appendectomy. *Ann Surg* 219(6):725–731, 1994.
9. Sosa JL, Sleeman D, McKenney MG, et al: A comparison of laparoscopic and traditional appendectomy. *J Laparosc Endosc Surg* 3(2):129–131, 1993.
10. Reddick EJ, Olsen DO: Laparoscopic laser cholecystectomy: A comparison with mini-lap cholecystectomy. *Surg Endosc* 3:34–39, 1989.
11. Brown JJ: Acute appendicitis: The radiologist's role. *Radiology* 180:13, 1991.
12. el Ferzli FG, Ozuner G, Davidson PG: Barium enema in the diagnosis of acute appendicitis. *SGO* 171:40, 1990.
13. Shapiro MP, Gale ME, Gerzof SG: CT or appendicitis. Diagnosis and treatment. *Radiol Clin North Am* 27:753, 1989.
14. Ooms HW, Koumans RK, Ho Kang, et al: Ultrasonography in the diagnosis of acute appendicitis. *Br J Surg* 78:315, 1991.
15. Kang WM, Lee CH, Chou YH: A clinical evaluation of ultrasonography in the diagnosis of acute appendicitis. *Surgery* 105:154, 1989.
16. Dueholm S, Bagi P, Bud M: Laboratory aid in the diagnosis of acute appendicitis. A blinded, prospective trial concerning diagnostic value of leukocyte count, neutrophil differential count and C-reactive protein. *Dis Colon Rectum* 32:855, 1989.
17. Schrenk P, Woisetschlager R, Wayand WU, et al: Diagnostic laparoscopy: A survey of 92 patients. *Am J Surg* 168:348–351, 1994.
18. Richards W, Watson D, Lynch G, et al: A review of the results of laparoscopic versus open appendectomy. *SGO* 177:473–480, 1993.
19. Valla JS, Limonne B, Valla V, et al: Laparoscopy appendectomy in children: Report of 465 cases. *Surg Laparosc Endosc* 1(3):166–172, 1991.
20. O'Reilly MJ, Mullins S: Unpublished data.
21. Nowzaradan Y, Barnes JP: Current techniques in laparoscopic appendectomy. *Surg Laparosc Endosc* 3(6):470–476, 1993.
22. Saye WB, Rives DA, Cochran EB: Laparoscopic appendectomy: Three years' experience. *Surg Laparosc Endosc* 1(2):109–115, 1991.
23. McAnena OJ, Austin O, Hederman WP, et al: Laparo-

scopic versus open appendicectomy. *Lancet* 338:693, 1991.

24. Kazarian KK, Roeder WJ, Mersheimer WL: Decreasing mortality and increasing morbidity from acute apendicitis. *Am J Surg* 119:681–685, 1970.
25. Lewis FR, Holcroft JW, Boey J, et al: Appendicitis. A critical review of diagnosis and treatment in 1000 cases. *Arch Surg* 110:677–684, 1975.
26. Cooperman M: Complications of appendectomy. *Surg Clin North Am* 63:1233–1247, 1983.
27. Hasson HM: A modified instrument and method for laparoscopy. *Am J Obstet Gynecol* 100:886–887, 1971.
28. Cohen MM, Dangleis K: The cost effectiveness of laparoscopic appendectomy. *J Laparosc Endosc Surg* 3(2): 93–97, 1993.
29. Schwerk WB, Wichtrup B, Ruschoff J, et al: Acute and perforated appendicitis: Current experience with ultrasound aided diagnosis. *World J Surg* 14:271, 1990.
30. Olak J, Christou NV, Stein LA, et al: Operative vs. percutaneous drainage of intra-abdominal abscesses. *Arch Surg* 121:141–146, 1986.
31. Devereaux DA, McDermott JP, Caushaj PF: Recurrent appendicitis following laparoscopic appendectomy. *Dis Colon Rectum* 37:719–720, 1994.

chapter twenty

Small Bowel Resection and Small Bowel Injuries

Joseph B. Petelin

INTRODUCTION

Laparoscopic surgery of the small intestine represents one of the advanced procedures that evolved naturally from the less demanding laparoscopic operations such as laparoscopic cholecystectomy. In the early 1990s, surgeons who had mastered the basic techniques of laparoscopic cholecystectomy were eager to extend the boundaries of the laparoscopic arena to treatment of other surgically correctable maladies of the abdomen. Surgeons first addressed one of the more common operations, appendectomy, in a laparoscopic fashion, and once the techniques of this operation became established, it was natural for surgical attention to be directed at other portions of the gastrointestinal tract.[1–20]

However, new challenges faced surgeons who wanted to operate on the intestines laparoscopically. Not only were problems of exposure and handling of the tissues to be solved, but also the challenges of repairing enterotomies and performing anastomoses demanded new equipment and new suturing skills.[21] These challenges have been met and have been successfully handled. The advanced laparoscopic surgeon of the 1990s should definitely consider operations on the small intestine to be not only doable but a first-order consideration in the treatment of patients with small bowel disorders.

In order to manage small intestinal pathology by laparoscopy safely and effectively, the surgeon must have the following:

- A firm grasp of the required technical skills.
- An understanding of the proper patient indications, contraindications, and preparation.
- Control of the operating room environment to the extent that the equipment and personnel are not only adequate but thoroughly prepared.

This chapter discusses the various aspects laparoscopic small intestinal surgery as they relate to these requirements.

PATIENT SELECTION AND PREPARATION

Indications

As in open surgery, there are a variety of situations which call for surgical treatment of the small intestine. These include:

- Foreign body removal
- Repair of perforation[22,23]
- Relief of obstruction after open or laparoscopic surgery[24–44]
- Polypectomy
- Diverticulectomy[5,6,45–47]
- Segmental resection of abnormalities (polyp, stricture, etc.) and anastomosis
- Bypass procedures.

Each of these clinical problems may be approached laparoscopically in the appropriate set of circumstances. First, the patient must be able to withstand general anesthesia. Second, the abdominal wall must be capable of distention beyond that which is present preoperatively. That is to say, laparoscopy by definition involves surgery in a closed space: the limits of the abdominal wall. If this space is maximally filled prior to surgery, for example with small bowel distention or with extensive diffuse adhesions or tumor, then the chances of successfully intervening laparoscopically are minimal. Third, such advanced laparoscopy requires that the surgeon be experienced in advanced techniques and that the team of assistants and ancillary personnel be prepared for the procedure.[21]

Contraindications

In addition to the same contraindications that apply to general basic laparoscopy, there are other conditions that apply to laparoscopic small bowel surgery. These include:

- A patient unwilling to undergo laparoscopic surgery
- A patient unsuitable for general anesthetic
- Severe, uncorrectable coagulopathy
- Septic shock
- Inadequate equipment
- Inadequate personnel staffing
- Inadequate surgeon training and preparation
- Massive distention precluding safe entry and laparoscopic manipulation
- Massive intra-abdominal metastatic disease precluding safe entry and laparoscopic manipulation

Most important, the surgeon must have clearly thought out his or her plans for the patient, both from a laparoscopic and an open surgical viewpoint. He or she must have a thorough understanding of the pathology involved, the extent to which a laparoscopic approach may be effective, the potential for a combined approach, and his or her own laparoscopic skill set. If any of these considerations suggest a high likelihood of an unsuccessful laparoscopic approach, then the surgeon should contemplate an alternative method.

Workup and Patient Preparation

Each clinical situation involves a somewhat different workup of the patient. There are certain common elements to the workup of any preoperative patient, such as a chest x-ray, electrocardiogram, complete blood count, and electrolyte measurements. Each of these should obviously be normalized as much as possible prior to surgical intervention. Imaging studies of the abdomen and intestines depend on the type of pathology suspected to be the cause of the patient's problem. These may include standard radiographs, oral contrast studies, barium enema, computed tomography, magnetic resonance imaging, endoscopy, or radionuclide imaging.

Additionally, in cases where there is significant distention of the intestine, a period of nasogastric decompression may convert a potentially inoperable laparoscopic case to one in which access can be achieved and surgery completed laparoscopically. The necessity for and the length of nasogastric decompression require surgical judgment that accrues with experience in managing patients with small bowel obstruction and experience with advanced laparoscopic procedures.

EQUIPMENT

General Laparoscopic Equipment

In order to perform small intestinal surgery laparoscopically, the standard set for basic laparoscopic surgery is mandatory. This obviously includes telescope, a camera, light source, monitor(s), basic laparoscopic hand instruments, and an electrosurgical generator. These materials should be in good working order because improperly maintained equipment not only makes advanced laparoscopy difficult, it can make it nearly impossible or hazardous.

One of the most important items in the standard set is the video system. Too many operating theaters claim to have state-of-the-art systems but in reality provide video cameras and monitors that display a true color picture in various shades of magenta. This can be easily checked by temporarily removing the camera from the laparoscope and looking directly into the scope. The difference in the view is often striking.

Laparoscopic intestinal surgery involves the manipulation of tissues that display very similar colors, unlike the difference in coloration displayed by the various structures of the biliary system. It is therefore imperative that the color rendition and spatial resolution of the video system be the best possible. When the view is distorted from its true color and when the resolution of the projected image is significantly lower than that perceived with the naked eye, it is difficult to imagine that safe laparoscopic dissection can be performed. The surgeon should demand that the video system not only be the best available, but also that it be maintained in the best possible working order. This will lay the groundwork for a successful approach to laparoscopic intestinal surgery.

Special Equipment

Manipulation of the intestine requires gentle handling of the tissues. Most of the grasping instruments used for basic laparoscopic surgery, such as cholecystectomy, are not suitable for advanced laparoscopic small intestinal surgery. Atraumatic graspers and/or Babcock clamps have been developed and are available from a variety of vendors. They should be used when handling the intestine and mesentery, especially when these tissues are diseased.

Retracting devices are often required during laparoscopic intestinal surgery. Many types of instruments with a variety of configurations are available in both 5-mm and 10-mm diameters. Some styles are less atraumatic than others, so caution should be used when selecting and applying them to the tissues.

Laparoscopic intestinal occlusion clamps (i.e., bulldog or Glassman types) should also be readily available. These are obviously necessary in situations in which an enterotomy is either planned or encountered. The bulldog-type clamps allow the surgeon to control an enterotomy without continually occupying a port with a clamp. They are easily applied and removed with a special applicator.

Laparoscopic needle holders are now available in a variety of configurations. They are usually an absolute necessity for anyone contemplating laparoscopic intestinal surgery. The surgeon should be skilled in using the type that is available, or should maintain a set with which he or she is familiar.

OPERATING ROOM SETUP

The Patient

Generally the patient is placed supine on the operating table and draped in the usual fashion for laparoscopic surgery. The low lithotomy position with the patient's legs spread apart is not usually necessary unless concomitant lower colonic surgery is planned. Pulsatile antiembolism stockings should be used in all of these cases. In most cases, a Foley catheter is necessary to decompress the bladder initially and to maintain decompression for longer operations. Nasogastric intubation is often already in place in patients with small bowel obstruction and should be considered in those in whom elective resectional small intestinal surgery is planned.

Equipment Placement

While most of the equipment should be placed in the same position as for laparoscopic cholecystectomy, the location of the video monitors requires special consideration. One monitor should be located on the patient's right side at the level of the shoulders. The other monitor should be located on the patient's left side at the foot of the table. This allows observation of the upper abdomen, lower abdomen, and pelvis from either side of the table, generally with proper retinal-camera chip orientation for all members of the team.

This latter point deserves some discussion. Laparoscopic video cameras acquire the image provided by the scope on a chip or series of three chips (for red-green-blue separation). This chip or collection of chips is oriented in the camera in the same plane that a surgeon's retina would be if he or she were to look directly into the scope without the camera. When the camera is placed on the scope, the view displayed on the monitor will perfectly match what the surgeon's occipital cortex expects to see as long as the surgeon's retina is in the same plane as the chip(s). If the surgeon's head is turned away from this plane, or if he or she is located opposite to the direction of the scope, then the view displayed and the movement of instruments in that view are not in a direct 1:1 relationship. Most laparoscopists have experienced this phenomenon but few have understood the reason for it. It is not the position of the monitors that directly causes it. Rather, it is the forced change in the surgeon's retinal position (caused by having to turn the head or by having the scope directed back at himself or herself) relative to the position of the chip, that causes the mental confusion surrounding the displayed image. So, it behooves the surgeon to arrange the monitors so that he or she may view either of them with the retina comfortably oriented in the same plane as the camera chip(s). This will allow the surgeon to manipulate instruments and tissues with greater dexterity and without having to calculate the direction of his or her movements.

Staff Placement

Assistant(s) and nursing personnel should be located in positions that make the most sense for the operation being performed. The scrub nurse is usually located on the opposite side of the table. The assistant should be located on the same side as the surgeon if possible. When this is not possible, the assistant should be instructed to view whichever monitor allows him or her to maintain the best retinal-chip orientation in order to maximize dexterity with tissue manipulation.

It is not uncommon for the surgeon and team members to have to change positions from one side of the table to the other in order to access all portions of the small intestine comfortably. The surgeon should not hesitate to do this if it appears that it will result in better visualization and manipulation of the tissues.

TECHNIQUE OF SMALL INTESTINAL SURGERY

Entry—Primary Port Placement

For elective small bowel surgery where no distention or adhesions are of concern, Veress needle insufflation and blind initial port introduction can be safely performed. In all other cases and when the surgeon's preference dictates, an open technique for establishing the initial port should be used. Generally, this port is placed at the umbilicus unless there is good reason to place it elsewhere. This might be the case when an ostomy is near that site or when attempts at open port placement there are unsuccessful.

Diagnostic Evaluation

Prior to placement of any secondary ports, the abdomen should be surveyed with the scope. This must be done carefully in order to avoid tearing adhesions that would result in bowel injury. If no adhesions are present, selection of secondary port sites will depend on the problem to be addressed.

Secondary Port Placement

In order to perform a more thorough diagnostic evaluation, at least one secondary port must be placed. I have found that the best site for this first secondary port is the right hemiabdomen at approximately the level of the umbilicus. This allows the camera to be controlled by the left hand of the surgeon while the right hand manipulates the tissues with an atraumatic grasper. I usually begin small intestinal investigation, i.e., "running the small bowel," at the ileocecal junction. This allows inspection of the appendix, ileum, mesentery, and jejunum in an organized fashion. Occasionally this maneuver requires placement of an additional port to provide retraction. My favorite second site is the left lower quadrant. Additional ports may be placed as necessary, depending on the operation to be performed. All of these secondary ports should be placed under direct laparoscopic vision.

When the patient harbors adhesions, it is important to first palpate the abdominal wall while viewing that site laparoscopically so that tissue injury may be avoided when secondary ports are placed. The location of adhesions often dictates where the initial secondary port must be located. If possible, it should be placed at least 10 cm away from the primary port. This will allow instrument manipulation without interference from the scope. After the abdominal wall adhesions are taken down in these cases, a subsequent port site location may be made at the discretion of the surgeon.

Maintaining the Field of View

Patient Position

In order to adequately access all portions of the small intestine laparoscopically, it is usually necessary to change the position of the operating table more than once. Initial inspection of the ileum is most easily accomplished with the patient in the Trendelenburg position. This allows delivery of the small bowel out of the pelvis. As the bowel is "run" and the jejunum is approached, returning the table to a neutral position facilitates more proximal exploration and manipulation. Occasionally, it is necessary to use a slight reverse Trendelenburg position to visualize the most proximal jejunum. Rotation of the table either to the right or the left is also often helpful in displacing small intestinal loops out of the field of view.

Retraction

Alteration of the patient's position is sometimes insufficient to maintain an adequate field of view. This is especially true when working with the proximal small intestine. Added exposure may be achieved here by employing a retractor. When inspecting and operating on the proximal jejunum, for example, the omentum and transverse colon may be retracted in a cephalad direction with an instrument inserted from a right-sided port. The breadth and configuration of the retracting device should be chosen for the situation at hand. In some cases, such as retraction of the transverse colon, a broad retractor works best. In other cases, where interloop dissection of adhesions may be required, a narrower retractor or atraumatic grasper often works best.

Irrigation

The importance of maintaining adequate hemostasis cannot be overemphasized. This implies that any collection of blood should be removed in a timely fashion and that the affected area be irrigated until tissue definition is once again restored. Failure to adhere to this principle is one of the major causes of surgeon frustration in these cases and can lead to tissue injury. Interestingly, it is often not the surgeon who is the first to recognize the need for irrigating the field. The laparoscopic intestinal surgeon should therefore continuously monitor the field of view with this in mind and should not allow interest in getting on with surgery to restrict the use of irrigation when necessary.

Bowel Resection

Laparoscopic versus Laparoscopic-Assisted Surgery

Prior to embarking on laparoscopic intestinal surgery, the surgeon should have a clear understanding of the role of a complete laparoscopic versus a laparoscopic-assisted procedure. Obviously, resectional surgery will usually involve enlargement of one of the port sites to allow removal of the specimen. That is not the issue here. What is important is the surgeon's grasp of the extent of the operation that may be safely and efficiently accomplished laparoscopically and what portion of the procedure, if any, would be better performed in an open fashion. Certainly laparoscopic division of the intestinal wall with an Endo-GIA device (U.S. Surgical Corp., Norwalk, Conn.) is feasible and efficient. Similarly, control and division of the mesentery with this device or with clips and scissors is feasible. Laparoscopic intestinal anastomosis may also be accomplished with the stapling devices or it may be hand sewn. If, however, after laparoscopic dissection and mobilization, the small bowel may be delivered to the abdominal wall in a relatively thin patient, then evisceration of the segment through a small extension of a port site incision, with resection and anastomosis on the surface, probably makes more sense than a prolonged laparoscopic adventure. It is this combination of laparoscopic and open techniques that requires judgment on the part of the surgeon.

Proximal and distal control

The Endo-GIA device provides the most efficient method of obtaining proximal and distal control of the segment to be removed. It is applied through a 12-mm port and not only staples but also divides the bowel at its application site. This device is very useful for resecting a Meckel's diverticulum; here it is applied to the base of the diverticulum, usually oriented at 90 degrees to the longitudinal axis of the ileum in order to avoid constricting the lumen.

The proximal and distal lines of resection may also be controlled with laparoscopic Glassman-type or bulldog-type clamps. The latter have the advantage of not occupying a port site while in position. These are most useful in cases where only a small enterotomy or "sleeve" resection of a proximal jejunal lesion is performed. In the latter case, the jejunal mesentary is usually not long enough to allow delivery of the intact bowel to the abdominal wall surface, thereby precluding a laparoscopic-assisted approach. Internal laparoscopic control and resection in this situation is preferred.

Controlling the mesentery

When performed laparoscopically, mesenteric division and control may be accomplished with scissors and clips, scissors and ligatures, or the harmonic scalpel. The last not only divides the mesentery but also seals all but the largest mesenteric vessels with its high-frequency oscillation. If any of these methods of control fail, then laparoscopic suture ligature of the bleeding vessel may be accomplished. If significant hemorrhage is present, however, then the case should be immediately converted to laparotomy.

Removing the Specimen

Completely resected specimens should be placed in a bag and removed through an enlarged port site. Small bowel segments that have been identified and mobilized but have not been divided, however, may be delivered through a somewhat larger port extension for resection and anastomosis on the surface. With the exception of proximal jejunal lesions and cases where the mesentery is so short so as to preclude delivery to the abdominal wall, the latter approach is preferred.

Reestablishing intestinal continuity

Laparoscopic anastomosis may be accomplished either with the automatic stapling devices, using a triangulation method as in open surgery, or by performing a hand-sewn anastomosis. The latter requires laparoscopic curved needle suturing skills and the ability to secure knots with intracorporeal tying techniques. If the surgeon chooses to hand-sew the anastomosis, a two-layer closure is generally preferred. The mucosal layer of suture is usually applied with absorbable material in a running fashion. This part of the anastomosis is usually the most difficult part of the procedure because of the length of suture material that must be handled laparoscopically. Nevertheless, with practice, the procedure may be accomplished effectively and efficiently. The serosal closure is generally performed with interrupted, nonabsorbable suture.

Closing the mesentery

As in open surgery, the integrity of the mesentery of small bowel should be restored prior to completion of surgery. This may be accomplished with either continuous running suture or interrupted suture. Closure of the mesentery with currently available staples and clips is not recommended. If the surgeon is not capable of suture closure of these tissues, then he or she should probably not attempt laparoscopic small intestinal surgery.

Examples of small bowel surgery

Examples of small bowel surgery include repair of enterotomy, Meckel's diverticulectomy, and Segmental small intestinal resection.

BOWEL INJURY

One of the most potentially devastating complications of any laparoscopic operation is intestinal injury.[48] This is not so much of a problem if it is recognized and repaired at the time it is caused. If, however, it goes undetected until the postoperative period, serious and potentially life-threatening problems with peritonitis may ensue.[49] In order to manage such problems successfully, an understanding of the sources of such injury, a low threshold for their detection, and immediate, definitive treatment are necessary. Adopting policies and procedures and developing techniques that minimize the risk of small intestinal injuries should be the ultimate goal.

Sources of Injury

Mechanical

Needles/trocars/scissors/scalpels Most sharp instrument injuries occur either upon initial blind insertion of the instrument into the abdomen or during its intraoperative manipulation outside the field of view of the scope. A high index of suspicion by the surgeon for these potential injuries should be maintained for any case in which multiple instrument passes or exchanges are made, any case that is prolonged, and any case in which difficult insertion has occurred. These injuries are usually so discrete and limited that they may be easily overlooked unless specific attention is directed to their detection.

Forceps, dissectors, and retractors These instruments usually cause blunt traction-type injuries which are generally more damaging than sharp injuries because the tissue is literally torn apart. Either the surgeon or the assistant(s) may cause such injuries by applying excessive traction on tissues either in the field of view or, more commonly, outside it. In order to avoid and/or quickly detect these problems, the surgeon should intermittently reassess the position and function of each retractor, especially during long or difficult cases. Gentle handling of the tissues with appropriately chosen atraumatic instruments will help lessen the likelihood of mishaps caused by these blunt instruments.

Thermal

Thermal injury may result from the application of energy from any of the following sources to the bowel wall: the light source, electrosurgical generators, lasers, harmonic oscillating instruments, and thermal coagulators.[50,51]

Light source Although uncommon, continued contact of the light source, i.e., the scope tip, with the bowel wall may result in a burn injury. This is more likely to occur in laproscopic-assisted cases where a significant amount of surgery is performed on the surface with the abdomen deflated. In such cases, injury may be avoided by temporarily removing the scope and/or turning off the light source during the open part of the procedure.

Electrosurgical equipment Injuries from this type of equipment are often difficult to detect unless they occur under the direct vision of the surgeon. This may occur when an electrically active element is placed in direct contact with tissue, or contacts another electrical conductor (such as a metal instrument) which itself is in contact with the small intestine. These injuries range from the very small, inconsequential serosal "burn" where the tissue barely changes color in a 1-mm area to the more serious injury where contact has been made for a prolonged period and more extensive damage has occurred. The latter injury usually occurs outside the field of view and therefore is often unlikely to be detected unless vigilant inspection occurs at the completion of the procedure.

Another type of electrical injury occurs not because of direct contact of an active element with tissue but because of a phenomenon labeled *capacitive coupling*. Here an insulated, electrically active element transfers its energy to another metal instrument (such as a metal sheath) despite the insulation that separates them. While this is a natural feature of electrical energy and normally causes no harm, it may cause injury to the small bowel if the metal sheath is itself insulated from the abdominal wall by a plastic connector. When this occurs, the charge that accumulates on the metal sheath is not allowed to discharge to the large surface of the abdominal wall (where it would have no damaging effect). Instead, the charge is transferred from the sheath to the nearest organ, likely the small bowel. The most worrisome problem with this type of injury is that it most commonly occurs outside the field of view and is totally unsuspected because all the instrumentation appears to be in good working order.

Laser Although popular for laparoscopic general surgery in the early 1990s, lasers have generally fallen into disuse. Generally, they are thought to be somewhat safer than electrosurgical energy sources, but they may still cause injury. This may occur with noncontact-type lasers, such as CO_2, KTP, Nd:YAG, or other varieties where the beam is directed accidentally to the small bowel or reflects off an instrument to the bowel wall. Direct-contact lasers, such as the contact tip Nd:YAG laser, may cause injury if the sapphire tip, which becomes extremely hot, comes into contact with the intestine.

Recognition and Treatment

Laparoscopic or open

The best time to detect an injury is at the time of the original operation. The laparoscope and camera provide an excellent way to do this. However, injuries can only be detected if the surgeon looks for them. This implies that at some time during surgery, preferably prior to removal of the ports, a general inspection is performed. This sounds rather simple, but this maneuver is often overlooked as the final laparoscopic step.

If an injury is detected at this time, the surgeon must determine its extent and decide the optimum treatment. It is also necessary to decide on the optimal method to repair and or resect the damaged segment—laparoscopic or open. For sharp injuries or others with limited damage, suture repair may be accomplished laparoscopically. For more extensive injuries, conversion to laparotomy is often necessary unless the surgeon feels confident that the intestinal defect can be controlled laparoscopically to prevent spillage, and that he or she can effectively repair and/or resect that segment expeditiously. If there is any question about the ability to repair the damage as well as in open surgery, then conversion to laparotomy should be performed.

Avoiding Bowel Injuries

It is obviously better to avoid injuries in the first place than to have to manage them after the fact. The surgeon can take a number of steps to decrease the likelihood of such injuries. First of all, the equipment and team for any laparoscopic surgery should be optimized. If either of these is not suited for the degree of difficulty of the case, then an alternative plan of treatment should be considered. This is more easily said than done, however, because the hospital managers who maintain the equipment and assign personnel to a given case are often unaware of the requirements of video laparoscopy. The surgeon must engage them in the dialogue so that they begin to understand that it is no more appropriate to provide inadequate video laparoscopic equipment or improperly trained personnel for such a case than it is to provide inexperienced nursing personnel or a malfunctioning cardiac bypass pump for open heart surgery.

Second, the surgeon must be keenly aware of the potential for small intestinal injury and the scenarios in which it is most likely to occur. This should result in not only greater caution with instrument manipulations but also greater vigilance for situations in which small intestinal injury is more likely to occur.

REFERENCES

1. Kurn CK, Yap CH, Goh PM: Palliation of advanced gastric cancer by laparoscopic gastrojejunostomy. *Sing Med J* 36(2):228–229, 1995.
2. Robles R, Lujan JA, Parrilla P, et al: Laparoscopic surgery in the treatment of small bowel obstruction by bezoar. *BJS* 82(4):520, 1995.
3. Greig JD, Miles WF, Nixon SJ, Laparoscopic technique for small bowel biopsy. *BJS* 82(3):363, 1995.
4. Panuel M, Campan N, Delarue A, et al: Ultrasonographic diagnosis and laparoscopic surgical treatment of Meckel's diverticulum. *Eur J Pediatr Surg* 4(6):344–345, 1994.
5. Catarci M, Zaraca F, Scaccia M, et al: Laparoscopic management of volvulated Meckel's diverticulum. *Surg Lap Endosc* 5(1):72–74, 1995.
6. Madsen MR: Laparoscopy in the diagnosis of bleeding Meckel's diverticulum. *Surg Endosc* 8(11):1346–1347, 1994.

7. Franklin ME, Dorman JP, Pharand D: Laparoscopic surgery in acute small bowel obstruction. *Surg Laparosc Endosc* 4(4):289–296, 1994.

8. Vara-Thorbeck C, Sanchez de Badajoz E: Laparoscopic illeal-loop conduit. *Surg Endosc* 8(2):114–115, 1994.

9. Duh QY: Laparoscopic procedures for small bowel disease. *Baillieres Clin Gastroenterol* 7(4):833–850, 1993.

10. Elkus RM: Laparoscopically assisted resection of small bowel injury during laparoscopic cholecystectomy. *Surg Laparosc Endosc* 3(4):349–350, 1993.

11. Milsom JW, Lavery IC, Bohm B, et al: Laparoscopically assisted ileocolectomy in Crohn's disease. *Surg Laparosc Endosc* 3(2):77–80, 1993.

12. Saw EC, Ramachandra S: Laparoscopically assisted resection of intussuscepted Meckel's diverticulum. *Surg Laparosc Endosc* 3(2):149–152, 1993.

13. Nathanson LK: Laparoscopic cholecyst-jejunostomy for malignant disease. *Surg Oncol* 1:19–24, 1993.

14. Nassar A: Laparoscopic mobilization and exteriorization for minimally invasive small bowel resection (letter; comment). *Br J Surg* 80(10):1351–1352, 1993.

15. Miller K, Hutter J: Videolaparoscopic treatment of Meckel's diverticulum. *Endoscopy* 25(5):373, 1993.

16. Echenique M, Domingues AS, Echenique I, et al: Laparoscopic diagnosis and treatment of Meckel's diverticulum complicated by gastrointestinal bleeding. *J Laparoendosc Surg* 3(2):145–148, 1993.

17. Nezhat C, Nezhat F, Ambroze W, et al: Laparoscopic repair of small bowel and colon: A report of 26 cases. *Surg Endosc* 7(2):88–89, 1993.

18. Cross MJ, Snyder SK: Laparoscopic-directed small bowel resection for jejunal diverticulitis with perforation. *J Laparoendosc Surg* 3(1):47–49, 1993.

19. Keating J, Hill A, Schroeder D, et al: Laparoscopy in the diagnosis and treatment of acute small bowel obstruction. *J Laparoendosc Surg* 2(5):239–244, 1992.

20. Bastug DF, Trammell SW, Boland JP, et al: Laparoscopic adhesiolysis for small bowel obstruction. *Surg Laparosc Endosc* 1(4):259–262, 1991.

21. Monson JR: Advanced techniques in abdominal surgery. *BMJ* 307(6915):1346–1350, 1993.

22. Westcott CJ, Westcott RJ, Kerstein MD: Perforation of Meckel's diverticulum during laparoscopic cholecystectomy. *South Med J* 88(6):661, 1995.

23. Eden CG, Williams TG: Duodenal perforation after laparoscopic cholecystectomy. *Endoscopy* 24(9):790–792, 1992.

24. Petersen TI, Qvist N, Wara P: Intestinal obstruction—a procedure related complication of laparoscopic inguinal hernia repair. *Surg Laparosc Endosc* 5(3):214–216, 1995.

25. Azurin DJ, Go LS, Arroyo LR, et al: Trocar site herniation following laparoscopic cholecystectomy and the significance of an incidental preexisting umbilical hernia. *Am Surg* 61(8):718–720, 1995.

26. Huntington TR, Klomp GR: Retained staples as a cause of mechanical small-bowel obstruction. *Surg Endosc* 9(3):353–354, 1995.

27. Puls LE, Henderson RC: Small bowel herniation after laparoscopically assisted vaginal hysterectomy. *Acta Obstet Gynecol Scand* 74(4):307–310, 1995.

28. Storms P, Stuyven G, Vanhemelen G, et al: Incarcerated trocar-wound hernia after laparoscopic hysterectomy. Is closure of large trocar fascia defects after laparoscopy necessary? *Surg Endosc* 8(8):901–902, 1994.

29. Kreutzer ER, Lemer SE, Kahan NZ, et al: Laparoscopic treatment of small bowel obstruction following laparoscopic lymphadenectomy. *Urology* 44(5):768–770, 1994.

30. Kopelman D, Schein M, Assalia A, et al: Small bowel obstruction following laparoscopic cholecystectomy: Diagnosis of incisional hernia by computed tomography. *Surg Laparosc Endosc* 4(4):325–326, 1994.

31. Reissman P, Shiloni E, Gofrit O, et al: Incarcerated hernia in a lateral trocar site—an unusual early postoperative complication of laparoscopic surgery: Case report. *Eur J Surg* 160(3):191–192, 1994.

32. Tsang S, Normand R, Karlin R: Small bowel obstruction: A morbid complication after laparoscopic herniorrhaphy. *Am Surg* 60(5):332–334, 1994.

33. Radcliffe AG: Richter's herniation of the small bowel through the trocar site following laparoscopic surgery. *J Laparoendosc Surg* 3(5):520–522, 1993.

34. Kumar S, Bremner DN: Herniation at the site of cannula insertion after laparoscopic cholecystectomy (letter; comment). *Br J Surg* 80(11):1488, 1993.

35. Jenkins DM, Paluzzi M, Scott TE: Postlaparoscopic small bowel obstruction. *Surg Laparosc Endosc* 3(2):139–141, 1993.

36. Watson SD, Saye W, Hollier PA: Combined laparoscopic incarcerated herniorrhaphy and small bowel resection. *Surg Laparosc Endosc* 3(2):106–108, 1993.

37. Hass BF, Schrager RE: Small bowel obstruction due to Richter's hernia after laparoscopic procedures. *J Laparoendosc Surg* 3(4):421–423, 1993.

38. Whiteley MS: Herniation at the site of cannula insertion after laparoscopic cholecystectomy (letter, comment). *Br J Surg* 80(11):1488, 1993.

39. Georgen, M, Azagra JS: Herniation at the site of cannula insertion after laparoscopic cholecystectomy (letter, comment). *Br J Surg* 80(11):1488, 1993.

40. Braithwaite BD, Gear MW: Herniation at the site of cannula insertion after laparoscopic cholecystectomy (letter, comment). *Br J Surg* 80(11):1488, 1993.

41. Kurtz BR, Daniell JF, Spaw AT: Incarcerated incisional hernia after laparoscopy: A case report. *J Reprod Med* 38(8):643–644, 1993.

42. McMillan J, Watt I: Herniation at the site of cannula insertion after laparoscopic cholecystectomy (see comments). *Br J Surg* 80(7):915, 1993.
43. Ballem RV, Kenny R, Giuliano M: Small bowel obstruction following laser laparoscopic cholecystectomy: A case study. *J Laparoendosc Surg* 3(3):313–314, 1993.
44. Wegener ME, Chung D, Crans C, et al: Small bowel obstruction secondary to incarcerated Richter's hernia from laparoscopic hernia repair. *J Laparoendosc Surg* 3(2):173–176, 1993.
45. Sessa R, Tricarico A, Tartaglia A, et al: New laparoscopic treatment of bleeding Meckel's diverticulum in adults. *Endoscopy* 26(7):629, 1994.
46. Teitelbaum DH, Polley TZ, Obeid F: Laparoscopic diagnosis and excision of Meckel's diverticulum. *J Pediatr Surg* 29(4):495–497, 1994.
47. Huang CS, Lin LH: Laparoscopic Meckel's diverticulectomy in infants: Report of three cases. *J Pediatr Surg* 28(11):1486 1489, 1993.
48. Ilebebrand D, Menningen R, Sommer H, et al: Small bowel necrosis following laparoscopic cholecystectomy: A clinically relevant complication? *Endoscopy* 27(3):281, 1995.
49. Talbot D, Miller IT, Miller IA: Fatal intestinal ischaemia following laparoscopic cholecystectomy (letter). *BJS* 82(8):1143, 1995.
50. Berry SM, Ose KJ, Bell RH, et al: Thermal injury of the posterior duodenum during laparoscopic cholecystectomy. *Surg Endosc* 8(3):197–200, 1994.
51. Ata AH, Bellemore TJ, Meisel JA, et al: Distal thermal injury from monopolar electrosurgery. *Surg Laparosc Endosc* 3(4):323–327, 1993.

chapter twenty-one

Management and Prevention of Complications in Laparoscopic Colectomy: Emphasis on Right Colon Resection

W. Peter Geis
Edward J. Brennan, Jr.

INTRODUCTION

Laparoscopic colectomy procedures have developed rapidly in spite of their mere 5-year history since the introduction of the first procedure.[1] Numerous complications are well known to occur following colectomy, the majority of which are preventable. Thus, the key to minimizing complications during and following laparoscopic colectomy is prevention. Complications specific to the laparoscopic approach to colon resection have been encountered by many investigators[2–5] and will be emphasized in this chapter. Since the video-assisted approach emphasizes an accurate and detailed view of the operative field and the important anatomic structures, emphasis will be placed on the appropriate, safe visualization of the entire surgical field laparoscopically. Further, the appropriate choice of cases to be treated by the laparoscopic approach to colon resection has an important role in minimizing operative and postoperative complications.[6]

Only approximately 5% of colon resections are currently performed laparoscopically. However, progressive expansion of the use of the minimally invasive approach to colectomy will depend largely on an organized and thoughtful learning process for each surgeon and each laparoscopic operating room team, as well as avoidance of complications by the operating room team during their experience with progressively more complex cases. Lastly, the laparoscopic approach to colon resection emphasizes early ambulation, rapid recovery, shortened hospitalization, and early return to activities for the patient. These dramatic benefits will only accrue in the absence of operative and postoperative complications. Therefore, the rate-limiting factor in the expanding utilization of laparoscopic procedures is successful outcomes in the absence of morbidity and mortality. The use of prudent, time-honored principles of surgical care must be transferred to the laparoscopic environment together with a structured, organized sequential experience with the unique factors engendered by the video-assisted approach and their unique potential complications.

CHOICE OF CASES

An appropriate choice of cases for the minimally invasive approach to colectomy will minimize complications. Factors which influence the use of laparoscopy include (1) prior abdominal surgery, (2) prior serious abdominal infection, (3) benign versus malignant disease of the colon, (4) laparoscopic complexity of the individual colectomy procedure, and (5) experience of the laparoscopic operating room team. Clearly, prior abdominal surgery and prior peritoneal infection increase the likelihood of abdominal adhesions which require adhesiolysis laparoscopically. The introduction of adhesiolysis, an additional procedure, increases the length of the operation and increases the likelihood of inadvertent injury to other vital structures, including the bowel, ureter, and major vascular structures.[7] Further, the use of monopolar cautery during adhesiolysis may increase injury to associated structures.[8] The ability of the operative team to manage adhesions quickly is learned and should be done in association with laparoscopic colectomy only after gaining a moderate amount of experience with adhesiolysis in less complex laparoscopic procedures. Further, other energy sources for adhesiolysis which have less chance of causing organ injury, including the ultrasonic scalpel,[8–11] bipolar cautery, or even appropriate laser energy, should be used appropriately.

Patients with benign disease of the colon seem to be at less risk for complications than those with malignant disease. Patients with malignant disease tend to have an increased risk of systemic postoperative complications.[13] Further, the use of laparoscopic colectomy in malignant disease has reportedly been associated with port site implantation of tumor cells reportedly.[5,14–19] While some investigators have considered malignant disease of the colon to be a major contraindication to laparoscopic colectomy due to port site implantation reports,[15,20] others have noted that this complication is extremely rare and that it occurs most often in patients with advanced malignancy involving malignant contamination of the serosa and peritoneal surface.[21] A few cases of port site recurrence have been reported in patients with malignancy confined to the colon. In these rare circumstances, technical aspects of manipulation of the tumor laparoscopically must be reassessed. If inappropriate manipulation of the intestine does cause port site implantation, then avoidance of this complication will occur only if colectomy for malignancy is performed by surgical teams with extensive experience with the laparoscopic approach. Principles which minimize complications should include (1) the use of laparoscopic operative teams who have extensive experience with laparoscopic colectomy, (2) irrigation of port sites with water, and (3) the use of a bag to cover the specimen as a wound protector during exteriorization and specimen removal.

Benign diseases of the right colon which might be treated laparoscopically include adenomatous polyps, bleeding arteriovenous malformations, cecal volvulus, ischemic bowel disease, colonic inertia, ulcerative colitis, and Crohn's disease. Since the last two diseases may occur in association with adhesions, thickened mesentery, and alteration of normal anatomic landmarks, the laparoscopic approach to these diseases should be limited to surgical teams with extensive experience.

Laparoscopic colectomy for malignant disease also requires a regional resection of the colon, with division of the regional vessel at its origin along with associated lymph node drainage. This requirement implies that the laparoscopic surgical team should be experienced in regional devascularization of the blood supply. The inexperienced laparoscopic surgical team should avoid these procedures since inadequate control or loss of control of a major vascular structure may result in a serious operative complication.

The issue of regional devascularization for colonic malignancy raises the issue of the complexity of laparoscopic colectomy procedures due to the three laparoscopic skills required to perform a variety of these procedures: mobilization, devascularization, and intracorporeal anastomosis. Surgery for benign disease of the cecum may be performed utilizing intracorporeal mobilization followed by exteriorization of the intestine and subsequent devascularization, resection, and anastomosis at the skin level through a mini-incision (Fig. 21.1 A,B). In contrast, laparoscopic right colon resection for malignant disease requires intracorporeal mobilization and devascularization (Fig. 21.2) to accomplish regional cancer resection prior to exteriorization of the resected specimen. Addition of the second intracorporeal skill adds complexity to the laparoscopic procedure. Figure 21.3 delineates the 13 common laparoscopic colectomy procedures based on progressive complexity ratings.[22] The complexity scale indicates procedures of low laparoscopic complexity on the left, moderate complexity in the center, and high complexity on the right. The complexity scale provides a road map that allows the surgeon and laparoscopic colectomy team to choose procedures of low complexity early in their experience, followed by procedures of moderate complexity as their experience increases and matures. Using this scale results in avoidance of inadvertent complications due to performance of highly complex laparoscopic colectomy procedures by an inexperienced team. Further, the complexity scale reiterates that the laparoscopic colectomy team may learn the three intracorporeal skills sequentially if cases are chosen carefully based on the expected skill or skills required for the individual procedure.[24] It should be noted that the only circumstance in which

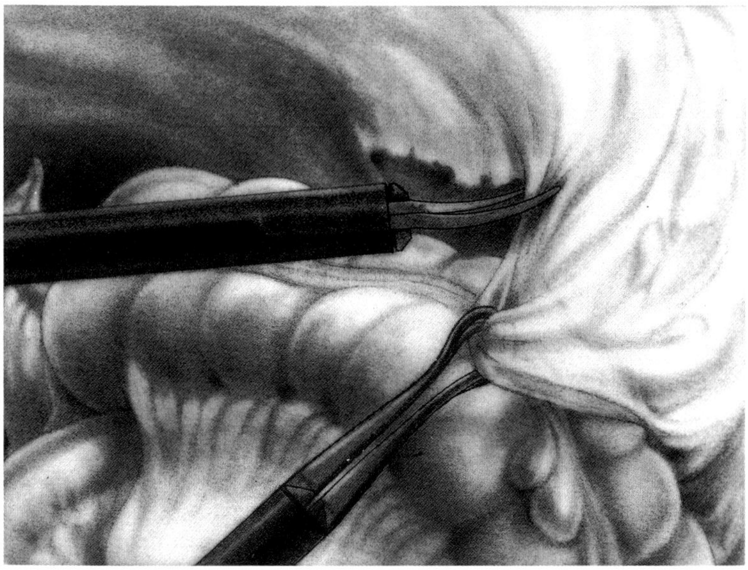

a

Figure 21.1. (a) Illustration delineates transection of lateral peritoneal attachment of cecum and ascending colon during laparoscopic mobilization of right colon. Traction and counter-traction are used to separate tissue layers. (b) Illustration delineates transection of transverse colon and ileum at skin level following exteriorization of right colon and distal ileum through mini-incision in right lower abdominal wall. The center illustration delineates side-to-side anastomosis of transverse colon to distal ileum at skin level through right lower quadrant mini-incision. The right photo identifies closure of ends of functional end-to-end anastomosis at skin level prior to re-insertion of anastomosis into abdominal cavity.

b

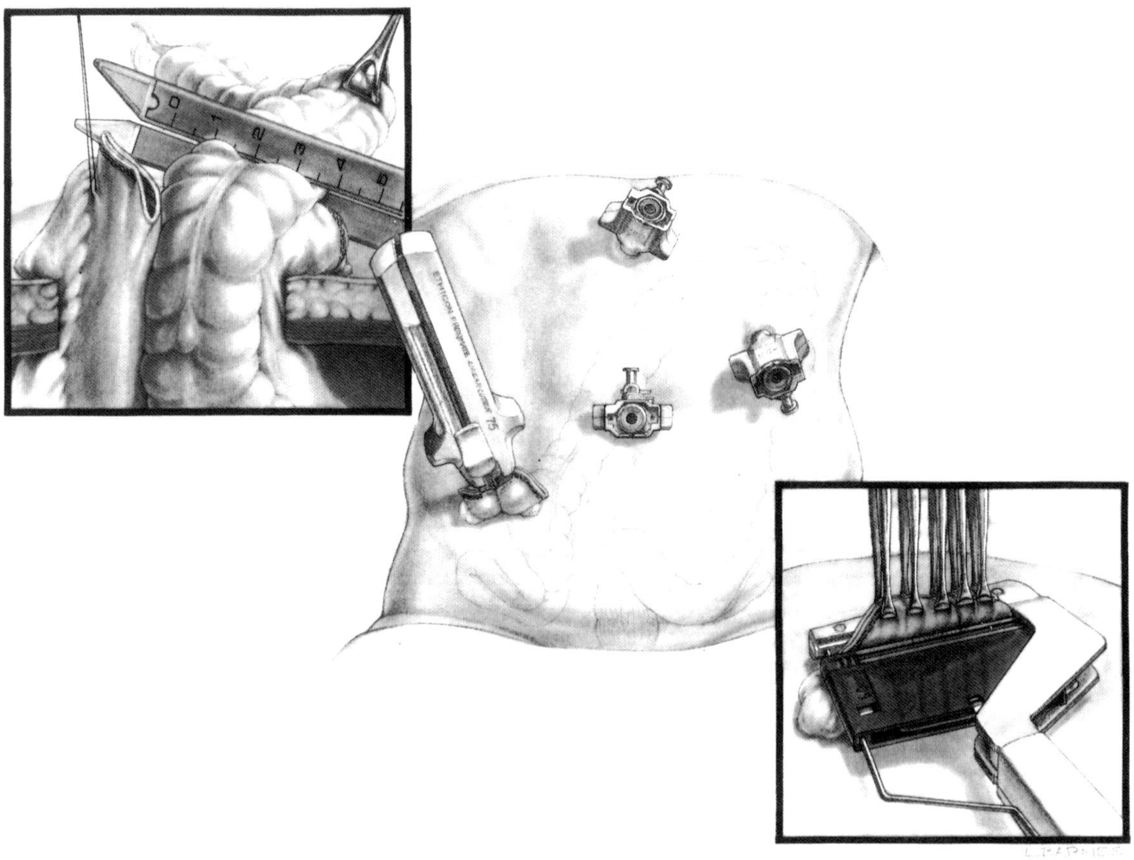

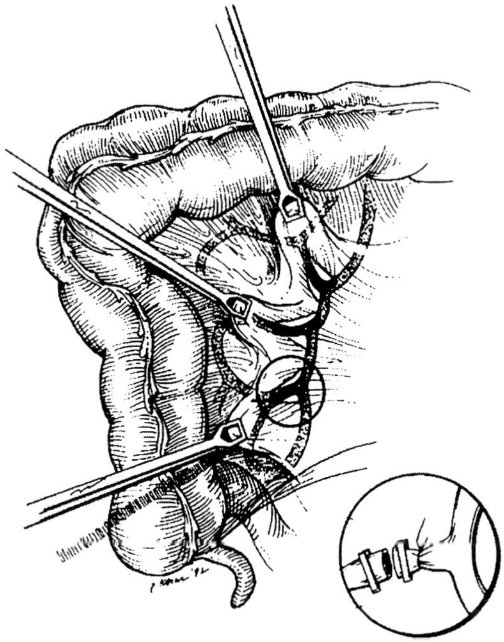

Figure 21.2. Retraction of mesentery of right colon opposite root of mesentery to delineate major regional vessels. Regional vessels are ligated with endoscopic clips and endoloops, or with endoscopic stapler.

an intracorporeal anastomosis is absolutely required occurs when both ends of the resected specimen do not reach the skin level through a mini-incision. Thus, intracorporeal anastomosis is largely restricted to sigmoid colon resection and low anterior resection, minimizing the risk and complexity of other laparoscopic colectomy anastomoses.

THE OPERATIVE FIELD AND VISIBILITY

Accurate visualization of the operative field and precise identification of vital structures is the key to avoiding of technical complications during laparoscopic colectomy. Exposure is provided by the location of laparoscopic ports, use of gravity as a retractor, location of the laparoscope and camera, position of the surgeon and first assistant, and position of the monitors in relation to the laparoscopic work and the surgeon. For right colon resection, two laparoscopic ports are placed far from the right colon to allow Babcock retractors a maximum radius of curvature and maximum versatility in retracting the colon in a variety of directions (Fig. 21.4). The two ports are placed in the epigastrium and the left upper quadrant of the abdomen. The umbilical port is used for the camera and laparoscope which provides the ability to view the pelvis, the right hemiabdomen, the root of the mesentery, the hepatic flexure, and the transverse colon and greater omentum with a single sweeping view. If a fourth port is placed in the

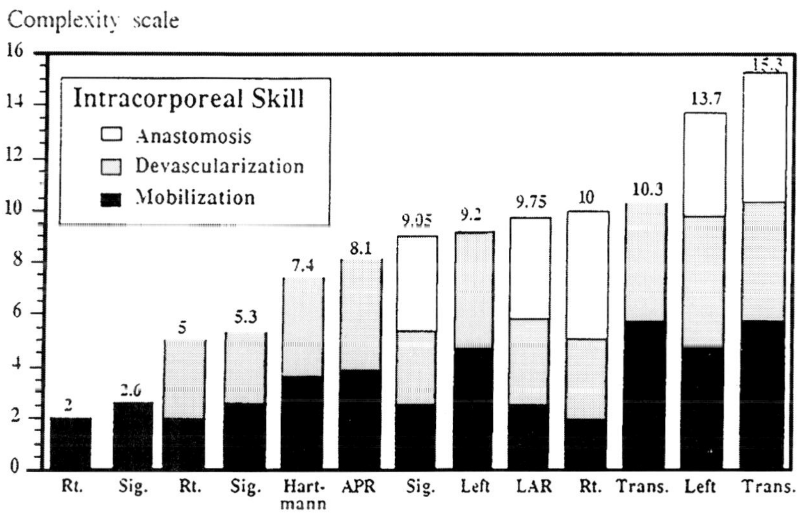

Figure 21.3. Colectomy complexity scale delineating laparoscopic complexity of 13 colectomy procedures based on use of three separate laparoscopic skills; mobilization, devascularization, and anastomosis.

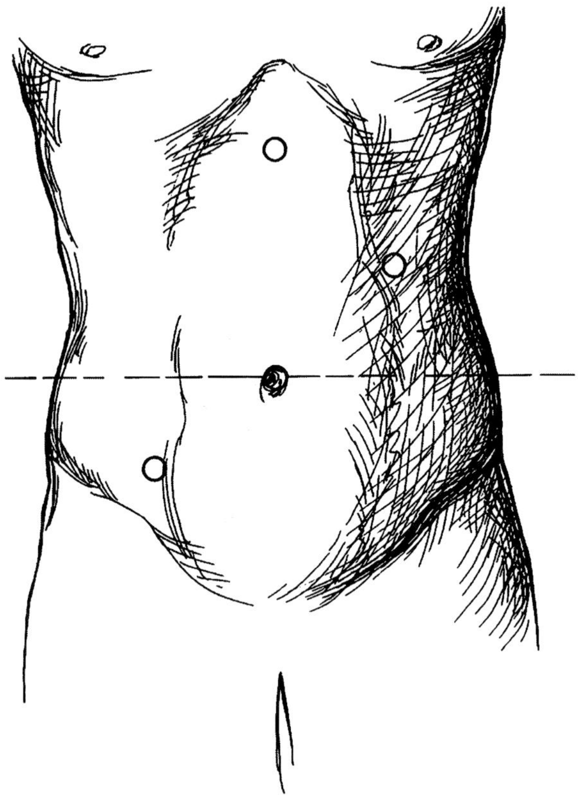

Figure 21.4. Illustration of anterior abdomen delineating four laparoscopic port sites recommended during laparoscopic right colon resection.

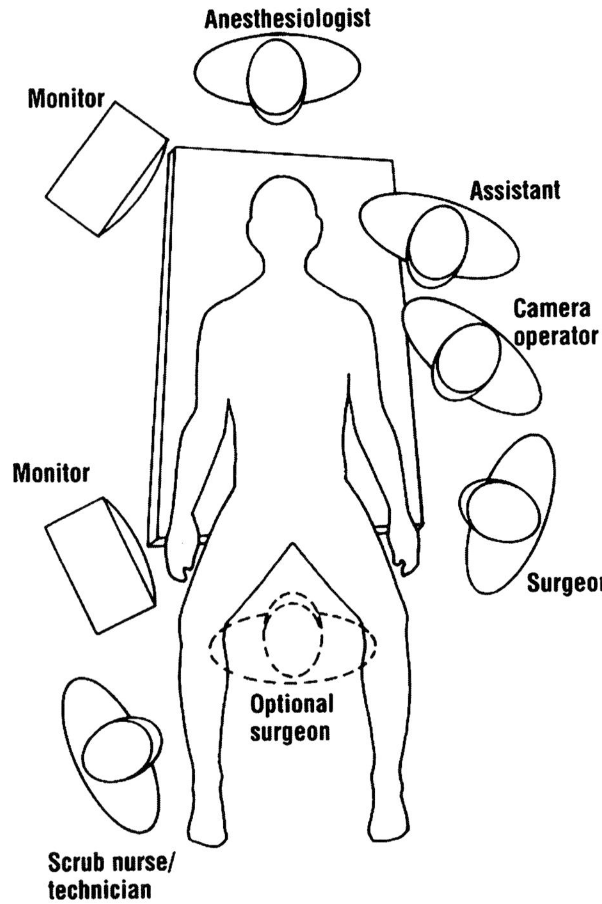

Figure 21.5. Illustration delineates room, equipment, and personnel distribution during right colon resection.

right lower abdomen under direct vision after retracting the cecum cephalad and to the left using a Babcock retractor from the left upper quadrant port, this manipulation will confirm the ability of the right lower quadrant port to act as working port in mobilizing the cecum and distal ileum caudad to the right colon.

All patients are placed in the modified lithotomy position for either the surgeon or scrub nurse to stand between the thighs (Fig. 21.5). The modified lithotomy position includes the use of rigid stirrups, with the anterior thighs parallel to the anterior abdominal wall. Flexion of the thighs anterior to the abdominal wall will result in competition for space by the laparoscopic instrumentation and the thigh.

Gravity is used as a retractor by placing the patient initially in the steep Trendelenburg position with the right side up. This is accomplished utilizing an electric operating room table with maximum three-dimensional versatility. In this position, all the small intestine will remain in the left upper abdomen following its placement by the surgeon. If the small bowel returns to the operative field and covers the right colon mesentery and/or the right colon and cecum, the table tilt must be increased. Occasionally, mild adhesions will hold the small intestine in the operative field. If this occurs, adhesiolysis should be performed prior to right colon mobilization. Mobilization of the right colon is begun in the safest area—the peritoneum lateral to the cecum. Traction is applied to the cecum, with countertraction on the lateral peritoneum. The peritoneum is incised lateral and caudad to the cecum, and is carried medial inferiorly into the pelvis to mobilize at least 10 cm of distal ileum. Care must be taken to transect the peritoneum only, since the right iliac vessels and the right ureter are immediately deep to this plane of dissection. The peritoneum is then transected in a cephalad direction lateral to the ascending colon to the hepatic flexure. The Babcocks then retract the cecum and ascending colon to the left and away from the right abdominal wall to provide traction on the soft tissue of the right retroperitoneum. Separation of the right mesocolon from the retroperitoneal structures is accomplished with sharp and blunt dissection under direct vision. The right ureter is identified as it crosses the right iliac vessels and enters the right retroperitoneal space. Separation of the right colon mesentery from the retroperitoneum is continued cephalad to the level of the mid-right kidney.

The reverse Trendelenburg position with the right side up is then used to gain access to the right upper abdomen. The midtransverse colon is identified, and the Babcocks retract the greater omentum cephalad and the transverse colon caucad. The avascular plane anterior to the transverse colon and the lesser sac are entered. Careful transection of the avascular plane between the greater omentum and the transverse colon is accomplished from the midtransverse colon to the hepatic flexure. The harmonic scalpel, endoscopic scissors, or a combination of scissors and endoscopic staples are used to provide hemostasis when vessels are encountered. Occasionally, an Endoloop is required to transfix a vessel which continues to bleed following transection. Cephalad retraction of the hepatocolic ligament by the epigastric Babcock, along with caudad retraction of the hepatic flexure of the colon by the second Babcock, allows appropriate tension and visibility of the hepatocolic ligament. Careful transection of the ligament will bring the hepatic flexure of the colon into the midabdomen. Continued separation of the mesocolon of the hepatic flexure and the transverse colon from the retroperitoneal structures allows identification of the second and third portions of the duodenum. Once this has occurred, the midcolic artery is identified as it emanates from the superior mesenteric artery along the third portion of the duodenum. Longitudinal traction on the mesentery identifies this vessel on both sides of the mesentery. The anterior surface of the pancreas is identified, and this organ is avoided. Following identification of these structures, generous mobilization of the right colon is performed. Mobilization may be demonstrated by retracting the ileocecal complex into the epigastrium, followed by retraction of the transverse colon and hepatic flexure into the pelvis.

Care should be taken to avoid grasping the bowel with Babcock retractors in the area of the disease process. The majority of the retraction should be performed by grasping the mesentery or peritoneum. If bowel must be grasped, the Babcocks should reach across the entire wall of the intestine rather than grasp an edge of the bowel and risk injury. If injury to the wall of the intestine occurs during mobilization, a seromuscular inverting suture must be placed. If the segment injured is part of the specimen to be removed, the injured area may often be approximated with an Endoloop, since it will be removed shortly. If the small intestine is injured, it is easily grasped and retracted through a dilated port site to inspect the injury above the skin level and subsequently to repair it. The small bowel is then returned to the abdominal cavity and the procedure is continued.

REGIONAL DEVASCULARIZATION WITHOUT INJURY

Following generous mobilization, the regional blood supply to the right colon should be freely accessible from both sides of its associated mesentery. Safe intracorporeal devascularization of the right colon includes accurate visualization, traction, proximal control, and a steep Trendelenburg position with the right side up to allow gravity to displace the small intestine. The mesentery of the ileocecal complex is grasped with a Babcock and retracted directly opposite the root of the mesentery. The mesenteric peritoneum will tent up as it resists lengthening, revealing the ileocolic vessel beneath the tented peritoneum (Fig. 21.6). An avascular window is present on both sides of the origin of the vessel. The peritoneum is transected along the avascular space, and the vessel is isolated. A Babcock or right-angle clamp is used to grasp the proximal vessel during this procedure. The vessel is ligated and divided either by using endoscopic clips followed by vessel transection and reinforcement of the ligature with an endoloop (Fig. 21.6) or by using the endoscopic stapling device with vascular staples. The stapling device should be used when the vessel and surrounding tissue are large enough to prevent the safe use of endoscopic clips. Following vessel transection, proximal control is maintained by the right-angle clamp until the surgeon is convinced that no bleeding is present. If bleeding occurs, reinforcement with an Endoloop under direct vision secures the vessel. If the vessel retracts into the mesenteric areolar tissue and bleeds, an expanding hematoma is present. We recommend open abdominal

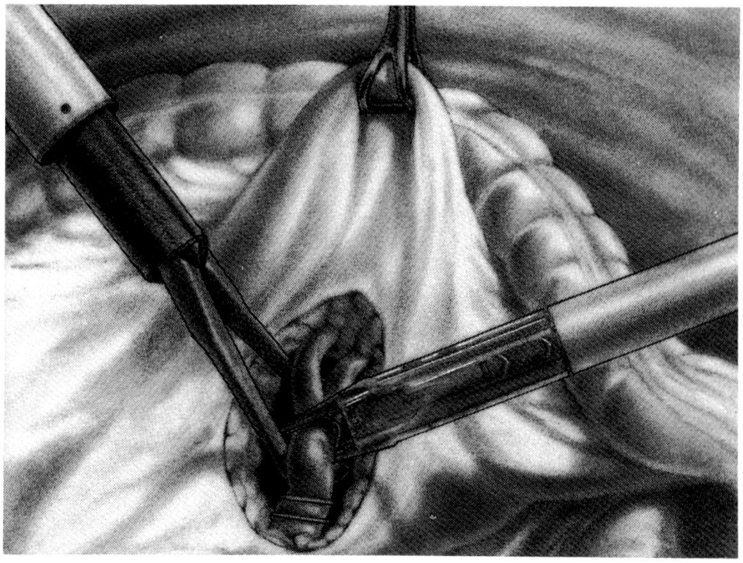

Figure 21.6. Illustration identifies longitudinal traction on mesentery of right colon opposite the direction of mesenteric base. Mesenteric peritoneum tents up at ileocolic vessel identifying its location prior to dissection, ligation, and transection.

exposure to gain control of the lost bleeding vessel in this circumstance.

Once the ileocolic vessel has been ligated and divided, a large window is present in the mesentery. Similar ligation and division of the right colic artery at its origin is easily accomplished. Access to the middle colic vessel is accomplished using the reverse Trendelenburg position, grasping the undersurface of the mesentery of the transverse colon and retracting cephalad and anteriorly. The origin of the middle colic vessel is identified by the tented mesenteric peritoneum. The avascular window is opened carefully on both sides of the vessels. Careful tension to avoid undue longitudinal tension on the middle colic vessel is necessary. Ligation and division of this vessel is accomplished utilizing the endoscopic clip or stapler techniques, followed by reinforcement with an Endoloop. Proximal control with a Babcock clamp is maintained until absolute hemostasis is ensured.

Occasionally, the visual field presented by the laparoscope through the umbilical port seems too close to the tissue for comfortable dissection. Special attention to retraction of the mesentery away from the scope usually increases the distance appropriately. If the scope continues to seem too close to the tissue, it may be placed in the left hemiabdominal port, which increases the distance between the scope view and the tissue.

It is possible to ligate and divide the regional blood supply to the right colon as the first step in the operative procedure if the surgeon believes that this process is beneficial. However, in this circumstance, the vessel must be isolated and carefully separated from surrounding tissue to ensure that no other vital structures are included in the ligation or stapling of the proximal vessel. The structures most vulnerable are the right ureter during dissection and ligation of the ileocolic vessel and the left ureter during dissection and ligation of the inferior mesenteric artery.

EXTERIORIZATION OF THE SPECIMEN

To date, a mini-incision in the abdominal cavity must be performed to remove the resected specimen from the abdominal cavity in nearly all cases of laparoscopic colectomy. The single exception is abdominoperineal resection, in which the specimen may be removed through the perineum. For this reason, the mini-abdominal incision may also be used simultaneously for completion of devascularization, completion of resection of the specimen, and for intestinal anastomosis (Fig. 21.1B). Therefore, the choice of location of the mini-abdominal incision should be made based partially on whether both ends of the resected segment of

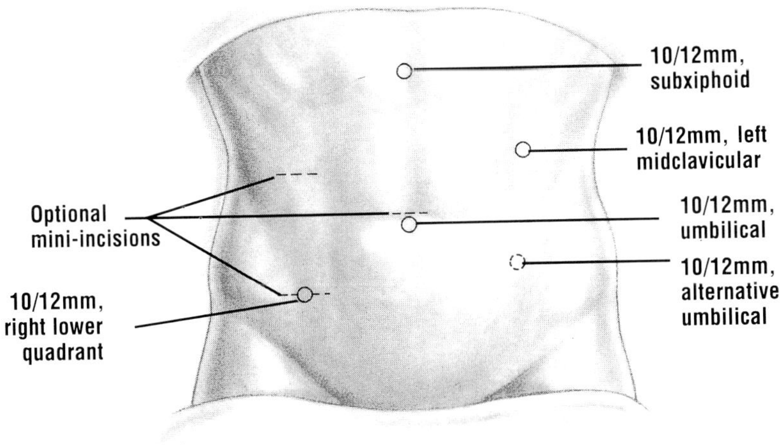

Figure 21.7. Illustration describes port sites utilized during laparoscopic right colon resection; also illustrated are optional locations for mini-incision depending on mobility of proximal and distal segments of specimen.

intestine will reach above the skin level through the incision.

Procedure

The location of the mini-incision will therefore be affected by (1) the ability to mobilize a generous segment of proximal and distal intestine adjacent to the resected segment, (2) the surgeon's preference regarding the most acceptable cosmetic incision, and (3) the least painful and least morbid location. As a result, most often, mini-abdominal incisions performed to extract the right colon are most often right lower quadrant muscle-splitting incisions or midline lower abdominal incisions (Fig. 21.7). Occasionally, however, mobility of the midtransverse colon will be limited due to adhesions, disease, and other factors, including prior surgery. In these circumstances, the transverse colon at the expected line of transection will not be mobile enough to reach an incision in the right lower abdomen. Therefore, an upper midline or muscle-splitting incision in the upper abdomen may be necessary (Fig. 21.8).

The right colon is often exteriorized as a long loop of intestine (Fig. 21.4). The loop method of extraction allows both segments of resected intestine to be extracted immediately adjacent to each other, and without possible *inadvertent torsion* of one of the bowel seg-

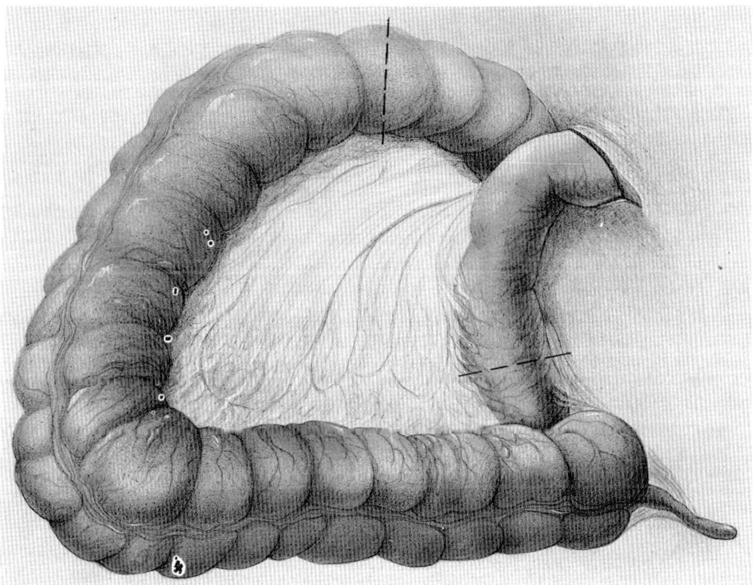

Figure 21.8. Illustration identifies exteriorization of the entire right colon and short segment of distal ileum in loop fashion through a right hemi-abdominal mini-incision prior to devascularization and prior to resection. Dotted lines describe lines of proposed resection.

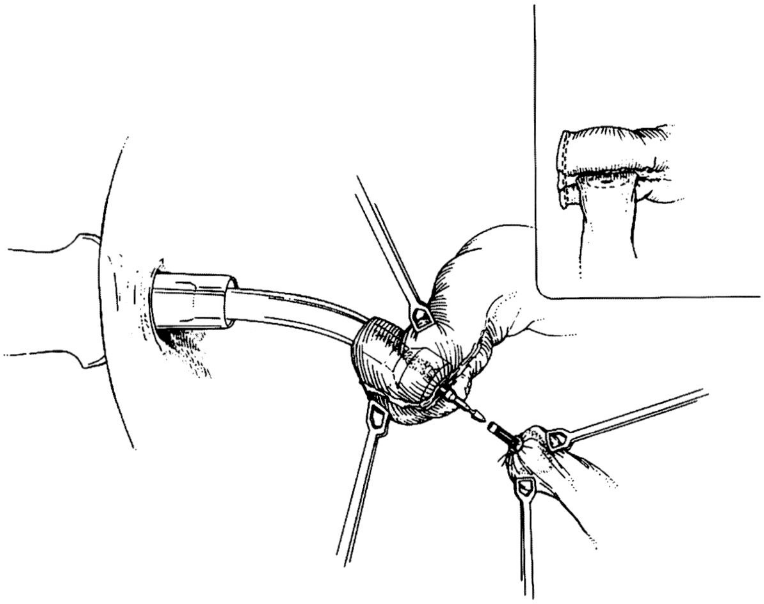

Figure 21.9. Illustration describes an end-to-side intracorporeal laparoscopic ileocolic anastomosis utilizing circular stapler. Following performance of anastomosis, circular stapler is removed and open end of transverse colon is closed with endoscopic linear stapler. Insert delineates completed anastomosis.

ments beneath the abdominal wall. The disadvantage of the method is that it requires a larger mini-incision to accommodate two limbs of intestine with mesentery. Further, extraction of the right colon by the loop method prior to devascularization of the specimen may involve undue traction and injury to the vascular regional vessels, especially the middle colic vein. Care must be taken to avoid this injury, which will result in a mesenteric hematoma and postoperative ileus, as well as post-operative blood loss.

To avoid the disadvantages of loop extraction, the right colon may be removed as a long tubular structure after first transecting the distal ileum and devascularizing the segment at vessel origins. Using this method, the transected distal ileum and cecum are removed through the mini-incision as a long tubular structure, with the last portion extracted being the midtransverse colon. The transverse colon is transected at the skin level, and the specimen is removed. The key to this approach is to have an atraumatic clamp fixed to the distal ileum within the right lower abdomen during the extraction process. Once the specimen has been extracted and resected, the distal ileum is carefully presented to the mini-incision by the atraumatic clamp. The transected transverse colon and transected ileum are then used for an ileocolic anastomosis at the skin level, and the anastomosis is replaced in the abdominal cavity. By this method, the size of the incision may be smaller, and the result in morbidity is more likely reduced. The surgeon must be certain that the intestine is not twisted 360° either proximally or distally.

Importantly, while this approach allows a smaller incision, it is important that the surgeon make the mini-incision large enough to accommodate the right colon mesentery and the bulk of the intestinal wall without the risk of damage to the specimen or contamination of the mini-incision wound. The choice of ileocolic anastomosis is left to the surgeon. We most often use a functional end-to-end (or side-to-side) anastomosis or an end-to-side anastomosis utilizing the circular stapling device (Fig. 21.9).

ANASTOMOSIS

Sigmoid colon resection and low anterior resection require intracorporeal anastomosis because the distal rectal or rectosigmoid segment will not reach a mini-incision in the anterior abdominal wall. However, right colon resection, transverse colon resection, and high left colon resection may almost invariably have their anastomoses performed extracorporeally by extracting both ends of transected intestine through a mini-incision. Rarely, however, one of the two ends of transected intestine will not reach the skin mini-incision because of adhesions or primary disease processes.

This situation has been encountered in cases of prior pelvic surgery resulting in severe adherence of the small intestine to the pelvis, prior upper abdominal surgery, prior trauma, or Crohn's disease, all of which have resulted in severe adhesions in the left upper abdomen transfixing the left transverse colon densely to surrounding tissues. In these uncommon circumstances, right colon resection is performed by intracorporeal mobilization, devascularization, and resection followed by extraction of the specimen then an intracorporeal anastomosis may be safely performed with either an end-to-side anastomosis or a side-to-side anastomosis utilizing the linear stapler. (Fig. 21.10A,B,C)

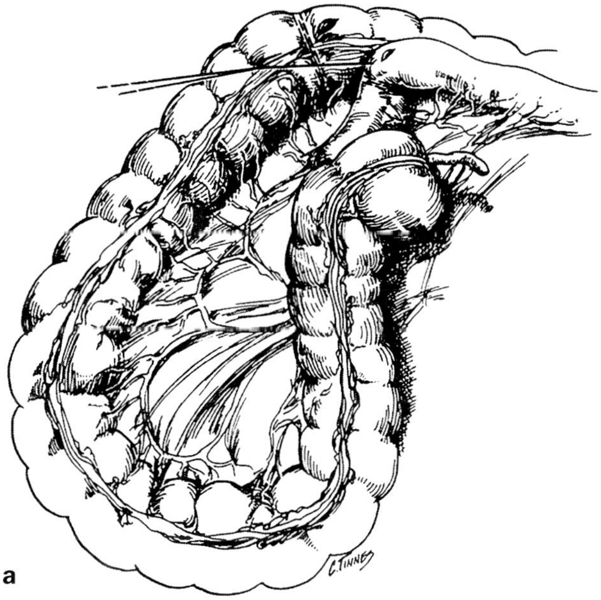

a

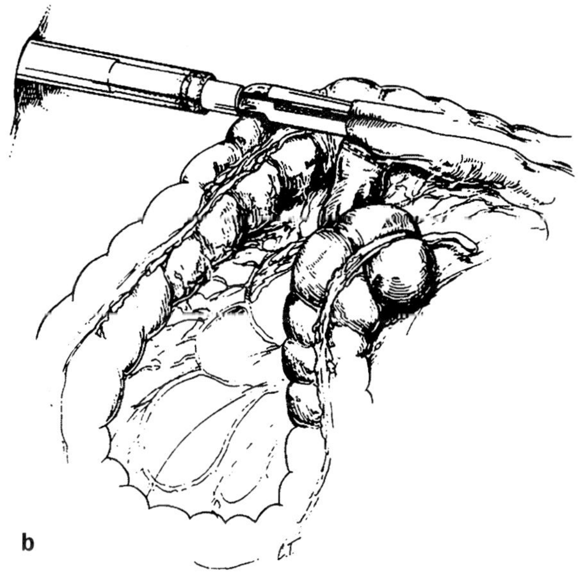

b

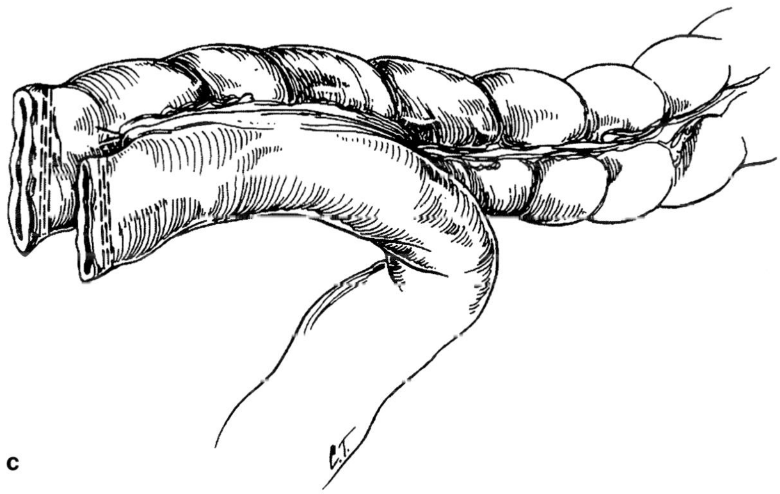

c

Figure 21.10. Three illustrations delineate intracorporeal laparoscopic side-to-side anastomosis of ileum to transverse colon during laparoscopic right colon resection. (a) Illustration delineates approximation of ileum to transverse colon and incision in distal ileum and transverse colon at location of planned anastomosis. (b) delineates intracorporeal linear stapler inserted during performance of functional end-to-end anastomosis; (c) identifies completed anastomosis following closure with resection utilizing linear stapler.

MESENTERIC REPAIR

Many surgeons believe that the mesentery must be approximated following colon resection—especially right colon resection and transverse colon resection, in which a large mesenteric opening may result in a loop of small intestine herniating through the mesenteric opening, followed by the risk of incarceration, strangulation, and bowel obstruction. Other surgeons have not closed the opening in the mesentery following colon resection for many years. There is no firm conclusion on whether closing the large defect in the mesentery versus allowing it to remain alters morbidity and outcome. Prudence dictates that the surgeon should deal with the mesenteric defect in exactly the same fashion as he or she would have in the open approach to the same colectomy procedure. A large opening in the mesentery may never become a significant hernia orifice and may never be a physiologic incarcerating mechanism. However, if the surgeon closes the mesenteric opening, it is of the utmost importance to close it completely, allowing no residual small mesentery defects. These small defects are much more likely to result in herniation, incarceration, and strangulation of the small intestine. Both extracorporeal and intracorporeal methods are used to close the mesenteric defect. The extracorporeal approach uses a running suture immediately following extracorporeal anastomosis. In this method, the first assistant pushes the anterior abdominal wall and mini-incision down toward the root of the mesentery, and the surgeon applies gentle traction in the opposite direction on the mesentery and intestinal anastomosis. The lowest portion of the mesenteric opening is identified, and a running suture is placed from the mesenteric base to the level of the anastomosis. Extracorporeal closure is performed under direct vision.

Intracorporeal closure of the mesentery may be performed with a running suture either laparoscopically or using an endoscopic hernia stapler. Gravity is used as a retractor to visualize the entire mesenteric opening (usually the Trendelenburg position with the right side up), and the mesenteric leafs are retracted opposite the root of the mesentery immediately adjacent to the anastomosis. Mesenteric approximation is performed using the hernia stapler under direct vision. Alternatively, running suture may be placed along the mesenteric defect intracorporeally. The most efficient way to transfix the running suture to the mesentery is to use PDS absorbable clips at both ends (Lapra-ty), which transfix each end of the suture to the mesentery without damaging the tensile strength of the suture. This process eliminates the need to tie at either end of the running suture intracorporeally.

COLECTOMY FOR MALIGNANCY

Colectomy for malignancy should be undertaken only by laparoscopic surgeons who have had enough experience with laparoscopic colon resection to perform the regional resection of colon laparoscopically exactly as it would have been performed using the open approach. We have already discussed the details of sequential progression of experience and prudent decision making regarding the choice of cases. The issue of port site implantation of tumor cells has also been discussed. Table 21.1 identifies appropriate technical details which are recommended during laparoscopic colectomy for malignancy.

DIAGNOSIS AND TREATMENT OF OPERATIVE INJURIES

Organs which may be at risk for injury during laparoscopic colectomy have been discussed. These are listed in Table 21.2, along with recommendations regarding the repairs of each injury. The emphasis should be on an appropriate choice of a strategically placed incision which will accommodate the repair. The same strategically placed mini-incision may then be used to complete the colectomy by extracting the specimen, devascularizing the segment, resecting the colon, and performing the anastomosis. The majority of these patients will have a postoperative course consistent with a laparoscopic colectomy rather than an open laparotomy.

Occult injuries to vital structures provide the greatest risk of morbidity and mortality following laparoscopic colectomy. Occult injuries which may likely occur during laparoscopic colectomy are listed in Table 21.3. This chapter has emphasized that careful technique and prudent judgment will avoid these injuries, focusing on prevention as the best treatment. If injuries do occur, however, Table 21.1 identifies the symptoms and findings. The common thread is always an unexpected adynamic ileus. Therefore, any patient who exhibits an unexpected fever or adynamic ileus in the

Table 21.1. Laparoscopic Colectomy: Right Colon Operative Injuries

Injury	Treatment
Intestine	Bring bowel to skin surface through port site or mini-incision and repair injury
Ureter	Make strategic mini-incision to accommodate ureteral repair and to allow extraction, resection, and anastomosis of the colon
Major vessel	
With proximal control	Endoloop
Without proximal control	Compress with endoscopic instrument, resuscitate, and make strategic mini-incision to accommodate vascular control and hemostasis, as well as to allow extraction, resection, and anastomosis of the colon
Stomach, duodenum	Make strategic mini-incision to accommodate repair of the injury and to allow extraction, resection, and anastomosis of the colon
Urinary bladder	Make strategic suprapubic incision to accommodate repair and to allow extraction resection, and anastomosis of the colon

Table 21.2. Laparoscopic Colectomy: Right Colon Occult Operative Injuries

Occult Injury	Postoperative Findings
Intestine, stomach, duodenum	Ileus, abdominal distention
Ureter	Ileus
Vascular, hematoma	Ileus, decline in hematocrit
Urinary bladder	Ileus, hematuria, oliguria, elevated blood urea nitrogen

Table 21.3. Laparoscopic Colectomy for Malignancy: Technical Aspects

Do not grasp diseased segment of colon; grasp mesentery or peritoneum during dissection.

Consider closure of proximal and distal margins of resection with endoscopic stapler early in the case.

Ligate regional vessels at their origin.

Extract specimen in a bag through the mini-incision.

Allow CO_2 to escape, and decompress abdomen prior to removal of laparoscopic ports.

Irrigate mini-incision, abdomen, and all port sites with water.

postoperative period should have an abdominal radiograph, complete blood count, including a white blood cell count differential and urinalysis. An emergent gastrograffin enema (low pressure) should also be performed to ascertain the integrity of the anastomosis, as well as to visualize the entire wall of the colon. Lastly, the use of a large closed-system drain in all laparoscopic colectomy procedures has a therapeutic as well as a diagnostic benefit, since most laparoscopic colectomy procedures involve a moderate amount of irrigation fluid in the abdomen. It is often time-consuming to irrigate and suction the entire abdomen laparoscopically at the end of the procedure. Therefore, placement of a drain for 12–24 hr will shorten the operative procedure and allow egress of the fluid. This drain will also function as a diagnostic tool in cases of occult injury to the intestine or, the ureter and in cases of delayed bleeding.

REFERENCES

1. Jacobs M, Verdeja JC, Goldstein HS: Minimally invasive colon resection (laparoscopic colectomy). *Surg Laparosc Endosc* 1:144–150, 1991.
2. Phillips EH, Franklin M, Carrol BJ, et al. Laparoscopic colectomy. *Ann Surg* 216:703–707, 1992.
3. Falk PM, Beart RW Jr, Wexner SD, et al: Laparoscopic colectomy: A critical appraisal. *Dis Colon Rectum* 36:28–34, 1993.
4. Beart RW Jr: Laparoscopic colectomy: status of the art. *Dis Colon Rectum* 37 (Suppl):S47–49, 1994.
5. Fusco MA, Paluzzi MW: Abdominal wall recurrence after laparoscopic-assisted colectomy for adenocarcinoma of the colon: report of a case. *Dis Colon Rectum* 341: 249–250, 1993.

6. Ramos JM, Beart RW Jr, Goes R, et al: Role of laparoscopy in colorectal surgery: A prospective evaluation of 200 cases. *Dis Colon Rectum* 38:494–501, 1995.
7. Plasencia G, Jacobs M, Verdeja JC, et al: Laparoscopic-assisted sigmoidolectomy and low anterior resection. *Dis Colon Rectum* 37:829–833, 1994.
8. Amaral JF: Ultrasonic dissection. *End Surg* 2:181–185, 1994.
9. Fowler DL, White SA: Laparoscopy-assisted sigmoid resection. *Surg Laparosc Endosc* 1:183–188, 1991.
10. Geis WP, Malago M: Improved efficiency in laparoscopic herniorrhaphy and appendectomy procedures. *J Soc Min Invas Ther* (In Press) 1995.
11. Brennan EJ, Kim HC, Geis WP: 110 Consecutive laparoscopic colectomies performed using the harmonic scalpel (LCS). Abstract presented Society Laparoendoscopic Surgeons 1995.
12. Fidler IJ, Hart IR: Principles of cancer biology: biology of cancer metastasis, in Devita VT, Hellmans, Rosenberg SA. (eds): Cancer: Principles and Practice of Oncology. Philadelphia, Lippincott, pp 80–92, 1982.
13. Nduka CC, Monson JRT, Menzies-Gow N, et al: Abdominal wall metastases following laparoscopy *Br J Surg* 81:648–652, 1994.
14. Cirocco WC, Schwartzman A, Golub RW: Abdominal wall recurrence after laparoscopic colectomy for colon cancer. *Surgery* 116:842–846, 1994.
15. Alexander RJT, Jaques BC, Mitchell KG: Laparoscopically assisted colectomy and wound recurrence. *Lancet* 341:249–50, 1993.
16. Walsh DCA, Wattchow DA, Wilson TG: Subcutaneous metastases after laparoscopic resection of malignancy. *Aust NZ J Surg* 63:563–565, 1993.
17. Salvalgi RS: Mechanism of abdominal wall recurrence after laparoscopic resection of colon cancers. *Semin Laparosc Surg* 2(3):158–162, 1995.
18. Mouiel J, Gugenheim J, Toouli J, et al: Port-Site recurrence of cancer associated with laparoscopic diagnosis and resection: The European experience. *Semin Laparosc Surg* 2(3):167–175, 1995.
19. Milson JW, Hammerhofer KA: Role of laparoscopic techniques in colorectal cancer surgery. *Oncology* 395–398, May 1995.
20. Beart RW, Ortega A: Review of Milson/Hammerhofer Article. *Oncology* 398–9; May 1995.
21. Beart RW: Wound and port-site recurrence. Letter to the Editor *Surgery* 117.6:719, June 1995.
22. Geis WP, Colletta AV, Jacobs M, et al: Benefits of complexity scales in laparoscopic colectomy. *Int Surg* 79:230–232, 1994.
23. Geis WP, Kim HC: Adoption of laparoscopic colectomy procedures: Relationship to local factors and preceptorships. *Int Surg* 79:228–229, 1994.
24. Geis WP, Coletta AV, Verdeja JC, et al: Sequential psychomotor skills development in laparoscopic colon surgery. *Arch Surg* 129:206–212, 1994.

chapter twenty-two

Left Colectomy and Surgery of the Rectosigmoid Colon

Frederick L. Greene

The techniques of left colectomy and extirpation of the rectosigmoid colon for both benign and malignant disease are standard fare in the armamentarium of the well-trained surgeon. With the advent of minimal access techniques, the principles of open procedures must now be translated to laparoscopic techniques with manipulation of the bowel allowed by accessories through 5- or 10-mm abdominal wall incisions.[1] While experienced surgeons have been confronted with both minor and major complications following bowel surgery, all colectomy procedures have been affected, including the possibility of more disturbing postoperative complications. Whether the colon is resected for benign polyps, diverticulosis, volvulus, or malignant lesions, the complications generally include septic processes, bleeding, ureteral injury, or wound problems. The addition of laparoscopic techniques has introduced potential complications created by CO_2 insufflation for pneumoperitoneum, increased deep vein thrombophlebitis, and other hypercoagulable states created by positioning on the operating table, as well as the systemic effects of abdominal distention. The specific complications related to removal of the left colon and rectosigmoid colon will be addressed in this chapter, but the systemic nature of minimal access techniques and possible complications must be remembered at all times[2] (Tables 22.1 and 22.2).

COMPLICATIONS

The traditional approach to any mortality-morbidity review is to list complications in terms of technical error, associated patient disease, or errors in management and judgment. Unfortunately, some errors in technique begin with faulty judgment, and it must be always remembered that the decision to perform laparoscopic colectomy should be clearly thought out, especially in relation to the patient's overall health and the possibility that previous abdominal procedures may obscure the laparoscopic approach to the colon. The technical issues involved in removal of the left colon and rectosigmoid colon center on the method of handling the bowel and the avoidance of inappropriate entry into the colon during manipulation. With the advent of newer and more "tissue-friendly" accessories, manipulation has become easier, but it still depends on the care of the surgeon in handling both normal and diseased bowel. Several series reporting left colon resection performed laparoscopically include data supporting the fact that instruments may be detrimental to bowel manipulation and that once bowel entry occurs, conversion to a traditional procedure may be indicated to reduce significant spillage even in the prepared colon.[3–5] Prior to the placement of graspers and other accessories in the colonic wall, trocar placement should be appropriate to avoid unusual angulation or tension on accessory instruments. Generally, a five-trocar technique is used for left colon and rectosigmoid colon resection. All trocars should be at least 10 mm in diameter to facilitate use of the laparoscopic camera in various locations. If camera placement is inappropriate, the chance of a misadventure through the use of misplaced accessories is increased.

The technical issues in left colectomy and rectosigmoid colon resection are basically the same. It is

Table 22.1. Prevention of Complications Related to Laparoscopic Left Colectomy and Rectosigmoid Colectomy

Complication	Prevention Strategy
Perforation of colon or small bowel	Use of atraumatic accessories Gentle manipulation Proper trocar and camera placement
Splenic injury	Table positioning in reverse Trendelenburg position Proper decompression and cleansing of bowel Gentle traction on splenic flexure
Ureteral injury	Identification of ureter(s) Avoid devascularization of ureter(s)
Mesenteric bleeding	Gentle creation of mesenteric window Double-clip technique with suture ligation (loop ties) as needed
Anastomotic leak	Proper suture or stapling technique Avoidance of tension
Wound or trocar site infection	Use of adequate bowel preparation and antibiotic prophylaxis Irrigation of trocar site Hemostasis of trocar site Use of protection bag for tissue extraction
Trocar site or wound metastasis	Use of specimen bag Hemostasis of trocar site ? Use of mechanical lift device

Table 22.2. Management of Complications Related to Laparoscopic Left Colectomy and Rectosigmoid Colectomy

Complication	Management Strategy
Perforation of colon or small bowel	Laparoscopic repair Conversion
Splenic injury	Control of capsular bleeding using topical hemostic agent ? Laparoscopic splenectomy Conversion
Ureteral injury	Laparoscopic repair over stent Conversion and conventional repair
Mesenteric bleeding	Laparoscopic clip or suture control Conversion
Anastomotic leak	Laparoscopic repair (intra-operative recognition) Conversion Open procedure and diversion (late recognition)
Wound or trocar site infection	Open drainage of site Debridement Packing
Trocar site or wound metastasis	Excision of metastasis ? Systemic chemotherapy Evaluation for systemic metastases

mandatory to visualize both ureters early in the procedure to minimize injury to these structures. In addition, the left and right external iliac artery and vein, inferior epigastric arteries and veins, and bladder should be clearly identified prior to beginning vascular division of the colon. While ureteral injury has been infrequent, several series have alluded to division of the ureter while mobilizing the left colon or sigmoid colon.[1,6]

It is imperative to localize the disease process in the left colon or rectosigmoid colon prior to beginning laparoscopy. If a small lesion such as a polypoid carcinoma is the reason for excision, additional techniques such as colonoscopy should be utilized intraoperatively to facilitate better localization. Prior staining with vital dyes through the colonoscope may also be important to allow the surgeon to include the proper area of colon in the dissection. One inherent drawback in minimal access surgical technique is the lack of full tactile sensation, which has been a traditional benefit for surgeons doing open procedures.

Once the appropriate structures are identified, the mesentery of the left colon or rectosigmoid colon should be freed completely before attempting to create windows in the mesenteric leaflet for identification of individual vessels. The possibility of causing a complication is enhanced when the patient's body habitus includes a significant amount of fat which obscures the mesenteric vessels. The proper technique of securing identified vessels may include metal clips, suture ligation, laparoscopic stapling devices, and intra-abdominal looping of vessels using a variety of suture materials. No matter what technique is utilized, secure closure and control of the mesenteric vessels will reduce the potential complication of immediate and delayed bleeding. If significant bleeding occurs and cannot be immediately controlled, conversion to an open procedure is warranted.

Following division of the mesentery and ligation of appropriate vessels, the bowel itself must be freed to allow complete dissection, which would ordinarily be performed if done in an open fashion. If less dissection is performed, the bowel will be under tension once an anastomosis is created, and this will lead to anastomotic leak. The anastomotic technique utilized following a left colectomy or sigmoid resection may be performed both intracorporeally and extra-abdominally, facilitated by suture techniques or staplers. If an intracorporeal anastomosis is used, the end-to-end stapler must be placed transanally to allow the anvil of the stapler to be positioned through the proximal colonic segment and brought down easily without tension. The possibility of an anastomotic leak will be increased if the stapler is not utilized properly and if a complete "doughnut" of tissue is not found after firing the end-to-end stapler. For this reason, several surgeons have reported experience with extra-abdominal techniques to create the anastomosis, which allow easier application of traditional suturing or placement of side-to-side anastomoses.

Division of the bowel is necessary in left colectomy and rectosigmoid colon resection. It must be done carefully to reduce spillage of colonic contents, which may be increased because of laparoscopic techniques. The preoperative preparation of the bowel is vitally important and should include the same mechanical and antibiotic approaches used in open surgery. Systemic antibiotics should be a routine part of the preparation for laparoscopic colectomy, and the continuation of the antibiotic postoperatively may be dictated by the findings at the same time of surgery.

The advent of laparoscopic abdominoperineal dissection allows complete dissection of the middle and lower rectum and control of the superior and middle hemorrhoidal vessels with clips. Although the magnification supplied by laparoscopic methods should minimize anatomic injuries, attention to every detail is needed to reduce trauma to the ureters and bladder. Complete dissection of the lower rectum to the level of the levator ani muscles is necessary to perform an unencumbered dissection from the perineal approach. Bleeding and colonic spillage are potential complications if dissection from the abdominal approach is not complete.

Laparoscopic resection of the anorectum also requires the creation of a technically correct end sigmoid or left colon colostomy. Positioning of the stoma in the left lower quadrant and fixation of the bowel wall at the peritoneal and fascial levels are mandatory in laparoscopic-assisted techniques and traditional open approaches alike.

One important technical issue which must be remembered is the method of applying electrocautery intra-abdominally. The standard cautery unit should be set at the lowest possible wattage which will allow both effective coagulation and cutting. If high energy is used, the possibility of contiguous spread of the cautery to adjacent structures will be heightened. The cautery should be routinely set at 25 to 30 watts, and the accessories should be tested for their cauterization effect on appropriate tissue to judge the cautery level prior to beginning dissection.

The potential for complications in completing laparoscopic left and rectosigmoid colectomy has been highlighted by the results of a prospective registry which included 1056 cases contributed by 118 surgeons.[7] Of the total number of cases, 763 were completed laparoscopically and included 294 patients (28%) with sigmoid resection and 82 patients (8%) with left colectomy. A variety of intraoperative and postoperative complications were reported in the registry data, including bleeding, perforation, and other forms of contamination. The complication rates were similar in colectomy and anastomosis performed either intra- or extracorporeally. The registry data support the finding of a 25% conversion rate to an open traditional technique, which reflected a very conservative approach by the group of surgeons as they began their experience with colectomy. As the learning curve matures, conversion rates below 15% should be expected.

THE ROLE OF LAPAROSCOPIC RESECTION FOR CANCER

As laparoscopic left colectomy and sigmoid colectomy are applied to neoplastic lesions of the colon, long-term potential complications of early recurrence of tumor and early death may surface. At this point in our collective experience, the role of minimal access techniques in the extirpation of colon cancer is unclear. One of the most significant recent findings is recurrence of tumor in trocar sites and small abdominal incisions used to extract portions of the colon.[8] It is clear that local contamination has probably resulted in the unusual formation of tumor foci, which may develop as early as 2 or 3 months postcolectomy. Recurrences, as noted in registry data, may be associated with advanced abdominal disease.[9] These are extremely unfortunate complications because abdominal wall recurrences may prove to be sites of further dissemination of tumor, resulting in systemic spread and early death. It is imperative that the potential complications secondary to colonic resection of cancer be minimized through gentle handing of tissue and control of specimens prior to manipulating them through the abdominal wall. Use of sterile bags during extraction of the colonic specimen should be routine. Even if the specimen is brought through a transanal approach, a bag should be used to reduce the possible dissemination and seeding of tumor cells in the distal colon and rectum.

The importance of tissue handling and avoidance of spilling tumor cells during laparoscopic colon resection cannot be overstated. Dissemination of tumor cells may be enhanced by tissue handling and blood loss during laparoscopic procedures.[10] This untoward effect is compounded by its occurrence in an already immunocompromised patient. The goal of the laparoscopic surgeon is to minimize bleeding, especially from vessels directly draining tumor sites.

While series have supported the fact that mesenteric dissection, nodal retrieval, and length of the colon removed are equal in both laparoscopic and open surgery for cancer,[11] there is concern about the overall effect of performing laparoscopic colon resection for cancer among the general population of surgeons, who may be performing inadequate cancer operations even when open techniques are used.[12] Current development of prospective trials for cancer patients utilizing appropriate randomization techniques will be the only way to judge the long-term consequences of colectomy for cancer therapy.

Reduction of complications following laparoscopic colon resection depends on both the expertise and the judgment of the surgeon. It is evident that appropriate training, credentialing, and involvement in continuing education will reduce complications following these techniques, whether they are performed laparoscopically or through a traditional abdominal incision. In addition, the well-trained laparoscopic colorectal or general surgeon should be expert in intra- and extracorporeal knot tying as well as suturing. These skills will diminish complications and should be honed in appropriate skill laboratories before being attempted in the operating room.

REFERENCES

1. Martin DT, Zucker KA: Laparoscopic surgery of the gastrointestinal tract. In Greene FL and Ponsky JL (eds). *Endoscopic Surgery*. Philadelphia, Saunders, 1994. pp 402–422.
2. Phillips JM: Complications in laparoscopy. *Int J Gynecol Obstet* 15:157–162, 1977.
3. Falk PM: Laparoscopic colectomy: a critical appraisal. *Dis Colon Rectum* 36:28–34, 1993.
4. Franklin ME: Laparoscopic colonic procedures. *World J Surg*. 17:51–56, 1993.

5. Jacobs M: Minimally invasive colon resection (laparoscopic colectomy). *Surg Laparosc Endosc* 1:144–150, 1991.
6. Guillou PJ, Darzi A, Monson JRT. Experience with laparoscopic colorectal surgery for malignant disease. *Surg Oncol* 2:43–49, Suppl 1, 1993.
7. Orteg BA, et al: Laparoscopic bowel surgery registry: Preliminary results. *Dis Colon Rectum* (In press).
8. Berends FJ, Kazemier G, Bonjer HJ. Subcutaneous metastases after laparoscopic colectomy. *Lancet* 344:58, 1994.
9. Ramos JM, et al: Laparoscopy and colon cancer. Is the port site at risk? A preliminary report. *Arch Surg* 129:897–899, 1994.
10. Greene FL. Principles of cancer biology in relation to minimal access techniques. *Semin Laparosc Surg* (In press).
11. Cohen SM, Wexner SD: Laparoscopic colorectal resection for cancer: The Cleveland clinic Florida experience. *Surg Oncol* 2:35–42, Suppl 1, 1993.
12. MacFadyen BV, Mathis CR: Laparoscopic colorectal resection of the colon and rectum. Greene FL and Rosin D. (eds). In *Minimal Access Surgical Oncology*, Radcliffe Med. Pub. 1995.

chapter twenty-three

Laparoscopic Nissen Fundoplication: Technique, Pitfalls, and Management of Complications

Namir Katkhouda
Adrian Ortega
Donald Waldrep
Jean Mouiel

INTRODUCTION

Gastroesophageal reflux disease (GERD) is the most common condition in the Western world. More than 80 million Americans suffer from heartburn, and it is estimated that about 20 million Americans have chronic GERD. This condition can be easily controlled medically in about 75% of cases. Unfortunately, in 25% of patients, medical treatment is not sufficient and the disease will progress to a more severe form (recurrent progressive disease).

Patients who do not respond to medical therapy may develop complications, such as stricture, ulceration, Barrett's esophagus, or pulmonary complications. In addition, the side effects of drugs such as proton pump blockers and the economic aspects have to be considered in long-term medical therapy. Surgery is therefore indicated for patients who are usually younger, present with recurrent severe reflux esophagitis, have complications, and/or are required to adhere to long-term medical management. Although there is no randomized study comparing long-term medical therapy to laparoscopic Nissen fundoplication, it is our belief that surgery is indicated to avoid end-stage disease that might require more aggressive surgical management.

Before performing the procedure, it is mandatory to perform an upper gastrointestinal (GI) endoscopy and biopsy, especially in the case of Barrett's esophagus, to rule out severe dysplasia or malignancy, an upper GI swallow, or, better, a video esophagogram. This will show dynamic aspects of gastroesophageal motility. A 24-hr pH monitoring study is needed to confirm that the symptoms are related to gastroesophageal reflux; esophageal manometry is also required. Manometry will answer three questions: Is the lower esophageal spincter incompetent? Is the propulsive force of the esophageal body adequate? Are any other motility disorders present which may cause symptoms of reflux disease? Usually a 24-hr pH study is considered positive when the score is above 14.8 (DeMeester's score). The competency of the lower esophageal sphincter (LES) is based on three manometric parameters: mean resting pressure, intra-abdominal length, and total length.

When all criteria have been met, the operation can be scheduled. The chances for success are high as long as the procedures as performed meticulously.

PURPOSES OF SURGICAL THERAPY

The purposes of surgery are as follows:

1. Reduce a hiatal hernia and resect the sac, when present.
2. Fix the lower esophageal sphincter in the abdomen, allowing it to function under positive intra-abdominal pressure.
3. Close the crura behind the esophagus to keep the wrap intra-abdominally.
4. Ensure adequate length of the intra-abdominal sphincter.
5. Restore the defective LES pressure and allow the LES to relax on swallowing. This fine balance between those two imperatives is critical to avoid postoperative complications such as dysphagia.

GENERAL TECHNICAL GUIDELINES

These guidelines have been described by DeMeester.[2,3] Technically, the goal is to close the crura and perform a fundoplication using a short, floppy wrap of 1.5 to 2 cm. The mobilization of the wrap is achieved by taking down the short gastric vessels, and calibration of the wrap is done around a No. 60 French bougie.

PATIENT PREPARATION AND POSITION OF THE TEAM

The procedure is carried out under general anesthesia. The surgeon is positioned between the patient's legs in order to have a direct view of the monitor placed at the head of the table. One assistant stands on either side of the patient; the camera assistant is on the left side of the surgeon, and the first assistant retracting the liver and the stomach is on the right. Once the trocars are inserted, the operating table is placed in the steep reverse Trendelenburg position, allowing the stomach and other organs to fall away from the diaphragm and providing access to the hiatus. The operation should be performed meticulously to avoid obscuring the view by blood or liquid that pools under the diaphragm. Irrigation should therefore be kept at a minimum (Fig. 23.1).

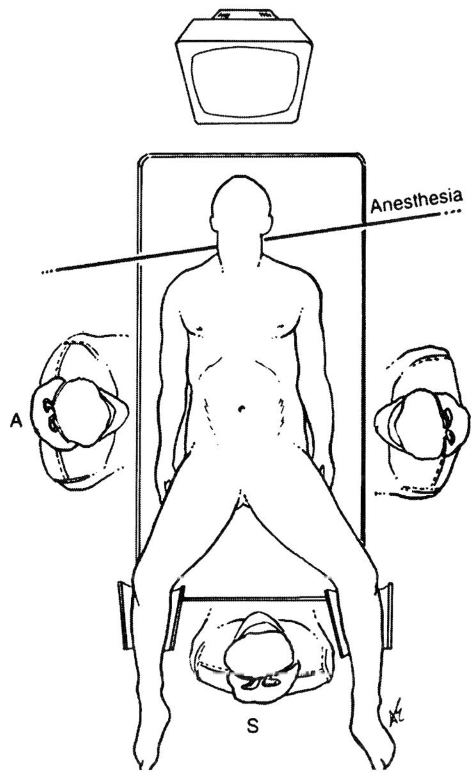

Figure 23.1. Position of surgeon and patient. S: surgeon; A: assistant.

TECHNIQUE

The pneumoperitoneum is established using a Veress needle. Once the security maneuvers are performed using a syringe, a decision is made on the position of the first and most important trocar (Ethicon Endoscopy, Inc., Cincinnati OH) that will allow insertion of the video laparoscope (Karl Storz, Inc., Tuttlingen, Germany). If the first trocar is inserted too low, the surgeon will have only a flat horizontal view of the hiatus, and the stomach will block his view at all times. If the trocars are inserted too high on the midline, the surgeon will not have the panoramic view necessary to evaluate the entire operative field. Insertion of the first trocar depends on the patient's habitus, but as a rule of thumb, the first trocar is inserted in the midline at about one-third, two-thirds, of a distance, separating the xiphoid process and the umbilicus. Once the first trocar is inserted, the second 10- to 12-mm trocar is placed just under the xiphoid, and care is taken not to injure branches of the superior epigastric vessels. This trocar will introduce the endo pool irrigation suction device (Davol, Inc.) and will also serve as a liver retractor, as the blunt, round tip presents less danger of traumatizing the left lobe. A standard fan retractor can also be used.

The next trocar to be inserted is the right lateral trocar for the grasping instruments of the surgeon and, more specifically, for the left hand. Then the left lateral trocar for the grasping instruments of the first assistant are placed in line with the right lateral trocar a few centimeters under the left costal margin. The last trocar to be inserted is the one for the operating instruments of the surgeon's right hand. This trocar is placed midway between the video laparoscope and the left lateral trocar.

All five trocars are triangulated with each other to enable a comfortable operation. They draw a pentagon shape (Fig. 23.2).

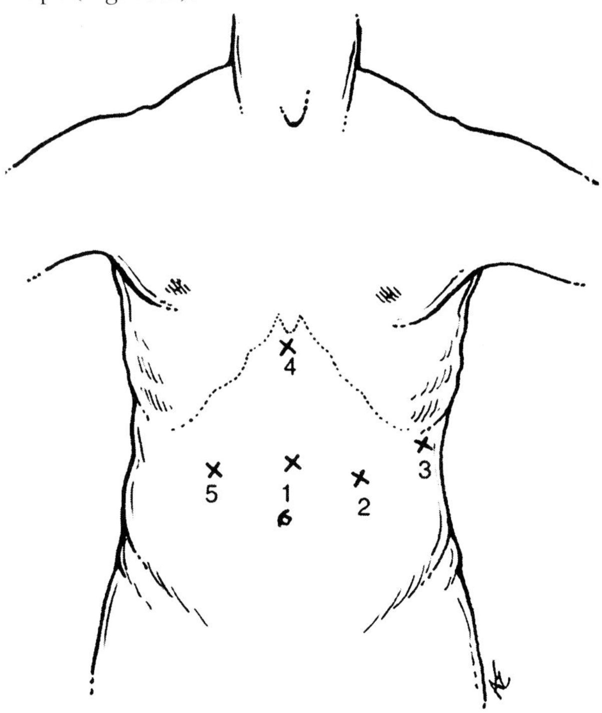

Figure 23.2. Trocar position. 1: supraumbilical videolaparoscope; 2: operating port; 3: grasper, 1st assistant; 4: xyphoid trocar for liver retractor; 5: grasper, left hand of surgeon.

The steps of the procedure are as follows:

1. Achieve access to the hiatus by opening the avascular aspect of the lesser sac, preserving the hepatic branch of the right vagus nerve when possible.
2. Identification of the important landmarks that will lead to the hiatus: caudate lobe and right crus to the left of the caudate lobe.
3. Dissection between the esophagus and right crus in an avascular plane and identification of the right vagus nerve.
4. Demonstration of the left crus from the right side, the left crus and the right crus forming a V.
5. Creation of a window below the left crus and under the esophagus that will allow the passage of the wrap.
6. Division of the phrenoesophageal membrane, preserving the branches of the left vagus nerve.
7. Demonstration of the left crus at the left side of the esophagus.
8. Completion of the window and passage of a Penrose drain around the esophagus.
9. Division of the short gastric vessels, starting at the midfundus and proceeding superiorly.
10. Reconstruction of a normal hiatus by closure of the crura and fundoplication calibrated around a No. 60 French bougie: sliding the posterior fundus behind the esophagus and fixing it to the anterior fundus, producing a short (1.5 to 2-cm) floppy wrap.

Steps of the Surgical Procedure

Access to the hiatus

After retraction of the left lobe, the avascular aspect of the lesser sac is demonstrated. It is grabbed by the left hand, using a traumatic grasper without a rachet (Fig. 23.3). An electrical scissor is used for this purpose. Care is taken to preserve the hepatic branch of the left vagus when possible. This will lead to identification of the caudate lobe at the right side. Just adjacent to the caudate lobe, one can see the pink color of the right crus (Fig. 23.4).

At this point, the anesthesiologist is advised to mobilize the nasogastric tube. This will help identify the esophagus. The dissection is then begun by grasping the right crus with the nontraumatic grasper and electrical scissor bluntly, finding an avascular plane be-

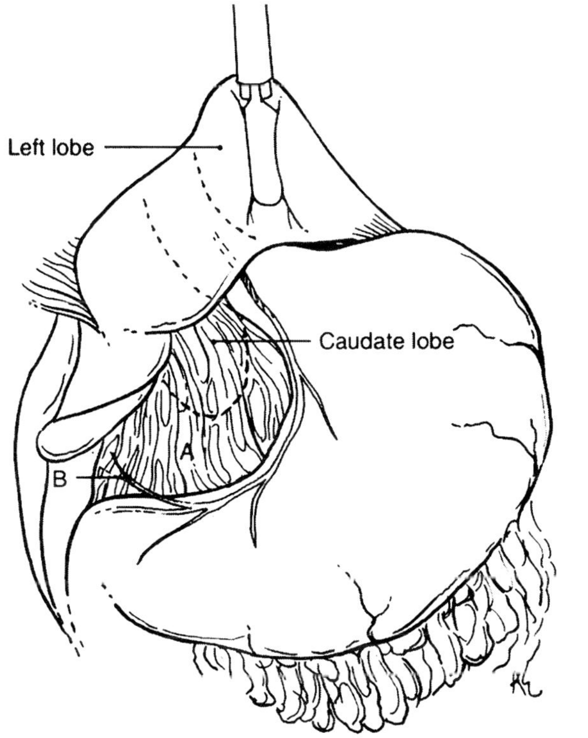

Figure 23.3. Approach to the hiatus. A: avascular aspect of the lesser sac; B: hepatic branch of the left vagus.

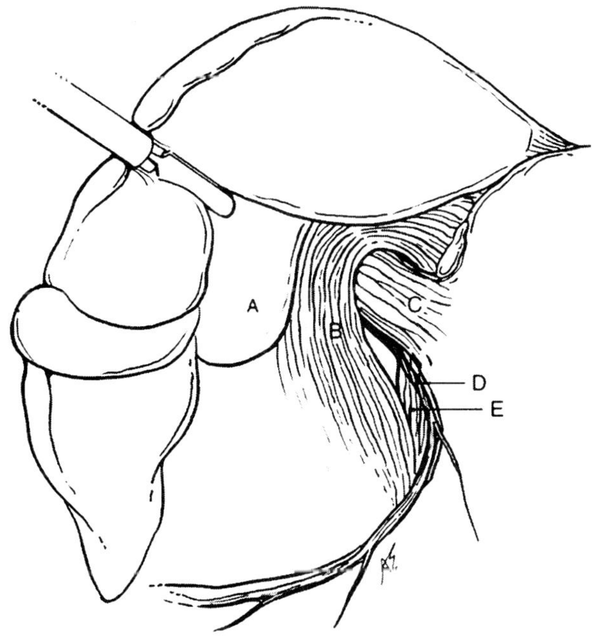

Figure 23.4. Critical landmarks of the hiatal dissection. A: caudate lobe; B: right crus; C: esophagus; D: right vagus nerve; E: left crus.

tween the esophagus and right crus. The plane is opened with a sweeping motion of the two instruments. The right trunk of the vagus nerve can usually be found easily, either along the right side of the esophagus or running on the left crus.

The right vagus is identified by its white color and by the small blue veins covering its surface. It is usually a very big trunk and will resist attempts to break it with a grasper.

Identification of the left crus

We believe that this is the key to hiatal dissection. It is mandatory to find the left crus at the right side of the esophagus. This will lead to a demonstration of the crural V that will help the creation of the retroesophageal window.

Creation of a window under the esophagus

The window is then created with a Babcock grasper (Ethicon Endoscopy, Cincinnati, OH), using gentle opening and closing motions of the jaws behind the esophagus without grasping it (Fig. 23.5). This will allow the creation of a space below the left crus and under the esophagus. This space will be utilized to pass the wrap.

It is not necessary to go all the way through blindly behind the esophagus. Rather, the surgeon should stop at this point and proceed to the next step.

Division of the phrenoesophageal membrane

Division of the phrenoesophageal membrane, preserving the terminal branches of the left vagus nerve, will allow the demonstration of the fat pad, indicating the position of its angle. At this point, it is useful to use a 30 degree angle laparoscope to identify the left vagus at the left side of the esophagus. That will allow the final creation of the passage behind the esophagus (Fig. 23.6). A right angle dissector passing from the right to the left side will allow safe insertion of a Penrose drain around the esophagus.

This clear dissection technique will prevent the blind creation of the retroesophageal window, avoiding potential injuries to the posterior aspect of the esophagus, as described in reported series, leading to perforation and delayed mediastinitis.

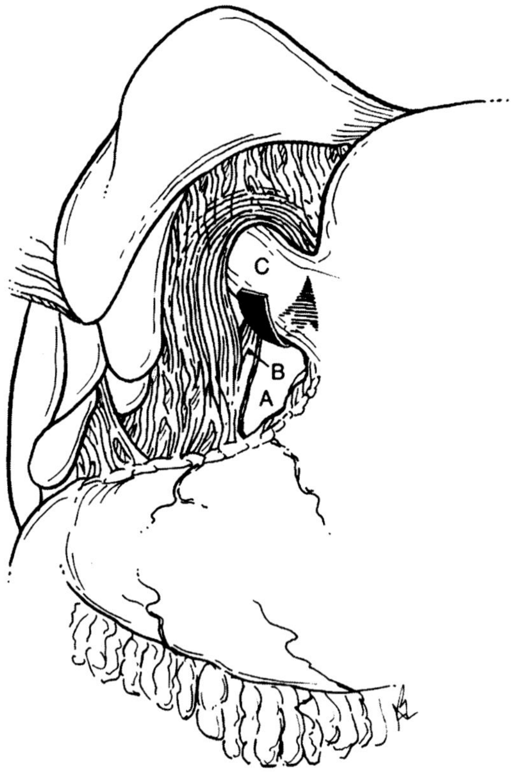

Figure 23.5. Creation of a window below the left crus. A: window; B: left crus; C: esophagus.

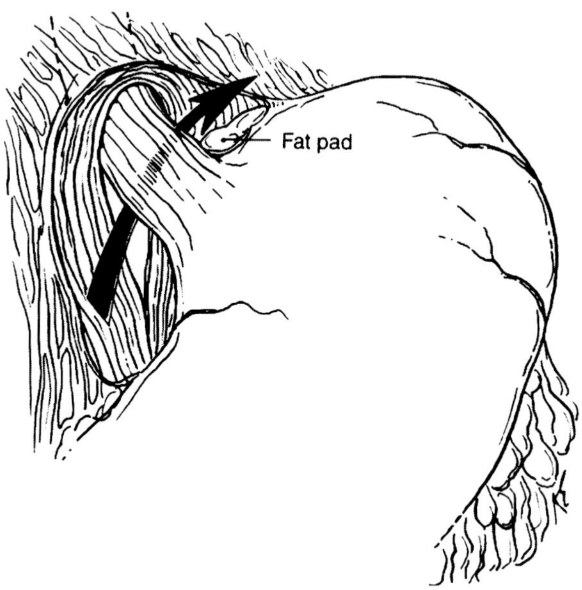

Figure 23.6. Completion of the window behind the esophagus.

Division of the short gastric vessels

Division of the short gastric vessels (Fig. 23.7) is a tedious step that many surgeons are reluctant to perform because of the potential threat of bleeding. Nevertheless, it can be done safely if simple rules are followed. The stomach is grabbed by the left grasper of the surgeon, and the lateral aspect of the gastrosplenic ligament is put under tension superiorly and laterally by the traumatic grasper of the first assistant. The surgeon then divides the short gastric vessels, starting at the midfundus and going superiorly, where the short gastric vessels are very short and close to the spleen. The electrical scissors (Ethicon Endoscopy, Cincinnati, OH) are then employed, using a scooping motion to create windows between the short gastrics. These vessels will then be divided between clips.

A better solution is to use the Harmonic scissors (Ethicon Endosurgery, Cincinnati, OH). The blades of these scissors oscillate at 50,000 cycles/sec, producing heat that seals the vessels by a coagulation process. This has become our instrument of choice, cutting OR time, increasing the safety, and simplifying the procedure.

The dissection proceeds superiorly until the final short gastric vessel is divided. One useful trick is to move the scope to the most lateral left trocar to look at the posterior aspect of the stomach in order to ensure that no short gastric vessels or posterior attachments to the peripancreatic fat are missed. This total division of all short gastric vessels and mobilization of the fundus will allow the creation of a very floppy wrap.

It is mandatory to recognize the posterior aspect of the fundus and differentiate it from the anterior fundus, as only the posterior fundus will be passed behind the esophagus. This is the concept of a "balanced wrap," in opposition to creating a sling mechanism by passing an inappropriate aspect of the fundus such as the anterior aspect, rolling it around the esophagus and suturing it to another anterior aspect of the stomach, usually the body, when all the anterior fundus has been utilized under tension. This creates an "unbalanced wrap," inducing lateral forces putting the gastroesophageal (GE) junction under tension and twisting the wrap.

Reconstruction and fundoplication

The crura are then closed behind the esophagus, using two or three stitches of O-Ethibond (Ethicon, Somerville, NJ) on an SH needle. The thread should be at least 33 in. long if knots are made extracorporeally (Fig. 23.8).

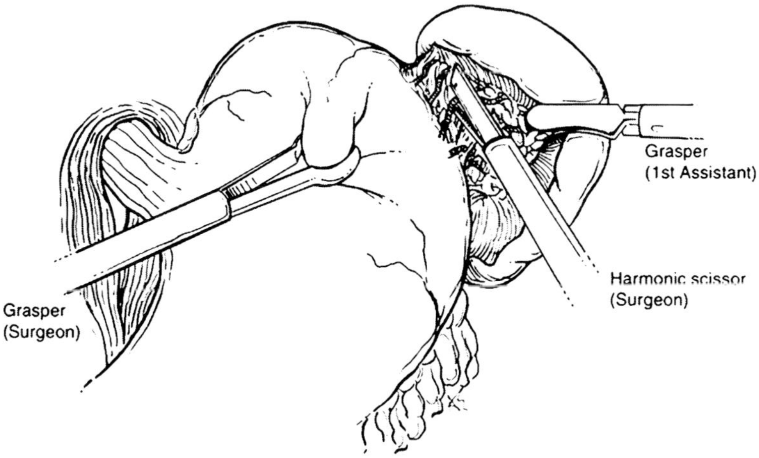

Figure 23.7. Division of the short vessels gastric.

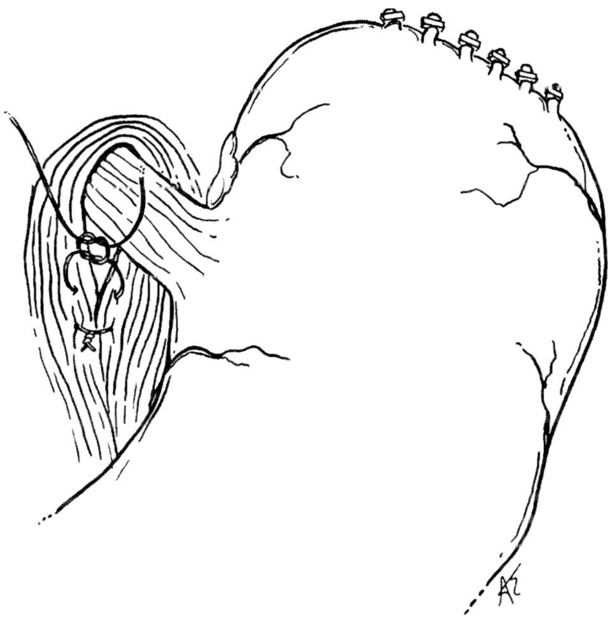

Figure 23.8. Closure of the crura behind the esophagus.

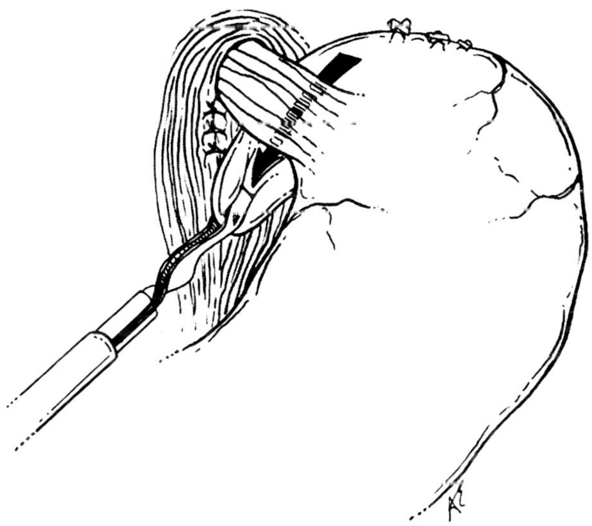

Figure 23.9. Babcok bringing posterior fudus behind the esophagus.

The knots are tied intracorporeally or extracorporeally, using either a Roeder's knot technique or sliding each half knot using a knot pusher. Both techniques are acceptable, and the surgeon should perform the knot he or she can do best.

After making sure that a Babcock grasper can pass between the esophagus and the last crural stitch, the wrap is passed in the created retroesophageal window. Care is taken to pass the appropriate part of the posterior fundus (Fig. 23.9).

One trick is to leave the passed fundus behind the esophagus. If it stays, the wrap is probably not under tension. If it slings back, another aspect of the fundus should be taken to ensure that the wrap is floppy and well constructed.

The next step is the passage of the No. 60 French

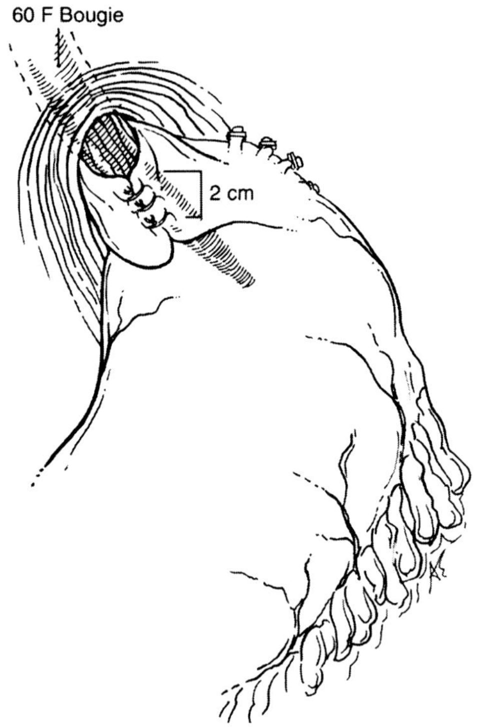

Figure 23.10. Short floppy fundoplication around a 60F bougie.

bougie by an experienced anesthesiologist. This is done by avoiding any cephalad esophageal retraction of the esophagus. The bougie is passed under direct scrutiny of the surgeon.

Once the bougie is passed, the wrap is sutured by placing two or three stitches of 2-0 prolene on an SH needle, again with a long thread if the knots are to be tied extracorporeally. Care is taken to pass the suture using a full thickness bite on the stomach but a seromuscular bite on the esophagus, so as not to contaminate the GE junction.

The final length of the wrap should be a maximum of 2 cm, as described by DeMeester. This calibration around the bougie in the creation of a very floppy wrap will allow not only restoration of the resting pressure of the sphincter, but also good relaxation of the sphincter on swallowing (Fig. 23.10).

The final step of the procedure is to irrigate the hiatal area and carefully check for hemostasis. The trocars are then extracted. All wounds are closed, including the fascia, to prevent any herniation of small bowel. All fluids must be aspirated with the patient in the Trendelenburg position to avoid any residual collection.

POSTOPERATIVE COURSE

We routinely leave the nasogastric tube in place for 24 hr, as some patients develop bloating, which puts the wrap under tension.

The patient is encouraged to ambulate on the night of surgery or the next morning. He or she is started on a fluid diet on the first postoperative day and is allowed a very soft diet on the second. If the patient has normal vital signs, can ambulate well, and tolerate fluids and a soft diet, he or she is authorized to leave the hospital as early as the second or third postoperative day.

Early in our experience, we studied all wraps with a gastrograffin swallow. This became unnecessary as we gained experience with this operation.

We do advise the patient that it is extremely important to continue a very soft diet for about 30 days, fractioning the meals into five meals a day. This will minimize the temporary swallowing discomfort that some patients may experience postoperatively.

PITFALLS AND COMPLICATIONS AND THEIR MANAGEMENT

Various problems occur during surgery, bleeding, esophageal perforations, and splenic injuries. Splenic injuries are most frequently reported in open surgery and have become rare incidents during laparoscopy.

During the postoperative course, two problems may be encountered: septic problems, such as mediastinitis or subphrenic abscesses due to delayed esophageal necrosis, and mechanical problems in relation to a tight wrap, a slipped wrap, or an early breakdown of repair.

Management of Bleeding During Surgery

During posterior dissection of the esophagus while creating the window, some bleeding may occur. It is dangerous to use electrocautery to stop the bleeding, especially in the blind area behind the esophagus. It is advisable to apply some compression using a laparoscopic 2 × 2 piece of gauze inserted through one of the trocars. This usually will take care of a small bleeder, generally a small branch of the phrenic vein.

More severe bleeding may occur during division of the short gastric vessels, forming a large hematoma in the gastrosplenic ligament that will render the dissection very difficult. It is therefore advisable to control the bleeder immediately using a nontraumatic clamp, clean and irrigate around the bleeding area, and apply clips to the bleeding site.

Bleeding from an injury to the spleen is more serious and difficult to control. Again, compression is best employed, using a 2 × 2 piece of gauze and alternating compression and high-current electrocautery. If the splenic injury is not very large, it is possible to finish by applying some collagen pads or other hemostatic agents. If the bleeding is not controllable, the decision to convert to an open procedure should be made promptly.

Esophageal Perforation During Insertion of the Large Bougie

Esophageal perforation (Fig. 23.11) is preventable if the bougie is inserted very slowly by an experienced anesthesiologist under the direct vision of the surgeon, avoiding cephalad retraction of the esophagus, which will angle the esophagus and lead to perforation. If perforation is clearly demonstrated and if it is possible to close it laparoscopically, this should be done if the surgeon is skilled. Otherwise, conversion should be the rule.

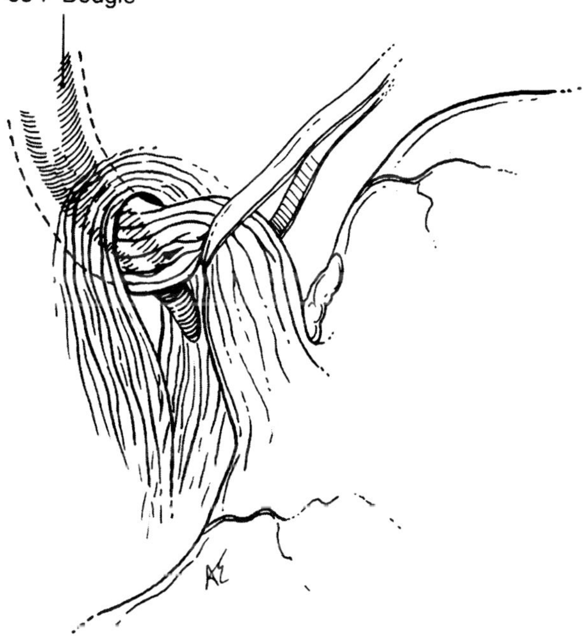

Figure 23.11. Common site of the esophageal perforations on the posterior aspect of the esophagus. Penrose drain retracting and tenting the esophagus superiorly.

During the postoperative period, any sign of sepsis or intra-abdominal abscess may indicate the possibility of an esophageal perforation with mediastinitis. This complication is severe and may lead to death. It should to be ruled out by a gastrograffin swallow, followed, if necessary, by a thorough upper GI endoscopy.

If the esophageal perforation is confirmed, and if repair is delayed and the patient's condition is septic, the only alternative is to reoperate immediately and divert the esophagus. Even though it is possible to perform a primary closure of the perforation, if the perforation is not diagnosed early enough, the safest way to save the patient's life is usually through diversion.

Mechanical Problems Related to a Tight, Slipped, or Broken Wrap

These complications are due to poor technique. The slipped Nissen is due to a failure to include the esophagus in the sutures. The tight Nissen is due to a nondivision of the short gastric vessels or noncalibration around the No. 60 French bougie. This condition will lead to dysphagia, and the wrap has to be taken down if dilation is not successful. This can be done laparoscopically if the surgeon has special expertise, but an open approach is safer.

The same remarks apply to the breakdown of repair due to improper suturing, with the wrap being under the tension. Again, if sufficient expertise is not available, the safest way to manage these problems is to use an open operation.

The Short Esophagus

One final comment should be made about the short esophagus. This is usually defined by a distance of more than 4 cm between the GE junction and the crura on endoscopy. The short esophagus is usually accompanied by complications such as a stricture or Barrett's esophagus. Technically, it is possible to bring the GE junction down by careful dissection of the esophagus in the mediastinum. However, with a very short esophagus, the only possible way is to use a thoracic approach and perform a Collis Belsey procedure through the chest. Even though the indication for such an operation is rare, it is probably safer to perform an antireflux procedure through a thoracic approach than to wrap inappropriately around the body of the stomach or around the esophageal body itself.

REFERENCES

1. Belsey MR: Gastroesophageal reflux. *Am J Surg* 139: 775–781, 1980.
2. DeMeester TR, Bonavina L, Albertucci M: Nissen fundoplication for gastroesophageal reflux disease. *Ann Surg* 204:9–20, 1986.
3. DeMeester TR, Wang GI, et al: Technique, indication and clinical use of 24 hour esophageal pH monitoring. *J Thorac Cardiovasc Surg* 79:656, 1980.
4. Hill LD, Tobias JA: An effective operation for hiatal hernia: An eight year appraisal. *Ann Surg* 166:681–692, 1967.
5. Lortat-Jacob JL, Robert F: Les joule cardiotuberositaires. *Arch Mal App Dig* 42:750–774, 1953.
6. Nissen R: Ein einfache operation zur beeinflussung der reflux esophagitis. *Schweiz Med Wochenschr* 86:590–592, 1956.
7. Rossetti M, Hall K: Fundoplication for the treatment of gastroesophageal reflux in hiatal hernia. *World J Surg* 1:439–444, 1977.
8. Thor KBA, Silander T: Long term randomized prospective trial of the Nissen procedure using a modified toupet technique. *Ann Surg* 210:719–724, 1989.
9. Toupet A: Technique d'oesophago-gastroplastie avec phrenogastropexie appliquee dans la cure radicale des hernie hiatales et comme complement de l'operation de Heller dans les cardiospasmes. *Mem Acad Chir* 89:386–389, 1963.
10. Katkhouda N: Laparoscopic treatment of gastroesophageal reflux disease defining a gold standard. *Surg Endosc* 9:765–768, 1995.

chapter twenty-four

Laparoscopic Resection of the Colon and Rectum

Joseph J. Pietrafitta

INTRODUCTION

Laparoscopy has been influencing all aspects of general surgery, at an increasing rate, since the introduction of laparoscopic cholecystectomy in 1987 by Moret in France. After climbing the learning curve associated with that procedure, a number of surgeons have incorporated a greater variety of surgical procedures into the armamentarium of the laparoscopic surgeon. The ability of the surgeon to perform different procedures laparoscopically has increased dramatically over a very short period of time and has revolutionized the way surgery is performed in a number of centers both in this country and in other parts of the world.

In addition to cholecystectomy we have seen the performance of a variety of other surgical procedures, including appendectomy, inguinal hernia repair, a variety of acid-reducing and antireflux procedures. In most of these procedures we have seen a reduction in cost, a reduction in the degree of postoperative pain, a decrease in the length of the postoperative hospital stay, and a more rapid recovery with earlier return to the preoperative levels of activity and productivity. In addition to a greater variety of procedures, the complexity of those procedures has increased. Certainly a laparoscopic colon resection is more challenging to the surgeon from a technical standpoint than a laparoscopic cholecystectomy. This procedure is not only technically more difficult, it is also one that the average general surgeon performs much less frequently.

A number of other procedures have been developed so that laparoscopy can be performed in a reproducible, reliable, and safe manner. In addition, many of the necessary tools have been developed and continue to be refined. From a technical standpoint, these tools have made the surgeon's job not only possible but also safe in terms of patient care. However, the surgeon who wishes to perform these new procedures must receive adequate training in order to deliver high-quality surgical care with a minimum number of postoperative complications.

The complications associated with open colon resection are well known (Table 24.1). Resection of the colon and rectum is one of the more difficult procedures, from a technical standpoint, and one which has the greatest potential for major postoperative complications. The reasons for this include the fact that the colon is not an end organ (in contrast to the gallbladder and appendix); it is large and bulky, and therefore more difficult to handle without injury, there is a rich supply of large blood vessels buried in fat that must be ligated while not interfering with the circulation to the cut ends of the bowel (affecting the viability of the anastomosis); transection of the bowel must be accomplished with instruments that will perform reliably and with little or no risk of leakage; specimen removal must

Table 24.1. Complications Associated with Open Resection of the Colon and Rectum

Complication
Bleeding
Intra-abdominal
Sacral
Anastomotic
Visceral injury
Spleen
Liver
Ureters
Major blood vessels
Other organs
Mesenteric twists
Deep venous thrombosis
Peroneal nerve injury
Acute wound breakdown
Prolonged postoperative ileus
Early small bowel obstruction
Acute wound breakdown
Intra-abdominal abscess formation
Wound infection
Anastomotic
Leaks
Strictures
Delayed wound breakdown (hernia)
Urinary tract infection
Bladder dysfunction
Sexual dysfunction
Erectile
Ejaculatory

be accomplished through relatively small incisions—otherwise, the value of the procedure would be questionable; reconstruction is usually necessary; the anastomosis must be performed securely; and finally, the possibility of infection (of the wound and intra-abdominal) is high even with the most meticulous open techniques (even with good-quality bowel preparation and prophylactic antibiotics).

All of these complications occur at a known rate. Individually, they are more or less likely to occur on the introduction of laparoscopic technology. Table 24.2 summarizes the likely change that will occur if good laparoscopic technique is employed to perform these procedures. This assumes that the "rules" regarding good technique are followed.

TOTALLY LAPAROSCOPIC VERSUS LAPAROSCOPICALLY ASSISTED SURGERY

We must distinguish between totally laparoscopic and laparoscopically assisted colon resection. In the completely laparoscopic colon resection, dissection, transection, and reanastomosis are all performed within the abdominal cavity. The specimen is removed either through the open rectum or through a small counter-incision. This incision is usually placed in the suprapubic area because of the relative lack of pain and postoperative complications (acute and delayed wound breakdown) associated with an incision in this location. Totally laparoscopic procedures are usually per-

Table 24.2. Change in the Open Complication Rate Associated with Good Laparoscopic Technique

Complication	Expected Change
Bleeding	No change
Intra-abdominal	No change
Sacral	No change
Anastomotic	No change
Visceral Injury	Decreased
Spleen	Decreased
Liver	Decreased
Ureters	No change
Major blood vessels	No change
Other organs	Decreased
Mesenteric twists	No change
Deep venous thrombosis	Increased
Peroneal nerve injury	Increased
Prolonged postoperative ileus	Decreased
Early small bowel obstruction	Decreased
Acute wound breakdown	Decreased
Wound infection	Decreased
Intra-abdominal abscess	No change
Anastomotic	No change
Leaks	No change
Strictures	No change
Delayed wound breakdown (hernia)	Decreased
Urinary tract infection	Decreased
Bladder dysfunction	Decreased
Sexual dysfunction	No change
Erectile	No change
Ejaculatory	No change

formed on the sigmoid colon and rectum. The proximal resection margin of the bowel is brought out through an enlarged trocar site in the left lower quadrant of the abdomen. The anvil of the circular stapler is placed in the bowel, and the bowel is then placed back within the peritoneal cavity for an intracorporeal anastomosis. The circular stapler is then introduced into the rectum through the anus and the anastomosis is completed. Totally laparoscopic procedures are also possible when performing abdominoperineal resections and fashioning either loop or end-descending colon colostomies.

Laparoscopically assisted colon resections, in contrast, are performed on other parts of the colon, usually above the level of the sigmoid colon. In these procedures the entire mobilization of the colon is done intracorporeally. The bowel is then exteriorized through an incision placed in the appropriate geographic location. The specimen is then amputated, and the anastomosis is performed outside of the peritoneal cavity.

A number of different techniques exist, and their details are continuously being reevaluated and refined. Considerable controversy exists as to whether or not laparoscopic resection of the colon and rectum is equal to or better than open surgery.

The purpose of this chapter is to help the surgeon avoid the many pitfalls associated with laparoscopic resection of the colon and rectum. In order to determine how to avoid these pitfalls, each section discusses the standard complications potentially associated with open colon resection as well as those that occur in laparoscopic bowel resection.

INDICATIONS FOR LAPAROSCOPIC RESECTION OF THE COLON AND RECTUM

Not all patients are candidates for laparoscopic resection of the colon and rectum. Procedures that would expose the patient to an undue risk when performed laparoscopically should be performed open in order to minimize the chances of either intraoperative or postoperative complications (Table 24.3).

Other colon operations that do not include resection of a segment of bowel include various types of colostomies. These can be performed in patients with end-stage cancer, in those who require radiation therapy of a rectal cancer prior to abdominoperineal resection; and in those with rectal or perineal trauma, fistulas, or severe infections that require temporary diversion. Colostomy formation is a simple, rapid procedure with results equivalent to those achieved using open techniques.

In some cases, the disease or associated conditions makes the patient an unsuitable candidate for a laparoscopic procedure (Table 24.4). There are no absolute contraindications to laparoscopic resection of the colon and rectum. All patients should be evaluated individually in order to determine whether they are candidates for that procedure. The degree of the associated condition, as well as the experience of the surgeon, will determine whether a laparoscopic procedure is possible.

Table 24.3. Indications for Resection of the Colon and Rectum

Benign lesions (colon polyps) not removable colonoscopically
Small colon cancers
Diverticular disease
Strictures of the sigmoid colon
Inflammatory bowel disease
Cecal or sigmoid volvulus
Rectal cancer

Table 24.4. Relative Contraindications to Laparoscopic Resection of the Colon and Rectum

Morbid obesity
Bleeding diathesis
Large cancers
Bowel obstruction with abdominal distention
Peritonitis
Acute diverticulitis with or without abscess formation
Stage D cancer
Previous abdominal surgery
Fistulas from the colon to other organs
Lack of adequate laparoscopic equipment
Inexperienced surgeon

CONTRAINDICATIONS TO RESECTION OF THE COLON AND RECTUM

In general, there are no absolute contraindications to laparoscopic or laparoscopically assisted resection of the colon and rectum. There are, however, a number of relative contraindications. Each patient must be individually evaluated with these in mind.

Morbid Obesity

The problems with the morbidly obese patient include the thickness and weight of the abdominal wall and the amount of fat in the mesentery of the bowel. With increased abdominal wall thickness comes a need for longer trocars. These are now available and can be of benefit in the obese patient. Access alone, however, is not the only problem associated with a thick abdominal wall. Instruments become much less functional because a relatively large percentage of their length is taken up within the trocar. Because of this reduction in the functional length of the instruments, access to remote areas of the abdomen is reduced. The only way to circumvent this problem is to increase the number of trocars that are utilized during the procedure. This, however, increases the cost as well as the complexity of the procedure. The weight of the abdominal wall also causes a significant problem in creating an adequate pneumoperitoneum. A standard operating pressure of 15 mmHg may not be adequate in the obese patient because of the lower-volume pneumoperitoneum that is obtained. It may be necessary to increase the inflation pressure to 18 to 25 mmHg. This is not without risk, however. There will be a concomitant interference with the maintenance of artificial respiration and adequate venous return. Close monitoring is mandatory, and the threshold for conversion to an open procedure should be low. Finally, there is increased difficulty with dissection of the mesentery because of the increased amount of fat.

Bleeding Diathesis

Patients with clotting abnormalities should not be considered good or ideal candidates for laparoscopic resection. The surgeon's ability to be hemostatically meticulous is reduced in totally laparoscopic procedures. There is a general inability to ligate tissue selectively, and the application of pressure and especially packing is extremely difficult. In laparoscopically assisted procedures where the bulk of the dissection and the reanastomosis are performed extracorporeally, the likelihood of bleeding is higher.

Large Cancers

Removing large cancers can be a formidable task from a number of standpoints. Because of their sheer size and weight, handling them can be difficult. Dissecting them from contiguous structures while maintaining adequate hemostasis can be extremely hazardous. Finally, removing them from the abdominal cavity intact may require a relatively large incision—larger than should be used to justify a laparoscopic procedure. In all of these instances, removing an intact specimen is the ultimate goal. Disrupting a specimen within the abdominal cavity, leaving tumor behind because of an inability to adequately dissect the specimen free, or spillage of tumor in the abdominal wall reduces the value of this procedure in patients who are good candidates for a laparoscopic approach. Good judgment concerning appropriate candidacy and conversion to an open procedure when necessary are critical to the success of these procedures.

Bowel Obstruction with Abdominal Distention

The reason for this is quite simple. The ability of the surgeon to create an adequate pneumoperitoneum is severely compromised in a patient who already has significant abdominal distention with stretching of the abdominal wall because of a bowel obstruction. In addition, the risk of organ injury is higher. Use of a Veress needle in these patients should be condemned. Open insertion of a Hassan cannula should be performed if an attempt will be made to perform bowel resection in a patient with significant bowel obstruction. In addition, the bowel tends to be somewhat friable and difficult to handle, and is injured easily with the instruments used by the laparoscopic surgeon.

Peritonitis

In patients with peritonitis, the identification of structures and safe dissection become extremely difficult. Identification of the site of perforation; separation of bowel loops from each other and from other structures; and cleansing of the abdominal cavity, especially if it contains solid material, may be all but impossible. Patients with perforation of the colon require the best possible procedure that can be performed, in terms of both technique and the length of time required to perform the surgery, to ensure the best possible outcome. There is no room in this situation for second-best procedures.

Acute Diverticulitis with or without Abscess Formation

A number of problems exist in the patient with acute diverticulitis with or without abscess formation. All of these problems have to do with thickening of tissue from the inflammatory reaction. The bowel may be thickened, making it difficult to transect it safely using the linear stapler. The mesentery may also be thickened, making it difficult to identify and ligate the blood supply. Identification of the ureter can be hazardous, resulting in an increased risk of injury. Intracorporeal anastomosis using a circular stapler may not be possible. All of these problems jeopardize the potential success of the procedure. The surgeon must assess these factors prior to beginning a procedure that has a high likelihood of conversion to an open procedure.

Stage D Cancer

In patients with extensive intra-abdominal cancer, there is usually a moderate adhesive process that also results in bowel loops with varying degrees of dilatation. In addition, a significant amount of ascitic fluid is usually present. In order to operate within this closed space, most if not all of the ascitic fluid must be evacuated either before or after the pneumoperitoneum is created. This adhesive process creates a number of problems, including an increased risk of injuries related to trocar placement, an increased risk of bleeding from metastatic deposits during dissection, and difficulty in identifying tissue planes, primarily those between individual bowel loops. Open placement of a Hassan cannula is probably indicated in these patients. Identification of stage D disease is not always possible. Up to 50% of patients with intra-abdominal carcinomatosis will have a negative computed tomography scan for extracolonic disease. In addition, specific anatomic landmarks may be difficult to identify with certainty.

Previous Abdominal Surgery

Extensive intra-abdominal adhesions can interfere significantly with laparoscopic bowel resection. The extent of adhesions is generally not known until the initial trocar has been placed. Some indication, however, can be inferred based on the number of previous abdominal operations, the types of procedures performed, and the reason for the operation. Until the initial trocar has been placed, one cannot know the severity of the adhesions and whether or not they would interfere with the safe, timely performance of a laparoscopic resection. Placement of a Hassan cannula through an open technique is advocated in these patients to avoid organ injury.

Fistulas from the Colon to Other Organs

The identification of fistulas laparoscopically is extremely difficult, and their closure laparoscopically is probably not warranted. Using currently available stapling and suturing techniques, the closure of fistulas by the average surgeon performing these procedures should be discouraged. It is unlikely that closure can be accomplished with enough certainty and therefore safety. When recognized, the presence of a fistula should probably result in conversion to an open procedure.

Lack of Adequate Laparoscopic Equipment

It goes without saying that the appropriate tools must be available. These procedures are difficult enough to perform even with the appropriate instruments. The essential hand instruments include Babcock clamps, endoscopic retractors and bipolar coagulating devices, ligating devices such as endoscopic linear staplers, two television monitors, a high-volume insufflator, and a second light source for transillumination, in addition to adequate assistance from both nurses and physicians.

Inexperienced Surgeon

An inexperienced surgeon attempting to perform a complicated laparoscopic procedure is a formula for disaster. Surgeons should increase their ability to perform these procedures in a stepwise fashion. First, they must be experienced with open procedures on the

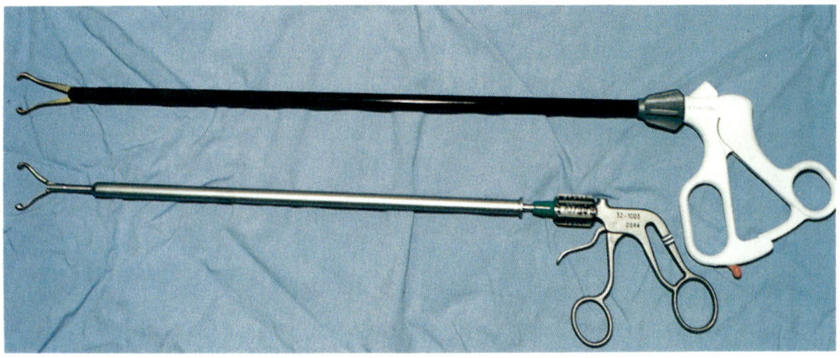

Figure 24.1. Babcock clamps (reusable and disposable) used for holding and manipulating the bowel. The disposable instruments tend to hold the bowel more securely yet are less traumatic to the tissues.

colon and rectum. They must know how to use standard laparoscopic equipment, as well as the more sophisticated tools now available. Firsthand experience in performing the more common laparoscopic procedures such as cholecystectomy, hernia repair, and appendectomy is mandatory. Having performed advanced procedures on other organs such as hiatus hernia repair and Nissen fundoplication will be of great value. The surgeon contemplating laparoscopic procedures on the large bowel must have a basic understanding of the tools as well as the techniques specific to these procedures. Taking a course in laparoscopic bowel resection should be considered mandatory.

INSTRUMENTATION

Tremendous improvement has occurred in the development of instruments for laparoscopic bowel resection. The most significant advances concern grasping instruments and staplers for ligation and anastomosis. The Babcock clamp has made it possible to hold and place traction on the bowel while dissecting. This instrument minimizes the possibility of injury to the wall of the bowel, which can either interfere with the blood supply in the area of the anastomosis or cause a remote injury that could result in an acute or delayed perforation with spillage of intestinal contents and infection. Many types of these instruments exist. Some of these have tips that are flat and smooth, while others have rather coarse serrations. Obviously, the strength with which the instrument will grasp the colon depends on the tip design. Each surgeon must determine which instrument is best. Generally, a design with some serrations will minimize trauma yet prevent the bowel from being released from the jaws unintentionally (Fig. 24.1).

Other instruments that have made this procedure possible include the laparoscopic linear stapler and the modified circular stapler. The linear staplers, like their open counterparts, apply two double or triple rows of staples to the bowel and cut between them, providing secure closure with little risk of leakage. As with open colon surgery, some bowel is not amenable to stapling because it is extremely thickened or edematous. This is also true for laparoscopic procedures. The same judgment must be made by the surgeon at the time of the operation. Can the bowel be stapled safely? In a low anterior resection, where bowel transection must be performed intracorporeally, the procedure may have to be converted to an open one (Fig. 24.2). The circular stapler has been modified to make it airtight; that is, it has been sealed in order to prevent carbon dioxide gas from leaking out through the handle. If this leakage were to occur, there would be loss of the pneumoperitoneum and loss of visualization while the anastomosis was being performed. This would make the completion of the anastomosis impossible or extremely difficult (Fig. 24.3).

High-pressure irrigators and aspiration devices are also of value in performing these procedures. They allow fluid dissection of the mesentery, copious irrigation, and large-bore aspiration. The last two are particularly important if there is spillage at the time of the procedure (Fig. 24.4).

Finally, retrieval bags for specimen removal allow the surgeon to remove a portion of the bowel from the peritoneal cavity without spillage of tissue, bowel contents, or tumor cells. This is also critical in preventing postoperative complications, including infection and tumor recurrence (Fig. 24.5).

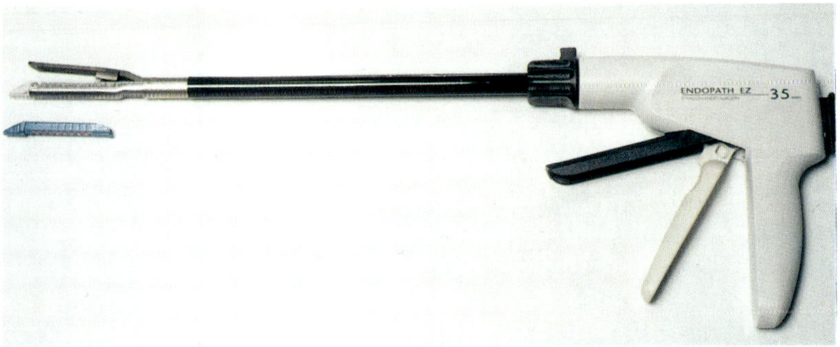

a

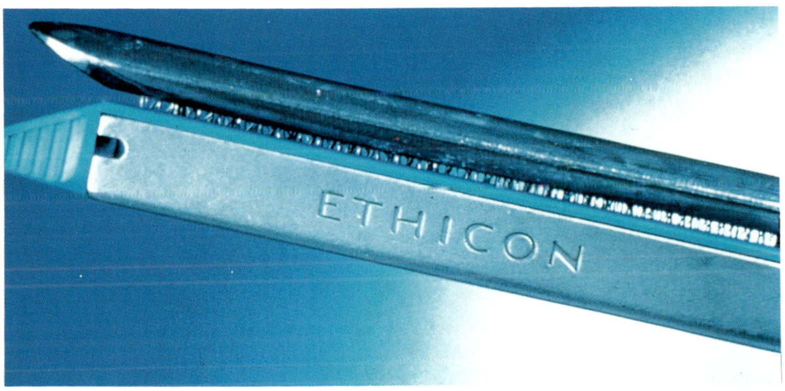

b

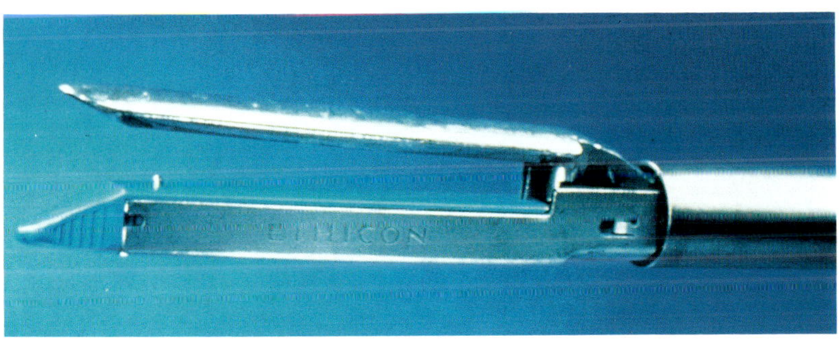

c

Figure 24.2. (a) Photo of the Ethicon linear cutter. Available in two staples heights (2.0 and 1.5 mm) for stapling different thicknesses of tissue. (b) Close-up of staple jaws closed. (c) Close-up of stapler jaws open.

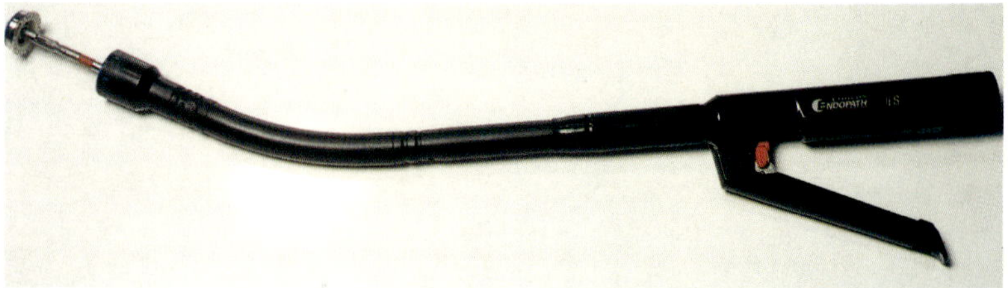

Figure 24.3. Ethicon stealth circular stapler. Length, curve, high ratio of anastomotic size relative to staple head size and airtight configuration, which prevents loss of pneumoperitoneum during a laparoscopic procedure, make it an ideal instrument for laparoscopic low colon anastomoses.

ACCESS

Entering the abdominal cavity safely and in the appropriate locations is critical in the prevention of technical difficulties. It allows the surgeon to perform these procedures expeditiously, without too much frustration.

Use of a Hassan cannula for the primary trocar is of value especially when the surgeon first begins performing these procedures (Fig. 24.6). It allows the surgeon to concentrate on the procedure rather than focusing on the trocars, i.e., preventing their dislodgment. Generally, when first performing laparoscopic colectomy, there is a great deal of telescope and instrument exchange down the trocars. Dislodgment is common, frustrating the surgeon and threatening the completion of the laparoscopic procedure. For the secondary punctures, some type of fascial gripper can also be of great value. As more expertise is gained these ancillary aids—especially the fascial grippers, which make larger holes and can potentially cause increased postoperative pain and an increased risk of trocar hernias—can be eliminated (Fig. 24.7).

The placement of trocars, both in number and in location, is critical. The following figures illustrate trocar placement for colostomy formation (Fig. 24.8), colostomy takedown (Fig. 24.9), left colon resection including sigmoid resection, low anterior resection and abdominoperineal resection (Fig. 24.10), and resection of the right colon. Trocar placement for transverse colectomy is the same for resection of the left colon.

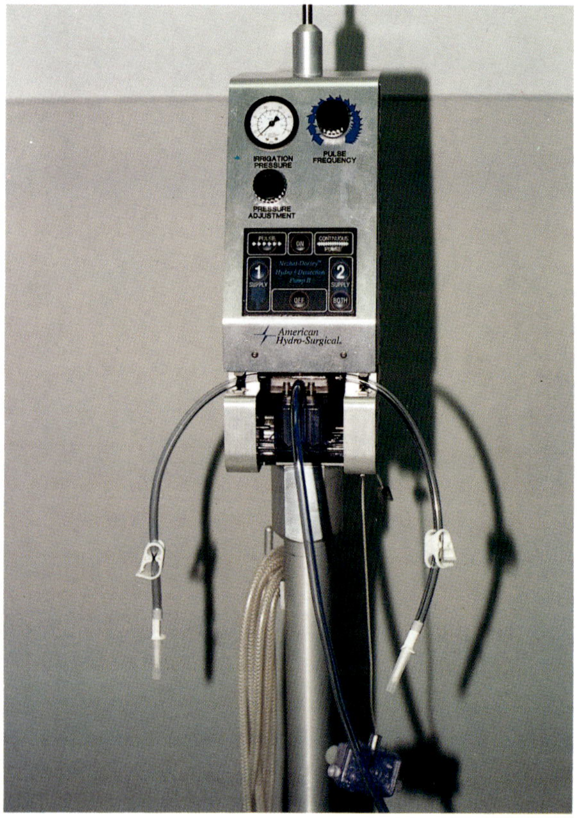

a

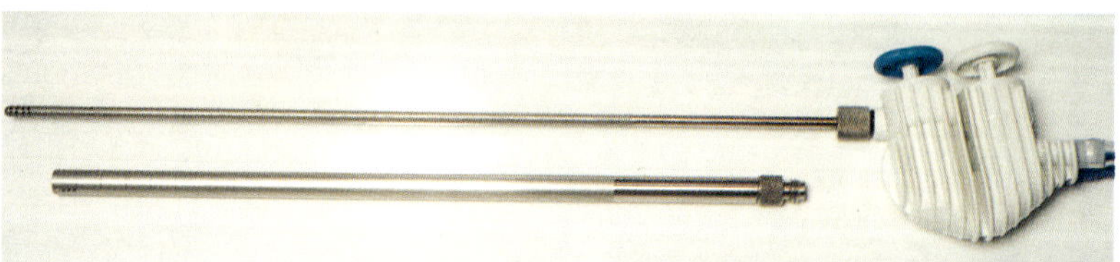

b

Figure 24.4. (a) High pressure pump of the Nezhat-Dorsey suction irrigation system from U.S. Hydrosurgical. (b) Disposable handpiece with interchangeable reusable wands up to 10 mm in size.

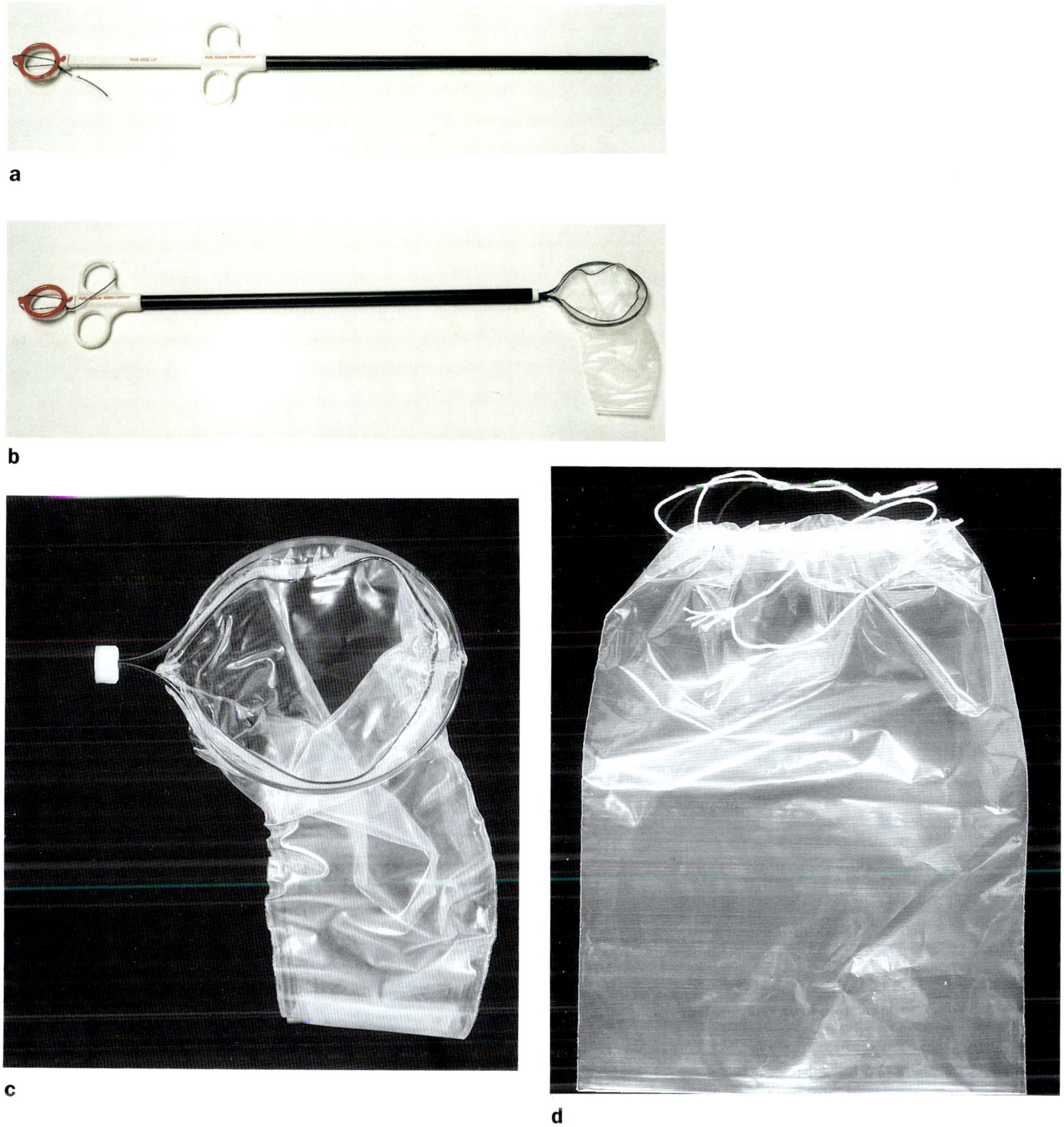

Figure 24.5. Retrieval bag with frame from Autosuture. Allows easy removal of smaller specimens. Larger specimens must be removed through counter incisions or through the open rectum. Larger specimens can be removed in larger extraction bags. (a) Device with bag closed. (b) Device with bag open. (c) Close up of bag showing frame that holds bag open to facilitate specimen insertion. (d) Large bag (9×12 inches) for use with larger specimens.

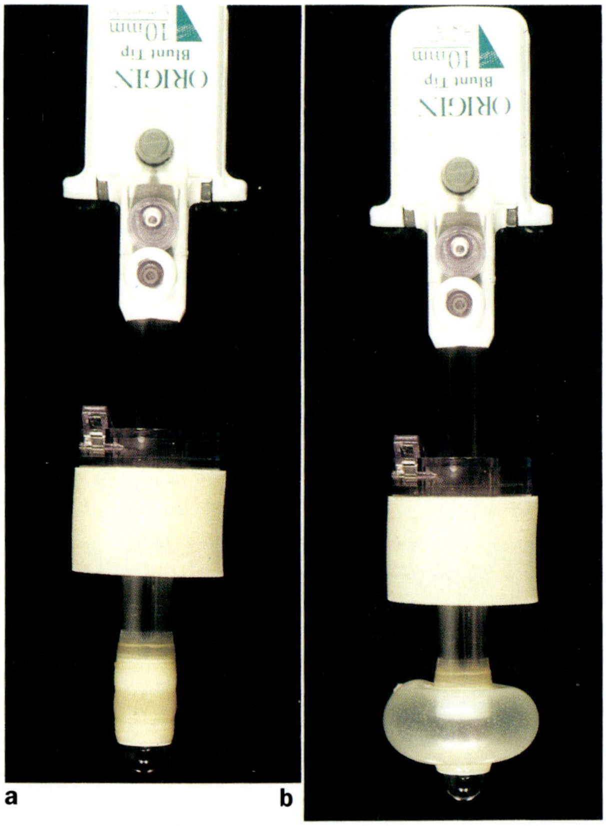

Figure 24.6. Hassan cannula from Origin Medsystems with locking balloon and cushion. Ideal mechanism to prevent dislodgement of the primary (umbilical) trocar during a laparoscopic procedure. It can be used in other locations. (a) Balloon deflated. (b) Balloon inflated.

However, it is infrequently performed because of the difficulty associated with the thickness of the transverse colon mesentery. Because of this anatomy, adequate exposure and visualization of the vascular supply in order to effect ligation are impaired.

AIDS TO RESECTION

Many colonic lesions are readily visible when the laparoscope is inserted into the peritoneal cavity. Others are visualized with minimal manipulation of the colon after introduction of the telescope. With laparoscopic resection, the surgeon cannot feel small lesions that are present within the colon. If these lesions cannot be felt, then it is necessary to perform the resection based on anatomic landmarks or use additional diagnostic tools to identify the lesion intraoperatively. If anatomic landmarks are used, the surgeon must be able to rely on the description of the location of the lesion by contrast study and/or by colonoscopy. This reemphasizes the need for surgeons to become more involved in surgical endoscopy and to perform their own colonoscopy preoperatively on the patients they will operate on. Intraoperative colonoscopy can be an invaluable aid to the surgeon who is performing laparoscopoic colon resections. It identifies the exact location of the lesion. The obvious disadvantage is the insufflatoin of air, which can interfere with the procedure. The benefits, however, outweigh the disadvantages. Precise localization of the lesion allows a more limited resection to be performed, with a reduction in operative time and cost.

BLEEDING

Abdominal Wall Bleeding

Vessels in the abdominal wall, especially the epigastric vessels, can cause considerable bleeding when injured. Injury to the larger vessels can be avoided by transilluminating the abdominal wall before placing each trocar. Bleeding that does occur from smaller blood vessels can be detected at the completion of the procedure and controlled by viewing each trocar puncture site with the laparoscope as the trocar is being removed. Bleeding that does occur can be controlled using electrocautery directed from inside the abdomen. The bipolar Kleppinger forceps are ideal for this maneuver. A hand-held cautery device directed from outside of the abdominal cavity can also be used. The air leak must obviously be controlled while the bleeding is being stopped. A Foley catheter can be inserted from the outside while the hand-held cautery device is being utilized from the outside, and a finger can be inserted. The trocar can be replaced in order to tamponade the bleeding while performing suture ligation from the outside. The 45 degree telescope is ideal, allowing en face visualization of the abdominal wall as the trocars are being removed. It also allows good visualization while attempting to control the bleeding.

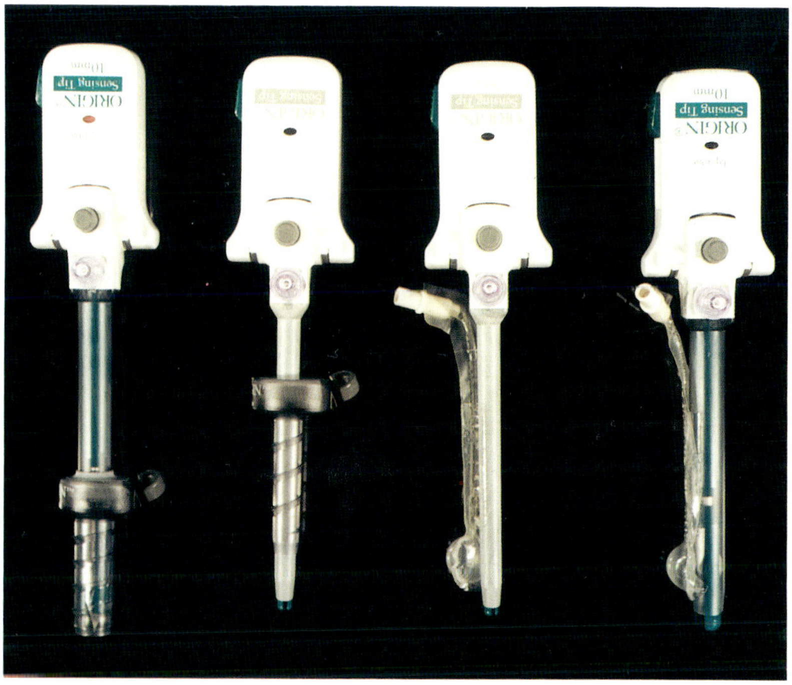

Figure 24.7. Trocars with gripping devices in rigid (threaded) and balloon configurations. Also used to prevent dislodgement during a laparoscopic procedure.

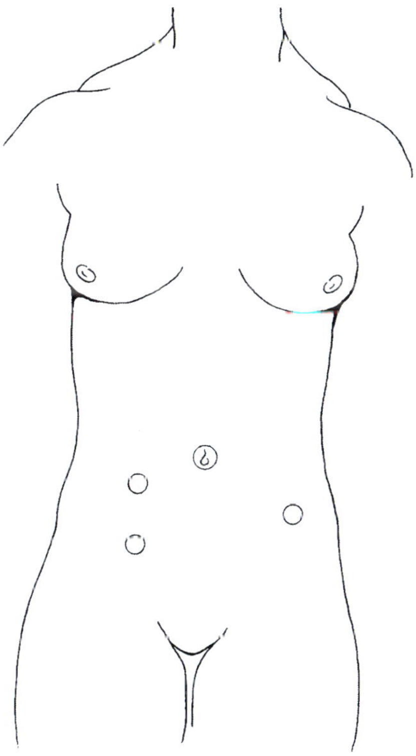

Figure 24.8. Trocar placement for formation of a laparoscopic end descending colon colostomy or for a sigmoid resection. The midline trocar is at the umbilicus. 12 mm trocars can be used at all locations to allow introduction of the linear stapler from a variety of angles. The end of the colon is brought out through the left lower quadrant trocar site which may need to be enlarged. The head of the circular stapler is inserted and the end of the colon is then returned to the abdominal cavity. That incision is then closed prior to fashioning the anastomosis.

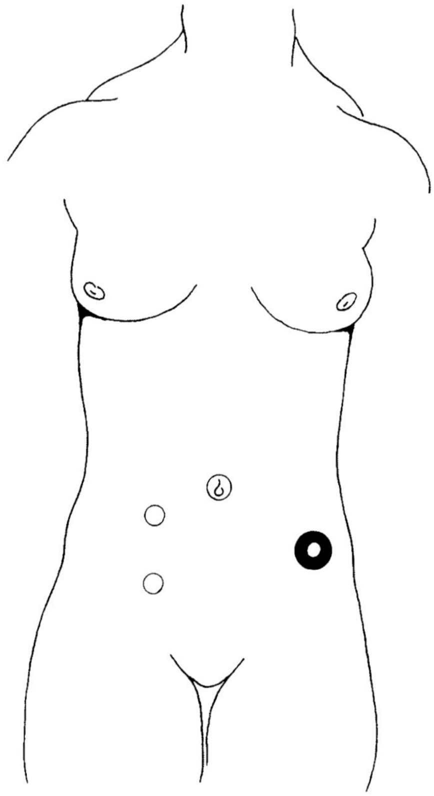

Figure 24.9. Trocar placement for end descending colon colostomy takedown. The midline trocar is at the umbilicus. 12 mm trocars are placed at all locations. The technique is the same as in end descending colon colostomy formation or sigmoid resection.

Figure 24.10. (facing page) (a) Trocar placement for left colectomy. The midline trocars are placed at the umbilicus in the epigastrium and in the suprapubic area. An additional trocar is placed in the left lower quadrant. 12 mm trocars are used at all locations. A counterincision placed in the left lower quadrant or alternatively in the suprapubic area is usually necessary for removal of the larger specimen. The anastomosis can be performed using the circular stapler through the counterincision or intracorporeally. (b) Trocar placement for a low anterior resection. 12 mm trocars are used at all locations. The smaller specimen can usually be removed through the trocar site in the left lower quadrant which can be enlarged if necessary. Unlike in the left colectomy a counterincision is usually not necessary. (c) Trocar placement for an abdominoperitoneal resection. 12 mm trocars are used at all locations. A counterincision is not always necessary. If the pelvic dissection can be performed laparoscopically deep into the pelvis, then the operation can be completed from the perineum and the counterincision is not necessary. (d) Trocar placement for right colectomy; 12 mm trocars are used at all locations. A counterincision is necessary in order to perform the extra corporeal anastomosis.

Mesenteric Intra-abdominal Bleeding

Intra-abdominal bleeding is a serious complication associated with laparoscopic colon resection, that may necessitate rapid conversion to an open procedure. The surgeon can handle bleeding in an open abdomen more easily and safely than during a laparoscopic procedure. The key to minimizing bleeding is to think in advance where the trouble spots might occur and use the appropriate technique in order to prevent bleeding from those areas.

The colon should always be mobilized along avascular tissue planes if possible. Mobilizing along the line of Toldt is commonly used during open procedures and should also be used when they are performed laparoscopically. This maneuver can be performed sharply and with little cause for concern.

When there is slightly thicker tissue, such as is found in the right colon mesentery, a different technique should be employed. Vessels that can be well visualized can be clipped using the endoclip applier. In addition, bipolar cautery is a safe and efficient method of controlling these vessels. When the vessels are not well visualized individually the bipolar cautery becomes extremely useful. The reusable Kleppinger bipolar forceps are an ideal instrument that is also very cost effective. The flat, solid paddles should be used, since they give the best coaptation and sealing of blood vessels. This device works well whether the vessels are individually seen or not. It is useful with vessels up to

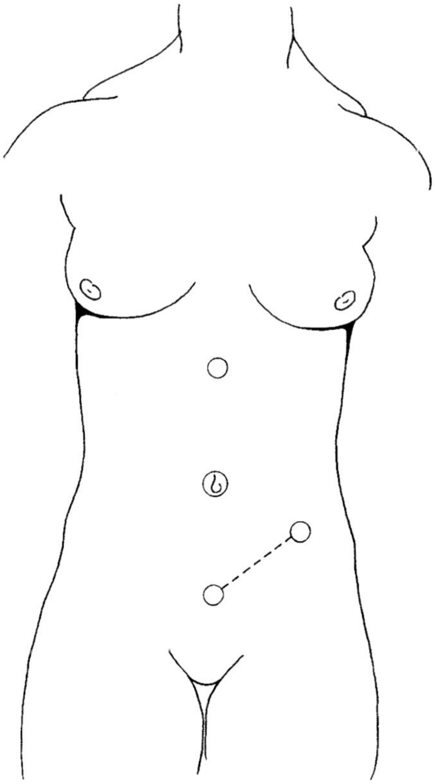

a

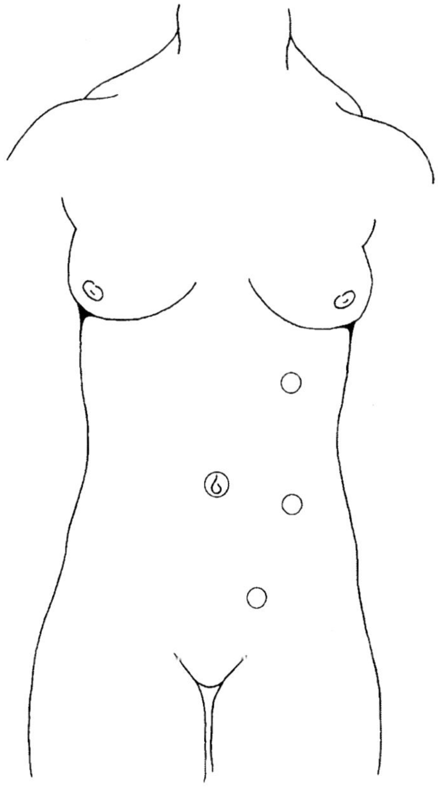

b

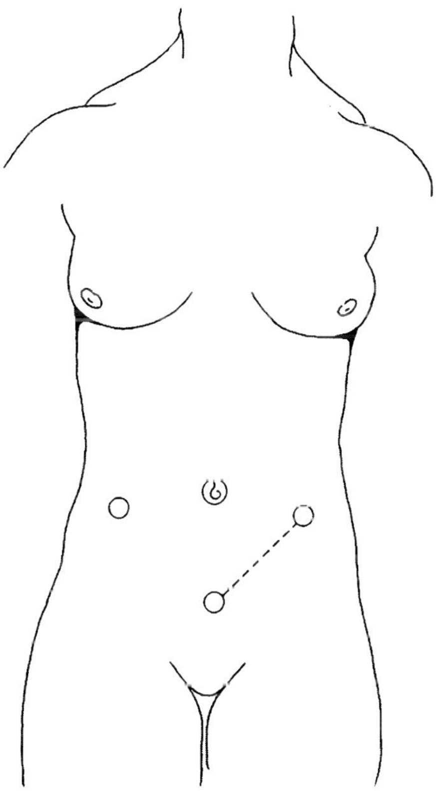

c

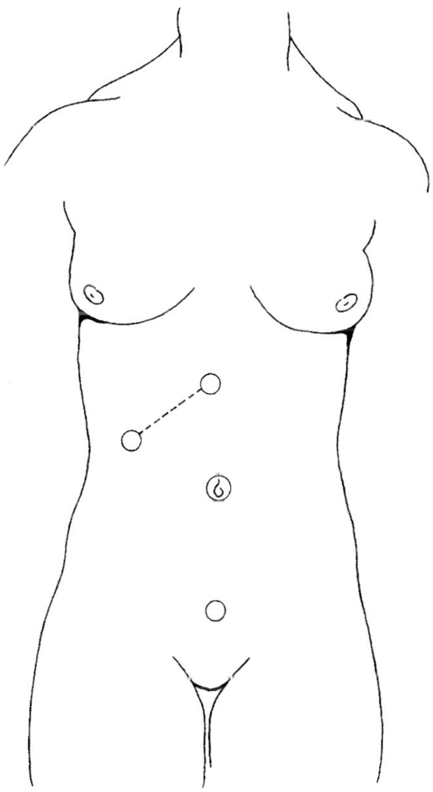

d

1–1.5 mm in diameter. It is important, however, to cauterize to the point of desiccation several paddle widths in diameter before the tissue and the blood vessel are transected in order to prevent bleeding.

In thicker tissue, such as in the deeper portions of the mesentery of the sigmoid colon, the mesentery of the transverse colon, and the perirectal tissue, the linear stapler is of considerable value. The stapler that is meant for vascular hemostasis will usually work quite reliably. Sequential firings allow rapid transection of these tissues. Trying to work in these fatty areas with other instruments is fraught with danger and the risk of uncontrollable bleeding. The disadvantage of these stapling devices is their relatively high cost.

Sacral Bleeding

In general this is not a problem, especially if the linear stapler is used to perform this portion of the mobilization, since with closure of the stapler there will always be a small cuff of tissue left on the sacrum. This type of bleeding is usually associated with denuding of the sacrum, with subsequent bleeding from the periosteum, bone, or vessels that have been avulsed and have retracted. The use of powdered Gelfoam mixed with thrombin is invaluable in this situation. The use of sterile toothpicks has also been advocated for this type of bleeding when it is not otherwise controllable.

Anastomotic Bleeding

Linear staplers have improved considerably since their introduction several years ago. In addition to having the luxury of choosing various staple heights, additional staple rows have been added (three) to ensure hemostasis. If there is minor bleeding after transection, light application of monopolar cautery can be extremely useful. Light application of the closed blunt forceps is as useful as any other available devices. Obviously, grasping the bleeding site and causing extensive coagulation and necrosis should be discouraged. This maneuver could result in subsequent leakage, with the development of intra-abdominal sepsis.

VISCERAL INJURY

Organ injury can occur with open abdominal surgery. Injury to the spleen can occur with mobilization of the splenic flexure of the colon; injury to the ureters can occur with mobilization of the rectosigmoid colon; and injury to the right ureter can occur with mobilization of the right colon. This is especially true when either inflammatory disease or a large, bulky tumor is present.

Spleen

Injury to the spleen during open colectomy occurs either with mechanical retraction by an assistant or with direct traction on the colon by the surgeon. With laparoscopic surgery, retractors are not utilized. This problem is therefore essentially eliminated. In addition, the spleen and its attachments to the colon can be more readily visualized than is possible with open surgery.

Traction injuries can still occur, potentially with increased frequency because of the lack of tactile sensation associated with open surgery. The surgeon must be extremely careful when pulling down on the splenic flexure while using instruments such as Babcock clamps because of this potential problem. He or she should key in on visual feedback and observe how much tension is being applied to the splenocolic ligament.

Care must be taken in introducing instruments down the trocars. When working around the spleen, introduction of instruments should be visualized in order to prevent inadvertent injury from instrument punctures. This type of injury can be extremely difficult to control and may result in the emergent opening of the abdominal cavity.

Ureters

The same care must be taken with laparoscopic surgery as with open abdominal surgery to avoid injury to the ureters. The ureters should be identified visually and followed if necessary. Initial identification is usually achieved by finding the ureter at the point where it crosses the iliac artery. The ureter is then followed distally or proximally by means of blunt dissection using either a blunt instrument or, ideally, a laparoscopic Kittner (Fig. 24.11). Care must be taken not to mobilize the ureter too vigorously or too extensively to avoid causing bleeding or devascularization.

Surgeons performing laparoscopic colon surgery should not hesitate to use ureteral stents. The use of traditional stents that the surgeon can feel is less useful in laparoscopic procedures. In any situation where a concern might arise, such as in the obese patient or the patient whose primary disease involves an inflamma-

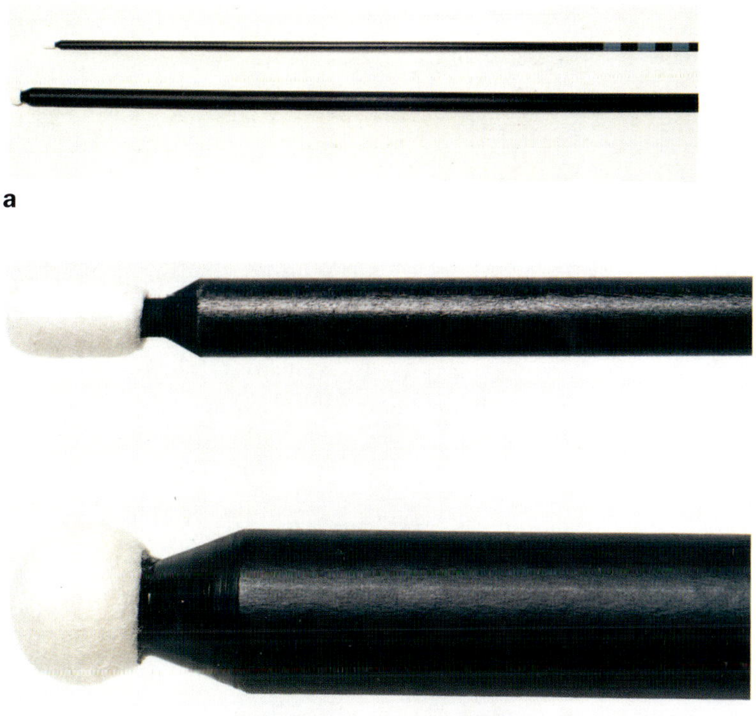

a

b

Figure 24.11. Laparoscopic Kittners useful for blunt dissection of the vessels, ureters. (a) 5 and 10 mm Kittner. Reverse end may also be used as a blunt probe. (b) Close-up of 5 and 10 mm Kittners.

tory process, stents should be placed preoperatively in one or both ureters. At a minimum, the use of conventional stents will allow immediate identification of an injury. When stents are not used, up to 30% of ureteral injuries are not identified during the original operation.

Lighted stents or stents that can be detected with an infrared detector can be of value. At any point during the procedure, the stents can be illuminated while laparoscopic illumination is reduced or the infrared camera can be utilized to show the exact location of the ureters. This can be extremely useful in facilitating identification periodically during the procedure, thereby preventing injury. Prior to completion of the procedure, vital dyes such as methylene blue can also be of value in verifying that no ureteral injury has occurred.

Major Blood Vessels

The most common mechanism of injuries to major blood vessels is a misadventure with trocar placement. As previously mentioned, the Hassan cannula is of value in placing the initial trocar. Major vascular injury cannot occur with initial placement of this trocar. All other trocars should then be placed under direct visualization after an adequate pneumoperitoneum has been obtained. This should eliminate most major vascular injuries.

Other injuries can occur during dissection of the colon. Careful attention should paid to pulsatile structures in the area of the dissection, and sharp or pointed instruments as well as electrocautery devices should be used with extreme care.

PROBLEMS WITH THE MESENTERY

Care must be taken to avoid mesenteric twists that can result in partial or complete postoperative bowel obstruction. Staple lines should always be placed from the antimesenteric to the mesenteric border of the bowel. Once the bowel is transected, one corner of it should always be held with an instrument in order to prevent twisting.

Rents in the mesentery should always be repaired. Several methods are now available. In low anterior resections, closure is generally not necessary. In other resections, the defect in the mesentery can often be closed extracorporeally prior to replacing the anastomosis in the peritoneal cavity. The defect can also be closed intracorporeally. Hernia staples can be used; however, closure using these staples can be somewhat tenuous and prone to disruption. The mesenteric defect can be sutured intracorporeally, either with free suture or using the new Endostitch that automatically passes the needle and suture back and forth between the jaws of the instrument.

DEEP VENOUS THROMBOSIS

In open abdominal surgery, deep venous thrombosis is related to the duration of the procedure and the position of the patient. When the same procedures are performed laparoscopically, there is potential for an increased incidence of deep venous thrombosis. There are a number of reasons for this.

First, the laparoscopic procedures takes longer to perform, especially when these procedures are performed for the first time. As more experience is gained, the operative time will undoubtedly decrease.

Positioning is the same with both open and laparoscopic colon resections. In operations that require the lithotomy position, deep venous thrombosis can increase because the patient is kept in this position for a longer period of time.

"Tension" pneumoperitoneum is peculiar to laparoscopic surgery. With a positive intra-abdominal pressure of approximately 15 mmHg, venous return is impeded. This tends to increase the incidence of deep venous thrombosis.

The use of sequential counterpulsation devices is important in any abdominal or pelvic procedure, especially when the lithotomy position is utilized and the procedure is performed laparoscopically using a tension pneumoperitoneum.

The small added advantage of laparoscopy is the early mobilization of the patient. Generally, patients will have less pain and earlier ambulation.

PERONEAL NERVE INJURIES

Peroneal nerve injuries are generally related to patient position. The stirrups used to place the patient in the lithotomy position are usually the culprit. Older stirrup devices generally placed the patient in a position with moderate flexion at both the hip and the knee, with some pressure resulting in nerve injury. Newer stirrups that minimize flexion at both joints and place most of the weight on the heel of the foot, coupled with better padding, minimize the problems associated with the lithotomy position.

PROLONGED POSTOPERATIVE ILEUS AND EARLY SMALL BOWEL OBSTRUCTION

Delayed resumption of bowel function has many causes, including the effects of anesthetic agents, manipulation of the bowel, and the presence of irritating intra-abdominal fluids. The most important causes are probably manipulation of the bowel and the presence of irritating fluids, especially blood. The postoperative ileus seen in patients undergoing laparoscopic procedures is considerably reduced. With laparoscopy, handling of the bowel is minimized and packing it away is unnecessary. The viscera are removed from the operative field by the effects of the CO_2 gas pressure and by the positioning of the patient.

ACUTE WOUND BREAKDOWN

Acute wound breakdown can occur in the forms of dehiscence and evisceration. Wound dehiscence is not uncommonly in open colon resections. Several factors predispose patients to this condition. The patient's overall medical condition is important in determining whether or not it occurs. Nutritional status is probably the most important factor in wound healing and the development of this postoperative complication. Unfortunately, there is little hard laboratory data that can be used for prediction. The best test is the patient's serum protein and albumin levels. Patients who have lost a large amount of weight and who are nutritionally depleted should be considered candidates for preoperative nutritional support in the form of total parenteral nutrition or enteral nutrition if possible. However, there is little evidence that preoperative use of intravenous feeding can reverse the metabolic abnormalities and alter the incidence of wound dehiscence and evisceration. The mortality associated with these operations rises dramatically when acute postoperative wound disruption occurs.

A completely different situation exists with respect to laparoscopic colon resection. In general, there are no long abdominal incisions that can break down. Most procedures can be performed through four to six trocar wounds that are 12 mm in size. In patients whose resection is above the rectum, it is necessary to make a small incision to remove the specimen. The incision can often be placed in a location that is not prone to breakdown, such as the upper quadrants of the abdomen or the suprapubic area (Fig. 24.10a,c,d). Placement of the incision should be determined by using the lighted telescope directed anteriorly to identify the location of the anastomosis. This will allow the smallest incision possible to accomplish transection of the bowel and reanastomosis. In general, the length of the incision required to complete the procedure is 10 cm or less. The key to utilizing the smallest incision possible is adequate mobilization of the bowel in order to bring the anastomotic lines easily up into the incision.

WOUND INFECTION

Postoperative wound infections are common in patients undergoing resection of the colon or rectum. Wound infections predispose to acute and delayed wound breakdown and increase the mortality rate associated with these procedures. There should be no increase in the postoperative wound infection rate in patients undergoing laparoscopic resection if good technique is utilized. The rate may in fact decrease because of the reduced incision length involved.

In patients undergoing laparoscopic procedures, the same precautions should be taken as are used in those undergoing open resection of the colon or rectum to prevent postoperative wound infections. All patients should have adequate mechanical cleansing of the bowel, with or without the use of nonabsorbable intraluminal antibiotics. Prophylactic perioperative intravenous antibiotics should be used in all patients. A broad-spectrum antibiotic that is effective against aerobic gram-positive and gram-negative organisms, as well as gram-negative anaerobes, is indicated. A second-generation cephalosporin offers effectiveness as well as economy.

ANASTOMOTIC PROBLEMS

Anastomotic Leaks

This is without doubt the most dreaded complication that can occur in patients undergoing resection of the colon or rectum. Leakage can be recognized early (i.e., within the first several days) when containment does not occur. Early leakage requires reoperation, with either resection of the anastomosis and diversion or drainage of the infection and diversion. Both of these procedures also require subsequent ostomy closure. Delayed leakage (i.e., occurring or, rather, recognized after the first several days) usually is associated with abscess formation. In this case, reoperation with drainage, diversion, and subsequent ostomy closure is generally required. At a minimum, percutaneous drainage of the abscess is necessary. In all situations where the anastomosis is not resected, there is a reasonable risk of stricture formation.

How can this complication be avoided? In general, the principles of open colon resection should be followed. Adequate circulation to the cut ends of the bowel should be maintained. The resection should be performed with anatomic considerations in mind. Major blood vessels should be left intact, circulation through long marginal vessels should be avoided, and overaggressive cleansing of the cut ends of the bowel should be avoided. Bleeding from the end of transected bowel should be controlled gingerly, using pressure with a Kittner sponge or gentle application of pressure together with the use of monopolar cautery.

Stricture

Stricture formation can occur in any anastomosis. Predisposing factors are ischemia and infection. Technical errors, such as an anastomosis that is too small, are extremely unusual. Adherence to the principles of reducing infection and preserving the blood supply to the bowel will all but eliminate this complication.

DELAYED WOUND BREAKDOWN

Hernias

Incisional hernias are relatively common after abdominal operations on the colon. They are largely related to the development of postoperative wound infections. They are also related to the location and length of the incision.

In laparoscopic colon resection the development of incisional hernias should be extremely uncommon. Their incidence should be the same as that of large (12 mm) trocar puncture sites. If a trocar site is enlarged (e.g., in a sigmoid resection or a low anterior resection where the specimen is brought out through a site in the left lower quadrant), there will undoubtedly be an increased risk of hernia development at that site. Obviously, the incision should be large enough to remove the specimen in order to maintain the integrity of the colon but not too large to minimize the risk of hernia formation.

In laparoscopically assisted colon resections there is obviously an increased risk of infection and subsequent hernia formation. Again, incisions should be made as small as possible and placed in locations that are less prone to the development of postoperative hernias (e.g., transverse suprapubic, lateral [flank], and subcostal).

BLADDER DYSFUNCTION

Retention

Bladder dysfunction in the postoperative patient, with either an open or a closed procedure, is related to a number of factors. These include creation of a pneumoperitoneum, with stretching of the abdominal wall musculature; excessive fluid administration, with overdistention of the bladder in the postoperative period; pain associated with large incisions, impairing the use of the Valsalva maneuver; and dissection around the bladder and the administration of anesthetics, both of which cause impairment of neuromuscular function. All of these factors are worsened by enlargement of the prostate in the male with mechanical obstruction at the bladder neck.

All of these factors are important in patients undergoing laparoscopic or laparoscopically assisted resection of the colon or rectum. Prolonged pneumoperitoneum is generally unavoidable. When surgeons first begin to perform these procedures, the pneumoperitoneum will be unavoidably long. As more experience is gained, this will decrease. It is unclear whether a brief pneumoperitoneum has any advantage over a longer one in terms of its effect on abdominal wall musculature. Catheter drainage of the bladder at the time of surgery is important in preventing postoperative urinary retention. Catheters should be left in place for an adequate period; when they are removed, excess fluid administration should be avoided.

URINARY TRACT INFECTION

Urinary tract infection in the postoperative patient is directly related to the presence of an indwelling catheter. Bladder catheterization is generally unavoidable in laparoscopic or laparoscopically assisted resection of the colon or rectum because of the factors mentioned above. The incidence of urinary tract infection increases with each day of catheterization and with urinary retention. The catheter must be removed as early as possible, yet not early enough to result in urinary retention.

The surgeon must evaluate all of the factors that predispose a patient to retention. These include the effects of the pneumoperitoneum on the abdominal wall musculature, the degree of pain associated with the incisions, the specific procedure (intra-abdominal or pelvic), the medications the patient was taking prior to the operation, and the presence and degree of prostatic enlargement. Prior operations that may also affect the patient's ability to urinate, such as a previous bladder suspension, may also increase the risk of postoperative urinary retention.

SEXUAL DYSFUNCTION

Postoperative erectile and ejaculatory dysfunction is common after resection of the colon and rectum. The functional abnormality depends on the specific injury that occurs (parasympathetic versus sympathetic nerves) during bowel resection. For the most part, these problems occur only with resection of the sigmoid colon and the rectum. The incidence of erectile and ejaculatory dysfunction after these operations varies directly with the age of the patient and the specific bowel segment removed. The incidence also varies with the status of the patient's sexual function prior to the operation.

The incidence is high in older patients, in those undergoing resection of the rectum, and in those with compromised or diminished sexual function prior to the operation. It is greatly reduced in younger patients, in those undergoing resection of the extrapelvic colon, and in those who had normal sexual function prior to the procedure. The incidence may also vary with the disease. There may be an increased incidence in patients undergoing resection for cancer, because of dissection closer to the sacrum and pelvic side walls, and a lower incidence in patients undergoing resection for inflammatory bowel disease, where dissection occurs closer to the bowel wall. The cause of this postoperative problem is not only injury to the sympathetic and parasympathetic nerves in and around the pelvis but also the interference with the blood supply to the pelvic organs.

The nerves can be injured by direct trauma as well as through traction. Theoretically, the incidence should be somewhat decreased with the laparoscopic approach because of the technique and instrumentation used. This should accrue because of a decreased ability to apply traction to the bowel and a relative inability to skeletonize the sacrum and pelvic side walls. A large series of patients will be needed to determine whether the incidence of these complications differs between the open and laparoscopic methods.

RESULTS OF LAPAROSCOPIC RESECTION OF THE COLON AND RECTUM

Several individual series, as well as many reviews of laparoscopic resection of the colon and rectum, have now been published. These have looked at a number of factors that are felt to be important when comparing laparoscopic or laparoscopically assisted procedures to standard or open colon resection (Table 24.5).

It has been shown that the operative time is considerably longer for laparoscopic procedures. Tate et al. looked prospectively at the operative times in open versus laparoscopic anterior resection of the colon. The mean operative time was 205 min for the laparoscopoic procedures versus 123 min for the conventional or open procedures. Increased operative time is also associated with increased operating room cost. This cost, however, is generally offset by the reduced hospital stay for patients who undergo laparoscopic or laparoscopically assisted resection. Fine et al. have looked at the total cost in patients undergoing laparoscopic and open resection of the colon. In the open group the total hospital cost was $11,010 and in the laparoscopic group it was $13,050—an insignificant difference.

Table 24.5. Factors Comparing Laparoscopic and Laparoscopically Assisted to Open Resection of the Colon and Rectum

Operative time
Operative blood loss
Conversion rates
Specimen length
Number of lymph nodes removed
Mortality
Morbidity
Length of hospital stay
Hospital cost
Time to return to normal activity

Conversion rates do drive costs up. The reasons for this are many. They include the use of laparoscopic as well as open surgical instruments, increased operating room time, and failure to realize the benefits of the laparoscopic procedure (reduced length of hospital stay). Conversion rates vary considerably between series, ranging from 0% in a series of 30 patients to 34.7% in a series of 95 patients. In the series that were evaluated, the average conversion rate was found to be 14%. The reasons for the discrepancy are not clear. Conversion is related to a number of factors, including the tools available, the experience and technical ability of the surgeon, the surgeon's patience, the surgeon's attitude toward prolonged operations and how long the attempted laparoscopic approach should be continued, the operation being performed, and the disease being treated. It is imperative that the surgeon assess the situation quickly and determine whether continuing the procedure laparoscopically will result in a successful outcome in a reasonable period of time.

Blood loss is significantly reduced in patients who undergo laparoscopic or laparoscopically assisted resection of the colon or rectum. Senagore et al. recently reported a more than 75% reduction in blood loss in patients undergoing successful laparoscopic resections. In patients undergoing open procedures, the total blood loss was 687 ± 54 ml. In patients undergoing successful laparoscopic procedures, the blood loss was reduced to 157 ± 19 ml. Even in the converted group where much of the dissection was initially performed laparoscopically, the blood loss was somewhat reduced over the open group, being 491 ± 50 ml.

Specimen length and the number of lymph nodes removed are of great concern in patients undergoing laparoscopic or laparoscopically assisted colon resection for colon cancer. A number of investigators have looked at these two factors. With regard to the length of the specimen removed at the time of surgery, the real question is whether there is a significant difference in the clinical outcome. The data in the literature vary somewhat among investigations. There appears to be a difference in the length of the specimens in some series. In others, however, this difference is not evident. Van Ye et al. looked at the length of the proximal and distal resection margins in patients who underwent laparoscopic resection for cancer and compared them to the resection margins in 20 patients who underwent open resection for cancer during the prior 6-month period. In the laparoscopic group the average proximal resection margin was 11.1 cm (range, 3–34 cm) and the average distal resection margin was 10.0 cm (range, 2–23 cm). In the open group the aver-

Table 24.6. Postoperative Morbidity and Mortality in Patients Undergoing Laparoscopic or Laparoscopically Assisted Resection of the Colon and Rectum

Author	No. of Patients	% Morbidity	% Mortality
Fine	30	24.0	0
Wexner	74	34.0	0
Senagore	38	—	0-11/C-17
Zucker	65	6.2	0
Jansen	51	20.5	1.9
Plasencia	30	10.0	0
Slim	40	25.0	3.2

O = open, C = converted.

age proximal resection margin was 7.4 cm (range, 1.5–20 cm) and the average distal resection margin was 14.2 cm (range, 2–30 cm). The differences between the two groups were not statistically significant. Van Ye et al. looked at the number of lymph nodes recovered with the specimen. In the laparoscopic group the average number was 10.5, with an average of 0.4 lymph nodes positive for metastatic cancer. In the open group the average number was 7.6, with an average of 0.5 lymph nodes positive for metastatic cancer. This was also not statistically significant.

Postoperative morbidity and in-hospital mortality are also extremely important in evaluating the value of laparoscopic and laparoscopically assisted resection of the colon and rectum. A number of published series have looked at these two factors (Table 24.6).

In general there is no difference between the open and laparoscopic groups. This assumes that the procedure is performed by a surgeon who is knowledgeable in open colon surgery; skillful in laparoscopic techniques, especially those related to laparoscopic colon resection; well versed in the use of the various instruments; and interested in performing these procedures expeditiously and with the patient's best interest (primarily safety) in mind.

The length of the patient's hospital stay is important but not of primary concern. In general, a significant reduction has been seen in virtually every series published to date. Patients resume a regular diet sooner and require much less pain medication during their hospitalization. The real benefit of laparoscopic surgery from the patient's point of view, however, occurs after the first week, when the patient returns to normal activity much earlier and with considerably less pain and disability. The fact that the hospital stay is reduced allows these procedures to be performed at an almost equivalent cost to their open counterparts.

BIBLIOGRAPHY

Asao T, Nagamachi Y: Intraoperative colonoscopy during laparoscopic bowel resection. *Lancet* 345(8957): 1123, 1995.

Darzi A, Super P, Guillou PJ, et al: Laparoscopic sigmoid colectomy: total laparoscopic approach. *Dis Colon Rectum* 37(3):268–271, 1994.

Finne AP, Lanasa S, Gannon MP, et al: Laparoscopic colon surgery. *Am Surg* 61(5):412–416, 1995.

Fowler DL, White SA: Laparoscopy assisted sigmoid resection. *Surg Laparosc Endosc* 1(3):183–188, 1991.

Fuhrman GM, Ota DM: Laparoscopic intestinal stomas. *Dis Colon Rectum* 37(5):444–449, 1994.

Geis WP, Coletta A, Verdeja JC, et al: Sequential psychomotor skills development in laparoendoscopic colon surgery. *Arch Surg* 129(2):206–212, 1994.

Gray D, Lee H, Schlinkert R: Adequacy of lymphadenectomy in laparoscopic-assisted colectomy for colorectal cancer: a preliminary report. *J Surg Oncol* 57(1):8–10, 1994.

Jansen A: Laparoscopic-assisted colon resection. Evolution from an experimental technique to a standardized surgical procedure. *Ann Chir Gynaecol* 83(2):86–91, 1994.

Kucker KA, Pitcher DE, Martin DT, et al: Laparoscopic-assisted colon resections. *Surg Endosc* 8(1): 12–17; discussion 18, 1994.

Lyerly HK, Mault JR: Laparoscopic ileostomy and colostomy. *Ann Surg* 219(3):317–322, 1994.

Plasencia G, Jacobs M, Verdeja JC, et al: Laparoscopic-assisted sigmoid colectomy and low anterior resection. *Dis Colon Rectum* 37(8):829–833, 1994.

Sackier JM: Visualization of the ureter during laparoscopic colonic resection. *Br J Surg* 80(10):1332, 1993.

Senagore AJ, Lutchefeld MA, Mackeigan JM, et al: Open colectomy versus laparoscopic colectomy: are there differences. *Am Surg* 59(8):549–553; discussion 553–554, 1993.

Shallman RW, Shaw TJ, Roach JM: Colonoscopically assisted intracorporeal laparoscopic wedge resection of a benign right colon lesion. *Surg Laparosc Endosc* 3(6):482–494, 1993.

Slim K, Pezet D, Stencl J Jr, et al: Prospective analysis of 40 initial laparoscopic colorectal resections: a plea for a randomized trial. *J Laparoendosc Surg* 4(4):241–245, 1994.

Tate JJ, Kwok S, Dawson JW, et al: Prospective comparison of laparoscopic and conventional anterior resection. *Br J Surg* 80(11):1396–1398, 1993.

Van Ye TM, Cattey RP, Henry LG: Laparoscopically assisted colon resections compare favorably with open technique. *Surg Laparosc Endosc* 4(1):25–31, 1994.

Wexner SD, Cohen SM, Johansen OB: Laparoscopic colorectal surgery: a prospective assessment and current perspective. *Br J Surg* 80(12):1602–1605, 1993.

Zinman LM, Libertino JA, Roth RA: Management of operative ureteral injury. *Urol* 12:290–303, 1978.

section six

Surgery of the Thorax

chapter twenty-five

Pulmonary Resection by Video-Assisted Techniques

Juan A. Sanchez
Utpal S. Desai

The recent revival of thoracoscopy as a diagnostic and therapeutic tool is a result of vastly improved instrumentation and the general trend toward less invasive approaches in surgery. New high-resolution video technology, refinements in surgical staplers and lasers, single-lung anesthesia, and improved hemodynamic monitoring have greatly expanded the use of what is now commonly referred to as *video-assisted thoracic surgery (VATS)*. As experience with these techniques has evolved, VATS is being increasingly employed for pulmonary resection including, occasionally, major anatomic pulmonary resections. There exists, almost invariably, a learning curve in the stereotaxic use of video-guided equipment made more difficult by the loss of depth perception as well as the loss of tactile discrimination of tissues. While improvements and experience have made these techniques safer, the potential for complications has not been eliminated.[1-3] The nature of the complications associated with pulmonary resections does not differ greatly between VATS and standard open approaches.

The issue of costs associated with the use of this or any other new technology has become an important one in today's health care environment. While shorter hospital stays may give VATS an advantage over standard thoracotomy, the use of disposable instruments, longer operations, and longer anesthesia times may mitigate this advantage. However, complications contribute significantly to costs, and prevention and efficient management are important factors.[4]

Comparison of pulmonary resection by VATS and by thoracotomy in terms of the incidence of complications is difficult given the general paucity of prospective randomized studies. Therefore, no definite conclusions can be drawn. Currently available data suffer from insufficient sample size or inherent biases in patient selection. Giudicelli et al., however, have reported on outcomes for lobectomy and have compared video-assisted minithoracotomy with muscle-sparing thoracotomy. They have concluded that while factors such as pain-related morbidity, duration of chest tubes, and hospital stay tended to favor the lesser approach, no statistically significant reduction in morbidity or improvement in pulmonary function was detected between the two groups.[5]

PATIENT SELECTION

The ideal patient for pulmonary resection using VATS technology has a small, peripherally located nodule in an easily accessible segment of the lung such as the lingula. In addition, no impairment of pulmonary function should be present, as well as no previous thoracic surgery on the involved side. In these patients, thoracoscopic examination of the pleural space and subsequent wedge resection is expected to carry an extremely low complication rate. More central lesions requiring larger degrees of resection incur higher morbidity. Patients who are critically ill may not be candidates for VATS despite the notion that less invasive procedures carry a smaller degree of risk in this group. Given a presumed longer operative time and an extended period of lung collapse with VATS, these patients may do better with an open approach in many circumstances.

As with open resection, identification of preexisting cardiopulmonary disease is an elemental part of the preoperative assessment due to the high prevalence of coronary and pulmonary disease in patients undergoing thoracic surgery.[6] An acceptable workup includes pulmonary function studies and quantitative ventilation and perfusion scans if a significant portion of lung will be resected. As with open approaches, severe impairment of pulmonary function precludes resection, although in some patients with stage I bronchogenic carcinoma, limited resection may provide acceptable results.[7] Pulmonary dysfunction should be optimized in the preoperative period by smoking cessation, use of bronchodilators, and improved bronchopulmonary hygiene.[6] Relative contraindications for pulmonary resection using VATS are outlined in Table 25.1. Paramount in the decision to employ VATS technology for resection is the result of frank discussions with the patient and the family with regard to expectations and the ability to accomplish the intended procedure, including the possibility of conversion to thoracotomy.

Conversion to thoracotomy should not be regarded as a complication of video-assisted procedures. It is performed either because the procedure cannot be accomplished safely or satisfactorily or because a complication cannot be managed due to limited exposure. The VATS Study Group has identified six reasons for conversion to thoracotomy (Table 25.2). With experience and proper patient selection, rates of conversion to thoracotomy are relatively low, although this depends greatly on the role played by this technology at a given institution for pulmonary resection.[8] Fortunately, conversion to an open surgery does not appear, in general, to be associated with increased costs.[4]

Table 25.1. Contraindications to VATS Pulmonary Resection

Hilar pulmonary lesions
Lung lesions invading upper mediastinum or posterior paravertebral area
Small thoracic cavities
Ventilator dependency
Noncompliant lung
Small, deep parenchymal lesions
Dense pleural symphysis

Source: Ref. 29

Table 25.2. Indications for Conversion to Thoracotomy

Further resection	50%
Unable to find lesion	15%
Lesion too large to remove	14%
Adhesion	13%
Equipment failure	6%
Bleeding	2%

Source: Ref. 22.

Wedge Resection

Wedge resection of nodules located in the outer third of the lung accounts for the majority of lung resections using VATS. If the nodule represents bronchogenic carcinoma, a thoracotomy is usually performed and standard anatomic resection is carried out. VATS represents adjunctive technology which avoids thoracotomy in patients with benign disease. In certain instances, a wedge resection for lung cancer in patients with extremely poor pulmonary function can be acceptable definitive treatment. However, it is exceedingly important not to regard VATS technology as a means of performing lesser resections as definitive treatment of lung cancer. The Lung Cancer Study Group has demonstrated an unacceptably high rate of local recurrence when limited resections were used to treat T1 (less than 3 cm) lesions.[9]

In resecting a pulmonary nodule, common reasons for conversion to thoracotomy are the need for further resection or the finding that the lesion is too large or too central to be removed by this approach. This decision depends to some degree on the familiarity and expertise of the surgeon with this technology. Unless VATS lobectomy is contemplated, preoperative identification of a lesion larger than 3 cm should preclude the use of video thoracoscopy for wedge resection because of the high probability that the lesion is malignant.[10]

The increasing number of transplant and otherwise immunocompromised patients has generated a demand for thoracoscopic lung biopsy, most commonly in the setting of diffuse lung infiltrates. In general, these patients present with debilitation due to poor nutrition and often serious pulmonary impairment. Critically ill patients may not be good candidates for this approach if pulmonary dysfunction prevents single-lung anesthesia or if longer operative time is anticipated with VATS.[11] An expeditiously performed open lung biopsy

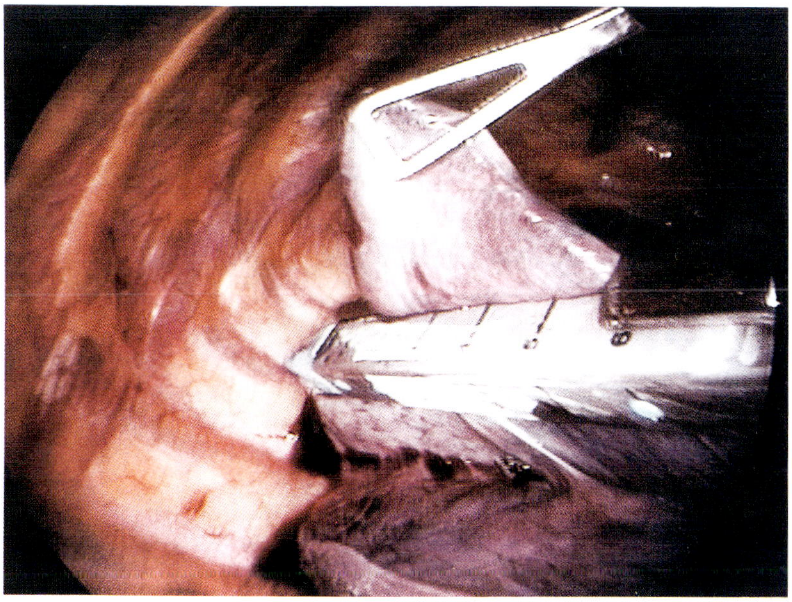

Figure 25.1. Video-assisted lung biopsy using endoscopic linear stapler.[29]

with ventilation of both lungs is more prudent under these circumstances. Otherwise, lung biopsy by video thoracoscopy is an excellent method in patients who can tolerate one-lung anesthesia (Fig. 25.1).

VATS has also proven practical in the evaluation of isolated metastatic disease to the lungs, both for diagnosis and as treatment in selected individuals.[12,13] However, a decrease in the surgeon's ability to evaluate the lung for additional lesions appears to limit the usefulness of this technique given the fact that the number of metastases is commonly underestimated by computed tomography (CT) scanning.[14] As well, trocar implantation of tumor following video-assisted resection of pulmonary metastases is known.[15]

Major pulmonary resections

Undoubtedly, major pulmonary resections including pneumonectomy are technically possible using VATS technology.[16-20] The long term benefits and disadvantages of anatomic resections using this approach have not been well delineated in a randomized fashion. While VATS lobectomy for cancer may have short-term advantages over conventional lobectomy with regard to postoperative pain, morphine consumption, and hospital stay, any anticipated compromise in the ability to resect sufficient tissue should prompt thoracotomy. In addition, reports of seeding of the port sites with carcinoma have raised grave concerns about the ability to control dissemination of malignant cells using this technique.[8,15,21]

The absence of a complete fissure between lobes presents a challenge in performing a lobectomy, regardless of the technique employed. Identification and ligation of the lobar vessels, followed by stapled transection of the pulmonary tissue to complete the interlobar fissure, is an accepted technique. However, a significant absence of fissurization should be approached with caution when contemplating VATS lobectomy, and strong consideration should be given to using the open technique.

COMPLICATIONS

Missed Lesions

Although video technology provides excellent visualization of the entire thoracic cavity, the loss of tactile discrimination can hamper efforts to locate a lesion detected on CT scan or another imaging modality. The incidence of this occurrence was 7.5% in the VAT Study Group data.[22] This appears to be a significant problem, especially in the case of small central lesions. In a series of 11 wedge resections, 3 were converted to thoracotomy because of an inability to find the lesion.[23]

Techniques used to help identify a lesion include careful inspection of the lung for discoloration or retraction of the visceral pleura, introduction of the surgeon's finger through a trocar hole for palpation, and the sweeping of smooth instruments over the parenchyma.[24,25] In addition, CO_2 insufflation of the pleural space, which promotes more complete and uniform collapse of all lung segments, may bring out lesions not previously seen. This should be done with caution so as not to produce tension within the thoracic cavity. In general, intrapleural pressures below 8 mmHg are safe.[26] Proper placement of the ports and proper positioning of the patient are fundamental to maximize the chances of locating a lesion.

Preoperative localization of lesions is being increasingly applied to lung pathology. Methylene blue applied to the area of the lesion preoperatively is often helpful at thoracoscopy, although it should be used in small amounts and as close to the time of surgery as possible to minimize diffusion of the dye, resulting in discoloration of the entire pleura. Needle localization, used extensively in the evaluation of breast lesions, has become an ideal method for locating difficult pulmonary lesions (Fig. 25.2).[24,25] Problems such as inexact placement, dislodgment, or submersion of the needle on collapse of the lung are known to occur. Pneumothorax is a well-known complication of this technique and occurs in 30% of all patients. Table 25.3 lists situations in which preoperative localization appears to be helpful.

Table 25.3. Use of Preoperative Needle Localization

Lesions less than 1 cm in diameter
Interstitial lung disease or emphysema
Extensive pleural disease
Previous chest radiation therapy
Limited experience with VATS

Source: Ref. 25.

Intraoperative ultrasound has also provided assistance not only in locating lesions but also in establishing margins and identifying vascular or airway involvement.[25] The inability to find a lesion by video can usually be resolved at thoracotomy when the surgeon feels the entire lung parenchyma. Persistent attempts to locate a lesion by thoracoscopy may result in excessive

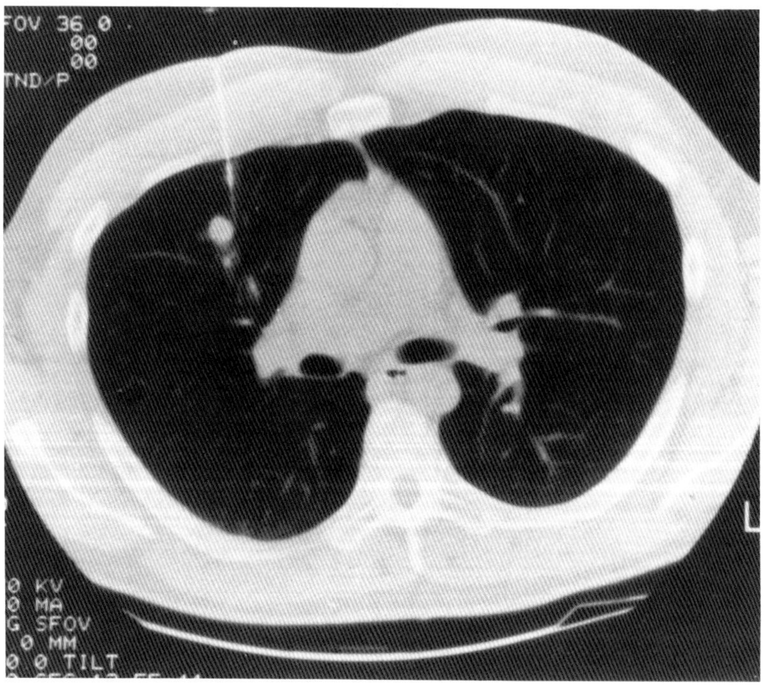

Figure 25.2. Preoperative wire localization of lung nodule by CT scan.[30]

prolongation of operative time, increased cost, and possibly increased morbidity.

Air Leak

Postoperative air leak following pulmonary resection is fairly common and usually resolves within the first few days after surgery. Leaks persisted after the first week in 4.7% of patients in the VATS Study Group.[22] Patients with a forced expiratory volume in 1 sec of under 1 L have a higher incidence of prolonged air leak following wedge resection than those with better lung function (2.3% versus 20.9%). Patients over 75 years of age also have a significantly increased incidence of air leaks. A 2.8% incidence of prolonged air leak was found following VATS for a pulmonary nodule versus a 10.5% incidence for diffuse parenchymal disease. Nonetheless, the higher incidence of prolonged air leaks did not appear to lengthen the hospital stay.

Initial management of air leaks involves watchful waiting. Often repositioning the chest tube or eliminating suction will resolve the leak. Persistent leaks may require repeat thoracoscopy and identification of the source. Occasionally, this can be difficult despite a variety of maneuvers, including ventilation of the involved lung in a fluid-filled pleural space. Once identified, leaks can be secured with the use of staplers, the directed application of fibrin glue, or direct suture. The use of the wide-field Nd:YAG laser and the argon beam electrocautery coagulator has been effective in relatively small areas of denuded visceral pleura. Electrocautery appears to be uniformly ineffective in the treatment of air leaks and should be avoided. In cases where air leaks are associated with significant bullous disease, use of the low-intensity argon beam coagulator results in shrinkage of the bullae, allowing limited resection of the involved lung. In these cases, a sleeve of bovine pericardium can be attached to the stapler to reinforce the staple line.[10] In certain instances, diffuse areas of air leakage in the presence of diseased lung tissue may require chemical sclerosants, mechanical abrasion of the pleurae, or partial pleurectomy. Caution should be employed, as these methods can result in significant bleeding or fibrothorax.[27]

Bleeding

Significant bleeding during pulmonary resection utilizing VATS has been the source of greatest concern given the dependence on good visualization. Brisk hemorrhage can obscure the camera lens, quickly resulting in inability to control the source. In experienced hands, significant bleeding is relatively rare, occurring in 2% of patients in the VATS Study Group.[3] Transfusion of blood was required in only 1% of these patients. However, the potential for catastrophic hemorrhage exists, especially in major lung resections, and the decision to convert to thoracotomy requires mature, decisive judgment.

Sources of bleeding in the chest vary from insignificant parenchymal capillaries to major pulmonary artery, veins, and bronchial arteries. Careful ligation of the larger vascular structures can be accomplished using a variety of methods, including direct suture ligature, large metal clips, and vascular staplers. Regardless of the method employed, it is essential that more than one ligature be applied precisely and securely, with no compromise of the visual field. When endoscopic linear staplers are used to ligate large vessels, the knife attachment within the instrument is often removed to prevent inadvertent cutting of the vessel without proper firing of the staples (Fig. 25.3). The vessel can then be divided under direct visualization.[27] In general, however, the use of endoscopic vascular stapling with simultaneous division of the vessel appears to be safe, as reported by McKenna in a series of 200 cases.[28]

A potential source of bleeding is the bronchial arterial network surrounding the bronchi. Bleeding from vessels at the severed end of the bronchus can generally be controlled with cautery or clips. These vessels are sometimes the source of bleeding in the postoperative period, and a thorough inspection of the bronchial staple line is warranted prior to completion of the procedure. In addition, bleeding from intercostal vessels can be voluminous if not recognized early (Fig. 25.4). With appropriate visualization, these vessels can often be ligated with metal clips thoracoscopically.[1]

Instrument Injury

Injury to the lung during insertion of trocars through the chest wall is rare, occurring in only 0.2%.[22] Current spring-loaded devices effectively prevent this complication. Since the rigid thorax allows thoracoscopy without insufflation of the pleural space, this space can be entered without the need for an airtight seal. Once the pleura is entered, the lung is allowed to collapse and the camera can be introduced. All other ports are then created under direct video visualization, with the lung well away from the chest wall. Nevertheless, injury to the parenchyma from trocars and other video instru-

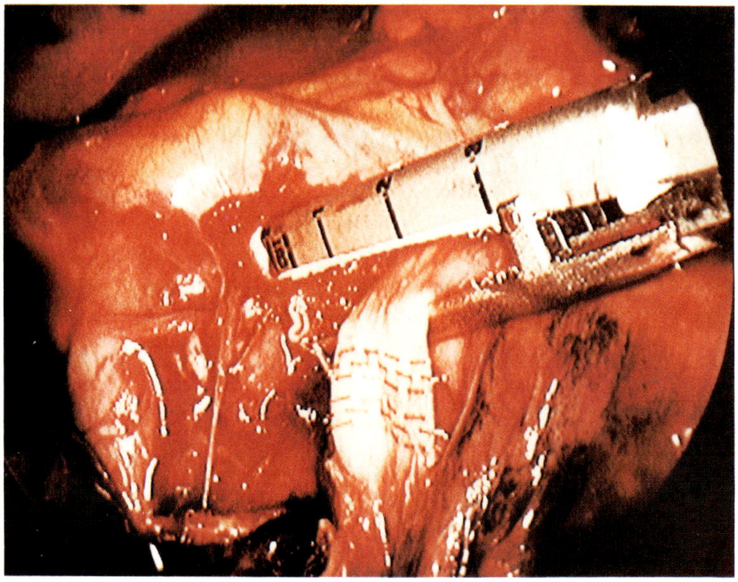

Figure 25.3. Ligation of the superior pulmonary vein after the knife blade has been removed from the stapler. The vessel is divided between staple lines with endoscopic scissors under direct visualization.[31]

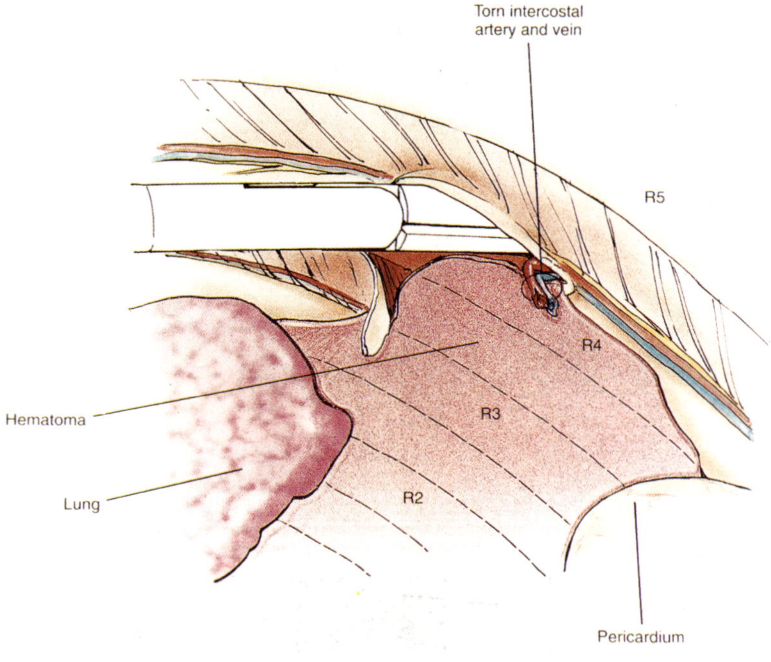

Figure 25.4. Instrument injury to intercostal vessels.[32]

ments is a known source of morbidity.[2] Bleeding from intercostal vessels and paresthesias from intercostal nerve injuries can occur at any time during the procedure. These complications usually follow repeated trauma caused by gyrating instruments when the ribs are used as a fulcrum. Anterior placement of the stapler, generally the culprit instrument, appears to decrease the incidence of chest wall injury and reduce the area of resulting paresthesia. Patients with adhesions of the lung to the chest wall are at particular risk of lung injury, regardless of the method employed to enter the chest. Patients with previous thoracotomy or known dense adhesions on the involved side are generally not candidates for VATS.

Instrument Failure

Locking of the stapler and failure to release tissue is an alarming occurrence, especially during video-assisted procedures.[22] While developments in stapler technology have made pulmonary resections easier and safer, steps to prevent misfiring should always be undertaken. Inadvertent bending of the instrument at any time can cause misfiring. The shaft of the stapler must be at least partly inside the chest cavity when firing. The stapler should be reloaded carefully and deliberately and should always involve thorough cleansing, with particular emphasis on the anvil. Deep pulmonary lesions are more likely to result in stapling mishaps as the tissue thickness involved increases. Instruments which gauge tissue thickness and dictate the staple size to employ are generally helpful. The Nd:YAG laser has become a useful adjunct to the stapler in deeper lesions.[23] With this technique, surrounding tissue is attenuated until the stapler can be safely applied.

Other Complications

Atrial tachyarrhythmias can occur following any type of major pulmonary resection. The VATS Study Group reported an incidence of 1.6% for all procedures.[22] This complication is most commonly observed in patients over 75 years of age. Particular emphasis on electrolyte levels, specifically potassium and magnesium, should be used in older patients or those with known heart disease. Atelectasis following thoracic procedures is a common source of postoperative fever. In this regard, lung resection by thoracoscopy minimizes the amount of postoperative pain and should minimize this complication. Early ambulation, incentive spirometry, and adequate postoperative analgesia are important preventive maneuvers. Significant or recurrent lung collapse may require fiberoptic bronchoscopy to clear the airway of thick secretions and to ensure that no mechanical obstruction of a bronchus exists.

Postoperative pneumonia is a serious and potentially lethal complication.[2] Frequently, these patients have preexisting pulmonary disease or are otherwise critically ill prior to surgery. Prompt recognition and institution of aggressive therapy is essential. Postoperative wound infection is uncommon following thoracoscopy, accounting for 0.4%, and aggressive interventions have not been necessary.[22] Other complications following VATS depend on the nature of the disease. While intraoperative mortality is uncommon, death following lung biopsy in critically ill patients can be significant as a result of the preexisting disease process.

SUMMARY

While it is difficult to predict the exact role of VATS technology in the future, current enthusiasm for it should lead to a rigorous assessment of its benefits, risks, and costs. Its success will ultimately depend on maintaining a superior safety profile and demonstrating continued effectiveness at low cost. This will require its judicious use and proper patient selection, as well as the prevention and expeditious management of complications in the hope that thoracoscopy will continue to be an invaluable tool in the thoracic surgeon's armamentarium.

REFERENCES

1. Kaiser D, Ennker IC, Hartz C: Video-assisted thoracoscopic surgery—indications, results, complications, and contraindications. *Thorac Cardiovasc Surg* 41:330–334, 1993.
2. Demmy TL, Curtis JJ, Boley TM et al: Diagnostic and therapeutic thoracoscopy: Lessons from the learning curve. *Am J Surg* 166:696–701, 1993.
3. Kaiser LR, Bavaria JE: Complications of thoracoscopy. *Ann Thorac Surg* 56:796–798, 1993.
4. Hazelrigg SR, Nunchuck SK, Landreneau RJ, et al: Cost analysis for thoracoscopy: Thoracoscopic wedge resection. *Ann Thorac Surg* 56:633–635, 1993.
5. Giudicelli R, Thomas P, Lonjon T, et al: Video assisted minithoracotomy for performing lobectomy. *Ann Thorac Surg* 58:712–718, 1994.

6. Horswell JL: Anesthetic techniques for thoracoscopy. *Ann Thorac Surg* 56:634–629, 1993.
7. Miller JI: Limited resection of bronchogenic carcinoma in the patient with limited pulmonary function. *Ann Thorac Surg* 56:769–771, 1993.
8. Allen MS, Pairolero PC: Inadequacy, mortality and thoracoscopy. *Ann Thorac Surg* 59(1):6, 1995.
9. Ginsberg RJ, Rubinstein L: Randomized trail of lobectomy versus limited resection for T1 NO non-small cell lung cancer. Lung cancer study group. *Ann Thorac Surg* 60(3):615–622, 1995.
10. Kaiser LR: Video-assisted thoracic surgery. *Ann Surg* 220(6):720–734, 1994.
11. Feins RH; The role of thoracoscopy in the AIDS/ immunocompromised patient. *Ann Thorac Surg* 56: 649–650, 1993.
12. Clair DG, Lautz DB, Brooks DC: Rapid development of umbilical metastasis after laparoscopic cholecystectomy for unsuspected gallbladder carcinoma. *Surgery* 113: 355–358, 1993.
13. Dowling RD, Keenan RJ, Ferson PF et al: Video-assisted thoracoscopic resection of pulmonary metastases. *Ann Thorac Surg* 56:772–775, 1993.
14. McCormack PM, Ginsberg KB, Bains MS, et al: Accuracy of lung imaging in metastases with implications for the role of thoracoscopy. *Ann Thorac Surg* 56:863–866, 1993.
15. Walsh GL, Nesbitt JC: Tumor implants after thoracoscopic resection of a metastatic sarcoma. *Ann Thorac Surg* 59:215–216, 1995.
16. Rovario G, Varoli F, Rebuffat C, et al: Major pulmonary resections: Pneumonectomies and lobectomies. *Ann Thorac Surg* 56:779–783, 1993.
17. Walker WS, Carnochan FM, Pugh GC: Thoracoscopic pulmonary lobectomy.*Thorac Cardiovasc Surg* 106: 1111–1117, 1993.
18. Lewis RJ, Sisler GE, Caccavale RJ: Imaged thoracic lobectomy: Should it be done? *Ann Thorac Surg* 54:80–83, 1992.
19. Walker WS, Carnochan FM, Tin M: Thoracoscopy assisted pulmonary lobectomy. *Thorax* 48:921–924, 1993.
20. Walker WS, Carnochan FM, Mattar S: Video assisted thoracoscopic pneumonectomy. *Br J Surg* 81:81–82, 1994.
21. Fry WA, Siddiqui A, Pensler JM, et al: Thoracoscopic implantation of cancer with a fatal outcome. *Ann Thorac Surg* 59:42–45, 1995.
22. Hazelrigg SR, Nunchuck SK, LoCicero J, et al: Video assisted thoracic surgery study group data. *Ann Thorac Surg* 56:1039–1044, 1993.
23. Rieger R, Woisetschlager R, Schinko H, et al: Thoracoscopic wedge resection of peripheral lung lesions. *Thorac Cardiovasc Surg* 31:152–155, 1993.
24. Daniel TM, Kern JA, Tribble CG, et al: Thoracoscopic surgery for diseases of the lung and pleura. *Ann Surg* 217(5):566–575, 1993.
25. Shennib H: Intraoperative localization techniques for pulmonary nodules. *Ann Thorac Surg* 56:745–748, 1993.
26. Sanchez JA, Baldwin JC: Diagnostic and therapeutic thoracoscopy. In Ballantyne GH, Leahy PF, Modlin IM (eds): *Textbook and Atlas of Laparascopic Surgery*. Philadelphia, Saunders, 1994, pp 345–350.
27. Bhatnagar NK, Berndt S: A solution to prolonged air leak after video-assisted thoracoscopic lobectomy. *Ann Thorac Surg* 59:260–261, 1995.
27. Kirby TJ, Rice TW: Thoracoscopic lobectomy. *Ann Thorac Surg* 56:784–786, 1993.
28. McKenna RJ: Lobectomy by video-assisted thoracic surgery with mediastinal node sampling for lung cancer. *J Thorac Cardiovasc Surg* 107:879–882, 1994.
29. Krasna MJ, Mack MJ: *Atlas of Thoracoscopic Surgery*. Quality Medical Publishing, Inc., St. Louis, 1995, p 95.
30. Mack MJ, Acuff TE: Localization techniques for pulmonary nodules. In Kaiser LR, Daniel TM (eds): *Thoracoscopic Surgery*. Boston, Little Brown, 1993, p 114.
31. Kirby TJ, Birnbaum PL: Thoracoscopic resection in the treatment of lung cancer. In Kaiser LR, Daniel TM (eds): *Thoracoscopic Surgery*. Boston, Little Brown, 1993, p 144.
32. Krasna MJ, Mack MJ: *Atlas of Thoracoscopic Surgery*. Quality Medical Publishing, Inc., St. Louis, 1995, p 49.

chapter twenty-six

Minimally Invasive Esophagogastric Surgery

Raymond J. Lanzafame

Although the detection of esophageal carcinoma at an early stage is increasing, the disease remains a serious condition with a poor prognosis, as well as significant operative morbidity and mortality. Surgery for palliation or cure remains the best therapy for these unfortunate patients.

The development and evolution of laparoscopic and thoracoscopic techniques and technologies have enabled many surgical procedures to be adapted and applied with minimally invasive approaches. The resultant potential benefits for the patient are great when one considers the morbidity from thoracotomy and thoracoabdominal incisions, particularly in the debilitated patient. It must be recognized, however, that these procedures are performed infrequently by the majority of surgeons and that the minimally invasive approach requires a high degree of technical skill, coupled with an excellent understanding of the relevant surgical anatomy and precise attention to detail. Both the stomach and the esophagus can be mobilized completely and manipulated by a combined laparoscopic and thoracoscopic approach. These procedures should be attempted only by the skilled surgical laparoscopist. A thorough understanding of the instrumentation is required, and the surgeon should be conversant with intracorporeal suturing and knot-tying techniques. Endostapling and ligating devices facilitate these procedures and should be readily available for use. This chapter will emphasize many of the technical details of these procedures, as well as the potential pitfalls.

THORACOSCOPIC ACCESS

The reader is referred to Chapters 25 and 28 for a discussion of the techniques and alternatives for gaining thoracoscopic access. The sites selected for trocar insertion will most often be the third, fourth, and sixth intercostal spaces. The precise locations for trocar insertion will depend on the size of the patient, the location of the lesion, and the type of instrumentation available. Many instruments are 30 cm long; therefore, port insertion in the lower interspaces is preferable. Specially designed, curved thoracoscopic instruments facilitate maneuverability and intrathoracic dissection if they are available. The surgeon must exercise caution to avoid injury to the liver or spleen as a result of traumatic insertion or inadvertent penetration of the diaphragm. The initial trocar should be placed in the midaxillary line rather than the anterior chest to avoid iatrogenic injury to the pericardium and heart. A Carlen's endotracheal tube should be used. This will facilitate preferential ventilation of the contralateral hemithorax and permit deflation and retraction of the lung at the surgical site.

Patient positioning should facilitate access to the thorax and abdomen. Many authors place the patient supine, with lateral rotation of the shoulders and with the thighs slightly flexed and abducted. This position facilitates simultaneous thoracic and abdominal surgery.

ESOPHAGEAL DISSECTION

The esophagus can be approached from either the right or the left hemithorax. Endoscopic ultrasound can assist the surgeon in delineating the anatomy of the lesion, as well as the adjacent structures of the mediastinum. The right-sided approach requires care in dissection, particularly in the areas of the azygous vein and the heart. The aorta and the heart must be protected during the left-sided approach.

The pleura are incised both anterior and posterior to the esophagus. This portion of dissection is accomplished with scissors, hook electrocautery, or laser technology. A curved atraumatic dissecting instrument is the safest type of device for this purpose. It enables the surgeon to carefully displace the esophagus medially and laterally without injury to the aorta or the esophagus.

The intrathoracic dissection should commence at the distalmost portion of the esophagus. The crura of the diaphragm and the left vagus nerve are identified. Care must be taken not to injure the aorta at this point in the dissection. The surgeon's viewing of the monitor is optimized by placing it near the patient's feet. The esophagus will be freed circumferentially and will be encircled with a Penrose drain or umbilical tape to provide countertraction for further dissection. Dissection is facilitated by using a two-handed technique. Hemoclips and cautery are used to control perforating vessels. The grasping and dissecting instruments are placed in the fifth and sixth intercostal space ports. The camera will be located in the third or fourth intercostal space ports during this phase of the dissection. The proximal esophageal dissection may be facilitated by placing the monitor near the patient's head. Alternatively, placement of the monitor on the side opposite the surgeon enables adequate visualization without the need to reposition the monitor or encroach on the abdominal operative team. The camera will be repositioned in the sixth intercostal space port.

Firm countertraction is applied via the Penrose drain or umbilical tape sling to distract the esophagus from the inferior pulmonary artery and vein. The surgeon must exercise extreme caution when dissecting near the pulmonary hilum. The inferior pulmonary artery and vein are gently elevated by a right angle clamp or hook dissector. The inferior pulmonary ligament is divided. The use of Pott's loops or silicone vessel loops around the pulmonary vasculature is recommended, as this permits rapid hemostatic control if inadvertent injury to these structures occurs during dissection.

Access to the cervical esophagus, when necessary, is obtained by making an incision along the anterior border of the sternocleidomastoid muscle. The trachea and recurrent laryngeal are carefully preserved as the esophagus is bluntly dissected and mobilized.

Recently, Buess and Lirici have reported on the use of endoscopic microsurgical dissection of the esophagus (EMDE). A key development for this technique was the creation of an operative mediastinoscope with a rotatable sleeve. The distal end of the mediastinoscope is fitted with a grooved "olive" which permits the instrument to maneuver along and around the esophagus. The instrument can be inserted via the cervical incision. It is crucial that vessels be coagulated as soon as they are encountered and prior to their division. This practice is also preferred for non-EMDE dissection.

GASTRIC DISSECTION

The mobilization and dissection of the stomach is accomplished via an abdominal approach. A two-team approach is preferred, as this will dramatically shorten the operative time. Trocar placement is similar to that for fundoplication (see Figure 23.2 in Chapter 23). The majority of gastric and esophageal dissections should be completed prior to incision of the diaphragm, as premature division of the diaphragm will obscure visualization and impair further laparoscopic dissection due to the loss of pneumoperitoneum. An additional problem is the potential for mediastinal shift and respiratory embarrassment resulting from positive-pressure abdominal insufflation.

Careful retraction of the liver is necessary to prevent iatrogenic injury to it. Curved, fan-shaped retractors or Nanticoke-type retractors are suggested for use as liver retractors. The curved portion of the fan should be directed away from the liver surface. Most minor liver lacerations will stop bleeding spontaneously if this occurs. However, gentle pressure with a sponge and/or the use of Surgi-cel or Avitene may be necessary for more persistent bleeding. The stomach should be grasped with a Babcock or atraumatic grasper and retracted in a downward (caudal) direction. The short gastric vessels and the lesser omental vessels are divided. A variety of methods have been described for this portion of the procedure. However, downward traction and the use of gravity to distract the spleen from the greater curvature will assist the surgeon as successive windows are made in the omentum and gastrosplenic ligaments to expose the vessels. The epiploic vessels and the short gastrics should be carefully identified and ligated near the wall of the stomach.

The midportion of the gastric body should then be grasped and retracted upward to allow the surgeon to create a window and incise the greater omentum. Once the gastrocolic membrane has been incised, the lesser sac is entered and any posterior adhesions between the stomach and pancreas are easily lysed. If the lesser omentum has not been separated and divided completely, the dissection is completed at this time. The left gastric artery and its branches are carefully identified and are doubly ligated both proximally and distally. The area for gastric transection is selected and cleared.

The anesthesiologist should withdraw the nasogastric tube prior to gastric division to prevent it from becoming trapped in the staple line. An endo-GIA or similar device can then be used to divide the stomach at the preselected site. Multiple firings of the stapler may be required. The surgeon must verify that each firing partially overlaps its predecessor to ensure that there are no gaps in the staple line.

Once the stomach has been divided, the peritoneum of the gastroesophageal junction is opened and the crura of the diaphragm are exposed. Careful blunt dissection in this area is necessary to free the esophagus from the adventitia. The surgeon must dissect in a deliberate but slow fashion to avert damage to the pleura. Pleural injury becomes manifest by the loss of pneumoperitoneum and the development of a pneumothorax and/or mediastinal shift.

The stomach will then be retracted laterally toward the patient's left to expose the periaortic fascia. It is crucial to properly identify the structures as the hiatus, including the aorta, the celiac axis, and the celiac plexus. The coronary vessels (i.e., arterial and venous supplies to the diaphragm) should be identified, and care must be taken to prevent their avulsion during the dissection. The risk of injury to these vessels is lessened by confining the dissection to the midline. Bleeding in this area can be extremely difficult to control.

The gastric segment is now prepared for displacement into the thorax. Division of the diaphragm is necessary to complete this portion of the procedure. The phrenic nerve and vessels must be identified and preserved. The relationship of the spleen, liver, and adjacent organs to the diaphragm should also be appreciated. The incision in the diaphragm should only be large enough to allow the gastric tube to be pulled easily into the thoracic cavity. An excessively large incision must be closed carefully. Several techniques for closure of the diaphragm have been described, including various suture closures as well as techniques which employ endoscopic hernia staplers and/or hemoclips.

Köcherization of the duodenum and pyloroplasty should be performed, particularly if a large segment of esophagus is to be resected and since resection of or injury to the vagus nerves is likely. These maneuvers are more easily accomplished prior to division of the stomach, as retraction and countertraction will be enhanced. Some authors have described the use of a pyloromyotomy rather than formal pyloroplasty. Both electrosurgical and laser techniques for the seromyotomy have been used successfully. A stapled pyloroplasty can be accomplished using multiple firings of the endo-GIA or a similar device.

Once the proximal stomach has been pushed into the thoracic cavity, the thoracoscopic surgeon transects the esophagus. The specimen can be removed through the cervical invision or a minithoracotomy, depending on the level at which the esophagus is transected. The distal stomach is then brought through the diaphragmatic window by gently pushing it cephalad with a Babcock clamp by the abdominal team.

Esophagogastric anastomosis may be performed in several ways. A side-to-side esophagogastrostomy can be fashioned using the endo-GIA device. A small enterotomy is made in the stomach and the adjacent esophagus. The instrument is placed into these openings, and the instrument is then closed and fired. The remaining opening is then closed by using the endo-GIA. The edges of the anastomosis are carefully grasped and approximated with Babcock or Allis clamps as the jaws of the stapler are closed and fired. Multiple firings may be necessary to ensure a complete closure of the anastomosis. A circular stapled anastomosis can be fashioned in cases where a lower esophageal anastomosis is necessary. Placement of the instrument is facilitated by placing the curved handle through a gastrotomy or the pyloroplasty site while the detachable head is inserted into the esophagus. This may be accomplished by opening the transected esophagus and using an endoloop as a "purse string". The gastrotomy is closed using the endo-GIA or via a hand-sewn technique. A hand-sewn thoracoscopic esophagogastrostomy is possible. However, this requires a high degree of skill. A conventional hand-sewn anastomosis can be accomplished via a thoracotomy.

The stomach is anchored to the diaphragm by the placement of interrupted silk sutures. The diaphragm is then closed with either interrupted sutures or by using endoscopic hernia staples to reapproximate the tissue.

A chest tube is placed in one of the lower thoracoscopic access sites and is tethered to the skin with 2-0 silk suture.

Meticulous attention to detail is the ideal way to prevent complications. The surgeon should proceed carefully and cautiously with the dissection and should not hesitate to convert the operation to an open procedure if any difficulties arise.

REFERENCES

1. Anbari MM, Levine MS, Cohen RB, et al: Delayed leaks and fistulas after esophagogastrectomy: Radiologic evaluation. *Am J Roentgenol* 160(6):1217–1220, 1993.
2. Buess G, Lirici MM: Perivisceral dissection of the esophagus. In Hunter JG, Sackier JM (eds): *Minimally Invasive Surgery*. New York, McGraw-Hill, 1993, pp 83–87.
3. Cadiére GB, Hinpens J, Bruyns J: How to avoid esophageal perforation while performing laparoscopic dissection of the hiatus. *Surg Endosc* 9:450–452, 1995.
4. Congreve, DP: Laparoscopic paraesophageal hernia repair. *J Laparoendosc Surg* 2(1):45–48, 1992.
5. DePaula AL, Hashiba K, Ferreira EAB, et al: Laparoscopic transhiatal esophagectomy with esophagogastroplasty. *Surg Laparosc Endosc* 5:1–5, 1995.
6. Deshmane VH, Sharma S, Shinde SR, et al: Functional results following esophagogastrectomy for carcinoma of the esophagus. *J Surg Oncol* 50(3):153–155, 1992.
7. Leahy PF, Pennino RP, Hinshaw JR, et al: Minimally invasive esophagogastrectomy: An approach to esophagogastrectomy through the left thorax. *J Laparoendosc Surg* 1:59–62, 1990.
8. Leahy PF: Esophagogastrectomy. In Ballantyne GH, Leahy PF, Modlin IM (eds): *Laparoscopic Surgery*. Philadelphia, Saunders, 1994, pp 397–399.
9. Leahy PF: *Complications of Laparoscopic Surgery*. St Louis: Quality Medical, 1995, pp 401–407.
10. Matory YL, Burt M: Esophagogastrectomy: Reoperation for complications. *J Surg Oncol* 54(1):29–33, 1993.
11. McKernan JB, Wolfe BM, MacFadyen BV Jr: Laparoscopic repair of duodenal ulcer and gastroesophageal reflux. *Surg Clin North Am* 72(5):1153–1167, 1992.
12. Moreira LF, Kamikawa Y, Naomoto Y, et al: Endoscopic mucusal resection for superficial carcinoma and high-grade dysplasia of the esophagus. *Surg Laparosc Endosc* 5:171–175, 1995.
13. Ohashi S: Laparoscopic intraluminal (intragastric) surgery for early gastric cancer: A new concept in laparoscopic surgery. *Surg Endosc* 9:169–171, 1995.
14. Pellegrini C, Wetter LA, Patti M, et al: Thorascopic esophagomyotomy. Initial experience with a new approach for the treatment of achalasia. *Ann Surg* 216(3): 291–299, 1992.
15. Peters JH, Hoeft SF, Heimbucher J, et al: Selection of patients for curative or palliative resection of esophageal cancer based on preoperative endoscopic ultrasonography. *Arch Surg* 129(5):534–539, 1994.
16. Shimi S, Nathanson LK, Cuschieri A: Laparoscopic cardiomyotomy for achalasia. *J R Coll Surg Edinb* 36(3): 152–154, 1991.
17. Slattery P, Hinder R, Gengler J, et al: Thoracoscopically assisted esophagectomy with gastric pull-up for esophageal cancer. *Surg Laparosc Endosc* 4:448–451, 1994.
18. Streitz JM Jr: Comparison of transhiatal and transthoracic esophagogastrectomy. *Semin Thorac Cardiovasc Surg* 4(4):300–306, 1992.
19. Zucker KA, Bailey RW, Reddick EJ (eds): *Surgical Laparoscopy Update*. St Louis: Quality Medical, 1993, pp 445–455.

chapter twenty-seven

Mediastinal and Pericardial Surgery Via Thoracoscopy

Robert McManus

INTRODUCTION

In 1910 Christian Jacobaeus first described the appearance of the lungs, pericardium, and mediastinum in two patients with exudative pleuritis as seen through a cystoscope placed through a trocar into the pleural space.[1] Jacobaeus recommended the procedure for its value in differentiating between tumor metastases and tuberculous changes. By 1925 he had initiated the era of thoracoscopic therapeutics by dividing pleural adhesions which prevented the accomplishment of a complete pneumothorax for the treatment of active cavitary tuberculosis. Effective drug therapy for tuberculosis and refinement of open thoracotomy led to virtual abandonment of thorasocopy by 1945 except for an occasional pleural biopsy.[2]

GENERAL COMPLICATIONS OF THORACOSCOPY

Bleeding, air embolism, subcutaneous emphysema, wound infections, empyema, spread of malignancy, arrhythmia, respiratory failure, persistent pneumothorax, and hypotension have been reported as complications of thoracoscopy. Braimbridge[2] enumerated "the five unacceptable disasters of thoracoscopy":

1. Performing the procedure on the wrong side.
2. Kebab lung syndrome (occurs when a trocar is inadvertently introduced into the pulmonary parenchyma).
3. Clotted hemothorax (occurs when the liver presenting through a diaphragmatic hernia is mistaken for a clotted hemothorax).
4. Artificial lunchothorax (occurs when the distended stomach in a paraesophageal hernia is mistaken for a hydropneumothorax).
5. Aortopleurocutaneous fistula (occurs when a mediastinal shift is not taken into account when an infected pneumonectomy space is drained).

Braimbridge recommended careful review of a recent chest x-ray and use of a blunt needle for entering the pleura.

Within the past decade, advances in endoscopic cameras and equipment have led to the rebirth of thoracoscopy as a diagnostic and therapeutic modality. Initial reports describe the wide range of applications for the new technology.[3–11] Small pulmonary lesions can be excised thoracoscopically in older patients with impaired cardiopulmonary reserve, with acceptable morbidity and mortality.[3] In an effort to reduce the major complications of hemorrhage and prolonged air leak, the neodymium: yttrium aluminum garnet (Nd:YAG) laser can be used in conjunction with video-assisted techniques to perform thoracoscopic lung biopsy. Air leak is the most frequent complication, followed by pneumonia[1] (Table 27.1). Persistent bleeding from an intercostal artery at the site of trocar insertion, requiring immediate reexploration in the immediate postoperative period, has been identified as a potentially avoidable complication of any thoracoscopic procedure. Initial entry into the pleural space should be made carefully above the rib, and all trocar insertion

Table 27.1. Complications in 16 Patients After Nd:YAG Laser Pulmonary Resection

Prolonged air leak (exceeding 7 days)	8
Pneumonia	4
Empyema	1
Pleural space problems	2
Bleeding	11

sites should be inspected for bleeding during the procedure. Fifty percent of patients have persistent air leaks (lasting longer than 7 days) after Nd:YAG laser pulmonary resections. A more liberal use of endostaplers to achieve aerostasis might reduce the incidence of this complication. "Down-lung" pneumonia can be attributed to the use of double-lumen tubes and the use of the lateral decubitus position. Its incidence might be reduced with more frequent endobronchial suctioning and intermittent reexpansion of the atelectatic lung. A documented local recurrence of carcinoma 18 months following laser wedge resection of a primary bronchogenic carcinoma underscores the need to confine wedge resections to patients with truly inadequate cardiopulmonary reserve.

Video-assisted thoracoscopy has been employed to create pericardial windows, as well as for bronchogenic cystectomy, aortopulmonary lymph node sampling, decortication, pleural scleroses, bullous ablations, explorations of the thorax, esophageal cystectomy, pleurectomy, excision of neurogenic tumor, and mediastinal exploration.[5]

Reexpansion pulmonary edema can occur with rapid drainage of a massive malignant pleural effusion in a patient with a double-lumen tube and a deflated lung. Gradual drainage with a chest tube prior to thoracoscopy for malignant pleural effusions might eliminate this complication.

Dense pleural adhesions and physiologic inability to tolerate one-lung anesthesia, as determined by unacceptable low oxygen saturations, are contraindications to thoracoscopy.[5] Lewis et al. cautioned that thoracoscopic procedures are more tedious and time-consuming than open procedures. They also reported that the approach to the pericardium is technically easier from the right side.[5]

Reports from Europe describe a variety of thoracoscopic procedures, with 15% requiring conversion to thoracotomy.[6,7] This percentage might be reduced with better patient selection.

Treatment of pneumothorax is greatly improved with the use of endostaplers for bleb resection.

Thoracoscopy has proven useful in the debilitated, immunocompromised patient.[8] Diminished lung compliance, high-pressure ventilation requirements, and diminished pulmonary reserve often do not allow single-lung ventilation in such patients. Open lung biopsy is still occasionally required.

Diagnostic thoracoscopy has been used in trauma patients to evaluate persistent bleeding, to confirm or negate the suspected diagnosis of diaphragmatic hernia, and to evaluate and localize tracheal or esophageal injuries.[9] Thoracoscopic evaluation in traumatic situations is limited by the overall instability of the injured patient and the presence of obscuring hematoma, and should not supplant careful endoscopic evaluation of the hollow viscera. Bleeding intercostal or internal mammary vessels can be controlled thoracoscopically, and a bleeding lung can occasionally be stapled. A clotted hemothorax can be fully evacuated thoracoscopically early after trauma before a fibrous peel prevents full expansion of the underlying lung and requires decortication.

Malignant pleural effusions can be managed with thoracoscopic drainage and talc insufflation with almost 100% success.[10,11] Dry talc may be a more effective sclerosant than other agents, and video imaging allows more even distribution. Pyogen testing must be rigorous to avoid inadvertent contamination. Underlying lung constriction by tumor can be recognized at thoracoscopy, giving better prognostic information on the likelihood of success with sclerosant therapy for malignant pleural effusions. No long-term construction has been identified in animals with a limited talc concentration, but there is no study in humans to prove that there is no long-term risk in the use of talc in younger patients with spontaneous pneumothorax.[11]

Careful preoperative planning, recognizing the dangers and limitations of single-lung ventilation, limitations in instrumentation, lack of tactile discrimination, loss of three-dimensional vision, and the risks of inadequate vascular control, can reduce the risks of major complications. Certain anatomic considerations limit the effectiveness of a thoracoscopic approach in general[12] (Table 27.2). Hilar pulmonary lesions can be difficult to visualize and are close to major vascular structures. The upper mediastinum and posterior paravertebral areas can be difficult to visualize using standard thoracoscopy ports. Small women and children may not have the thoracic capacity to allow introduction of thoracoscopic instruments. Lungs in patients

Table 27.2. Complicating Anatomic Features

Hilar pulmonary lesions
Pulmonary parenchymal lesions abutting the upper mediastinum or posterior paravertebral area
Small thoracic cavities
Severe emphysema
Ventilator dependency
Noncompliant lung
Small, deep parenchymal lesions identified by CT scan of the chest
Dense pleural symphysis

with severe emphysema may not deflate readily with a double-lumen endotracheal tube. Patients with low oxygen saturation dependent on a ventilator may not tolerate single-lung ventilation, and noncompliant lungs may remain expanded. Small, deep parenchymal lesions may be difficult to locate during thoracoscopy, requiring preoperative needle placement. Pleural adhesions can obscure landmarks and lead to inadvertent entry into visceral or vascular structures.

Numerous cautions have been expressed about the potential drawbacks of thoracoscopy, including overapplication of the modality when simpler procedures exist and misapplication in oncologic disease.[13,14] Length of the hospital stay in patients who undergo diagnostic or therapeutic pulmonary procedures is more dependent on the persistence of air leaks than on the length of the incision. Patients who can tolerate lobectomy or other procedures with a proven record of cure should not be subjected to lesser wedge resections for the sake of a smaller incision. The potential for uncontrolled bleeding or inadvertent, undetected organ injury demands constant vigilance.

Although thoracoscopic procedures lead to less postoperative pain, there may be a slightly increased incidence of minor complications, such as air leak or superficial wound infection, compared with what is seen after analogous open cases.[14]

THORACOSCOPIC SURGERY OF THE ANTERIOR MEDIASTINUM

Mediastinal Lymph Node Staging

Mediastinal lymph node sampling is directed at abnormally enlarged lymph nodes identified by chest x-ray, computed tomography (CT), or magnetic resonance imaging (MRI) in patients with known or suspected malignancy. Histologic examination of mediastinal lymph nodes, documenting the presence or absence of metastatic disease, determines the stage of the disease and offers important prognostic information. Rational therapeutic modalities can be designed based on such information.

Suprasternal mediastinoscopy has been extensively used for more than 35 years to stage lung cancer.[15] Although it is a very safe procedure, 2.1% of patients suffer a complication and 0.3% require emergency thoracotomy[16] (Table 27.3). The major complications of hemorrhage, tracheal injury, esophageal injury, and recurrent laryngeal nerve injury occur from inadvertent application of the bioptome to the pulmonary artery, azygous vein, or hollow viscus or nerve or from traction injury when an adherent lymph node leads to an avulsion injury.

Complete knowledge of the anatomic relationships of mediastinal structures is the key to avoiding complications. Meticulous dissection of the lymph nodes prior to biopsy will avoid most injuries. When doubt exists about the identity of a structure, particularly with very large lymph nodes, a small needle can be used for exploration. Excessive traction should be avoided, and a bloodless field should be maintained.

Table 27.3. Morbidity and Mortality Associated With 2259 Mediastinoscopies for Staging of Bronchogenic Carcinoma

Mortality	0
Morbidity	
Major Complications	
Hemorrhage	3
Tracheal injury	2
Esophageal injury	2
Total	7 (0.3%)
Minor Complications	
Pneumothorax	14
Wound infection	5
Recurrent nerve injury	7
Other	13
Total	39 (1.73%)
Total (all complications)	46 (2.04%)

Management of massive hemorrhage includes (1) immediate packing and pressure until blood is available for transfusion, (2) packing removal and use of topical hemostasis aids, and (3) thoracotomy if these measures fail. Median sternotomy may be preferable with innominate artery injuries. Airway injuries can usually be managed with a red rubber catheter left at the site of airway entry until the air leak stops.

Video-assisted thoracoscopy is useful in staging patients with primary lung cancer following CT scanning, bronchoscopy, and mediastinoscopy.[17] Pleural metastases not identified on CT scan can be visualized thoracoscopically, precluding a curative exploratory thoracotomy. Thoracoscopy can also identify visceral pleural invasion. Anatomic limitations of thoracoscopy preclude access to 50% of N-1 lymph nodes.[17]

Esophageal cancer carries such a poor prognosis that most esophagectomies are performed for palliation. Adjunctive chemotherapy and radiotherapy are frequently employed. Protocols using preoperative adjunctive therapy depend on accurate staging to gauge the effectiveness of the therapy. Krasha reported on 14 patients with biopsy-proven cancer of the thoracic esophagus who underwent left thoracoscopic mediastinal lymph node biopsies for staging prior to resection.[18] In two patients with enlarged lymph nodes and suspected locally metastatic disease, no cancer was seen on histologic examination of the lymph nodes. Two patients were found to have previously unrecognized pulmonary metastases on staging thoracoscopy.

No morbidity or mortality was noted in 49 patients who underwent thoracoscopic staging for lung cancer. One patient out of 14 who underwent thoracoscopic staging for esophageal cancer developed a methicillin-resistant *Staphylococcus aureus* pulmonary infection postoperatively.[17,18]

Thoracoscopic lymph node sampling has been found to be useful for examining nodes inaccessible by cervical mediastinoscopy. Aortopulmonary, anterior mediastinal, periazygous, and subcarinal lymph nodes are inaccessible by mediastinoscopy. Landreneau et al. described 40 patients who underwent thoracoscopic lymph node sampling as an adjunct to cervical mediastinoscopy in the staging of bronchogenic carcinoma.[19] The sensitivity and specificity were 100%, and the authors recommend the procedure over the limited visibility available through parasternal mediastinotomy (Chamberlain procedure). Morbidity was minimal. No patient had postoperative bronchopleural fistual or significant bleeding, but one patient had a chylous fistual which sealed spontaneously after 4 days of chest tube drainage. Liberal use of endoscopic clips to control the lymphatics during lymphadenectomy is recommended, as well as constant awareness of the vagus and phrenic nerves, the pulmonary artery, and the aorta.

Rendina et al. compared thoracoscopy, mediastinoscopy, and mediastinotomy for mediastinal biopsy in 51 patients with an unknown mediastinal mass.[20] Three out of 26 mediastinoscopy procedures failed to yield a diagnosis, which was subsequently obtained by thoracoscopy. Three patients suffered complications. One patient with non-Hodgkin's lymphoma compressing the airway developed airway collapse following single-lumen intubation for a parasternal mediastinotomy. A second patient required open thoracotomy for control of bleeding after thoracoscopic biopsy of hilar lymphadenopathy. The third patient developed a wound infection after mediastinotomy. Subjective comparison suggests less postoperative pain with mediastinoscopy compared to the other procedures, but thoracoscopy has a superior diagnostic yield, allows better operative exposure, and reduces the hospital stay compared to mediastinotomy. Mediastinoscopy requires simpler airway management and is still the procedure of choice for biopsy of anterior peritracheal lymph nodes.

Mediastinal masses

Lymphoma is a common mediastinal mass which requires a tissue diagnosis but is best treated with nonexcisional therapy. Traditional surgical approaches for biopsy include thoracotomy, mediastinotomy, and partial and complete median sternotomy.[21] With satisfactory nonoperative therapy available, the sole justification for an operation is to obtain diagnostic tissue. Preferential consideration of thoracoscopy is indicated.

Kern et al. reported on thoracoscopic biopsy of suspected mediastinal malignancies in 22 patients.[22] Accurate tissue diagnosis was obtained in 86%. Only one patient required thoracotomy to confirm suspected histoplasmosis. No procedure-related complications were reported, but the procedure could not be performed on an 11-month-old baby because of inability to perform single-lung ventilation.

Mediastinal cysts

The cystic nature of a mediastinal mass can readily be identified by CT scan. Mediastinal cysts should be excised when symptomatic or when a suspicion of malignancy exists. Multiple reports have demonstrated the feasibility of resection of enteric or bronchogenic cysts thoracoscopically.[23–25] Few complications occurred, but occasionally cyst walls were left behind when they were adjacent to vital structures. Argon beam coagulation has been recommended to ablate any residual mucosa. No recurrences were reported after short (6-month) follow-up periods. Early aspiration for large cysts allow easier resection and manipulation, but surgical judgment is required when complete excision risks major hemorrhage.

Thymic masses

Thoracoscopic thymectomy has been performed for new-onset myasthenia gravis and for resection of encapsulated thymoma.[26,27] Maximal thymectomy via median sternotomy and anterior mediastinal exenteration has been recommended as the most reliable treatment for generalized myasthenia gravis. Less radical procedures risk leaving microscopic foci of thymus in pericapsular mediastinal fat, leading to incomplete disease remission.[28] Although thoracoscopic thymectomy for new-onset myasthenia gravis can be technically performed if the CT scan does not demonstrate thymic hyperplasia or thymoma, there is no evidence that this less radical approach is an efficacious as maximal thymectomy.[26]

Recurrent thymoma occurring 2 months to 18 years following thymectomy has led to the recommendation that "thymectomy alone (enucleation) or incomplete thymectomy should be abandoned in favor of 'complete' thymectomy. Wide operative exposure is necessary." Kirschner recommended "complete sternal splitting with opening of both pleural cavities in all patients with thymoma to accomplish as complete a thymectomy as possible."[29] Thoracoscopic resection of a stage 1 (encapsulated) thymoma can be performed as long as no intrathoracic metastases or local invasion are seen.[27] Because of the good prognosis with excision and the good results with reoperation for recurrence, thoracoscopic excision for stage 1 thymoma can be justified, but the risks of inadequate excision are significant.

Thoracoscopic Surgery of the Posterior Mediastinum

Posterior mediastinal masses derive from nerve tissue, lymphatic tissue, trachea or esophagus, and pleura, or the spine itself[30] (Table 27.4). Thoracoscopy can be used for diagnosis or treatment of the various conditions listed in Table 27.4. The age of the patient is an important consideration in the preoperative differential diagnosis. According to Naunheim, "3% of posterior mediastinal neurogenic tumors are found to be malignant in the adult; 60% of those diagnosed in children under the age of 16 years are found to be cancerous."[30] A thoracoscopic approach to a suspected neurogenic tumor may be more justifiable in an adult. An additional consideration with neurogenic tumors is the propensity for extension into the intradural space. Such extension should be discernible preoperatively with CT scan or high-resolution MRI and represent a contraindication to attempted thoracoscopic resection. Endoscopic bags should be used during resection of unknown mediastinal masses to avoid the spread of malignancy to the trocar site.

Table 27.4. Lesions Diagnosed or Treated by Thoracoscopy

Neurogenic tumor	Lymphoma
Nerve sheath	Pleural tumor
Autonomic ganglia	Bronchogenic
Paraganglionic	Esophageal anomalies
Neuroectodermic stem cell	Diverticulum
Anterior meningomyelocele	Duplication cyst
Paravertebral abscess	Leiomyoma

Esophageal Surgery

Thoracoscopic approaches have been used successfully for distal esophageal cardiomyotomy in achalasia and for enucleation of esophageal leiomyomas.[31,32] Pellegrini et al. reported on 22 patients with achalasia who underwent successful thoracoscopic myotomy. Two patients required a thoracotomy to repair a mucosal laceration, but a third patient underwent thoracoscopic repair of the laceration. Incomplete myotomy in three patients necessitated subsequent myotomy when the esophagogastric junction was not clearly seen. Performance of concomitant flexible esophagoscopy allows accurate verification that the myotomy is complete and provides visualization of mucosal defects, which is important for accurate thoracoscopic repair. The most vulnerable area of the mucosa is at the cardio esophageal junction. The hook cautery should be avoided in favor of bipolar scissors.[31] Sharp endoscopic forceps should not be used on the external surface of the denuded mucosal layer. Blunt grasping instruments should be applied only to the muscular layer.

Concomitant video esophagoscopy has also been found to be a valuable adjunct to thoracoscopic enucleation of esophageal leiomyomas. Mucosal injury can be more easily avoided and repaired. Traction sutures placed through the leiomyoma facilitate dissection.[32] Endoscopic insufflation and illumination can make difficult dissection easier to accomplish. The right side is the best approach for an uncomplicated leiomyoma. After enucleation, the split esophageal muscle should be reapproximated to prevent mucusal bulging.

EXPOSURE OF THE THORACIC SPINE

Surgical access to the anterior thoracic spine is necessary for drainage of spinal abscess, vertebral body biopsy in cases of suspected malignancy, discectomy for herniated nucleus pulposus, stabilization for destructive lesions, and anterior release for kyphoscoliosis. Traditionally, postero-lateral thoracotomy has been required for exposure. Improved thoracoscopic instrumentation allows these procedures to be performed using a minimally invasive approach.[33] Mack et al. describe a thoracoscopic approach for exposure of the thoracic spine in 10 patients (Table 27.5). The optimal position of thoracoscopic ports depends on the anatomic level of the spinal pathology. A 30 degree angled scope "provides enhanced visualization into the disc space without crowding the surgical instrumentation."[33]

Exact localization of the appropriate vertebral body or disc space must be ascertained by counting ribs, but an exploratory needle can be placed preoperatively or intraoperatively for radiographic confirmation of the level prior to dissection. A right-sided approach to the vertebral body may require careful thoracoscopic division of a large azygous vein, and the left-sided approach to the upper thoracic vertebrae will be obscured by the aortic arch. The exact relationship of the esophagus must be known, as it is sometimes necessary to dissect well above and below the level of spinal pathology to provide adequate, safe exposure. Left-sided exposure requires intimate knowledge of the anatomy of the descending aorta and its vertebral branches. Inflammatory conditions may obscure the location of vertebral vessels. An open approach may be safer in such circumstances. Longer operating times may result in more postoperative pneumonia in the deflated lung, but a reduced postoperative hospital stay and decreased pain requiring narcotics are clear advantages of the thoracoscopic approach to surgically correctable thoracic spinal pathology.

Table 27.5. Thorascopic Spinal Procedures

Procedure	Number
Anterior release (discectomy) with fusion for correction of kyphosis/scoliosis plus thoracoplasty (one case)	3
Discectomy for herniated nucleus pulposus	3
Biopsy/debride collapsed vertebral body/discectomy	1
Drain disc space abscess	1
Biopsy collapsed vertebral body	1
Fusion of disc space	1
Total	10

THORACOSCOPY FOR PERICARDIAL DISEASE

Benign or malignant pericardial effusions, pericardial cysts, and congenital constrictive pericardial defects can be treated thoracoscopically.[34,35] Pericardiectomy can be relatively easily performed or a pericardial window created thoracoscopically. Hazelrigg et al. reported on a series of 35 patients with purely effusive disorders of the pericardium unresponsive to medical therapy or pericardiocentesis who underwent thoracoscopic pericardiectomy.[34] Patients with advanced malignancy, generalized poor health, and a limited expected life span can undergo an alternative drainage procedure via a subxyphoid approach. This requires a single incision and can be performed in patients with tamponade who cannot tolerate single-lung anesthesia. More than 90% of patients with symptomatic pericardial effusions can obtain relief with the simpler approach.

Long-term relief of effusion depends on the creation of an inflammatory fusion of epicardium to pericardium by prolonged tube drainage (3 to 5 days).[36] Recurrent pericardial effusions and concerns about the eventual evolution of a constrictive process has led some authors to abandon the pericardial window in favor of total pericardiectomy.[37] Inflammatory pericardial conditions and venous engorgement from tamponade can lead to significant bleeding. The location of the phrenic nerve must be known at all times to avoid a subsequent paralytic diaphragm from electrocautery injury, and extreme care must be exercised to avoid inducing ventricular or atrial arrhythmias during pericardiectomy. An external defibrillator with patches in place or sterile paddles should always be available during thoracoscopic pericardiectomy. The presence of adhesions to the heart or the development of constrictive pericarditis, with its thin, restrictive epicardial component, dictates conversion to an open approach. Trocar placement should be more posterior and superior to avoid encroachment by an enlarged pericardium. Resection anterior to the phrenic nerve should be performed in all cases. Resection posterior to the phrenic nerve should be reserved for patients with posterior loculations.[34]

Pericardiocentesis under local anesthesia should precede the induction of general anesthesia in cases where preoperative echocardiography demonstrates early diastolic collapse of the right atrium or ventricle. Thoracoscopic pericardiectomy for symptomatic pericardial effusive disease may provide more complete, long-lasting relief than simple subxyphoid drainage, but it requires more complex anesthetic management and may be most useful in patients with combined pericardial and pleural effusions or in those with concomitant parenchymal or mediastinal lesions that require a tissue diagnosis. Thoracoscopic pericardiectomy and talc pleurodesis can be an effective treatment for combined pericardial and pleural effusive disease.

THORACOSCOPY FOR CHYLOTHORAX

Thoracoscopy has been used for localization and surgical control of chylothorax following open thoracic procedures.[38–40] Conservative management with chest tube drainage and elimination of dietary fat will resolve most postoperative chyle leaks nonoperatively, but 20% of such complications will require surgical intervention.[38] Administration of heavy cream into the gastrointestinal tract at the time of thoracoscopy can help to pinpoint the site of the chylous leak, allowing direct control using clips or sutures. Fibrin glue application to the exact site of leakage is an important adjunct. As little as 2–3 mL of fibrin glue can control leaks of 400–700 cc/day.[39,40]

THORACOSCOPIC CARDIOVASCULAR PROCEDURES

Few cardiovascular procedures have been clinically performed using a thoracoscopic approach. Thoracoscopic closure of a patient ductus arteriosus (PDA) using titanium clips has been reported.[41,42] Incomplete closure can be avoided with the use of two clips instead of one. Complete dissection of the PDA and surrounding tissues must be done to avoid damage to the recurrent laryngeal nerve. The use of a small chest tube for a few hours postoperatively helps to avoid pneumothorax. Ductal tissue is known to be friable, and potentially disastrous hemorrhage can result from faulty clip application. Since the duct is not divided, the possibility of persistent PDA will be present with the use of clips. Because of difficulties in maintaining a sufficient pneumothorax, some authors have cautioned against the use of thoracoscopy in children weighing less than 8 kg.[43]

REFERENCES

1. Thomas PA: A thoracoscopic peek: What did Jacobaeus see? *Ann Thorac Surg* 57:770–771, 1994.
2. Braimbridge MV: The history of thoracoscopic surgery. *Ann Thorac Surg* 56:610–614, 1993.
3. Landreneau RJ, Hazelrigg SR, Ferson PF, et al: Thoracoscopic resection of 85 pulmonary lesions. *Ann Thorac Surg* 54:415–420, 1992.
4. Landreneau RJ, Keenan RJ, Hazelrigg SR, et al: VATS wedge resection of the lung using the Neodymum:Yttrium-Aluminum Garnet laser. *Ann Thorac Surg* 56:758–761, 1993.
5. Lewis RJ, Caccavale RJ, Sisler GE, et al: One hundred consecutive patients undergoing video-assisted thoracic operations. *Ann Thorac Surg* 54:421–426, 1992.
6. Coosemans W, Lerut TE, Van Raemdonck DM: Thoracoscopic surgery: The Belgian experience. *Ann Thorac Surg* 56:721–730, 1993.
7. Mulder DS: Thoracoscopy in Europe: Views from North America. *Ann Thorac Surg* 56:731–733, 1993.
8. Feins RH: The role of thoracoscopy in the AIDS/immunocompromised patient. *Ann Thorac Surg* 56:649–650, 1993.
9. Graeber GM, Jones DR. The role of thoracoscopy in thoracic trauma. *Ann Thorac Surg* 56:646–648, 1993.
10. LoCicero J III: Thoracoscopic management of malignant pleural effusion. *Ann Thorac Surg* 56:641–643, 1993.
11. Daniel TM: Diagnostic thoracoscopy for pleural disease. *Ann Thorac Surg* 56:639–640, 1993.
12. Landreneau RJ, Mack MJ, Keenan RJ et al: Strategic planning for video-assisted thoracic surgery. *Ann Thorac Surg* 56:615–619, 1993.
13. Ginsberg RJ: Thoracoscopy: A cautionary note. *Ann Thorac Surg* 56:801–803, 1993.

14. Kaiser LR, Bavaria JE: Complications of thoracoscopy. *Ann Thorac Surg* 56:796–798, 1993.
15. Carlens E: Mediastinoscopy: A method for inspection and tissue biopsy in the superior mediastinum. *Dis Chest* 36:343, 1959.
16. Waldhausen JA, Orringer MB: *Complications in Cardiothoracic Surgery*. St Louis, Mosby-Year Book, 1991, p 325.
17. Wain JC: Video-assisted thoracoscopy and the staging of lung cancer. *Ann Thorac Surg* 56:776–778, 1993.
18. Krasna MJ: Thoracoscopic lymph node staging for esophageal cancer. *Ann Thorac Surg* 56:671–674, 1993.
19. Landreneau RJ, Hazelrigg SR, Mack MJ, et al: Thoracoscopic mediastinal lymph node sampling: Useful for mediastinal lymph node stations inaccessible by cervical mediastinoscopy. *J Thorac Cardiovasc Surg* 106:554–558, 1993.
20. Rendina EA, Venuta F, DeGiacomo T, et al: Comparative merits of thoracoscopy, mediastinoscopy, and mediastinotomy for mediastinal biopsy. *Ann Thorac Surg* 57:992–995, 1994.
21. Ricci C, Rendina EA, Venuta F, et al: Surgical approach to isolated mediastinal lymphoma. *J Thorac Cardiovasc Surg* 99:691–695, 1990.
22. Kern JA, Daniel TM, Tribble CG, et al: Thoracoscopic diagnosis and treatment of mediastinal masses. *Ann Thorac Surg* 56:92–96, 1993.
23. Lewis RJ, Caccavale RJ, Sisler GE: Imaged thoracoscopic surgery: A new thoracic technique for resection of mediastinal cysts. *Ann Thorac Surg* 53:318–320, 1992.
24. Naunheim KS, Andrus CH: Thoracoscopic drainage and resection of giant mediastinal cyst. *Ann Thorac Surg* 55:156–158, 1993.
25. Hazelrigg SR, Landreneau RJ, Mack MJ, et al: Thoracoscopic resection of mediastinal cysts. *Ann Thorac Surg* 56:659–660, 1993.
26. Sugarbaker DJ: Thoracoscopy in the management of anterior mediastinal masses. *Ann Thorac Surg* 56: 653–656, 1993.
27. Landreneau RJ, Dowling RD, Castillo WM, et al: Thoracoscopic resection of an anterior mediastinal tumor. *Ann Thorac Surg* 54:142–144, 1992.
28. Jaretzki A III, Penn AS, Younger DS, et al: "Maximal" thymectomy for myasthenia gravis. *J Thorac Cardiovasc Surg* 95:747–757, 1988.
29. Kirschner PA: Reoperation for thymoma: Report of 23 cases. *Ann Thorac Surg* 49:550–555, 1990.
30. Naunheim KS: Video thoracoscopy for masses of the posterior mediastinum. *Ann Thorac Surg* 56:657–658, 1993.
31. Pellegrini CA, Leichter R, Patti M, et al: Thoracoscopic esophageal myotomy in the treatment of achalasia. *Ann Thorac Surg* 56:680–682, 1993.
32. Bardini R, Segalin A, Ruol A, et al: Videothoracoscopic enucleation of esophageal leiomyoma. *Ann Thorac Surg* 54:576–577, 1992.
33. Mack MJ, Regan JJ, Bobechko WP, et al: Application of thoracoscopy for diseases of the spine. *Ann Thorac Surg* 56:736–738, 1993.
34. Hazelrigg SR, Mack MJ, Landreneau RJ, et al: Thoracoscopic pericardiectomy for effusive pericardial disease. *Ann Thorac Surg* 56:792–795, 1993.
35. Rischer WH, Rees AP, Ochsner JL, et al: Thoracoscopic resection of pericardium for symptomatic congenital pericardial defect. *Ann Thorac Surg* 56:1390–1391, 1993.
36. Sugimoto JT, Little AG, Ferguson MK, et al: Pericardial window: Mechanisms of efficacy. *Ann Thorac Surg* 50: 442–445, 1990.
37. Miller JI, Mansour KA, Hatcher CR: Jr: Pericardiectomy: Current indications, concepts and results in a university center. *Ann Thorac Surg* 34:40–45, 1982.
38. Ferguson MK: Thoracoscopy for empyema, bronchopleural fistula and chylothorax. *Ann Thorac Surg* 56:644–645, 1993.
39. Shirai T, Amano J, Takabe K: Thoracoscopic diagnosis and treatment of chylothorax after pneumonectomy. *Ann Thorac Surg* 52:306–307, 1991.
40. Inderbitzi RG, Krebs T, Stirnemann P, et al: Treatment of post-operative chylothorax by fibrin glue application under thoracoscopic view with use of local anesthesia. *J Thorac Cardiovasc Surg* 104:201–210, 1992.
41. Laborde F, Noirhomme P, Karam J, et al: A new video-assisted thoracoscopic surgical technique for interruption of patent ductus arteriosus in infants and children. *J Thorac Cardiovasc Surg* 105:278–280, 1993.
42. Alvarez-Tostado RA, Millan MA, Tovar LA, et al: Thoracoscopic clipping and ligation of a patent ductus arteriosus. *Ann Thorac Surg* 57:755–757, 1994.
43. Rodgers BM: Pediatric thoracoscopy: Where have we come and what have we learned? *Ann Thorac Surg* 56:704–707, 1993.

chapter twenty-eight

The Management and Prevention of Complications in Minimally Invasive Surgery of the Pleura

Kenneth L. Franco

The pleural space separates the thoracic wall from the lungs. A small amount of fluid is normally present which acts as a lubricant to facilitate movement of the lung within the thoracic cavity, but changes in the pleural space secondary to fluid accumulation or tumor account for most diseases. Diseases of the pleura provided the first indication for thoracoscopy by the Swedish medical professor Jacobaeus in 1910.[1] Recent advances in instrumentation for thoracoscopy have expanded the indications for this procedure, and now approximately 25% of operations performed are for diseases of the pleura.[2] Recent indications include effusions, undiagnosed masses, mesothelioma, empyemas, hemothorax, and chylothorax. Thoracoscopy can be used to biopsy a mass, drain an effusion or empyema, achieve pleurodesis, ligate a thoracic duct, or explore the thoracic cavity for hemorrhage.

Thoracoscopic procedures are performed in the operating room, which allows the thoracic surgeon to convert immediately to an open thoracotomy if necessary. All procedures are performed under general anesthesia using a double-lumen endotracheal tube or a bronchial blocker. Most thoracic surgeons use a 0° 10-mm rigid operating thoracoscope with a 5-mm biopsy channel and two video monitors, one on each side of the table, to allow an unobstructed view for all operators. Placement of incisions depends on the location of the pathology and the procedure planned. Initial trocar placement is usually in the fifth or sixth intercostal space in the midaxillary line, which provides an unobstructed view of the entire hemithorax.[3] A 10-mm incision is made and the dissection continued through the subcutaneous tissue and intercostal muscle with a hemostat until the pleural cavity is entered. The pleura is entered bluntly and probed with a finger to make sure that the pleural surfaces are not fused and the lungs have dropped away to allow free access for trocar insertions (Fig. 28.1). Disposable plastic or nondisposable metal thoracoports of 10 mm or 12 mm provide excellent access for most instruments, and they are more maneuverable than the usual laparoscopic trocars. After the thoracoscopic lens is warmed and covered with defogging solution, the thoracoscope is introduced through the port and the pleural space is explored. Subsequent incisions are made and additional trocars are placed under direct visualization to ensure that no injury occurs to intrathoracic organs. An attempt should be made to keep trocar incisions in line with the standard thoracotomy incision so that if opening is required, the incisions can be incorporated into one. When the procedure is completed, a chest tube is inserted through one of the trocar sites and all sites are closed with absorbable suture. Major complications of thoracoscopy are uncommon and can be avoided by using proper technique and equipment.

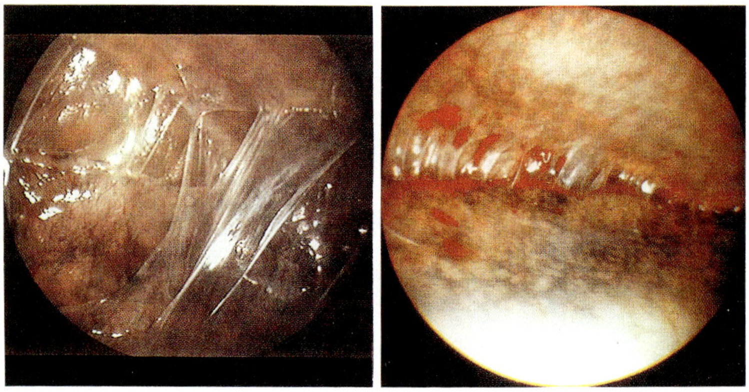

Figure 28.1. Examples of filmy and dense adhesions as seen through a thoracoscope. (From Inderbitzi R: *Surgical Thoracoscopy.* New York, Springer-Verlag, 1994, p 40. Reprinted by permission.)

HEMORRHAGE

Bleeding can occur from an intercostal vessel, injury to the lung, or tearing of vascular adhesions, but transfusion is rarely required.[4] Injury to the intercostal vessels can be prevented by placing the initial trocar incision above the rib, not below the rib where the narrow vascular bundle is located. Should bleeding occur, one should apply pressure to the bleeding artery by pressing on the exterior chest wall with an index finger. This can be done under visual control because the outline of the finger on the parietal pleura can clearly be seen on the video screen. Injury of the lung during placement of trocars occurs mainly in patients with pleural adhesions. This complication can be avoided by initially placing the finger within the pleural space to rule out significant pleural adhesions and then placing the trocar after the lung has dropped away from the chest wall. Once the thoracoscopic camera has been placed into the pleural space, any adhesions should be removed with the use of a coagulating instrument, and they should be resected as close to the chest wall as possible. Bleeding after a pleural biopsy is rare, but if it does occur, it can usually be controlled with electrocautery or laser.

REEXPANSION PULMONARY EDEMA

Pulmonary edema is a possible complication of overly rapid reexpansion of the lung at the end of thoracoscopy. To prevent this complication, the lung should be reexpanded gently. The suction tube may be pinched between the fingers for a few minutes until fluid or blood starts exiting, a sign that the lung has completely reexpanded.

EMPYEMA

The best protection against infection is to maintain aseptic conditions during the thoracoscopic procedure. In addition, prophylactic antibiotics may be helpful. More important, complete reexpansion of the lung against the chest wall will prevent infection after thoracoscopy.

TUMOR SEEDING

Patients with mesothelioma pose a particular problem, with tumor recurrence developing at the site of the thoracoscopic incision. Several reports in the literature state that the incidence is 1.5–4.3%[5] This complication does not appear to occur in cases of metastatic carcinoma to the pleura. In cases of mesothelioma, many advocate prophylactic radiotherapy following thoracoscopy. They recommend administering 2000 rads on the 10th postoperative day to prevent this complication.[6] The incidence of this complication may increase as the indications for thoracoscopy are extended to more debilitated patients.

Thoracoscopy for pleural disease remains a straightforward procedure associated with low morbidity and high benefit. Major complications are uncommon and can be avoided by using proper technique and equipment.

REFERENCES

1. Jacobaeus HC: Possibility of the use of the cystoscope for investigation of serous cavities. *Munch Med Wochenschr* 59:2090–2092, 1910.
2. Miller DL, Allen MS: Set-up and present indications for video-assisted thoracic surgery. *Semin Thorac Cardiovasc Surg* 5:280–283, 1993.
3. Landreneau RJ, Mack MJ, Hazelrigg SR, et al: Video-assisted thoracic surgery—Basic technical concepts and intercostal approach strategies. *Ann Thorac Surg* 54: 800–807, 1992.
4. Cultharp WH, Arnold JH, Alford WC, et al: Videothoracoscopy—Improved technique and expanded indications. *Ann Thorac Surg* 53:776–779, 1992.
5. Macha HN, Reichle G, VonZwehl D, et al: The role of ultrasound assisted thoracoscopy in the diagnosis of pleural disease. *Eur J Cardiol Thorac Surg* 7:19–25, 1993.
6. Law MR, Hodson ME, Turner-Warwick M: Malignant mesothelioma of pleura—clinical aspects and symptomatic treatment. *Eur J Respir Dis* 65:162–168, 1985.

section seven

Special Techniques/ Miscellaneous Procedures

chapter twenty-nine

Diagnostic and Therapeutic Laparoscopy in Trauma

Rao R. Ivatury
Ronald J. Simon

The current approach to abdominal trauma in the hemodynamically stable patient is the judicious use of available investigative techniques to determine the need for operation. This selective management has the objectives of maximizing the value of surgical intervention and minimizing the rate of negative exploration. Serial physical examination is supplemented by peritoneal lavage, ultrasonography, computed tomography (CT), and, in some cases, magnetic resonance imaging (MRI). The recent technical advances in video endoscopy have caused renewed interest in laparoscopy for trauma. This chapter will review the current status of this modality in the evaluation of abdominal trauma.

HISTORICAL ASPECTS

Diagnostic laparoscopy was recommended by Ruddock[1] for general surgeons in 1937. Heselson in 1963 through 1970,[2] Gazzaniga et al. in 1976,[3] and Carnevale and colleagues[4] in 1977 noted that laparoscopy was useful in determining the need for laparotomy. In the 1980s, a series of articles by Berci and coauthors described the advantages of minilaparoscopy in the emergency department in patients with blunt trauma.[5-8] Other reports,[9,10] also using nonvideo endoscopy, supported this enthusiasm for the procedure.

THE ROLE OF DIAGNOSTIC LAPAROSCOPY IN BLUNT TRAUMA

Laparoscopy appears to have a very limited role in the evaluation of blunt trauma. Several reasons account for this fact: the accuracy and reliability of peritoneal lavage and CT scanning, the emergence of ultrasonography as a screening technique in the emergency department, and the recent finding that pneumoperitoneum with CO_2 may have adverse effects on intracranial pressure.[11] Salvino and associates prospectively compared peritoneal lavage and laparoscopy in 59 patients with blunt abdominal trauma and concluded that laparoscopy offered no advantage over lavage as the *primary* diagnostic tool.[12] Others concurred with this conclusion.[13,14]

Laparoscopy may, however, have a role as an adjunct to CT in nonoperative management of blunt abdominal trauma. Townsend and coauthors employed laparoscopy in 15 patients with CT-documented solid organ injuries with the objectives of evaluating the injury, detecting occult lesions, and selecting patients for nonoperative treatment.[15] Laparoscopy demonstrated gross hemoperitoneum in 14 of these patients. All eight hepatic lacerations and seven of the nine splenic lacerations could be inspected. Laparoscopic visualization prompted an "upgrading" of the CT grading of the solid organ injury in eight patients and lowering of the grade in one patient. Of great import, occult bowel injuries (to the sigmoid colon and jejunum) were detected in two patients. We also recommend laparoscopy in stable patients with hemoperitoneum diagnosed by peritoneal lavage or ultrasonography who are taken to the operating room for other reasons. Minor injuries of the liver and spleen may be diagnosed and treated without a laparotomy.

THE ROLE OF DIAGNOSTIC LAPAROSCOPY IN PENETRATING TRAUMA

Laparoscopy appears to offer a greater "scope" for penetrating trauma. It is potentially useful in the evaluation of peritoneal penetration, in the diagnosis of occult diaphragmatic injury, and in avoiding a nontherapeutic laparotomy. Each of these areas will now be discussed in detail.

Laparoscopy in the Evaluation of Peritoneal Penetration

Stab Wounds

A majority of trauma centers perform local wound exploration to confirm peritoneal penetration by stab wounds. This, however, may be difficult in the intercostal spaces and the back in muscular patients who are uncooperative. We have documented the difficulty in evaluating peritoneal penetration in lower chest stab wounds and the efficacy of laparoscopy.[16,17] These patients had absent or equivocal peritoneal signs and, in the majority, the wound was judged to have penetrated the peritoneum on clinical examination. Laparoscopy documented nonpenetration in a one-third of these patients, and they were managed nonoperatively. Fabian and associates, in a series of 99 patients with stab wounds, found nonpenetration in 41 (49%). These authors, based on their protocol for fascial penetration, would have done a negative laparotomy had a laparoscopy not been performed.[14] The importance of this approach is obvious: one-third to one-half of patients with stab wounds will not have peritoneal violation and can be identified with certainty by laparoscopy.

Gunshot Wounds

Most trauma centers recommend mandatory celiotomy for gunshot wounds (GSW) that have penetrated the peritoneal cavity. *The difficulty is to establish peritoneal penetration* in patients with wounds of exit and entry but without diffuse peritoneal signs or hemodynamic instability[18] (Fig. 29.1). While some centers would do a peritoneal lavage and consider a red blood cell count of $>10{,}000/cm^3$ as an indication for a celiotomy,[19] the majority would perform celiotomy in any case.

We have found laparoscopy to be of value in identifying these patients with an extraperitoneal missile trajectory. In our series, 38 patients had questionable penetration of peritoneum by the bullet.[18] Twenty-three (60.5%) of them had no peritoneal penetration on laparoscopy and avoided a laparotomy. Thirteen of the remaining 15 patients had a therapeutic celiotomy. Sosa et al. recently confirmed the value of this

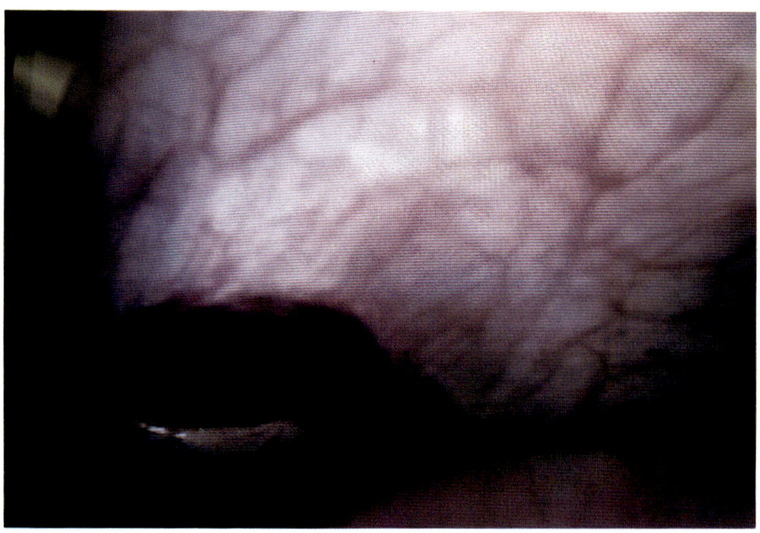

Figure 29.1. Laparoscopic appearance of a diaphragmatic laceration.

approach in 100 patients with GSW to the abdomen and flank.[20] Fabian and colleagues noted negative laparoscopy (no penetration) in 62%.[14] These data and the experience of others confirm the utility of laparoscopy in *selected* patients with abdominal GSW.[21-23]

Laparoscopy may also help avoid an unnecessary celiotomy in thoracoabdominal GSW. Missiles entering the lower chest (below the nipple line) are traditionally considered to have entered the abdomen but may indeed have an extra-abdominal trajectory. In such cases, if the patient is hemodynamically stable, laparoscopy may confirm the true track of the bullet. This was illustrated by two of our patients. In one, the bullet was completely extraperitoneal in its course. The second patient also had an extraperitoneal tract, but had a contusion of the diaphragm and of the adjacent portion of the superior surface of the liver, an example of intra-abdominal injury from an extra-abdominal missile.

The benefits of avoiding a negative laparotomy for nonpenetrating GSW of the abdomen are a reduction in the hospital stay and a reduction in morbidity from a negative celiotomy. We recently compared groups of patients with negative laparotomy (no laparoscopy, negative laparotomy for nonpenetrating GSW) and negative laparoscopy (nonpenetration on laparoscopy, no laparotomy). The negative laparoscopy group had a significantly shorter hospital stay and a lower incidence of complications than the negative laparotomy group.[17,18] A similar benefit from laparoscopy was noted by Sosa and associates.[20]

Laparoscopy in the Evaluation of the Diaphragm

Isolated penetrating diaphragmatic injury is an extremely difficult lesion to detect. The associated hemoperitoneum may be minimal, and the associated physical signs may be completely nonspecific. If the lesion is missed, it may lead to the subsequent development of a diaphragmatic hernia with the potential for significant morbidity and mortality. Currently, there are no data available to estimate the incidence of the complication. The risk factors that lead to herniation are not known. Therefore, we believe that the presence of a penetrating injury to the intrathoracic abdomen, especially on the left, should lead to a search for an occult diaphragmatic injury.

Laparoscopy has proved to be extremely useful in this regard. We have documented diaphragmatic injury in 17 (47.2%) of 36 patients with penetrating thoracoabdominal wounds.[17] A similar incidence (32%) was noted by Fabian et al.[14] in a direct comparison of laparoscopy with diagnostic peritoneal lavage (DPL), Salvino and associates noted that three patients with red blood cell counts <10,000/cm^3 on DPL were found to have injuries to the diaphragm on laparoscopy.[12] These would have been missed if only lavage was performed. These data confirmed the observations of Merlotti and coauthors,[24] as well as those of Madden et al.[25] that diaphragmatic injury may exist with red blood cell counts on DPL ranging from 0 to 8400/cm^3. At this time, none of the available diagnostic modalities are as specific as laparoscopy or thoracoscopy for the detection of diaphragmatic lacerations (Figs. 29.2 and 29.3). In addition, these techniques offer the possibility of endoscopic repair of the diaphragm.

Laparoscopy in Avoiding a Nontherapeutic Laparotomy

There is a significant incidence of nontherapeutic celiotomies with lower chest wounds from minor low-grade lacerations of the liver and spleen that result in a positive DPL but have stopped bleeding. Laparoscopy has a potential application in such patients. The lacerations can be visualized, the extent of bleeding assessed, and hemoperitoneum evacuated. The liver and spleen can be mobilized for a more complete evaluation. In the absence of significant bleeding, these patients may be managed without laparotomy. Successful management of such cases was documented by us,[17] Fabian et al.[14] and Sosa and associates.[20]

The majority of trauma centers consider omental herniation through an anterior abdominal stab wound an indication for celiotomy because of the frequent presence of significant injuries, 85% in one series.[26] In stable patients, laparoscopy may be employed to evaluate the need for a laparotomy. In the operating room, the omentum is excised, the wound is temporarily closed with towel clips, and laparoscopy is performed. Some of these patients may have no other significant injuries and can be managed without laparotomy.

Laparoscopy in Lower Precordial Penetration

Lower precordial wounds have a potential for causing thoracic as well as abdominal injury. Specifically, the incidence of occult cardiac injury is significant in these patients. In our series of 88 stable patients with precordial penetrating wounds,[27] 23% had cardiac injury on the subxiphoid pericardial window. Interestingly,

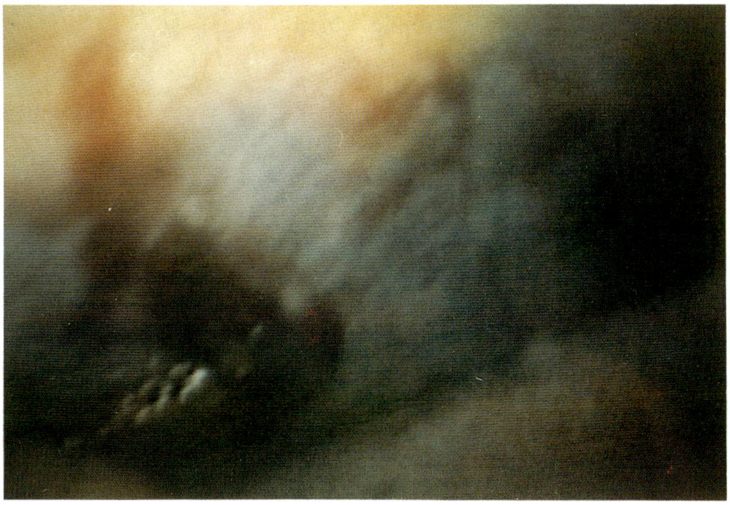

Figure 29.2. Laparoscopic view of GSW of the diaphragm. A large area of contusion and a small full-thickness laceration are evident.

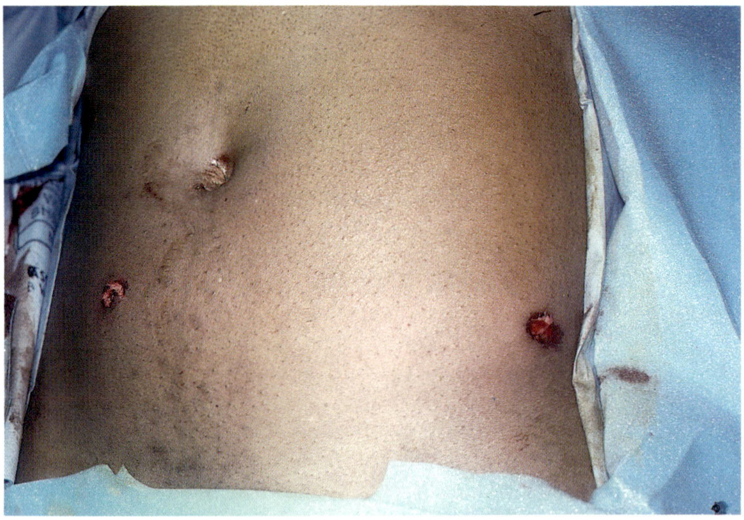

Figure 29.3. GSW of entry and exit in the anterior abdominal wall. Has the bullet penetrated the peritoneum? Laparoscopy is helpful in making this assessment.

none of the clinical criteria (elevated central venous pressure, pulsus paradoxus, etc.) was successful in predicting the presence or absence of cardiac injury. We inspected the pericardium laparoscopically in 9 of the 88 patients. The pericardial area was seen to be sharp and nondistended in seven. All of these patients had a negative subxiphoid window. In two patients it appeared to be dull and opaque, leading to a suspicion of pericardial blood. Both of these patients did have hemopericardium from an occult cardiac injury on subsequent subxiphoid window. The obvious advantage of this approach is that the thoracic as well as abdominal cavities may be evaluated for significant injury. We caution that these are preliminary observations that need to be verified by greater experience.

Results of Laparoscopy According to the Site of Penetration

Laparoscopy, as discussed above, is most important in the region of the intrathoracic abdomen, bounded by the costal margins and the tips of the scapulae. In the areas of the epigastrium and flanks, however, laparoscopy had a sensitivity of only 43% compared to

Table 29.1. Laparoscopy: Applications in Trauma

Diagnostic	Therapeutic
Thoracoabdominal wounds	Thoracoabdominal wounds
Diaphragmatic injury*	Minor liver and spleen lacerations*
Liver, spleen injuries*	
Nonpenetrating wounds*	
Anterior wounds†	Diaphragmatic repair†
Precordial wounds†	Autotransfusion†
Isolated gastric wounds†	Isolated bowel perforations†
Back and flank wounds‡	Bowel perforations‡
Multiple bowel perforations‡	Retroperitoneal injuries‡

* Definitely helpful.
† Potentially helpful.
‡ Not helpful.

97% in the intrathoracic abdomen.[17] Even though nonpenetration may be ruled out with certainty in flank wounds, the difficulty of excluding bowel perforations and the inadequate visualization of the retroperitoneum makes laparoscopy unreliable. This low sensitivity in anterior and flank wounds is a result of missed bowel injuries and the difficulty in evaluating retroperitoneal hematomas.

These conclusions are confirmed by a recent study from Los Angeles by Ortega and colleagues.[28] The authors studied 24 patients (11 GSW and 13 SW) with laparoscopy and compared the results with those of subsequent laparotomy in the same group of patients. Laparoscopy had a sensitivity of 83% for diaphragmatic injury (negative predictive value [NPV] 95%), 88% for liver and spleen lacerations (NPV 94%), 50% for pancreas and kidney trauma (NPV 91%), and 25% (NPV 57%) for hollow viscus perforations. The specificity and positive predictive value were 100% for all of these injuries. These investigators concluded that laparoscopy could have avoided an unnecessary laparotomy in 38% of cases.

In summary, the best indications for laparoscopy are hemodynamically stable patients with lower chest penetration and patients with GSW of the abdomen where peritoneal penetration is doubtful (Table 29.1). *We caution against relying on laparoscopy to exclude bowel or retroperitoneal injuries.*[17,18]

TECHNICAL CONSIDERATIONS

Laparoscopy may be performed in the emergency department under local anesthesia and sedation with intravenous midazolam or morphine.[12,13] The 5-mm scope is particularly applicable for emergency department laparoscopy, even though the 10-mm scope offers better visualization. Significant findings (hemoperitoneum, organ injuries) should prompt transport to the operating room for further evaluation. We prefer to perform the procedure under general anesthesia in the operating room. This facilitates positioning the operating table for optimal viewing and makes laparoscopic instrumentation much easier. The obvious drawback is that the cost of the procedure is increased.

Pneumoperitoneum may be induced either by a Veress needle or by using an open technique. We prefer the open method, a view supported by Ballem and Rudomanski.[29] These authors compared the two techniques in over 300 cases of laparoscopy and found that the open method was quicker, less expensive, and with a zero complication rate. The choice, however, depends on the surgeon's preference.

The patient must be monitored carefully during induction of pneumoperitoneum. It is very important to monitor the abdominal pressure and maintain it below 15 mmHg. Special attention must be directed to airway and systemic pressures, oxygen saturation, and end-tidal CO_2 to facilitate the early detection of pneumothorax (see below).

Excellent visualization of the major portion of the liver, spleen, and diaphragm is obtained. The posterior recesses of the diaphragm may not be seen well and may require a 30° scope and proper positioning of the patient. The pericardium can be inspected for lack of lustre. The colon may be mobilized for inspection of the flexures and the retroperitonal area. The small bowel may be "run" with the currently available endoscopic Babcock forceps. One must keep in mind, however, that it is easy to miss small bowel perforations and retroperitoneal injuries to the colon. The key to success is an extremely disciplined appraisal of the findings. The surgeon should not hesitate to do a celiotomy if he or she is not *100% certain* of the lack of missed injuries.

THERAPEUTIC LAPAROSCOPY

Laparoscopy offers the exciting potential to be therapeutic. Examples of therapeutic laparoscopy include repair of diaphragmatic lacerations with sutures,[30] staples, or the application of prosthetic mesh, suturing of gastrointestinal perforations[31]; and hemostasis of low-grade liver and splenic lacerations.

We have successfully applied hemostatic agents to control minor bleeding from the liver and spleen. Agents such as Gelfoam soaked in thrombin solution or sheets of Oxycel may be introduced through the accessory ports, grasped intracorporeally, and placed in the lacerations. Minor lacerations of the liver and spleen lend themselves to laparoscopic suture.

Autotransfusion of collected blood from the hemoperitoneum is another potential application, as illustrated by Smith and associates.[32] Their patient had a splenic laceration with significant hemoperitoneum seen on laparoscopy. The blood was retrieved via a bronchoscopic suction device, processed through a cell saver, and retransfused to the patient. The splenic injury was carefully visualized to confirm the absence of active bleeding.

Diaphragmatic lacerations from penetrating trauma are usually small and may be repaired by laparoscopic suturing. Even though some authors advocate stapling for repair of such lesions, the long-term results in a mobile organ such as the diaphragm are unknown. Suturing, in our opinion, is the method of choice.

Sporadic reports of laparoscopic repair of hollow viscus lacerations have appeared in the literature. These examples are the forerunners of therapeutic laparoscopy in trauma and illustrate the utility of the technique in *highly selected* patients.

PITFALLS OF LAPAROSCOPY

Laparoscopy is not without pitfalls (Table 29.2). Direct morbidity from laparoscopy usually is related to improper insertion of the Veress needle or a trocar, leading to preperitoneal insufflation, tension pneumothorax, accidental enterotomy, and vascular injuries. Other complications, such as CO_2 embolism and cardiac dysrhythmia, have not (yet) been reported in trauma patients but may become more frequent with more widespread use of the technique.

Tension Pneumothorax

Tension pneumothorax must be guarded against whenever the possibility of injury to the diaphragm is suspected. In our experience with more than 150 patients with penetrating trauma, this complication occurred in 3. Pneumoperitoneum may enter the pleural space through the diaphragmatic laceration and cause a tension pneumothorax. The onset of this complication should be suspected by a sudden deterioration of O_2 saturation or a rise in airway pressures during insufflation. In later stages, hypotension may result. The complication should be carefully looked for. If suspected,

Table 29.2. Potential Complications of Laparoscopy

Procedure	Complication
Related to trocar insertion	Injury to bowel, bladder, epigastric vessels, etc.
	Extraperitoneal insufflation of CO_2
Related to pneumoperitoneum	Tension pneumothorax
	Adverse effects on cardiac function, ICP
	Air embolism
Related to manipulation	Injury to bowel by graspers, cautery
	Mesenteric injury with bleeding
Related to solid organ injury	Underestimation of injury severity
Related to hollow viscus	Missed bowel perforations
Related to closure of port sites	Bowel incarceration, herniation

induction of pneumoperitoneum is stopped, the trocar is withdrawn and an immediate needle thoracentesis is performed on the side at risk to relieve the tension pneumothorax. This may be followed by a tube thoracostomy. Routine prophylactic placement of a thoracostomy tube, in our opinion, is not needed as long as the patient is closely monitored.

Hemodynamic Consequences of Laparoscopy

Pneumoperitoneum with CO_2 insufflation and increased intra-abdominal pressure, along with changes in the patient's position, may cause a significant deterioration in cardiovascular hemodynamics. In a recent presentation, Dorsay and associates studied cardiac function during laparoscopic cholecystectomy using biplane transesophageal echocardiography.[33] They observed that with an intra-abdominal pressure of 15 mmHg the cardiac index decreased by 3%, the mean arterial pressure increased by 16%, and the heart rate rose by 7%. Head-up tilting further decreased the cardiac index and the stroke volume index. Similar but more dramatic changes in these cardiovascular parameters were noted by McLaughlin et al.[34] The exact pathophysiology of these changes remains unclear.[35] While these reductions in cardiac output are well tolerated by patients undergoing elective cholecystectomy, they may be a significant insult to the trauma patient who is hemodynamically compromised. These facts underscore the importance of careful selection of patients for laparoscopy after trauma.

Intracranial Pressure (ICP) and Laparoscopy

In a provocative experimental study on the effects of laparoscopy on ICP, Josephs et al. noted that induction of pneumoperitoneum to a pressure of 15 mmHg with CO_2 elevated the ICP from a mean of 13.5 to 18.7 mmHg ($p < 0.0001$).[11]This change was found to be independent of changes in arterial pH, mean arterial pressure, arterial O_2 pressure, or arterial CO_2 pressure, indicating a direct effect on the cerebral circulation. Furthermore, the authors artificially elevated the IPC to 22 mmHg (mean) by inflating an epidural balloon. Pneumoperitoneum in these animals elevated the ICP to 27 mmHg ($p < 0.0001$). Based on these results, these authors cautioned against the use of pneumoperitoneum and laparoscopy in patients with head trauma, speculating that in patients with an ICP > 25 mmHg, small increases in intra-abdominal pressure may lead to an exponential increase in ICP. Further trials are clearly needed to validate these observations in the clinical situation. However, it seems prudent to avoid laparoscopy in patients with significant head trauma.

Missed Injuries

Missed injuries can be a disastrous complication of laparoscopy. Intestinal perforations, splenic lacerations, and retroperitoneal injuries may be missed.[18,23] Laparoscopy, in its current stage of evolution, cannot be relied on to exclude these lesions with 100% certainty 100% of the time. Extreme caution, therefore, is urged to avoid these mistakes.

Intestinal Herniation Through Trocar Sites

This complication is being recognized more frequently. In a recent communication, Williams et al. reviewed its reported incidence.[36] Describing three cases of Richter's hernia (herniation of a circumference of bowel), these authors noted four reported cases of incisional hernia following laparoscopic cholecystectomy and one instance of Richter's hernia following laparoscopic herniorrhaphy. We recently saw this complication in a 57-year-old man who had laparoscopic splenorrhaphy after trauma. After initial discharge from the hospital, he returned 2 weeks after the injury with crampy abdominal pain and multiple air-fluid levels on abdominal radiographs (Fig. 29.4). A CT scan confirmed the suspicion of a Richter's hernia (Fig. 29.5). As noted by other authors,[36] the hernia was not evident on clinical examination. Operative exploration (Figs. 29.6 and 29.7) confirmed the diagnosis. The herniation had occurred through the site of a 10-mm port that was sutured at the initial operation. The fascial suture had apparently broken down.

Prevention of this complication is crucial. All port sites of trocars larger than 10 mm should be securely and meticulously sutured. As emphasized by Williams and coauthors,[36] any patient with delayed bowel function, postoperative ileus, or abdominal distention and pain must be investigated for a possible intestinal herniation. Richter's hernia is an extremely difficult diagnosis by clinical examination. An early CT scan based on a high index of suspicion will help minimize delay and reduce the morbidity of this complication.

Cost Ineffectiveness

The cost ineffectiveness of laparoscopy in trauma is a matter of concern. Fabian et al.[14] noted that there were

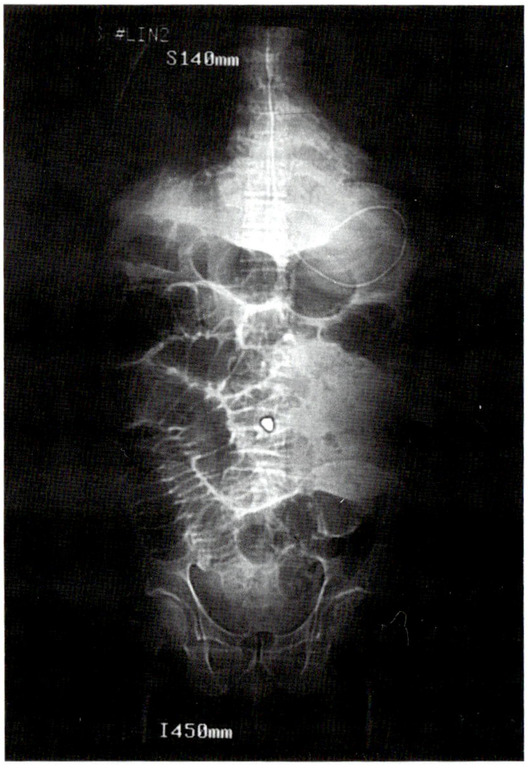

Figure 29.4. Abdominal radiograph following laparoscopy demonstrating multiple air-fluid levels and dilated bowel loops.

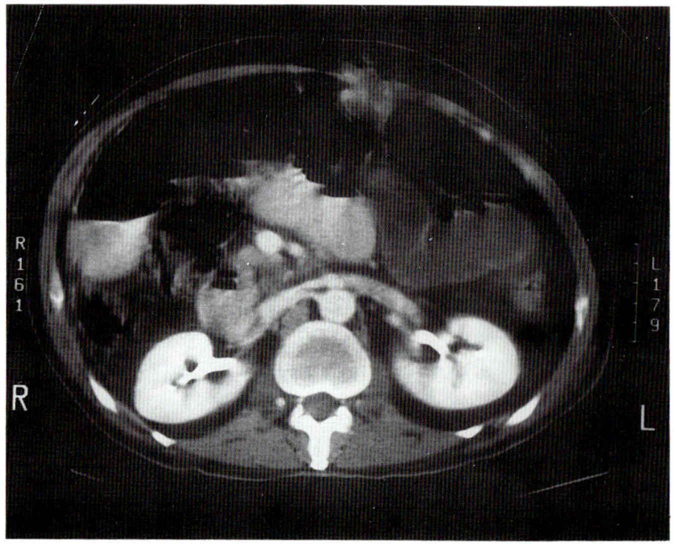

Figure 29.5. CT scan of the abdomen clearly shows herniation of a circumference of bowel through the fascia.

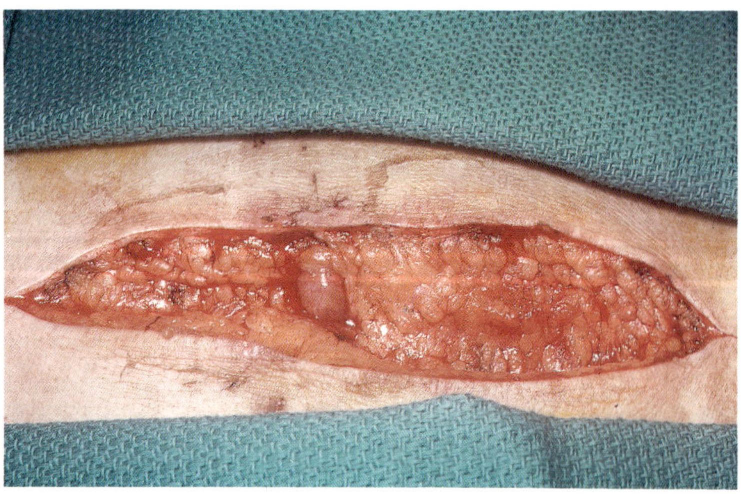

Figure 29.6. Operative appearance of the Richter's herniation through the fascia.

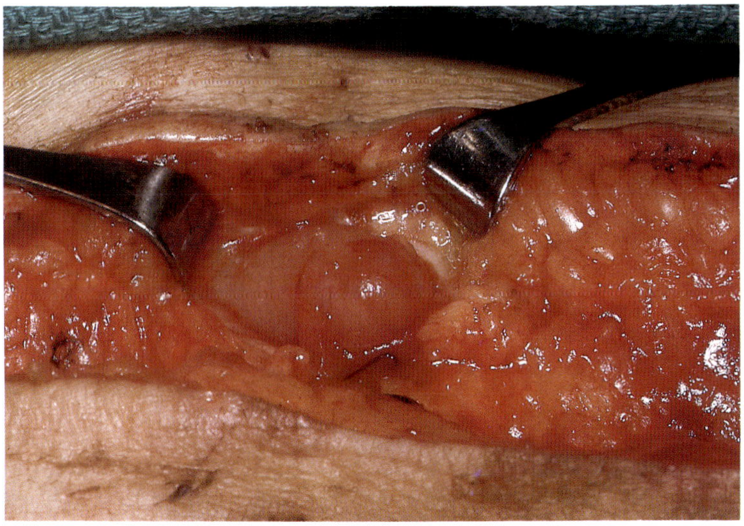

Figure 29.7. Operative appearance of the Richter's herniation through the fascia.

no significant savings in hospital costs despite a reduction in hospital stay when laparoscopy was used to select patients for laparotomy. The cost of the equipment and the need for an operating room, anesthesia, and anesthesiologists are some of the factors that increase the cost of laparoscopy compared to peritoneal lavage. Future technical innovations and modifications of the procedure (small-diameter scopes, surgery in the emergency department under local anesthesia, etc.) may help reduce the cost of laparoscopy.

GASLESS LAPAROSCOPY

The potential problems of laparoscopy, as discussed in the previous sections, have stimulated interest in performing "gasless" laparoscopy.[37] This method is based on expansion of the peritoneal cavity from without by mechanical retractors. In addition to avoiding the risks of pneumoperitoneum, this apneumic laparoscopy facilitates the use of conventional instruments such as hemostats, needles, and sutures. Conventional electrocautery and Yancouver suction may be used effectively, resulting in significant cost savings.

Technical Details

As described by Smith and Fry,[37] under general endotracheal anesthesia a fan-shaped retractor is inserted into the peritoneal cavity through a periumbilical or infraumbilical incision. Care is taken to avoid entrapment of bowel between the abdominal wall and the retractor. The retractor is attached to a mechanically powered arm attached to the table. The laparoscope is passed through the same umbilical incision, behind the crotch of the fan retractor. Accessory ports may be introduced through skin incisions at sites that are similar to those of standard laparoscopy. Since there is no need for airtight ports, conventional instruments may be passed directly intraperitoneally. For bowel exploration, the umbilical incision is enlarged, and the bowel is eviscerated in segments and inspected. If enteric perforations are identified, they can be repaired extracorporeally.

Smith and Fry[37] summarized their initial experience in the evaluation of 36 patients with abdominal trauma (GSW 13, SW 17, and blunt 6). In 31 patients, the examination was negative. Four patients had diaphragmatic lacerations that were repaired laparoscopically but with conventional instruments. Examination of the small bowel by adjunctive minilaparotomy and evisceration facilitated the diagnosis and repair of enteric perforations in three patients.

The major disadvantage of gasless laparoscopy is the excessive cost of the powered mechanical arm. Less expensive ways to lift the abdominal wall are under development.

REFERENCES

1. Ruddock JC: Peritoneoscopy. *Surg Gynecol Obstet* 65:623–638, 1937.

2. Heselson J: Peritoneoscopy in abdominal trauma. *S Afr J Surg* 8:53–60, 1970.
3. Gazzaniga AB, Stanton WW, Bartlett RH: Laparoscopy in the diagnosis of blunt and penetrating injuries to the abdomen. *Am J Surg* 131:315–318, 1976.
4. Carnevale N, Baron N, Delany HM: Peritoneoscopy as an aid in the diagnosis of abdominal trauma: A preliminary report. *J Trauma* 17:634–641, 1977.
5. Berci G, Dunkelman D, Michael SL, et al: Emergency minilaparoscopy in abdominal trauma. *Am J Surg* 146: 261, 1983.
6. Sherwood R, Berci G, Austin E, et al: Minilaparoscopy for blunt abdominal trauma. *Arch Surg* 115:672, 1980.
7. Wood D, Berci G, Morgenstern L, et al: Minilaparoscopy in blunt abdominal trauma. *Surg Endosc* 2:184, 1988.
8. Berci G, Sacker JM, Pas MP: Emergency laparoscopy. *Am J Surg* 161:332–335, 1991.
9. Nagy AG, James D: Diagnostic laparoscopy. *Am J Surg* 157:490, 1989.
10. Cuschieri A, Hennessy TP, Stephens RB, et al: Diagnosis of significant abdominal trauma after road traffic accidents: Preliminary results of a multicenter clinical trial comparing minilaparoscopy with peritoneal lavage. *Ann R Coll Surg Engl* 70:153, 1988.
11. Josephs LG, Este-McDonald JR, Rosiello AP, et al: Changes in intracranial hemodynamics during standard pneumoperitoneum for laparoscopy. *J Trauma* 36: 815–819, 1994.
12. Salvino CK, Esposito TJ, Marshall WJ, et al: The role of diagnostic laparoscopy in the management of trauma patients: A preliminary assessment. *J Trauma* 34: 506–515, 1993.
13. Esposito TJ: Laparoscopy in blunt trauma. *Trauma Q: Cavitary Endosc* 10:260–272, 1994.
14. Fabian TC, Croce MA, Stewart RM, et al: A prospective analysis of diagnostic laparoscopy in trauma. *Ann Surg* 217:557–565, 1993.
15. Townsend MS, Flancbaum L, Choban PS, et al: Diagnostic laparoscopy as an adjunct to selective conservative management of solid organ injuries after blunt abdominal trauma. *J Trauma* 35:647–653, 1993.
16. Ivatury RR, Simon RJ, Weksler B, et al: Laparoscopy in the evaluation of the intrathoracic abdomen after penetrating injury. *J Trauma* 33:101–109, 1992.
17. Ivatury RR, Simon RJ, Stahl WM: A critical evaluation of laparoscopy in penetrating abdominal trauma. *J Trauma* 34:822–828, 1992.
18. Ivatury RR, Simon RJ, Stahl WM: Selective celiotomy for missile wounds of the abdomen based on laparoscopy. *Surg Endosc*
19. Merlotti GJ, Marcet E, Sheaff CM, et al: Use of peritoneal lavage to evaluate abdominal penetration. *J Trauma* 25:228, 1985.
20. Sosa JL, Puente I, Arrillaga A, et al: Laparoscopy in 100 consecutive patients with abdominal gunshot wounds (abstract). *J Trauma* 37:159, 1994.
21. Livingston DH, Tortella BJ, Blackwood J, et al: The role of laparoscopy in abdominal trauma. *J Trauma* 33:471–475, 1992.
22. Smith RS, Tsoi EKM, Fry WR, et al: Laparoscopic evaluation of abdominal trauma: A preliminary report. *Contemp Surg* 42:13–18, 1993.
23. Zantut LFC, Rodrigues AJ JR, Birolini D: Laparoscopy as a diagnostic tool in the evaluation of trauma. *Pan Am J Trauma* 2:6–11, 1990.
24. Merlotti GJ, Dillon BC, Lange DA, et al: Peritoneal lavage in penetrating thoracoabdominal trauma. *J Trauma* 28:17–23, 1988.
25. Madden MR, Paull DE, Finklestein JL, et al: Occult diaphragmatic injury from stab wounds to the lower chest and abdomen. *J Trauma* 29:292–298, 1989.
26. Medina M, Ivatury RR, Stahl WM: Omental evisceration through an abdominal stab wound: Is exploratory laparotomy mandatory? *Can J Surg* 118:57, 1983.
27. Grewal H, Ivatury RR, Divakar M, et al: A critical evaluation of diagnostic modalities used in the detection of occult cardiac injury. *J Trauma* 35:986, 1993.
28. Ortega AE, Tang E, Froes ET, et al: Laparoscopic evaluation of penetrating thoracoabdominal trauma. *Surg Endosc* 9:211, 1995.
29. Ballem RV, Rudomanski JR: Techniques of pneumoperitoneum. *Surg Laparosc Endosc* 3:42–43, 1993.
30. Fabian TC, McCord S: Therapeutic laparoscopy in trauma. *Trauma Q* 10:285–290, 1994.
31. Frantzides CT, Ludwig KA, Aprahamian C, et al: Laparoscopic closure of gastric stab wounds: A case report. *Surg Laparosc Endosc* 3:63–66, 1993.
32. Smith RS, Meister RK, Tsoi EKM, et al: Laparoscopically guided blood salvage and autotransfusion in splenic trauma: A case report. *J Trauma* 34:313–314, 1993.
33. Dorsay DA, Greene FL, Baysinger CL: Hemodynamic changes during laparoscopic cholecystectomy monitored with transesophageal echocardiography. *Surg Endosc* 9:128–134, 1995.
34. McLaughlin JG, Scheeres DE, Dean RJ, et al: The adverse hemodynamic effects of laparoscopic cholecystectomy. *Surg Endosc* 9:121–124, 1995.
35. Schauer PR, Schwesinger WH: Hemodynamic effects of laparoscopy. *Surg Endosc* 9:119–120, 1995.
36. Williams MD, Flowers SS, Fenoglio ME, et al: Richter's hernia following laparoscopy. *Surg Rounds* 61–65, 1995.
37. Smith RS, Fry WR: Alternative techniques in laparoscopy for trauma. *Trauma Q* 10:291–300, 1994.

chapter thirty

Endoscopic Complications in Plastic Surgery: Endoscopic Carpal Tunnel Release

Ralph P. Pennino

Carpal tunnel syndrome is caused by compression of the median nerve as it passes under the transverse carpal ligament. It is estimated to affect 1% of the general population in the United States and is the most common form of nerve entrapment of the extremities. It can affect 10% of the population over age 40 and up to 5% of those in certain occupations. Initial management consists of splints, steroid injections, ergonomic review of the workplace, and review of the patient's interaction with the workplace.[1]

Surgery is indicated in those patients who fail to respond to conservative therapy. The time-honored gold standard is open carpal tunnel release. This is usually done under a local or regional anesthetic. A short axial-based curvilinear incision is made over the transverse carpal ligament in line with the ring finger. The transverse carpal ligament is then divided under direct visualization. Postoperatively, these patients have excellent relief of median paresthesias. The advantages of open carpal tunnel release are its reported safety and its ability to visualize the median nerve and flexor tendons for other pathology. It requires no special equipment.

However, the disadvantages include prolonged postoperative palmar tenderness, stiffness, delayed return of pinch and grip strength, and a prolonged period of convalescence and long-delayed normalization of the activities of daily living. Cotton[2] reported that up to one-third patients had palmar tenderness and stiffness 2 years postoperatively. Recently, the safety of this procedure has also been questioned. Numerous authors have reported injuries to the median, ulnar, and radial nerves during open carpal tunnel release.[14] Kuschner[3] reviewed 14 studies of open carpal tunnel release, including 3035 hands. He found a surprising 9.2% complication rate. Complications included those previously listed, as well as injuries to nerves, arteries, tendons, and incomplete ligament division. However, Schneck[4] further analyzed this report and found that 6% of the complications were to due painful scars. Further, if transient nerve complications (e.g., neuropraxia) were omitted, the complication rate was reduced to 0.8%. This included 24 nerve injuries (palmar cutaneous nerve, thenar motor branch, digital nerve) and two arterial injuries.

Various authors have reported using endoscopic techniques to release the transverse carpal ligament.[4–21] These techniques all divide the ligament alone and avoid cutting the overlying skin, subcutaneous fat, palmaris fascia, and palmaris brevis. This results in decreased postoperative palmar tenderness, less scarring, quicker return to preoperative grip and pinch strength, faster recovery, and more rapid return to the activities of daily living and work. Initial studies showed an earlier return to work in noncompensation cases. Recent reports show a similar trend for compensation cases.[7,8] This has a potentially significant financial savings in the Worker's Compensation System. One study in Minnesota calculated a potential savings of almost $5 million for loss of time in 3596 workers' compensation injuries due to carpal tunnel syndrome.

Despite these reported benefits, there is considerable debate over the value of endoscopic procedures due to reported complications. Complication rates and severity vary widely. Earlier reports were sometimes related to equipment or techniques which were subsequently modified. Complications include incomplete release of the transverse carpal ligament, neurologic and vascular recurrence of symptoms, tendon injury, and wound infection. Neurologic injury includes temporary neuropraxia (ulnar or median nerve—reported in most studies) and partial or complete nerve (median, ulnar, common digital) division.

Endoscopic carpal tunnel release is initially a demanding procedure. Complications are related to the technique used, lack of attention to the anatomy, specific details of the procedure, and experience of the surgeon. There are presently three endoscopic procedures that have been proposed by different surgeons and employ different equipment. They are briefly outlined.

Agee[8] describes a one-portal technique utilizing a pistol grip device that incorporates a 3-mm video endoscope and a trigger-activated retractable blade. The technique is as follows:

1. A tourniquet block, regional anesthesia, or general anesthesia is used.
2. A 2-cm transverse incision is made between the flexor carpi ulnaris and flexor carpi radialis in the distal wrist flexion crease.
3. Care is taken to protect the palmar cutaneous branch of the median nerve.
4. A distally based, U-shaped incision is made in the forearm fascia.
5. A probe is inserted to define a path along the ulnar side of the carpal tunnel.
6. The probe is removed.
7. A synovial elevator is used to clear any adherent flexor synovium.
8. The transverse carpal ligament is identified; its distal edge is then identified and cleared.
9. The cutting device is placed into the carpal tunnel.
10. Device alignment is checked along the ring finger axis.
11. The trigger is pulled elevating the blade.
12. Upward pressure is used to hold the cutting device against the transverse carpal ligament, and the device is then gently withdrawn under endoscopic visualization.
13. The carpal canal is then checked endoscopically to ensure that the ligament is completely divided.
14. If necessary, the procedure is repeated until the ligament is totally divided.
15. The distal 2 cm of the flexor retinaculum is divided to ensure that the median nerve is not pinched with wrist flexion.

Chow[5,16] described a two-portal technique which utilizes a metal tube opened on the palmar surface against the transverse carpal ligament, along with an endoscope and various knives. The technique has been modified from the original transbursal to an extrabursal technique. It consists of the following steps:

1. Regional anesthesia is used.
2. The hand and forearm are placed on a special holder with the wrist extended.
3. A 1-cm incision is made in the proximal volar wrist crease ulnar to the palmaris longus tendon.
4. The distal forearm fascia is opened.
5. The trocar tip is introduced along the radial side of the hook of the hamate in line with the ring finger axis.
6. The trocar will exit through a small transverse incision in the palm of the hand.
7. This exit point is determined by the intersection of two lines drawn at right angles, one from the third web space proximally and the other from the volar surface of a fully abducted thumb (Kaplan's cardinal line).
8. The obturator is removed.
9. A 30 degree endoscope is placed proximally and the transverse carpal ligament is identified.
10. Initial transection is performed distally with a probe knife inserted through the distal portal.
11. A vertical incision in the center of the ligament is made with a triangular knife placed from the distal port, followed by the hook knife, which divides the remaining distal ligament by pulling distally.
12. The endoscope and knife are removed.
13. The endoscope is placed through the distal end, and the proximal half of the ligament is transected using the same technique. Endoscopic visualization of the transverse carpal ligament is done to ensure complete transection.

Menon[15] described a technique utilizing a hollowed-out plastic cannula, a series of dilators, a 30 degree arthroscope, and a concave tip knife to divide the carpal ligament. His technique is as follows:

1. Regional anesthesia is used.

2. Skin markings consist of Kaplan's cardinal line drawn from the first web space to a point .5 cm distal to the pisiform second line drawn proximally from the ulnar aspect of the ring finger. This intersection is used to mark the distal border of the transverse carpal ligament at its attachment to the hook of the hamate.
3. The single-port entry is marked by an oblique line drawn from the ulnar side of the palmaris longus at a 45 degree angle proximally.
4. A 1-cm incision is made.
5. The antebrachial fascia is dissected and opened.
6. An obturator is initially passed into the carpal canal.
7. The obturator is removed, followed by insertion of a 5.5- and then a 7-mm dilator.
8. The cannula is inserted into the canal and advanced until it is palpated at the distal margin of the transverse carpal ligament. Care is taken to ensure that it remains in the axis of the ring finger.
9. A 25-gauge needle is inserted at the distal end of the ligament.
10. A 30 degree endoscope and a double-guarded concave endoscopic knife are introduced down the cannula.
11. The ligament is divided by pushing the knife in a proximal-to-distal direction under full visualization.
12. The distal extent is determined by the previously placed needle tip.

AVOIDING COMPLICATIONS

It is clear that endoscopic release of the transverse carpal ligament by any of the previously described methods is a technically demanding procedure. It should not be undertaken lightly. Following are suggestions to avoid complications.

Anatomy

In-depth knowledge and understanding of the hand and wrist anatomy and its relationship to topographic landmarks is especially important for success with minimal experience. One should be particularly concerned with the following structures and topical anatomy: transverse carpal ligament, pisiform, hook of the hamate, median and ulnar nerves, palmar cutaneous branch of the median nerve, common digital nerve branches of the median nerve, and the superficial palmar arch and its relation to the transverse carpal ligament.

In one cadaver study,[20] the transverse carpal ligament averaged 2.9 cm in length (range, 1.9–5.5 cm) and 1.3 cm in width (ranges 1.0–1.9 cm). It begins proximally as the continuation of the antebrachial fascia and ends distally with the fibers of the midpalmar fascia.

Open and endoscopic carpal tunnel release are approached in the line of the ring finger axis. This avoids injury to the palmar cutaneous nerve branches of the median or ulnar nerves. Endoscopically, this axis avoids placement of the device under the median nerve. Also, most variations of median nerve anatomy occur on either the radial or volar side of the nerve and should be out of harm's way with this approach.

Kaplan et al. describes a fat pad which invests the superficial palmar arch, common digital nerves, and synovial bursa of the flexor tendons. Rotman et al. showed that this fat pad extends proximal to the distal edge of the transverse carpal ligament in the ring finger axis, a distance of 2–3.5 mm. It is important to incise the ligament beyond this fat encroachment; otherwise, there will be an incomplete release. Rotman et al. also reported that the superficial palmar arch is approximately 5 mm away from the distal edge of the transverse carpal ligament. Therefore, with good endoscopic visualization, it should be safe from harm when using a one-portal technique (i.e., that of Agee).

Cobbs et al. reported a cadaver study which used various topographic markings as reference points, aiding the surgeon in placing the Agee device for distal release of the transverse carpal ligament. They reported no incomplete releases in 30 procedures using this system, which is based on using the hook of the hamate as a reference point. The hook of the hamate is localized by the intersection of two lines—one along the ring finger axis continued proximally to the distal wrist crease and the other from the proximal palmar crease over the index finger central axis drawn to the pisiform. Once this point is known, the following can be assumed:

- The distal edge of the transverse carpal ligament is 1 cm distal.
- The transverse carpal ligament should be incised just radial to this point, as the median nerve occupies the other side of the carpal canal.
- Inadvertent entry into Guyon's canal would pass ulnar to this point and be easily noted by the surgeon.

- The superficial palmar artery should be 2.5 cm distal to the hook of the hamate.

The last point is basically in agreement with the results of Nagle,[21] who noted that the superficial palmar arch was approximately 1–1.5 cm from the edge of the transverse carpal ligament, or about 2.5 cm from the hook of the hamate.

A common problem using the Agee technique[7] is difficulty passing the device (blade assembly) into the carpal tunnel entrance. This is more frequent in small-framed (4.5%) versus large-framed (8.8%) patients. Entry is facilitated by lubrication with normal saline and by aiming the device slightly dorsally at the carpal tunnel entrance.

Many reported complications using the two-portal technique (Chow) were secondary to injuries of the superficial palmar arch.[5] Anatomic studies have shown the average distance between the distal palmar incision (distal port) and the superficial palmar artery to be 0.4 cm, with a range of −1.1 cm (distal incision located distal to the level of the superficial palmar artery) to 1.5 cm (distal incision located proximal to the superficial palmar artery). The surgeon should be aware of these potential anatomic differences. Adequate wrist extension can help ensure exit of the cannula superficial to the arch. This, coupled with blunt dissection to visualize the arch directly, should help reduce the incidence of this complication.

Cadaver Laboratory

Anatomy is best learned from the cadaveric specimen. If a cadaver hand is available, actual procedures should be performed on it to gain experience in the technical details of the chosen endoscopic technique. The surgeon must understand the anatomic relationship between the endoscopic device and the surrounding structures (transverse carpal ligament, nerves, tendons, etc.). Various authors have reported using cadaver hands to learn the technique prior to clinical practice.[20–25] Numerous authors have reported many complications and technical errors in these preclinical studies, demonstrating the importance of prior study before clinical use. Lee et al.[20] noted incomplete release in 12 of 24 specimens. This included one release of Guyon's canal, five incomplete releases of the distal transverse carpal ligament, and six incomplete central superficial releases. Rowlan et al.,[24] using a two-portal technique, had only 12 of 24 specimens released without complications. Complications included ulnar artery laceration, fracture of the hook of the hamate, median nerve division, and partial flexor tendon laceration. Many of these complications occurred when the techniques and equipment were being developed. Recent studies[24] on cadavers show significantly fewer complications, with a better understanding of topographic anatomy. However, it is to the surgeon's benefit to practice the procedure of his or her choice in the anatomy lab. This will help lessen the number and seriousness of potential complications until experience is gained.

Contraindications

Complications include the following:

- Proliferative or septic tenosynovitis
- Mass in the carpal canal
- Significant anatomic anomalies (traumatic or developmental)
- Previous carpal tunnel surgery
- Concomitant ulnar nerve entrapment in Guyon's canal
- Moderate to severe rheumatoid arthritis
- Stiff wrist joint, which prevents adequate wrist hyperextension

With experience, some of these may be reduced or eliminated.

Equipment

The surgeon should be thoroughly familiar with the equipment for the endoscopic procedure performed. This includes not only the instrumentation but also the video endoscope. Endoscopic release depends on clear visualization of the transverse carpal ligament. Many reported cases were converted to open carpal tunnel release secondary to poor visualization. Sometimes this is due to technical problems such as fogging. The surgeon should be knowledgeable about techniques to prevent and/or treat this problem.

Initial Training

No surgeon should undertake this procedure without a basic hands-on training workshop in the technique that he or she will use. If possible, this should be followed with cadaver studies. If a cadaver lab is not available, the initial operations should be performed with a surgeon experienced in the technique. Most authors report a learning curve. With experience the number of complications decreases. Surgeons employing one of these new techniques would clearly benefit by the assistance of a more experienced surgeon until they are familiar and comfortable with the procedure and equipment. Obviously, the number of cases will vary depending on the surgeon.

In summary, the various techniques of endoscopic carpal tunnel release have proven effective, with considerable benefit compared to the open technique. However, their major drawbacks at this time are the reported complications associated with gaining experience. The complication rate should fall in the future due to better equipment, modification of technique with regard to anatomic structures, and experience of the surgeon. Surgeons in practice have had to attend a workshop to learn the technique and then start immediately in clinical practice. They did not have the benefit of an experienced surgeon to help them avoid complications. Young surgeons in training will avoid this problem. They should be trained by surgeons experienced in this technique and therefore should avoid the learning curve, where most complications occur. Once this transition occurs, endoscopic carpal tunnel release should become a more established procedure.

REFERENCES

1. Szabo RN: Carpal tunnel syndrome—general. In Gelberman RH (ed): *Operative Nerve Repair and Reconstruction*, Vol II:60. Philadelphia, JB Lippincott, 1991, pp 869–888.
2. Cotton P: Symptoms may return after carpal tunnel surgery. *JAMA* 265(15):1922–1925, 1991.
3. Kuschner SH, Brien WW, et al: Complications associated with carpal tunnel release. *Orthop Rev* 20:346–351, 1991.
4. Schneck RR: *The Role of Endoscopic Surgery in Treatment of Carpal Tunnel Syndrome. Advances in Plastic and Reconstructive Surgery*, Vol 11. Mosby Year Book, 1995.
5. Chow JC: Endoscopic release of the carpal ligament: A new technique for carpal tunnel syndrome. *Arthroscopy* 5(1):19–21, 1989.
6. McDonough JW, et al: A comparison of endoscopic and open carpal tunnel releases. *Wis Med J* 675–677, 1993.
7. Agee JM, et al: Endoscopic release of the carpal tunnel: A randomized prospective multicenter study. *J Hand Surg* 17A(6):987–995, 1992.
8. Agee JM, et al: Endoscopic carpal tunnel release: A prospectus study of complications and surgical experience. *J Hand Surg* 20A(2):165–171, 1995.
9. Menon J: Endoscopic carpal tunnel release: A preliminary report. *Arthroscopy* 10(1):31–38, 1994.
10. Viegas SF, et al: Carpal arch alteration and related clinical status after endoscopic carpal tunnel release. *J Hand Surg* 17A(6):1012–1016, 1992.
11. Palmer DH, et al: Endoscopic carpal tunnel release: A comparison of two techniques with open release. *Arthroscopy* 9(5):498–508, 1993.
12. Brown RA, et al: Carpal tunnel release. *J Bone Joint Surg* 75A(9):1265–1275, 1993.
13. Erdmann MW: Endoscopic carpal tunnel decompression. *J Hand Surg* 19B(1):5–13, 1994.
14. Murphy RX, et al: Major neurovascular complications of endoscopic carpal tunnel release. *J Hand Surg* 19(1): 114–118, 1994.
15. Menon J: Endoscopic carpal tunnel release: A single portal technique. *Contemp Orthop* 26:109–115, 1993.
16. Chow JC: Endoscopic release of the carpal ligament for carpal tunnel syndrome: 22 month clinical result. *Arthroscopy* 6:288–296, 1990.
18. Resnick CT, Miller BW: Endoscopic carpal tunnel release using the subligamentous two portal technique. *Contemp Orthop* 22:269–277, 1991.
19. Brown MG, et al: Endoscopic carpal tunnel release. *J Hand Surg* 17A(6):1009–1011, 1992.
20. Lee DH, et al: Endoscopic carpal tunnel release: A cadaveric study. *J Hand Surg* 17A(6):1003–1008, 1992.
21. Nagle D, et al: A review of 279 endoscopic carpal tunnel releases using the modified chow technique. *Arthroscopy* in press.
22. Rothman MB, Manske PR: Anatomic relationships of endoscopic carpal tunnel device to surrounding structures. *J Hand Surg* 18A:442–450, 1993.
23. Kaplan EB, Milford LW: The retinacular system of the hand. In Spinner M (ed): *Kaplan's Functional and Surgical Anatomy of the Hand*, ed 3. Philadelphia, JB Lippincott, 1984, pp 245–282.
24. Rowlan E, Kleinert JM: Endoscopic carpal tunnel release in cadavers: Investigation of the results of twelve surgeons with this training model. *J Bone Joint Surg* 76:226–268, 1994.
25. Cobb TK, et al: Relationship of deep structures of the hand and wrist to topographical landmarks. *Clin Anat* 6:300–307, 1993.

Index